EXPERT GUIDE TO

INFECTIOUS
DISEASES

For a catalogue of publications available from ACP–ASIM, contact:

Customer Service Center
American College of Physicians–American Society of Internal Medicine
190 N. Independence Mall West
Philadelphia, PA 19106-1572
215-351-2600
800-523-1546, ext. 2600

Visit our Web site at www. acponline.org

Expert Guide to

INFECTIOUS
DISEASES

James S. Tan, MD, MACP, FCCP

Professor and Vice Chairman, Department of Internal Medicine
Northeastern Ohio Universities College of Medicine;
Head, Infectious Disease Section
Chairman, Department of Internal Medicine
Summa Health System
Akron, Ohio

American College of Physicians
Philadelphia

Clinical Consultant: David R. Goldmann, MD
Acquisitions Editor: Mary K. Ruff
Manager, Book Publishing: David Myers
Developmental Editor: Victoria Hoenigke
Production Supervisor: Allan S. Kleinberg
Production Editor: Scott Thomas Hurd
Editorial Coordinator: Alicia Dillihay
Cover and Interior Design: Patrick Whelan
Indexer: Nelle Garrecht

Manufactured in the United States of America
Composition by Fulcrum Data Services, Inc.
Printing/binding by Versa Press

American College of Physicians (ACP) became an imprint of the American College of Physicians–American Society of Internal Medicine in July 1998.

Library of Congress Cataloging-in-Publication Data

Expert guide to infectious diseases / edited by James S. Tan
     p. ; cm. – (ACP expert guides series)
    Includes bibliographical references and index.
    ISBN 0-943126-98-3
      1. Communicable diseases. 2. Evidence-based medicine. I. Tan, James S.
    II. American College of Physicians–American Society of Internal Medicine.
    III. Series.
      [DNLM: 1. Communicable Diseases–diagnosis. 2. Communicable
    Diseases–therapy. 3. Evidence-Based Medicine. 4. Primary Health Care.
    WC 100 E96 2000]
    RC112.E97 2000
    616.9–dc21

                             00-069964

---

02 03 04 05 06 / 9 8 7 6 5 4 3 2 1

Contributors

Keith B. Armitage, MD
Vice Chair for Education
Associate Professor of Medicine
Department of Medicine
Division of Infectious Diseases
University Hospitals of Cleveland
Case Western Reserve University
Cleveland, Ohio

William Bonnez, MD, FACP
Associate Professor of Medicine
Infectious Diseases Unit
Department of Medicine
University of Rochester School of Medicine
    and Dentistry
Rochester, New York

Robert A. Bonomo, MD
Assistant Professor of Medicine
Department of Medicine
Division of Infectious Disease and Geriatric
    Medicine
University Hospitals of Cleveland
Geriatric Care Center
Cleveland, Ohio

W. Henry Boom, MD
Professor of Medicine
Director, Tuberculosis Research Unit
Vice Chair for Research
Department of Medicine
Case Western Reserve University School of
    Medicine and University Hospitals of
    Cleveland
Cleveland, Ohio

Itzhak Brook, MD, MSc
Professor of Pediatrics
Georgetown University School of Medicine
Washington, DC;
Consultant
Infectious Disease Naval Hospital and
    Georgetown University Hospital
Bethesda, Maryland

Jason Calhoun, MD
Professor and Director
Department of Orthopedic Surgery
Adjunctive Member
Marine Biomedical Institute
University of Texas Medical Branch
Galveston, Texas

David H. Canaday, MD
Senior Instructor
Division of Infectious Diseases
Case Western Reserve University School of
    Medicine
University Hospitals of Cleveland
Cleveland, Ohio

Jason W. Chien, MD
Acting Instructor
Division of Pulmonary and Critical Care
    Medicine
Fred Hutchison Cancer Research Center
University of Washington
Seattle, Washington

Catherine Markin Colecraft, MD
Fellow
Division of Infectious Diseases
Case Western Reserve University
  School of Medicine
University Hospitals of Cleveland
Cleveland, Ohio

Blaise L. Congeni, MD
Professor of Pediatrics
Professor of Microbiology and Immunology
Northeastern Ohio Universities
  College of Medicine;
Division of Infectious Disease
Children's Hospital Medical Center of
  Akron
Akron, Ohio

Curtis J. Donskey, MD
Assistant Professor of Medicine
Case Western Reserve University
  School of Medicine
Infectious Diseases Section
Louis Stokes Cleveland Veterans Affairs
  Medical Center
Cleveland, Ohio

Thomas M. File Jr., MD, MS, FACP
Professor of Medicine
Northeastern Ohio Universities
  College of Medicine;
Chief, Infectious Disease Section
Summa Health System
Akron, Ohio

Robert F. Flora, MD, FACOG
Director, Residency Program in Obstetrics
  and Gynecology
Head, Section of Urogynecology and
  Reconstructive Pelvic Surgery
Summa Health System
Akron, Ohio;
Assistant Professor
Northeastern Ohio Universities College
  of Medicine
Rootstown, Ohio

Scott A. Fulton, MD
Assistant Professor of Medicine
Division of Infectious Diseases
Case Western Reserve University School
  of Medicine
University Hospitals of Cleveland
Cleveland, Ohio

William G. Gardner, MD, FACP
Professor and Chairman
Department of Internal Medicine
Northeastern Ohio Universities College
  of Medicine
Rootstown, Ohio;
Chairman, Department of Medicine
Akron General Medicine Center
Akron, Ohio

K.V. Gopalakrishna, MD, FACP
Associate Professor of Medicine
Case Western Reserve University;
Clinical Professor of Medicine
Ohio State University College of Medicine;
Chairman and Program Director
Department of Internal Medicine
Infectious Disease Section
Fairview General Hospital
Cleveland, Ohio

Barbara M. Gripshover, MD
Assistant Professor of Medicine
Director, HIV Clinical Programs
Division of Infectious Diseases
Case Western Reserve University School
  of Medicine
University Hospitals of Cleveland
Cleveland, Ohio

Daniel P. Guyton, MD, FACS
Professor of Surgery
Chairman, Department of Surgery
Northeastern Ohio Universities College
  of Medicine
Rootstown, Ohio

Jennifer A. Hanrahan, DO
Assistant Clinical Professor of Medicine
Division of Infectious Diseases
Case Western Reserve University School
  of Medicine
University Hospitals of Cleveland
Cleveland, Ohio

Amy S. Indorf, MD
Assistant Professor of Internal Medicine
Northeastern Ohio Universities College
  of Medicine
Rootstown, Ohio;
Infectious Disease Service
Summa Health System
Akron, Ohio

John L. Johnson, MD, FACP
Assistant Professor of Medicine
Division of Infectious Diseases
Case Western Reserve University School
    of Medicine
Tuberculosis Research Unit
Cleveland, Ohio

Kathleen T. Jordan, MD
Baynet LTC Medical Group
San Francisco, California

Charles H. King, MD, FACP
Associate Professor of Medicine
Division of Infectious Diseases
Case Western Reserve University School
    of Medicine
University Hospitals of Cleveland
Cleveland, Ohio

Richard B. Kohler, MD, FACP
Professor of Medicine
Department of Medicine
Indiana University School of Medicine
Indianapolis, Indiana

Jon T. Mader, MD, FACP
Professor
Department of Internal Medicine and
    Pathology
Division of Infectious Diseases
Adjunct Professor
Department of Orthopaedic Surgery
Chief of Marine Medicine
Marine Biomedical Institute
University of Texas Medical Branch
Galveston, Texas

Thomas J. Marrie, MD, FACP, FRCP
Professor and Chair
Department of Medicine
University of Alberta
Edmonton, Alberta, Canada

Donald K. Maxwell, DO
Critical Care Medicine Subspecialty
    Resident
St. John's Mercy Medical Center
St Louis University School of Medicine
Chesterfield, Missouri

Farid F. Muakkassa, MD, FACS
Associate Professor of Surgery
Northeastern Ohio Universities College of
    Medicine;
Chief, Trauma/Surgical Care
Akron General Medical Center
Akron, Ohio

Joseph P. Myers, MD, FACP
Program Director
Internal Medicine - Pediatrics and
    Transitional Residencies;
Summa Health System
Professor of Internal Medicine
Vice Chairperson, Infectious Disease Section
Northern Ohio Universities College of
    Medicine
Akron, Ohio

William C. Papouras, MD
Chief Resident in Surgery
Akron General Medical Center
Akron, Ohio

Carlos R. Ramirez-Ramirez, MD
Instructor of Medicine
University of Puerto Rico School of
    Medicine;
Chief Resident
Department of Medicine
San Juan Veterans Affairs Medical Center
San Juan, Puerto Rico

Carlos H. Ramirez-Ronda, MD, FACP
Professor of Medicine
University of Puerto Rico School of
    Medicine;
Department of Medicine
San Juan Veterans Affairs Medical Center
San Juan, Puerto Rico

Louis B. Rice, MD, FACP
Chief, Medicine Service
Louis Stokes Cleveland Veterans
    Administration Medical Center
Case Western Reserve University School of
    Medicine
Chief, Infectious Diseases Section
Veterans Administration Medical Center
Cleveland, Ohio

Allan R. Ronald, OC, MD, FACP, FRCP
Consultant
Section of Infectious Diseases
St. Boniface General Hospital;
Professor Emeritus
University of Manitoba
Winnipeg, Manitoba, Canada

Robert A. Salata, MD, FACP
Professor of Medicine
Chief, Division of Infectious Diseases
Case Western Reserve University School
   of Medicine
University Hospitals of Cleveland
Cleveland, Ohio

Francisco L. Sapico, MD, FACP
Professor of Medicine
USC School of Medicine
University of Southern California;
Chief of Infectious Diseases
Rancho Los Amigos National
   Rehabilitation Center
Downey, California

Louis D. Saravolatz, MD, FACP
Professor of Medicine
Wayne State University School of Medicine;
Chairman, Department of Internal Medicine
St. John Hospital
Detroit, Michigan

Stephen M. Seink, MD
Fellow
Pulmonary Critical Care
University of Illinois
Chicago, Illinois

Mark E. Shirtliff, PhD
Post-Doctoral Fellow
Center for Biofilm Engineering
Montana State University
Bozemon, Montana;
Department of Microbiology and
   Immunology
University of Texas Medical Branch
Galveston, Texas

Denise J. Signs, MD, MS, FACP
Assistant Professor of Medicine
Northeastern Ohio Universities College
   of Medicine;
Department of Infectious Disease
Summa Health System
Akron, Ohio

Gary I. Sinclair, MD, FACP
Assistant Professor of Medicine
Division of Infectious Diseases
University of Texas Southwestern
Dallas, Texas

J.D. Sobel, MD, FACP
Professor of Internal Medicine
Wayne State University School of Medicine;
Chief, Division of Infectious Diseases
Harper Hospital
Detroit Medical Center
Detroit, Michigan

James S. Tan, MD, MACP, FCCP
Professor and Vice Chairman
Department of Internal Medicine
Northeastern Ohio Universities College
   of Medicine;
Head, Infectious Disease Section
Chairman, Department of Internal Medicine
Summa Health System
Akron, Ohio

Richard B. Thomson Jr., PhD
Associate Professor of Pathology
Northwestern University Medical School;
Director
Microbiology and Virology Laboratory
Department of Pathology and Laboratory
   Medicine
Evanston Hospital
Evanston Northwestern Healthcare
Evanston, Illinois

Hernan Valdez, MD
Assistant Professor of Medicine
Department of Medicine
Division of Infectious Diseases
Case Western Reserve University School
   of Medicine
University Hospitals of Cleveland
Cleveland, Ohio

Arjun Venkataramani, MD, MPH
Assistant Professor of Medicine
Northeastern Ohio Universities College of
   Medicine;
Summa Health System
Akron, Ohio

Jue Wang, MD
Fellow, Hyperbaric Medicine
University of Texas Medical Branch
Galveston, Texas

Chatrchai Watanakunakorn, MD, MACP, FCCP†
Professor of Internal Medicine
Northeastern Ohio Universities College
   of Medicine;
Director, Infectious Disease Section
Department of Internal Medicine
St. Elizabeth Health Center
Youngstown, Ohio

Sharon B. Weissman, MD
Assistant Professor of Medicine
Department of Medicine
Division of Infectious Diseases
Veterans Affairs Medical Center;
University Hospitals of Cleveland
Case Western Reserve University
Cleveland, Ohio

Burton C. West, MD, FACP
Department Of Medicine
Huron Hospital
East Cleveland, Ohio

L. Joseph Wheat, MD, FACP
Professor of Medicine
Histoplasmosis Reference Laboratory
Indiana University School of Medicine
Indiana Veterans Hospital
Indianapolis, Indiana

Ian Woolley, MD, MB, FRACP
Director
Infectious Diseases/Infection Control Units
Peninsula Health
Frankston Hospital;
Physician and Honorary Senior Lecturer
Infectious Diseases Unit/Department
   of Medicine
Alfred Hospital/Monash University
   Medical School
Victoria, Australia

† Deceased.

Preface

The purpose of this newest volume in the ACP Expert Guide series is to provide up-to-date information on common infectious diseases encountered in the office of the primary care physician. Infections comprise a sizable proportion of the common, and less common, diseases seen in the office as well as in the hospital. Physicians are expected to know not only the basic clinical manifestations of each infection but also the names of the etiologic agents, the new diagnostic tests, and the new therapies. With the number of new antimicrobial agents increasing yearly, it has been ever more difficult for practicing physicians to distinguish and master all the treatments and therapies that could be useful to their patients.

Many physicians have not kept up with advances in clinical microbiology since their graduation from medical school. The first chapter introduces the proper use of clinical microbiology and discusses some of the recent advances in diagnostic techniques. The most appropriate and practical diagnostic tests for the more commonly encountered diseases are reviewed. Richard Thomson, a clinical microbiologist with extensive experience, was asked to write this chapter because of his ability to clearly convey clinical microbiology information to the practicing physician.

The discussion of individual diseases begins with common central nervous system infections, with emphasis on bacterial infections such as meningitis and brain abscess. Two chapters are then devoted to heart and vascular infections. The first, on endocarditis, was written by Chatrchai Watanakunakorn, one of the most active researchers in this field. Sadly, this close friend and colleague passed away in July 2001. Because of the increased use of vascular devices, the second chapter in this section considers native vascular and device-associated infections.

Infections in the gastrointestinal tract, including diarrhea, hepatitis, and surgical diseases, continue to be commonly encountered in the primary care practice, and five chapters are devoted to them here. The following section focuses on genitourinary infections, including sexually transmitted diseases and papillomavirus, the latter meriting a separate chapter because of its increasing importance in the detection of cervical cancer.

Respiratory tract infections are one of the most common reasons for prescription of antimicrobial agents in the United States. Itzhak Brook, Thomas Marrie, and Thomas File, all members of guidelines committees of important medical societies, were among the contributors to this section, the longest in the book.

Bone infections and skin infections are commonly seen in patients; however, diagnosis does not always come easy. Without intending to be exhaustive, the chapters in these two sections provide important principles that will guide physicians in their management of these problems.

HIV infection is one of leading causes of death in the world. Because of rapid advances in the diagnostic and therapeutic fields, the clinician is urged to consult the most recent literature and specialists in treating HIV patients. Our purpose herein has been to give the basic information the physician needs to manage the patient with this infection. Opportunistic fungal, mycobacterial, viral, and *Pneumocystis* infections are next reviewed.

The final two chapters discuss Lyme disease (included because of its prevalence in certain geographic areas of the United States) and malaria (representing the parasitic infections).

The authors have written with clarity and conciseness. For the convenience of the reader, helpful tables on diagnosis and treatment recommendations have been provided throughout the text. *Expert Guide to Infectious Diseases* cannot be the final word on a subject so vast. Its aim is more modest but of equal importance: to be the best source for the *essential* information sought by the primary care physician.

James S. Tan, MD

Contents

SECTION III   GASTROINTESTINAL INFECTIONS

SECTION IV   GENITOURINARY INFECTIONS

SECTION V RESPIRATORY TRACT INFECTIONS

1

Use of Microbiology Laboratory Tests in the Diagnosis of Infectious Diseases

Richard B. Thomson Jr., PhD

The laboratory diagnosis of infectious diseases requires the detection of etiologic microorganisms or antibodies specific for the etiologies. Microorganisms can be detected by staining and recognition of characteristic morphology, by culture and identification of the isolate, and by detection of antigens or nucleic acid (RNA or DNA) unique to the pathogen. Serologic testing for specific antibodies can be performed by many different methods, all of which are designed to detect the presence or absence of antibody, the relative amount of specific antibody, and the class of antibody (immunoglobulin [Ig]M, IgG, etc.) present. Table 1.1 summarizes the use of microbiology tests in the diagnosis of infectious diseases.

Regardless of the diagnostic approach used, communication between the laboratory professional and clinician is essential to proper selection and interpretation of tests and results (1). Evolving technology, emerging infectious diseases, and the need to provide rapid, economical testing fuel the need for new methods of communication. Communication can be accomplished by well-organized test requisitions and clearly formatted computer or "hard copy" written reports but often requires verbal or detailed, written exchange to convey important nuances. The need for a primary care physician to discuss personally a radiograph with a radiologist or for a surgeon to review a surgical pathology slide and report in conjunction with a pathologist are well-established practices that improve the clinician's understanding of diagnostic and treatment options. Reviewing specific laboratory data with a laboratory pro-

Table 1.1 Summary of Laboratory Tests for the Detection of Infectious Disease

Test	Detects	Use	TAT	Relative Cost*
Microscopic examination of fluid, exudate, or minced specimen	Inflammatory cells and morphology of microorganisms present	Rapid, presumptive identification of acute inflammatory process (pus), adequacy of sample and microorganism present	Minutes–hours	Low
Histopathologic examinations of biopsy tissue, curettings	Inflammatory reaction and morphology of microorganisms present	Detection of abnormal tissue, presence and type of inflammation and microorganism in relatively high quantity	Hours–days	High
Culture	Growth of microorganism	Confirms presence and identity of pathogen with antimicrobial testing results and allows typing if epidemiologically necessary	1 Day–many days	Medium
Antigen detection (EIA, FA)	Unique portion of microorganism	Establish presence of microorganism	Hours	Low–medium
Nucleic acid detection (probe, PCR, LCR)	RNA or DNA unique to microorganism or groups	Establish presence of viable or nonviable microorganism	Hours–days	Medium–high
Serology	Antibody specific for a microorganism or groups of microorganisms	Establish presence of past disease, immune status, or acute current disease	Hours–days	Low–medium

EIA = enzyme immunoassay; FA = fluorescent antibody; PCR = polymerase chain reaction; LCR = ligase chain reaction; TAT = turn-around time.
* Cost, not charge. Low = $10 to $20; Medium = $20 to $30; High = >$30.

fessional, beyond checking normal values, is a step in the diagnostic process that has been lost during recent years as laboratories have moved off site and as schedules have become more hectic. The responsibility for establishing new channels of communication lies with both the clinician and the laboratory technician. Computers, e-mail, Web sites, pagers, and voice mail offer simple and effective avenues for exchanging information essential to patient care. Table 1.2 lists issues in the laboratory diagnosis of infectious diseases that are enhanced by communication over and above the usual test requisitions and the preliminary and final written reports.

Principles of Culture

Culture represents the century-old "gold standard" for detecting microorganisms and remains essentially unchanged except for nutritional modifications that allow for growing a wider variety of bacterial species. Bacteria grow by binary fission, with average strains requiring 30 to 60 minutes for one cell to become two cells or for the total organism count to double. This process,

Table 1.2   Importance of Communication Between Clinician and Laboratory Diagnosis of Infectious Diseases

Process	Examples of Issues To Discuss
Test selection	Unusual pathogen suspected (e.g., *Letospira*). Multiple tests available (e.g., influenza virus).
Specimen collection and transport	Review of appropriate specimen (e.g., urethral vs cervical vs vaginal discharge vs urine for *Chlamydia* detection). Review of appropriate transport medium and holding conditions (e.g., urine).
Quality of specimen	Review of microscopic screening results and need for replacement specimen.
Interpretation of results	Does "positive" result represent contaminating normal flora, or presence of potential pathogen?
Antibiotic testing	Is antibiotic test necessary? What antibiotics are appropriate for potential pathogen? Interpretation of resistance mechanism requiring unique therapeutic approach or infection-control precautions.
Laboratory trends	Antibiogram (% of bacteria susceptible to usual antimicrobial agents). Common pathogens from important specimens (e.g., blood). Epidemiologic investigation required.

which cannot be accelerated, results in at least an overnight delay before growing bacteria are detected by colony formation. Some microorganisms, such as the mycobacteria, have doubling times that approach 24 hours, resulting in detection times of many weeks. Viruses grow only within other living cells and therefore are isolated in cell cultures that consist of living, metabolizing cells. Cell cultures serve as hosts for the propagation and detection of pathogenic viruses. The average turnaround times or times to detection of microbial colonies for common cultures and virus isolation tests are listed in Table 1.3.

Although culture and virus isolation tests can delay the detection or confirmation of an infectious disease, they have many important advantages. Positive cultures provide 1) definitive proof of the presence of a pathogen, 2) organisms for typing in cases of suspected outbreaks, and most importantly 3) isolates for antimicrobial testing. Surrogate markers for the presence of a pathogen (e.g., antigen detection by enzyme or fluorescence methods, antibody detection in serum) are subject to misleading false-positive and -negative results. Diagnosis by molecular methods (e.g., detection of pathogen nucleic acid by polymerase chain reaction [PCR]) provides results nearly similar to those of culture but cannot provide antimicrobial susceptibility test results. It is for these reasons that culture remains the gold standard for the diagnosis of infectious diseases.

Specimens for Culture

Specimens for culture require specific clinical material collected, stabilized, and transported according to exacting specifications to ensure valid results (2). Table 1.4 lists appropriate and inappropriate microbiology specimens for the diagnosis of different types of diseases. Table 1.5 lists specimen holding and transportation conditions that are required to maintain viable microorganisms in the relative quantities in which they are found at the time of collection. It may seem surprising that common specimens and conditions of specimen transport from the inpatient bedside and outpatient office or clinic to the laboratory violate requirements shown in these tables. Poor specimen quality is the single greatest obstacle to the accurate diagnosis of infectious diseases. Diagnoses are missed, and overdiagnoses are made from inaccurate culture reports that stem from improper specimen collection methods or transport conditions.

In general, specimens for culture should be collected as soon as possible after the onset of acute disease and before the initiation of antibiotic therapy. Collecting a second specimen for culture may be necessary because of poor specimen quality or inadequate transport conditions that affect a first speci-

Table 1.3   Average Turn-Around Times for Microbial Cultures and Virus Isolation*

Test	Average Time to Detection	Comment
Routine bacterial culture	16 – 24 hours	May be longer if few bacteria are present and inhibitory substances, such as antibiotics, are present in specimen
Anaerobic bacterial culture	24 – 48 hours	Occasional anaerobes, such as *Actinomyces* spp., require 1–2 weeks before growth can be detected
Mycobacterial culture		
Slow growers (e.g., *Mycobacterium tuberculosis*)	1 – 2 days	Molecular methods
	3 – 14 days	By rapid, broth culture method
	3 – 6 weeks	By conventional, solid medium method
Rapid growers (e.g., *Mycobacterium fortuitum* complex)	2 – 7 days	May grow on routine bacterial culture media
Fungal culture		
Yeasts and most molds	1 – 5 days	May grow on bacterial and mycobacterial culture media
Dimorphic pathogens (e.g., *Histoplasma, Blastomyces, Coccidioides*)	3 days – 2 weeks	Occasional strains require 2 – 4 weeks
Virus isolation	1 day – 1 week	Strains of cytomegalovirus and varicella-zoster virus may require 2 – 4 weeks for detection

*Time until colonies appear or virus replication in cell culture can be detected.

men, but it is rarely required in other situations. Exceptions include the collection of 1) multiple blood specimens for culture, 2) additional stool cultures from patients with chronic diarrhea, and 3) additional specimens if unusual or fastidious pathogens need to be added to the list of suspected causes.

Table 1.4   Selection of Common Clinical Specimens for Microbiologic Culture

Disease	Clinical Specimen	
	Appropriate	Inappropriate
Lower respiratory tract infection (especially bronchitis and pneumonia)	Freshly expectorated mucus and inflammatory cells (pus), sputum.	Saliva, oropharyngeal secretions, sinus drainage from nasopharynx.
Sinusitis	Secretions collected by direct sinus aspiration, or washes, curettage and biopsy material collected during endoscopy. Pus freshly "blown" into clean tissue from infected sinus.	Nasal or nasophayngeal swab, nasopharyngeal secretions, sputum, and saliva.
Urinary tract infection	Midstream urine. Urine collected by "straight" catheterization. Urine collected by suprapubic aspiration. Urine collected during cystoscopy or other surgical procedure.	Urine from Foley catheter collection bag.
Superficial wound infection	Aspirations of pus or local irrigation fluid (nonbacteriostatic saline). Swab of purulence originating from beneath the dermis.	Swab of surface material or specimen contaminated with surface material. Irrigation with saline containing preservative.
Gastrointestinal infection (diarrhea)	Freshly passed stool. Washes, feces collected during endoscopy.	Rectal swab. Specimen for bacterial culture if diarrhea developed after patient in hospitalization for ≥ 3 days.
Bacteremia/sepsis	2-3 blood specimens collected from separate venipunctures, before initiation of antibiotics, each containing ~20 mL of blood. Antisepsis with iodine-containing compound.	Clotted blood. One or more than three blood specimens collected within a 24-hour period. Volume of blood <10 mL per culture (i.e., per venipuncture). Antisepsis with alcohol only.

Screening To Ensure Specimen Quality

Most specimens that are submitted for bacterial culture can be "screened" to check for quality (3). Important questions in such screening are: 1) Does the material originate from the site of infection?, and 2) Is the material

Table 1.5   Specimen Holding and Transportation Conditions Required for Microbial Cultures

| Specimen | Holding and Transportation Conditions | |
	Appropriate	Inappropriate
Sputum	Transport to laboratory within 1 hour. Refrigerate (store on ice) specimen for longer delays. Use sterile or clean container with leakproof top.	Room temperature >1 hour. Excessive heat during transport, freezing during transport; exposure to sunlight.
Purulence or secretions on swab	Keep moist in sterile container. Use of holding medium to maintain viability and halt overgrowth of normal flora or contaminants. Room or refrigeration temperatures.	Dry container. No holding medium. Excessive heat or freezing temperatures. Delay of >24–48 hours before culture.
Fluid or purulent aspirate	Same as for swab, except that holding medium should be in vial rather than in swab holder. Holding media and vial commonly support maintenance of anaerobes. Hold at room temperature if anaerobes suspected.	Do not send to laboratory in syringe with needle. No anaerobic conditions if anaerobic bacteria suspected. Excessive heat or freezing temperatures. Delay of >24–48 hours before culture.
Urine	Transport to laboratory within 1 hour. Refrigerate (store on ice) specimen for longer delays or use boric acid-containing transport tube to stabilize bacteria.	Room temperature holding and transport without using boric acid preservative. Excessive heat or freezing during transport.
Stool	Transport to laboratory within 1 hour. Use holding medium for longer transport.	No holding medium used. Excessive heat or freezing during transport.
Blood for culture	Inoculate culture bottle directly with blood from venipuncture. Hold in incubator or at room temperature, or collect into sterile tubes containing SPS anticoagulant. Hold at room temperature.	Blood transported in syringe. Clotted blood. Blood in collection tube containing anticoagulant other than SPS. Excessive heat or freezing during transport.
Blood for serology tests	Clotted blood in sterile tube. Transport to laboratory within 1 hour. Refrigerate (store on ice) for delay of 1–4 hours. Separate serum if delay >4 hour. Keep serum refrigerated.	Blood in nonsterile tube. Blood hemolyzed. Blood stored at room temperature for >1 hour. Excessive heat or freezing during transport.

likely to contain a suspected pathogen in the absence of contaminating flora? An ideal specimen is full of inflammatory cells (usually polymorphonuclear leukocytes) and is devoid of squamous epithelial cells that indicate superficial contamination. Specimens without inflammation are unlikely to contain the specific etiologic agent being sought. Specimens with squamous epithelial cells are likely to contain contaminating bacteria that will be misinterpreted as the likely pathogen, leading to unnecessary treatment and oversight of the true cause. Specimens that fail a screening examination for quality should be discarded and replaced with acceptable specimens if possible. Table 1.6 lists common specimens and results of screens performed to ensure quality.

Laboratory Processing

Laboratory processing includes verifying the appropriateness of requested tests, selecting appropriate culture media and incubation conditions, and identifying potentially pathogenic bacteria that grow in culture. Efficient and appropriate laboratory processing requires proper labeling of the specimen, clear indication of the test(s) that have been requested, the clinical diagnosis or code according to the *International Classification of Diseases, 9th Edition*, and complete billing information. All laboratories have procedures that must be followed for unlabeled specimens to ensure compliance with licensing regulations (4). Specimens that are not labeled with patient-identifying characters or have been mislabeled cannot be processed. Additionally, it is illegal for laboratories to perform tests that have not been requested. Improper test requests cannot be changed without a physician's written order.

The clinical diagnosis helps the laboratory technician to select the appropriate medium for a requested culture. Although standard media with inocula from a specific site grow pathogens typical for that site, unusual or fastidious microorganisms can be missed unless specific tests for them are requested or are indicated by the clinical diagnosis. Enterohemorrhagic *Escherichia coli*, *Vibrio* species other than *V. cholerae*, and *Cyclospora cayetanensis* are examples of causes of enterocolitis that can go undetected by most laboratories if clinical suspicion is not conveyed to the laboratory.

Interpreting Culture Results

Because there are no "normal values" for most microbial culture results, interpretation of positive cultures is a challenge. Methods used to review the "significance" of results are, as a rule, not standardized or evidence based.

Table 1.6 Screening Specimens Requested for Culture To Ensure Quality

Specimen	Screening Method	Results of Screen		Action If Unacceptable
		Acceptable	Unacceptable	
Sputum, routine bacterial culture	Microscopic examination (stained or unstained) of smear	<25 SEC per average 10× field.	>25 SEC per average 10× field.	Do not culture.
Endotracheal aspirate, routine bacterial culture	Microscopic examination of Gram-stained smear	<25 SEC per average 10× field and bacteria detected in at least 1 of 20 fields (100×).	>25 SEC per average 10× field or no bacteria detected in 20 fields (100×).	Do not culture.
Bronchoalveolar lavage fluid, routine bacterial culture	Microscopic examination of Gram-stained smear	<1% of cells present are SEC.	>1% of cells present are SEC.	Interpret culture results with potential for contamination in mind.
Urine	Urinalysis, Gram stain of urine sediment	<3+ SEC by on urinalysis. Positive LE test result with >10 polymorphonuclear leukocytes/mm³ from symptomatic patient (patients with asymptomatic bacteriuria may not have increased number of leukocytes).	>3+ SEC on urinalysis or more than 2 potential pathogens by Gram stain. Implies grossly contaminated. Negative LE test result from symptomatic patient.	Do not culture urine. Resubmit if grossly contaminated.
Superficial wound	Microscopic examination of Gram-stained smear	<1 SEC per oil field, polymorphonuclear leukocytes present.	<1 SEC per oil field and no polymorphonuclear neutrophils.	Culture results more misleading than helpful. Submit new specimen using different collection procedure.
Stool for bacterial pathogens (Salmonella, Shigella, Campylobacter)	Location of patient/duration of hospitalization	Outpatient or inpatient ≤ 3 days.	In hospital >3 days, or diarrhea developed while in hospital.	Do not perform culture without consultation between clinician and laboratorian.
Other specimens	Screening methods unavailable or unproven			

LE = leukocyte esterase; SEC = squamous epithelial cells.

Table 1.7   Routine Bacterial Culture Results

Specimen*	Likely To Be Significant	Not Likely To Be Significant	Additional Data Suggesting Isolate Is Significant
Specimens Expected To Contain Normal Flora			
Sputum and endotracheal aspirate	Predominant potential pathogen by both Gram stain and culture. Neutrophils abundant on Gram stain.	Potential pathogen not present in Gram stain and only scant (1–2+) growth in culture. Neutrophils not abundant.	Presence of potential pathogen in neutrophils (intracellular bacteria)
Bronchoalveolar lavage	Predominant potential pathogen seen in every oil immersion field of Gram stain. Quantitative culture grows more than 10^5 cfu/mL of potential pathogen.	Potential pathogen not present in Gram stain. Culture grows less than 10^4 cfu/mL of potential pathogen.	Presence of potential pathogen in neutrophils (intracellular bacteria). In patients with prior antibiotics, clinical judgment rather than quantitative counts may be necessary.
Urine–midstream, female with cystitis	> 10^2 cfu/mL of potential pathogen and urine leukocyte esterase test is positive.	Quantity of potential pathogen equal to or less than contaminating flora.	
Midstream urine, female with pyelonephritis	> 10^5 cfu/mL of potential pathogen and urine leukocyte esterase test is positive.	Same or smaller quantity of potential pathogen as of contaminating flora.	Gram stain demonstrates potential pathogens in neutrophils and/or casts.
Midstream urine from patient with asymptomatic bacteriuria.	> 10^5 cfu/mL of potential pathogen. Urine leukocyte esterase test is usually negative.	< 10^5 cfu/mL of potential pathogen. Quantity of potential pathogen less than or equal to that of contaminating flora.	Confirm asymptomatic bacteria (by repeating urine culture when clinically necessary).
Midstream urine from male with UTI	> 10^3 cfu/mL of potential pathogen. Urine leukocyte esterase test is positive.	< 10^3 cfu/mL of potential pathogen. Quantity of potential pathogen less than or equal to that of contaminating flora.	Gram stain demonstrates potential pathogen in neutrophils or casts.
Straight catheter urine, all patients	> 10^2 or 10^3 cfu/ml of potential pathogen. Urine leukocyte esterase test is positive in symptomatic patients.	< 10^2–10^3 cfu/mL of potential pathogen. Urine leukocyte esterase test is negative.	Gram stain demonstrates potential pathogen in neutrophils or casts.

Foley catheter urine, all patients	>10³ cfu/mL of potential pathogens (multiple pathogens may be present). Urine leukocyte esterase test is positive.	Bacteria detected in asymptomatic patients. Urine leukocyte esterase test may be positive or negative.	No reason to culture unless patient is symptomatic.
Superficial wound	Predominant potential pathogens in both Gram stain and culture. Neutrophils abundant.	Absence of neutrophils. Abundance of squamous epithelial cells.	Intracellular bacteria seen on Gram stain.
Specimens from Normally Sterile Sites			
Fluids (e.g., cerebrospinal fluid) and tissue from deep sources (e.g., liver)	Neutrophils present. Potential pathogen in both Gram stain and culture, or if direct smear is negative, multiple colonies of potential pathogen present on multiple culture plates.	Absence of neutrophils. Single colony on one culture plate or growth in broth culture† only.	Intracellular bacteria seen on Gram stain.
Blood	Detection of potential pathogen in one or more cultures.	Detection of coagulase-negative staphylococci, Corynebacterium spp., Propionibacterium spp., Bacillus spp., and saprophytic Neisseria spp. in one culture only.	Detection of blood isolate at site of primary infection (e.g., sputum wound, urine, intravascular catheter, etc.).

* Assumes screens indicate acceptable specimen.
† Broth culture alone implies very few microorganisms in specimen. Broth media are inoculated with a larger volume of specimen than are agar media, resulting in broth-only positive results when very low numbers of microorganisms are present. In addition, anaerobic bacteria may grow in broth culture only, since many broth media are more reduced than are agar plates incubated aerobically.

Circumstances in which scientific evidence, common sense, and understanding of the pathogenesis of infection can be used to guide the interpretation of culture results are listed in Table 1.7 (5). Proper interpretation of culture results requires an understanding of laboratory information and the patient's clinical presentation. Many correct interpretations can be made only if direct communication occurs between the clinician and laboratory professional. Better patient care, along with clinician satisfaction and confidence, follows. Table 1.8 lists critical values for microbiology tests (i.e., those results that are likely to have an immediate effect on patient care and that require rapid communication to the patient's physician or caregiver).

Principles of Rapid and Non–Culture-Based Testing

Although culture remains the gold standard for detecting most microorganisms, non–culture-based detection methods offer more rapid results, and in some cases are more sensitive than culture-based methods. However, non–culture-based methods suffer from the inability to provide information about antimicrobial susceptibility and do not provide isolates for bacterial strain typing when epidemiologic studies are needed.

Non–culture-based detection methods can be divided into three categories: 1) microscopic examination of stained smears; 2) microbial antigen detection by FA, EIA, or LA testing; and 3) detection by molecular methods such as nucleic acid probing or amplification.

The easiest and fastest non–culture-based detection method is the microscopic examination of wet mounts and stained smears. Bacterial infection is best detected with the Gram stain; mycobacterial infection with the auramine–rhodamine fluorescent acid-fast stain; fungal infections with the KOH/Calcofluor wet mount; and parasitic infections with Giemsa stain for intracellular and blood parasites, iodine wet mount for helminths, trichrome stain for protozoans, and Kinyoun acid-fast stain for stool coccidians. Tables 1.9 to 1.11 summarize the use and interpretation of microbial stains and wet mounts.

Microbial antigen detection is nearly as quick as conventional bright-field microscopic examination and is more specific, because microorganisms can be identified by unique antigens. However, microbial antigen detection does not allow the examination of specimen cellularity (e.g., neutrophils, contaminating epithelial cells) that is inherent in conventional microscopy. Antigen can be detected with FA, EIA, and LA methods. FA stains require the use of an expensive fluorescence microscope and a trained microscopist. Moreover, smear preparation for fluorescent staining requires centrifugation to concentrate the specimen as well as specimen washing to eliminate nonspecific fluo-

Table 1.8   Summary of Critical Values in Clinical Microbiology

Observation / Critical Value	Rapid Communication Helpful	Immediate Verbal Communication Required
Positive blood culture		X
All positive findings for normally sterile body fluids (e.g., cerebrospinal fluid), including stains, molecular tests, antigen screens, and cultures (all microorganisms)		X
Detection of unusual or highly significant microorganism (e.g., *Listeria monocytogenes*, *Brucella*, malarial parasites, *Mycobacterium tuberculosis*, etc.)		X
Gram stain result suggesting gas gangrene		X
Physician request for immediate communication of positive result (especially surgery)		X
Any smear result strongly suggestive of pneumonia	X	
Detection of group A or B streptococcus from patient in labor and delivery status or a newborn	X	
Detection of group A streptococcus from surgical wound infections	X	
Detection of microorganism with unusual antimicrobial resistance (e.g., multidrug-resistant Gram-negative bacillus)	X	
Detection or confirmation of a communicable disease requiring immediate notification of public health laboratory	X	

rescence. Fluorescent stains are 40% to 100% as sensitive as are cultures but require only 2 to 4 hours to complete. Table 1.12 summarizes the performance of common FA tests.

Enzyme immunoassays are available as conventional and membrane tests. Conventional tests must be performed by trained personnel, require expensive instrumentation, and are best for testing large batches of specimens at one time. Membrane tests, such as the rapid *Streptococcus* tests available for detecting *S. pyogenes*, can be performed by personnel with minimal training and are designed for individual rather than batch use. Both testing formats are well suited to the detection of microorganisms that cannot be easily detected by culture.

Latex agglutination testing in modern laboratories is limited to testing for bacterial antigens in body fluids (especially cerebrospinal fluid) and for

Table 1.9   Microscopic Examination of Stained Smears: Interpretation of the Gram Stain

Morphology Observed/Reported	Interpretation
Gram-positive cocci, clusters	Straphylococci
Gram-positive cocci, chains	Streptococci
Gram-positive diplococci	Pneumococci
Gram-negative diplococci	*Neisseria/Moraxella*
Gram-negative coccobacilli	*Haemophilus*
Gram-positive rod, diphtheroid	*Corynebacterium/Propionibacterium*
Gram-positive rod, boxcar	*Clostridum/Bacillus*
Gram-positive rod, branching	*Nocardia/Actinomyces*
Gram-positive rod	Other Gram-positive rods (*Listeria, Lactobacillus,* etc.)
Gram-negative rod	Enteric and *Pseudomonas*-like Gram-negative rods
Yeast cells	Yeast (e.g., *Candida, Torulopsis,* and *Cryptococcus*)
Yeast cells with pseudohyphae	*Candida* species
Hyphae	Mold (e.g., *Aspergillus*)

Clostridium difficile in stool specimens. Bacterial antigens, including those of *S. pneumoniae, Haemophilus influenzae, Neisseria meningitidis,* and *S. agalactiae* (group B *Streptococcus*), have diminished the usefulness in today's hospitals. Laboratory evaluations show antigen-testing results to be equivalent to those of the Gram stain, and clinical evaluations show that, in the overwhelming majority of instances, no change in antibiotic therapy occurs until culture results are available. In a climate of limited testing resources, bacterial antigen tests should be used infrequently (6). An approach to limiting the use of antigen tests is to test only specimens of cerebrospinal fluid with abnormal glucose and/or protein concentrations or those with abnormal cell counts *or* to test only specimens from patients who have taken antibiotics that might interfere with culture results. Table 1.13 summarizes the performance of common EIAs and LA tests.

Molecular methods for detecting pathogenic organisms are emerging as essential components of the diagnosis of some infectious diseases (7). Common molecular methods include detection without amplification, using nucleic acid probes, and detection with amplification through the PCR and ligase chain reaction. Amplification increases the sensitivity of detection and is required for most assays. Molecular methods are suited for the detection of microorganisms in cases in which 1) antimicrobial susceptibility testing is not needed, 2)

Table 1.10   Microscopic Examination of Stained Smears: Interpretation of the KOH/Calcofluor Stain for Fungi

Morphology Observed/Reported	Interpretation
Yeasts	
Budding yeast cells	Yeast, including *Candida* spp., *Torulopsis* (*Candida*) *glabrata*, *Cryptococcus* spp., etc.
Budding yeast cells with pseudohyphae	*Candida* spp.
Filamentous fungi (molds)	
Septate dematiaceous (brown) hyphae	Dematiaceous fungi, including *Curvularia*, *Cladosporium*, *Phialophora*, *Exophiala*, *Alternaria*, etc.
Hyaline septate hyphae with or without arthroconidia in hair, skin, or nail	Dematiaceous fungi, including *Trichophyton*, *Microsporum*, *Epidermophyton*, etc.
Hyaline, septate hyphae	*Aspergillus*, *Fusarium*, *Pseudallescheria*, etc.
Nonseptate ribbon-like hyphae	Zygomycetes, including *Rhizopus* etc.
Other fungal structures	See Table 1.24.

strains of an infecting organism are not required for epidemiologic analysis, and 3) culture methods are not available. Although molecular testing is relatively expensive, it permits rapid diagnosis in cases in which detection by culture was previously unavailable. Table 1.14 summarizes molecular tests and their uses. New molecular methods and commercially available instruments that allow all laboratories to perform sophisticated assays should not be used without caution. The extreme sensitivity of molecular tests necessitates vigilance for false-positive results. Interlaboratory surveys have shown that contamination of testing equipment with amplified DNA contributes to spurious results. Laboratory professionals and clinicians alike must evaluate every case with this pitfall in mind.

Principles of Identification

Bacteria

Isolated bacteria are identified by immunologic testing, which reveals the presence of unique antigens, and biochemical testing, in which a characteristic pattern of substrate utilization is compiled (8). Identification by immunologic

Table 1.11   Microscopic Examination of Stained Smears: Use of Stains for Mycobacteria and Parasites

Stain	Use	Example of Specific Microorganisms Detected
Auramine-rhodamine stain	Acid-fast bacilli	All mycobacteria *Nocardia* species
Giemsa stain	Intracellular blood and tissue parasites	Malarial parasites *Babesia* *Toxoplasma* *Leishmania* Trypansomes
Trichrome	Stool protozoas	*Entamoeba histolytica* *Giardia lamblia* *Strongyloides stercoralis* Schistosomes
Iodine wet mount	Helminth eggs, larvae and adult worms (helminths) in stool	
Kinyoun acid-fast stain	Oocysts of coccidians in stool	*Cryptosporidium parvum* *Cyclospora cayetanensis* *Isospora belli*

Table 1.12   Performance of Common Fluorescent Antibody Tests

Microorganism Detected	Sensitivity (%)	Specificity (%)
Bordetella pertussis	60–90% (Good)	80–90% (Poor-good)
Respiratory syncytial virus	85–100% (Excellent)	90–100% (Good-excellent)
Influenza and other respiratory viruses	50–70% (Poor-good)	90–100% (Good-excellent)
Giardia and *Cryptosporidium*	90–100% (Excellent)	95–100% (Excellent)
Legionella pneumophila	40–70% (Poor-good)	90–100% (Good-excellent)

methods, such as latex agglutination (LA), can be accomplished in minutes but is restricted to *Staphylococcus aureus*, beta-hemolytic streptococci, the *Salmonella* and *Shigella* groups, and a few other organisms. Biochemical testing is the mainstay of bacterial identification, and is accomplished by "spot," same-day, or overnight testing. Spot testing requires only minutes to complete, and involves rubbing the unknown microorganism on a substrate-impregnated paper. Large amounts of preformed bacterial enzyme degrade the substrate,

Table 1.13   Performance of Common Enzyme Immunoassays and Latex Agglutination Tests

Microorganism Detected	Format*	Sensitivity	TAT
Streptococcus pyogences (streptococcal pharyngitis)	Membrane EIA	60%–90%	Minutes
Clostridium difficile (antibiotic-associated diarrhea)	Conventional and membrane EIAs	70%–95%	Minutes–hours
	Latex agglutination	60%–80%	Minutes
Rotavirus (pediatric diarrhea)	Conventional and membrane EIAs	90%–100%	Minutes–hours
Respiratory syncytial virus	Conventional and membrane EIAs	85%–100%	Minutes–hours
Influenza virus	Membrane EIA	60%–80%	Minutes
Bacterial antigens of *Streptococcus pneumoniae, Haemophilus influenzae, Neisseria meningitidis,* and *Streptococcus agalactiae*	Latex agglutination	50%–90%	Hours

EIA = enzyme immunoassay; TAT = turn–around time.
* *See text for description of EIA formats.*

which is signaled by a color indicator mixed with the reagent-containing substrate. Spot testing is inexpensive and rapid but works only with bacteria that produce excessive amounts of enzyme and have unique substrate patterns. Same-day testing works with bacteria that have sufficient amounts of preformed enzyme to degrade a substrate without prolonged incubation. It requires hours to complete but no overnight incubation. The advantage of same-day testing is the relative speed of identification. Overnight testing is required for bacteria that produce small quantities of enzyme or whose enzymes require induction before detectable substrate degradation occurs. Overnight testing is, in general, costly and time consuming but more comprehensive and accurate than is same-day testing.

Automated identification of bacterial isolates is accomplished by biochemical testing that uses unique signals to identify substrate utilization. For example, the Vitek System (bioMerieux Vitek, Hazelwood, MO) detects early growth and substrate utilization through the use of colorimetry and nephelometry (light scattering). The Microscan System (Dade Microscan, Inc., West Sacramento, CA) uses colorimetry and spectrophotometry (light trans-

Table 1.14   Molecular Tests for the Diagnosis of Infectious Disease

Microorganism Detected	Method	Common Uses (Specimens)
Neisseria gonorrhoeae	PCR/LCR	Genital
Chlamydia trachomatis	PCR/LCR	Genital
Bordetella pertussis	PCR	Nasopharyngeal
Mycobacterium tuberculosis	rRNA target amplification /PCR	Respiratory/CSF
Herpes simplex virus	PCR	CSF
Other herpes viruses (EBV, VZV)	PCR	CSF
HIV	RT–PCR	Blood (viral load)
Hepatitis C virus	RT–PCR	Blood (viral load)
Jakob–Creutzfeldt virus	PCR	CSF/brain tissue
Parovirus	PCR	Amniotic fluid fetal blood
Human papilloma virus	DNA probe (In situ by hybridization)	Skin biopsy

CSF = cerebrospinal fluid; EBV = Epstein–Barr virus; HIV = human immunodeficiency virus; PCR = polymerase chain reaction; LCR = ligase chain reaction; rRNA = ribosomal ribonucleic acid; RT–PCR = reverse transcriptase PCR; VZV = Varicella-Zoster virus.

mission) to detect growth and reactions that involve a color change. In both instruments, identification is accomplished by computer software that matches the substrate-utilization profiles of unknown organisms with databases of known utilization profiles (9).

Terminology is common among all microbiology laboratories and is used to characterize bacteria before their definitive identification. In some instances, it is helpful for the clinician to understand this terminology to better interpret preliminary culture results. Tables 1.15 and 1.16 organize common and important bacteria according to official classification schemes and current jargon.

Mycobacteria

The mycobacteria are identified by molecular probe technology and by substrate utilization studies that are similar in principle to those used with the common bacteria discussed above. Commercially available nucleic acid probes can be used to rapidly identify *Mycobacterium tuberculosis*, *M. avium*, *M. kansasii*, and *M. gordonae*. Once in vitro growth occurs, probe identification requires 2 to 4 hours. Other mycobacteria are identified by biochemical utilization studies, which may require 2 weeks or longer to complete. The terminology used to classify the clinically significant mycobacteria is summarized in Table 1.17 (10).

Fungi

The fungi are identified by morphologic analysis and, occasionally, by physical or biochemical tests. The fungi are divided into yeasts (single-celled organisms that reproduce by budding) and molds or filamentous fungi (organisms that grow by producing multicellular filaments and aerial growth). Identification can be completed on the same day on which growth occurs but may require weeks in circumstances in which identifying characteristics are not produced readily during growth on agar plates. Colonies that represent common yeasts, such as *Candida albicans* and *C. (Torulopsis) glabrata*, can be identified with rapid tests that require only 1 to 3 hours. The terminology used to classify the clinically significant fungi is summarized in Table 1.18 (11).

Parasites

Parasites are identified by morphologic studies and, in cases of intestinal infection with *Giardia, Cryptosporidium,* or *Entamoeba histolytica,* by enzyme immunoassay (EIA; immunologic detection). The terminology used to classify human parasites is summarized in Table 1.19 (12).

Viruses

The gold standard for identifying viruses in clinical specimens is cell culture (13). Viruses cannot grow on or in artificial media (e.g., agar); they require living cells for their growth. The viral infectious cycle, which represents the sequence of events that begins with viral recognition of a susceptible cell and ends with the release of tens of thousands of new infectious virions, results in dead and dying cells in cell culture. Although viruses are too small to be seen with bright-field microscopy, the morphologic changes they produce in dying cells can be recognized and are referred to as cytopathic effect (CPE). The presence of virus in a cell culture can be recognized by the presence of CPE. In fact, the CPE of each virus is unique and can be used to identify the infecting virus.

A CPE may require days or weeks before appearing. To overcome this delay inherent in conventional cell culture, the rapid cell culture (or shell-vial culture) was developed. Rapid cell culture uses the same principle of viral detection as does conventional culture, with the infection of living cells by a virus. However, rather than await the development of a CPE, the cell monolayer is stained after 24 to 48 hours with an antibody directed at early proteins specific to the suspected infecting virus. Once the virus has infected a cell, viral genes and host cell transcription and translation machinery direct the production of viral gene-encoded proteins. The advantage of the rapid shell-vial cell culture is the rapid production and detection of viral antigen as compared with the more time-consuming detection of a CPE.

Table 1.15   Classification and Terminology Used To Describe Common Aerobic and Facultative Bacteria

Gram-Positive Cocci
    Streptococci, enterococci, *Abiotrophia*
        Beta-hemolytic streptococci
            Group A (*Streptococcus pyogenes*)
            Group B (*Streptococcus agalactiae*)
            Group C
            Group G
            Group F (*Streptococcus milleri /anginosus*)
        Group D
            Enterococci (*Enterococcus faecalis, Enterococcus faecium*)
            Streptococcus bovis
        Streptococcus pneumoniae (pneumococcus) more than 80 capsular serotypes
            viridans group streptococcus
                Streptococcus mutans
                Streptococcus salivarius
                Streptococcus sanguis
                Streptococcus milleri /anginosus
        Nutrionally variant streptococci (*Abiotrophia*)
            Abiotrophia defectiva
            Abiotrophia adiacens
    Staphylococci
        Staphylococcus aureus (coagulase positive)
        Coagulase-negative staphylococci (CNS)
        Staphylococcus saprophyticus
        Staphylococcus epidermidis
        Staphylococcus haemolyticus
        Staphylococcus hominis
        Staphylococcus capitis
Gram-Negative Cocci
    Neisseria–Moraxella
        Neisseria gonorrhoeae (gonococcus)
        Neisseria meningitidis (meningococcus)
        Neisseria catarrhalis (formerly *Branhamella*)
Gram-Positive Bacilli
    Corynebacterium species (diphtheroids)
        Corynebacterium diphtheriae
        Corynebacterium jeikeium
        Corynebacterium urealyticum
    Lactobacillus species (lactobacilli)
    Bacillus species (produce endospores)
        Bacillus anthracis
        Bacillus cereus
    Listeria monocytogenes
    Erysipelothrix rhusiopathiae
    Arcanobacterium haemolyticus

Table 1.15   Classification and Terminology Used To Describe Common Aerobic and Facultative Bacteria (Continued)

Gram-Negative Bacilli
 Fermentative
  Glucose fermenting oxidase negative
   Enterobacteriaceae
   Lactose ferment
   Escherichia coli
   Klebsiella pneumoniae
   Non-lactose-fermenting
   Proteus mirabilis
   Salmonella species
   Shigella species
   Lactose or non-lactose fermenters
   Enterobacter species
   Serratia species
   Citrobacter species
  Glucose fermenting oxidase positive
   Vibrio–Aeromonas–Pleisomonas
   V. chlorae
   V. parahaemolyticus
   V. vulnificus
   Vibrio species—other
   A. hydrophila
   Aeromonas species—other
   Plesiomonas species
 Nonfermentative
  Glucose-nonfermenting oxidase negative
   Acinetobacter species
   Stenotrophomonas maltophilia (formerly *Xanthomonas*)
  Glucose nonfermenting oxidase positive
   Pseudomonas aeruginosa
   Pseudomonas species—other
Fastidious Gram-Negative Bacteria (fastidious implies no growth on selective medium for Gram-negative organisms; i.e., MacConkey's or EMB agar)
 Haemophilus influenzae ("H. flu")
 HACEK (*Haemophilus aphrophilus, Actinobacillus, Cardiobacterium, Eikenella, Kingella*)
 Bordetella species
 Pasteurella species
 Legionella pneumophila
Uncultivatable or Difficult To Cultivate Bacteria
 Ehrlichia species
 Rickettsia species
 Tropheryma whippelii

Table 1.16   Classification and Terminology Used To Describe Common Anaerobic Bacteria

Anaerobic Cocci	Anaerobic Gram-Negative Rods
Gram-negative cocci	*Bacteroides fragilis* groups
Veillonella	*B. fragilis*
Gram-positive cocci	*B. thetaiotaomicron*
Peptostreptococcus	*B. vulgatus*
Peptococcus	*B. distasonis*
	B. ovatus
Anaerobic Gram-Positive Rods	*B. uniformis*
(Non-Spore-Forming)	*B. fragilis* group—other species
Actinomyces	
Propionibacterium	*Bacteroides* species, not *B. fragilis* group
P. acnes	*B. ureolyticus*
Eubacterium	*Bilophila*
Lactobacillus	*Porphyromonas*
Bifidobacterium	*Prevotella*
	Fusobacterium group
Anaerobic Gram-Positive Rods	*F. nucleatum*
(Spore-Forming)	*F. mortiferum*
Clostridium	*F. necrophorum*
C. perfringens	
C. ramosum	
C. septicum	
C. difficile	
C. botulinum	
C. tetani	

Viruses can be detected directly in clinical specimens within hours by EIA and fluorescent antibody (FA) staining. These methods are especially useful for viruses that do not grow in cell culture. Although direct enzyme or FA detection of viruses is rapid, these methods lack sensitivity, generally detecting only 50% to 80% of the viruses that can be detected by cell culture.

Molecular methods (e.g., PCR) are fast becoming the gold standard for the detection of many viruses. Table 1.20 summarizes tests used to detect viruses in clinical specimens.

Principles of Serologic Tests

Serologic tests, which detect antibody in serum, can be used both to establish immunity or susceptibility to infectious disease and to diagnose such disease (14). In general, exposure to and infection with a microorganism is followed

Table 1.17   Classification and Terminology Used To Describe Common Mycobacteria

Category	Mycobacterium
Mycobacterium complex	M. tuberculosis
	M. bovis
Photochromogens (colony pigment produced following exposure to light)	M. kansasii
	M. marinum
	M. simiae
Scotochromogens (colony pigment produced in light and dark)	M. szulgai
	M. xenopi
	M. scrofulaceum
	M. thermoresistible
Nonchromogens (no colony pigment)	M. avium-intracellulare (MAI)
	M. ulcerans
	M. malmoense
	M. haemophilum
	M. genavence
Rapid growers (Mycobacterium fortuitum complex)	M. fortuitum
	M. chelonei
	M. abscessus
Not able to cultivate in vitro	M. leprae

within 1 to 2 weeks by the formation of acute-phase IgM and lifelong IgG antibodies. These antibodies are specific to the infecting microorganism and continue to increase in titer for weeks to months, depending on the microorganism and the severity of disease. As the patient convalesces, the titer of microorganism-specific IgM antibody wanes and, as a rule, becomes undetectable from 1 to 4 months after the onset of infection. Although the titer of microorganism-specific IgG antibody also wanes, it is usually detectable for the remainder of that patient's life. Reinfection by an antigenically similar microorganism results in a spike in the titer of this specific IgG and occasionally a spike to detectable levels of specific IgM. Titers then once again diminish to undetectable levels of IgM and detectable but lower levels of IgG.

Serum specimens are collected by venipuncture into a sterile tube that contains no anticoagulant. Specimens should be stored on ice or refrigerated until clots are removed. Clots should be removed as soon as possible, preferably within hours, to prevent hemolysis and subsequent interference with assays.

Table 1.18   Classification and Terminology Used To Describe Common Fungi

Yeasts and Yeast-Like Fungi	Filamentous Fungi (Molds)	Dimophic Fungi
Candida albicans	Hyaline, Septate Hyphae	Histoplasma capsulatum
C. tropicalis	Aspergillus fumigatus	Blastomyces dermatitidis
C. parapsilosis	A. flavus	Coccidioides immitis
C. krusei	A. niger	Sporothrix schenckii
C. lusitaniae	A. terreus	Paracoccidioides
C. (Torulopsis) glabrata	Fusarium	brasiliensis
Cryptococcus neoformans	Pseudallescheria	
Saccharomyces	Nonseptate, Ribbon-like Hyphae	
Rhodotorula	Rhizopus	
Malassezia	Mucor	
Trichosporon	Absidia	
Blastoschizomyces	Dematiaceous Fungi	
Geotrichum	Curvularia	
	Cladosporium	
	Phialophora	
	Exophiala	
	Alternaria	
	Dermatophytes	
	Trichophyton	
	Microsporum	
	Epidermorphyton	
	Branching Filamentous Bacteria	
	Nocardia	
	Actinomyces	

Serum separator tubes can be stored for longer periods without drawing off the serum. Serum can be stored for days to years before testing.

Storage for a few days should be at refrigeration temperatures (4°C). Storage for longer periods should be at freezer temperatures (colder than –12°C). Prolonged storage (>1 month) should be at –70°C. Serum specimens should not be stored in frost-free freezers or with repeated freezing and thawing, because this can aggregate IgM-type antibodies and denature all antibodies and result in false-negative tests. Specimens that are frozen and need to be transported to another office or laboratory for analysis should be sent in the frozen state.

Immunity, especially to viral diseases, can be established by detecting antibody—an indication that infection has occurred sometime in the past. Serologic tests for immunity must be performed with sensitive methods that detect IgG-type antibodies (e.g., enzyme-based assays rather than complement fixation-type assays).

Serologic diagnosis of disease can be accomplished by detecting either pathogen-specific IgM or a rise in the titer of pathogen-specific IgG. IgM can

Table 1.19   Classification and Terminology Used To Describe Common Parasites

| Protozoa | Helminths | |
	Intestinal	Tissue
Intestinal and urogenital	Cestodes (flat worms)	Cestodes (flat worms)
Amebae	*Diphyllobothrium* (fish tapeworm)	*Cysticercus* (Taenia solium)
Blastocystis	*Hymenolepis* (dwarf tapeworm)	*Echinococcus*
Endolimax	*Taenia* (beef and pork tapeworms)	
Entamoeba		
Iodamoeba	Nematodes (round worms)	Nematodes (round worms)
Ciliate	*Ancylostoma* (Old World hook-	*Ancylostoma* (dog or cat
Balantidium	worm)	hookworm)
Coccidia	*Ascaris* (roundworm)	*Anisakis*
Cryptosoridium	*Enterobius* (pinworm)	*Brugia* (lymphatic filaria)
Cyclospora	Nematodes (round worms)	*Capillaria* (visceral larva
Isospora	*Strongyloides* (threadworm)	migrans)
Flagellates	*Trichuris* (whipworm)	*Dirofilaria* (dog heartworm)
Dientamoeba		*Dracunculus* (Guinea worm;
Giardia		subcutaneous tissue)
Trichomonas		*Loa* (eye worm;
Microsporidia		subcutaneous tissue)
Encephalitozoon		*Mansonella* (dermal filaria)
Enterocytozoon		*Onchocerca* (subcutaneous
Nosema		tissue filaria)
Pleistophora		*Strongyloides*
Septata		*Toxocara* (dog or cat
		ascaris)
		Trichinella
		Wuchereria (lymphatic filaria)
Blood and tissue		
Babesia	Trematodes (flukes)	Trematodes (flukes)
Leishmania	*Clonorchis* (liver fluke)	*Clonorchis* (liver fluke)
Plasmodium	*Fasciola* (liver fluke)	*Fasciola* (liver fluke)
Toxoplasma	*Fasciolopsis* (intestinal fluke)	*Paragonimus* (lung fluke)
Trypanosoma	*Metagonimus* (intestinal fluke)	*Schistosoma* (blood fluke)
	Opisthorchis (liver fluke)	
Free-living amebae	*Paragonimus* (lung fluke)	
Acanthamoeba	*Schistosoma* (blood fluke)	
Hartmannella		
Naegleria		

be detected as early as 1 week after the onset of disease. The presence of pathogen-specific IgM in a single serum specimen suggests current or very recent infection by that particular pathogen. Rising IgG titers are detected by collecting and assaying acute and convalescent serum specimens. The acute

Table 1.20   Tests for the Detection of Common Viruses

Virus	Specimen	Diagnostic Test
Viruses causing respiratory tract disease	Throat swab, respiratory secretion	
Influenza A and B virus		FA stain, EIA, culture
Adenovirus virus		FA stain, culture
Respiratory syncytial virus		FA stain, EIA, culture
Parainfluenza virus		FA stain, culture
Viruses causing central nervous system disease	Cerebrospinal fluid or brain tissue	
Enteroviruses		PCR, culture
Herpes simplex virus		PCR
Varicella-zoster virus		PCR
Jakob–Creutzfeldt virus (polyoma)		PCR, EM
Cytomegalovirus		PCR
Viruses causing cutaneous disease		
Herpes simplex virus	Cells for Tzanck smear, vesicle fluid	Tzanck for FA, fluid for culture
Varicella-zoster virus	Cells for Tzanck smear	Tzanck for FA
Enteroviruses	Vesicle fluid, throat or, rectal swab	Culture
Parvovirus	Serum	Serology (virus-specific IgM test)
Viruses causing multisystem disease		
Cytomegalovirus	Blood (white blood cells), tissue	Antigenemia for blood, rapid shell vial culture for blood and tissue

FA = fluorescent antibody; EIA = enzyme immunoassay; culture = cell culture; PCR = polymerase chain reaction; EM = electron microscopy.

specimen is collected as soon as possible after the onset of disease, and the convalescent specimen is collected 3 to 6 weeks later. A significantly greater antibody titer in the convalescent specimen than that detected in the acute specimen suggests current infection by the specifically infecting pathogen. In some clinical situations, both convalescent and postconvalescent serum specimens are collected. In such instances, a significant decrease in serum antibody titer from the convalescent to the postconvalescent specimen may indicate recent infection. This approach and interpretation should be confirmed with the laboratory performing the test. Serologic diagnosis of infection by detection of IgM or IgG antibody is more effective for some infectious agents than for others. Drawbacks to serologic testing include the persistence of IgM for months after acute infection, the need to wait for a convalescent specimen when test-

Table 1.21   Serologic Test Used To Detect Immunity and Diagnose Disease

Disease	Microorganism	Test/Antibody
Amoebic dysentary	*Entamoeba histolytica*	IgG/Acute only
Cytomegalovirus disease	Cytomegalovirus	Immune status
		IgM/Acute only
		IgG/Acute, convalescent
Gastritris, ulcer	*Helicobacter pylori*	Immune status
HIV diseases	HIV	Immune status
Infectious mononucleosis	Epstein-Barr Virus (EBV)	Immune status
		IgM/Acute only
		IgG (multiple antigens used)/Acute only or acute, convalescent
Fungal disease (systemic)	*Histoplasma capsulatum*	IgG/Acute, convalescent
	Blastomyces dermatitidis	IgG/Acute, convalescent
	Coccidiodes immitis	IgG/Acute, convalescent
Hepatitis	Hepatitis A virus	Immune status
		IgM/Acute only
		IgG/Acute, convalescent
	Hepatitis B virus	IgG (multiple antigens used)
	Hepatitis C virus	Immune status with confirmation
Leptospirosis	*Leptospira*-multiple serotypes	IgG/Acute, convalescent
Lyme disease	*Borrelia burgdorferi*	IgG/Acute, convalescent
Measles	Measles virus	Immune status
		IgM/Acute only
Mycoplasma respiratory disease	*Mycoplasma pneumoniae*	Immune status
		IgM/Acute only
Parvovirus disease	Parvovirus	Immune status
		IgM/Acute only (diagnosis)
		IgG/Acute, convalescent
Rubella	Rubella virus	Immune status
		IgM/Acute only (diagnosis)
		IgG/Acute, convalescent
Syphilis	*Treponema pallidum*	Non-treponemal test (e.g., RPR/VDRL)
		Treponemal tests (e.g., FTA-ABS)
Varicella and zoster	Varicella–zoster virus	Immune status

RPR = rapid plasma reagin test; VDRL = veneral disease research laboratory test; FTA-ABS = fluorescent treponemal antibody absorption test.

ing for IgG, and interference with diagnostic antibody levels after vaccination. Table 1.21 lists the common serology tests that are used to detect immunity and diagnose disease.

Interpreting Biopsy Specimens

Microorganisms can be detected in thin sections of biopsy tissue through characteristic histopathologic reactions and by identifying microbial morphology with histologic stains. In either case, unfixed tissue from the same biopsy specimen as the tissue that was submitted for microscopic examination by the pathologist should be aseptically dissected and submitted to the microbiology laboratory for culture. Detecting microorganisms in culture is 1) more sensitive than is microscopic examination, 2) serves to confirm morphologic findings and to provide more complete identification of an organism, and 3) provides cells of the organism for antimicrobial susceptibility testing or microbial typing in epidemiologically related cases.

Histopathologic Reactions

Histopathologic inflammatory responses to infection depend on both the pathogenic properties of the infectious agent and the immune status of the host and can be divided into the following categories as reviewed by Woods and Walker (15):

- Acute inflammation characterized by an exudative and suppurative response, which may result in abscess formation
- Caseating and noncaseating granulomatous inflammation
- Mixed suppurative and granulomatous inflammation
- Nonorganizing, mixed acute and chronic or chronic inflammation
- Histiocyte aggregates or diffuse infiltrates

Tables 1.22 to 1.26 summarize histopathologic inflammatory responses, tissue-stain findings, and the morphologic appearance of the causative microorganisms in tissue.

Interpreting In Vitro Antimicrobial Susceptibility Tests

In vitro antimicrobial susceptibility tests are used to help predict whether a specific antimicrobial agent will eradicate a pathogen from a site of infection. Laboratories perform in vitro susceptibility tests when they isolate a likely pathogen that has an unpredictable antimicrobial profile, and proven methods exist for determining the pathogen's susceptibility and resistance. The methods used to test antimicrobial susceptibility are established by the National Committee for Clinical Laboratory Standards (NCCLS), a consensus group

Table 1.22   Microorganisms That Cause Acute Inflammation With or Without Abscess Formation

Organism	Tissue Stains	Organism Appearance
Pyogenic bacteria*	Brown–Brenn, Brown–Hopps	GPC, GNDC, GNB
Actinomycetes	Brown–Brenn, GMS, Fite[†]	Beaded, gram-positive filaments (1 μm in diameter), may fragment and form what appears to be chains or clusters of gram-positive bacilli or coccobacilli.
Candida species	H&E, PAS, GMS	Budding yeasts (3–5 μm diameter), pseudohyphae, occasionally septate hyphae.
Aspergillus species**	H&E, PAS, GMS	Septate hyphae (3–8 μm diameter) with parallel walls, often showing repeated, dichotomous branching at 45 degree angle.
Zygomycetes	H&E, PAS, GMS[††]	Broad (8–24 μm in diameter), nonseptate (or sparsely septate) ribbon-like, often distorted hyphae with nonparallel walls.

GMS = Gomori's methenamine silver stain; GNB, Gram-negative bacilli; GNDC = Gram-negative diplococci; GPC = Gram-positive cocci; H&E = hematoxylin and eosin; PAS = periodic acid–Schiff stain.
* Includes many bacteria, such as staphylocci, streptococci, *Neisseria* species, most members of the *Enterobacteriaceae*, *Pseudomonas aeruginosa*, *Haemophilus influenzae*, and many other gram-negative bacilli.
[†] *Nocardia* positive; *Actinomyces* negative (may be weakly positive with Putt's modification of Fite's stain).
** Hyphae of other hyaline molds, such as *Pseudallescheria boydii* and *Fusarium* species, have a similar apperance in tissue.
[††] Zygomycetes stain weakly with GMS.
Republished with permission from Woods GL, Walker DH. Detection of infection or infectious agents by use of cytologic and histologic stains. Clin Microbiol Rev. 1996; 9:382-404.

composed of representatives from industry, government, clinical laboratories, and appropriate medical societies. The NCCLS publishes updated procedures yearly, and all laboratories are required by licensing regulations to follow NCCLS methods. The antimicrobial agents to be tested by the laboratory should be determined by local resistance patterns, cost, and the preferences of physicians who are knowledgeable in antimicrobial therapy. Physician, pharmacy, and laboratory representatives commonly form the nucleus of the committee responsible for determining the batteries of antimicrobials to be tested. These batteries of tests need to be reviewed and changed on a periodic basis.

Table 1.23   Microorganisms That Cause Granulomatous Inflammation

Microorganism	Tissue Stains	Morphology
Formation of Noncaseating "Mature" Granulomas*		
Mycobacterium tuberculosis	Auramine–rhodamine, Kinyoun, Ziehl–Neelsen	Yellow fluorescent (fluorochrome) or red (with carbolfuchsin) beaded bacilli
Nontuberculous mycobacteria	As above	As above. Primarily Mycobacterium marinum (skin lesions), Mycobacterium szulgai (most commonly chronic pulmonary disease), and Mycobacterium leprae (tuberculoid leprosy)
Histoplasma capsulatum	GMS, PAS	Small yeast cells (2–5 µm in diameter) with single buds, often in macrophages
Brucella spp.	NA	NA
Toxoplasma gondii	H&E, PAS	Spherical cysts (up to 30 µm); crescentic tachyzoites (2–3 µm by 4–8 µm)
Coxiella burnetti	NA	NA
Ehrlichia spp.	NA	NA
Cytomegalovirus	NA	NA
Schistosoma spp.	H&E	Eggs in different stages of destruction and calcification
Dirofilaria immitis	H&E	Worm in pulmonary artery, diameter 140–200 µm (male) to 300 µm (female), smooth cuticle
Formation of Caseating Granulomas†		
Mycobacterium tuberculosis	Auramine–rhodamine, Kinyoun, Ziehl–Neelsen	Yellow fluorescent (with fluorochrome) or red (with carbolfuchsin)
Nontuberculous mycobacteria**	As above	As above. M. kansasii usually larger than M. tuberculosis (resembles "shepherd's crook"), with broad bands
Histoplasma capsulatum	GMS, PAS	Round to oval yeast cells (2–5 µm) with single buds
Coccidioides immitis	H&E, GMS, PAS	Spherules (20–200 µm) with or without internal endospores (2–5 µm)
Cryptococcus neoformans	H&E, GMS, PAS, mucicarmine, Fontana–Masson	Variably sized yeast cells (2–15 µm) with single buds

H&E = hematoxylin and eosin; GMS = Gomori's methenamine silver stain; NA, not applicable because organisms typically are not seen in tissue; PAS = periodic acid–Schiff stain.

* Other organisms that may (but usually do not) cause noncaseating granulomas are Pneumocystis, Candida spp., Treponema pallidum (secondary syphilis; granulomas rarely in skin lesions, liver lymph node), Trypanosoma cruzi (placenta), Epstein–Barr virus, hepatitis virus, Strongyloides stercoralis, and Ascaris lumbricoides (ova). Organisms that cause noncaseating granulomas but are less commonly (or rarely) seen in the United States are Leishmania (cutaneous leishmaniasis), Toxocara spp., and Loboa loboi.

† Other organisms that may cause caseating granulomas are Blastomyces dermatitidis, Sporothrix schenckii (systemic disease), Brucella, Aspergillus, and rarely Nocardia spp.

** Most commonly Mycobacterium kansasii, Mycobacterium avium complex (immune competent host), and Mycobacterium scrofulaceum.

Republished with permission from Woods GL, Walker DH. Detection of infection or infectious agents by use of cytologic and histologic stains. Clin Microbiol Rev. 1996; 9:382-404.

The Minimum Inhibitory Concentration Test and Its Interpretation

The backbone of in vitro antimicrobial susceptibility testing is the minimum inhibitory concentration (MIC) test (16), which determines the lowest concentration of an antimicrobial agent needed to inhibit the growth of a microorganism. MIC values are reported in micrograms per milliliter (μg/mL) of antimicrobial agent and are established at concentrations that range from 0.1 μg/mL to as high as 64 μg/mL, depending on the antimicrobial agent being tested. The MIC value is compared with the quantity of antimicrobial agent that can be achieved in vivo at the site of infection. In general, when the MIC is lower than the concentration achievable at the infected site, the infecting organism is considered "susceptible" to the antimicrobial agent being tested. When the MIC is higher, the microorganism is considered "resistant." The specific concentration of antimicrobial agent at the infection site that is used to differentiate between susceptible and resistant organisms is referred to as the *breakpoint.*

Every antimicrobial agent can have a different breakpoint. These drugs are used in varying dosages and dosing schedules because they have different pharamacologic properties in the body. In practice, the breakpoint for a particular antimicrobial agent is set with many different criteria, such as the results of clinical trials, resistance mechanisms of bacteria, animal studies, pharmacokinetic and pharmacodynamic properties, and concentrations of the agent at important sites of infection (e.g., cerebrospinal fluid). It should be clear that selecting an antimicrobial agent from a list of MIC values is not simply a matter of selecting the drug with the lowest MIC. One must know the breakpoint concentration for each antimicrobial agent to ensure that the MIC value of the agent for a particular pathogen is below this concentration.

The goal of antimicrobial therapy is to kill a patient's pathogen. Can an inhibitory test be used in the laboratory to predict the killing of a pathogen in the patient? The answer is "Yes." Although methods for bactericidal (agents that kill bacteria) testing are available to the laboratory, the MIC test has proven to be an accurate predictor of clinical response through decades of trial and clinical use. In most patients, a susceptible MIC test result implies that the pathogen is likely to be eradicated from the site of infection, increasing the likelihood of a favorable outcome. A resistant MIC test result suggests that the pathogen will not be eradicated. A laboratory report indicating an "intermediate" result means that the concentration of antimicrobial agent at the infected site is at or near the MIC of the infecting pathogen. In most such cases, an alternative drug that yields a susceptible MIC test result is selected. The term *intermediate* as applied to an MIC test result also implies that the infecting organism can be interpreted as susceptible if higher-than-normal doses of the

Table 1.24   Microorganisms That Cause Mixed Suppurative and Granulomatous* Inflammation

Microorganism or Disease	Tissue Stain	Morphology of Microorganism and Unique Inflammation Response
Nontuberculous mycobacteria[†]	Auramine–rhodamine, Kinyoun, Ziehl–Neelsen	Yellow fluorescent (with fluorochrome) or red (with carbolfuchsin) beaded bacilli. *Mycobacterium fortuitum* complex may not stain with fluorochrome technique.
Blastomyces dermatitidis	H&E, PAS, GMS	Spherical multinucleate yeast (8–15 μm) with thick (double contour) walls and single, broad-based buds.
Sporothrix schenckii	PAS, GMS	Pleomorphic, spherical, oval, or cigar-shaped yeasts (2–10 μm) with single buds. Yeast cells often are not detected in tissue.
Paracoccidiodes brasiliensis	H&E, PAS, GMS	Large spherical yeasts (5–60 μm) with multiple buds attached by narrow necks ("mariner's wheel").
Chromoblastomycosis**	H&E, Fontana–Masson	Large (6–12 μm), spherical to polyhedral, thick-walled, dark brown muriform cells (sclerotic bodies) with septations along one or two planes in subcutaneous tissue ± pigmented hyphae.
Systemic phaeohyphomycosis[††]	H&E, Fontana–Masson	Brown pigmented hyphae (2–6 μm wide) branched or unbranched, often constricted at prominent septations.
Acanthamoeba spp.	H&E, PAS	Trophozoites (22 μm in diameter) with large nucleolus and vacuolated cytoplasm; cysts have thick ectocyst containing endocyst, often shrunken.
Yersinia enterocolitica, Yersinia pseudotuberculosis	Brown–Hopps	Clumps of Gram-negative bacilli (necrotizing granulomas with stellate abscesses usual).
Francisella tularensis	NA	Necrotizing granulomas with stellate abscesses usual.

**Table 1.24   Microorganisms That Cause Mixed Suppurative and Gran-
ulomatous* Inflammation (Continued)**

Microorganism or Disease	Tissue Stain	Morphology of Microorganism and Unique Inflammation Response
Bartonella henselae	Brown–Hopps, Warthin–Starry, Dieterle	Gram-negative bacilli (Warthin-Starry and Dieterle positive bacilli) in cluster of necrotic cells (early lesion), spectrum of histologic changes is usual; early lesions show focal necrosis and small abscesses; with disease progression, polymorphonuclear leukocytes become fragmented and macrophages surround the area; finally, areas of inflammation coalesce and are surrounded by epithelioid macrophages.
Chlamydia trachomatis, serotypes L_1–L_3	NA	Necrotizing granulomas with stellate abscesses usual.

GMS = Gomori's methenamine silver stain; GNB = Gram-negative bacilli; H&E = hematoxylin and eosin; ± = may or may not be present; NA = not applicable because organisms typically are not detected in tissue, although tissue is stained with H&E; PAS = periodic acid–Schiff stain.

* An uncommon infectious cause of necrotizing granulomas is *Protochea* spp. (olecranon bursitis).

† Especially *Mycobacterium fortuitum-chelonei* complex and early cutaneous lesions caused by *Mycobacterium marinum.*

** Most often *Fonsecaea pedrosoi* or *Cladosporium carrionii.*

†† Most often *Exophiala jeanselmei, Curvularia, Bipolaris,* and *Xylohypha* spp., *Phaeoannellomyces werneckii,* or *Wangiella dermatitidis.*

Republished with permission from Woods GL, Walker DH. Detection of infection or infectious agents by use of cytologic and histologic stains. Clin Microbiol Rev. 1996; 9:382-404.

specific antimicrobial agent are used or if the antimicrobial agent is concentrated at the site of infection (e.g., in the urinary tract, where drugs excreted by the kidneys become concentrated). Increasing the dose and concentration of an antimicrobial agent at various body sites increases the breakpoint of the agent for a particular pathogen, transforming intermediate MIC test results into susceptible ones.

Methods Used To Determine Minimum Inhibitory Concentration

Laboratories use many manual and automated methods to determine the MICs of antimicrobial agents for various pathogens. The microbroth dilution

Table 1.25   Microorganisms That Cause Nonorganizing Mixed Acute and Chronic or Chronic Inflammation

Microorganism	Tissue Stains	Morphology of Microorganism
Legionella species (pneumonia)	Warthin–Starry, Dieterle, or Steiner; ± Brown–Hopps; Wolbach modification of Giemsa; Kinyoun or Fite*; specific antibodies for IFA or DFA	Pleomorphic, tapered and centrally constricted bacilli (0.3–0.7 by 2–4 μm), predominantly intracellular, in polymorphonuclear leukocytes and macrophages; rare filamentous forms; appear as short, blunt rods with Dieterle stain (or other silver impregnation method)
Helicobacter pylori	Warthin–Starry, Dieterle, or Steiner; Giemsa; toluidine O; acridine orange; H&E†; "triple stain" (Steiner, H&E, alcian blue)	Curved bacteria in mucus layer
Cryptosporidium spp.	H&E, Fite	Rows or clusters of basophilic spherical structures (2–4 μm in diameter) attached to microvillous border of epithelial cells
Microsporidia	H&E, Brown–Brenn or Brown–Hopps, Warthin–Starry, modified trichrome	Organisms and round to oval spores (2–5 μm in diameter) located in cytoplasm of enterocytes (or other ciliated cells) between microvillous border and nucleus
Treponema pallidum	Warthin–Starry, Dieterle, or Steiner	Thin, spiral bacilli

DFA = direct immunofluorescence assay; H&E = hematoxylin and eosin; IFA = indirect immunofluorescence assay.
* *Legionella micdadei* positive.
† May or may not stain.
Republished with permission from Wood GL, Walker DH. Detection of infection or infectious agents by use of cytologic and histologic stains. Clin Microbiol Rev. 1996, 9:382-404.

method is the commonly used gold standard. In this technique, dilutions of antimicrobial agent prepared in a 96-well microtiter tray are inoculated with a standard concentration of the microorganism whose susceptibility is to be tested. After overnight incubation, quantitative MIC results are determined and reported in micrograms per milliliter (μg/mL), with a qualitative interpretation of susceptible, resistant, or intermediate susceptibility. Commercially

Table 1.26   Microorganisms That Cause Aggregate or Diffuse Infiltrates of Histiocytes

Microorganisms	Tissue Stains	Morphology
Mycobacterium avium complex*	Auramine–rhodamine, Kinyuon, Ziehl–Neelsen	Yellow fluorescent (with fluorochrome) or red (with carbolfuchin) beaded bacilli
Mycobacterium genavense	As above	As above
Mycobacterium leprae	Fite	Red, beaded bacilli
Leishmania spp.	H&E, Giemsa	Ovoid amastigotes (2–4 μm in diameter) within macrophages
Listeria monocytogenes	Brown–Brenn, Brown–Hopps	Short Gram-positive bacilli

H&E = hematoxylin and eosin.
* In patients with acquired immune deficiency syndrome.
Republished with permission from Wood GL, Walker DH. Detection of infection or infectious agents by use of cytologic and histologic stains. Clin Microbiol Rev. 1996, 9:382-404.

available automated methods are adjusted to meet the microbroth dilution standard.

The agar disk diffusion test is used by nearly every laboratory as a supplementary testing method. The disk-diffusion test is an MIC test performed on the surface of an agar plate. Disks containing the antimicrobial agent to be tested are placed on the surface of a standard agar plate that has been inoculated with a carefully adjusted "lawn" of bacteria. The antimicrobial agent diffuses into and across the agar surface, creating a concentration gradient that mimics the dilutions one uses in the broth microdilution procedure, with a high concentration near the disk and progressively lower concentrations at increasing distances from the disk. Bacteria grow toward the disk until they reach the surrounding region that contains the test antibiotic at their MIC value, producing a circular zone of inhibited growth around the disk. Statistical analysis has been used to determine MIC and breakpoint equivalents for disk diffusion with most antimicrobial–organism combinations. Results of disk-diffusion testing are reported as being susceptible, intermediate, or resistant, without including the MIC equivalent value.

The E-test is an agar-gradient method that uses an antimicrobial agent applied in gradient concentrations to a strip. The strip is marked to show the exact decreasing concentrations of the antimicrobial agent from one end to the other. The strip is placed onto an agar surface that has been inoculated with

the bacterium to be tested. Bacterial growth occurs around the strip in an el-
liptical pattern, with a larger area of growth inhibition at the high-concentra-
tion end of the strip and a narrowing area of inhibition toward the
low-concentration end. The MIC value is read from the concentration mark-
ing on the strip at the point at which the concentration of antimicrobial agent
is low enough to permit growth of bacteria right up to the strip. Results are reported as quantitative MIC values with a susceptible, resistant, or intermediate interpretation.

Special Methods Used To Detect Specific Resistance

Standard MIC and disk-diffusion methods do not detect all resistant bacteria
accurately (17). Supplementary methods are used to ensure accurate results.
Table 1.27 lists combinations of bacteria and antimicrobials that require supplementary testing.

Synergy Testing

The term *synergy* describes an inhibitory or microbicidal result from a combination of two antimicrobial agents that exceeds the expected result from the
effects of each agent added together. Combinations of antimicrobial agents are
commonly used with the expectation that synergy will occur, although laboratory testing is rarely needed to prove that synergy is present. Even if synergy
does not occur, the two antimicrobial agents in a particular combination may
be necessary either to broaden the spectrum of organisms covered by antimicrobial therapy in a particular case or to ensure that mutant organisms that
are resistant to one antimicrobial agent will be inhibited by the second agent.
Synergy is expected with the following regimens: 1) a β-lactam drug plus an
aminoglycoside in treating infections caused by many gram-negative bacilli,
especially *Pseudomonas aeruginosa*, 2) an antistaphylococcal β-lactam drug plus
an aminoglycoside when treating *S. aureus*, and 3) ampicillin (or an equivalent
drug) or vancomycin plus an aminoglycoside when treating enterococci or *S.
viridans*. Only the combinations of antimicrobials that are needed to treat enterococcal infections require laboratory testing to confirm synergy.

Enterococci are not routinely killed by therapy with a single antimicrobial
agent. Enterococcal endocarditis requires bactericidal therapy to ensure a high
probability of bacteriologic cure. Combinations of inhibitory, cell wall–active
antimicrobials (e.g., ampicillin or vancomycin plus gentamicin) are synergistic
because the cell wall–destroying antimicrobial agent augments the penetration
of gentamicin into the cytoplasm of the enterococcal pathogen; this is where

Table 1.27 Bacterial-Antimicrobial Combinations That Require Supplementary Testing To Confirm In Vitro Susceptibility

Microorganism	Antimicrobial	Mechanism of Resistance	Supplementary Test
Gram-Positive Cocci			
Staphylococcus aureus	Penicillin	Beta-lactamase production	Beta-lactamase assay
All Staphylococci	Methicillin and related drugs	Altered penicillin-binding proteins	MEC-A gene analysis or a combination of agar and broth dilution testing with increased concentrations of NaCl.
	Vancomycin	Altered cell wall morphology that consumes excess drug	Broth dilution MIC or agar dilution. Disk diffusion should not be used.
Enterococci	Vancomycin	Altered cell wall morphology that consumes excess drug	Broth dilution MIC or agar dilution. Disk diffusion should not be used.
Gram-Negative Bacilli			
Escherichia coli/Klebsiella	Cephalosporins	Extended-spectrum beta-lactamase production (ESBL)	Review overall antimicrobial pattern. Compare cephalosporin (e.q., ceftazidime) MIC or zone diameter to cephalosporin plus clavulanate MIC or zone diameter.
Haemophilus influenzae	Ampicillin	Beta-lactamase production	Beta-lactamase assay
Gram-Negative Cocci			
Moraxella catarrhalis	Ampicillin	Beta-lactamase production	Beta-lactamase assay
Neisseria gonorrhoeae	Penicillin	Beta-lactamase production	Beta-lactamase assay

MIC = minimum inhibitory concentration.

Table 1.28   Collection of Specimens and Interpretation of Results for Aminoglycocide and Vancomycin Assays*

Antimicrobial	Infusion	Timing of Blood Specimen	Interpretation
Vancomycin	At least 60 minutes for <1 g dose or 90–120 minutes if >1 g dose	*Peak:* 60 minutes after end of infusion	25–40 µg/mL
		Trough: Before next dose	5–15 µg/mL
		Random Level: Anytime	Redose if <5–15 µg/mL
Gentamicin or tobramycin	30 minutes	*Peak Conventional Dosing:* 30 minutes after end of transfusion	4.0–8.0 µg/mL
		Trough: Before next dose or 18 hours after q 24 h dose	<2 µg/mL
		Peak Synergy Dosing: Same as Peak Conventional Dosing	3–5 µg/mL
		Trough Synergy Dosing: Same as Trough Dosing	<1 µg/mL
		Random Level: Anytime	Redose if <2 µg/mL
Amikacin	30–60 minutes	*Peak Conventional Dosing:* 30 minutes after end of transfusion	15–30 µg/mL
		Trough: Before next dose	≤10 µg/mL
		Random Level: Anytime	Redose if <1 µg/mL

* Levels should be monitored after the third dose. Frequency of testing varies with patient conditions. In many patients, assay testing can be minimized. Consult regimens for particular diseases. Synergy dose refers to lower doses used to treat enterococci in combination with a second antimicrobial.

the gentamicin binds to ribosomes and kills the bacterial cell. A surrogate test for synergy in this instance is to perform a MIC test at a single concentration of gentamicin. The *Enterococcus* sample to be tested is inoculated into an agar plate or into broth medium that contains 500 µg/mL of gentamicin, a concentration so high that gentamicin is forced across the enterococcal cell wall and into the cell's cytoplasm. If the gentamicin is not inactivated by enterococcal aminoglycoside–inactivating enzymes, the organism will be inhibited (i.e., will be susceptible to the 500 µg/mL concentration of the drug) and synergy can

Table 1.29 Penicillin Antibiogram for Viridans Group Streptococci

Organism (n)	Cumulative Percent Inhibited at Penicillin MIC (μg/mL) of										
	0.007	0.015	0.030	0.06	0.12	0.25	0.5	1.0	2.0	4.0	8.0
Streptococcus milleri (anginosus) (115)	2	7	45	94	98	99	100	100	100	100	100
Streptococcus mitis (163)	1	10	26	41	60	71	78	80	85	92	100
Streptococcus mutans (15)	11	27	100	100	100	100	100	100	100	100	100
Streptococcus salivarius (32)	-	-	6	31	47	53	75	88	91	94	100
Streptococcus sanguis (39)	8	21	28	39	62	80	90	95	97	100	100

MIC = minimum inhibitory concentration.

be expected. If the gentamicin is inactivated by enterococcal enzymes, growth is not inhibited, the isolate is resistant to the 500 µg/mL concentration of gentamicin, and synergy will not occur. This high-level gentamicin test should be performed whenever combination antimicrobial therapy is used for the treatment of enterococcal infection.

Antimicrobial Assays

Assays of antimicrobial agents are used to measure the concentrations of these drugs in the blood. These assays can be used to document compliance with a prescribed regimen, to ensure that concentrations of a drug are adequate to effectively treat a serious infection, and to document that concentrations are not at toxic levels. In practice, measurements of aminoglycoside and vancomycin concentrations are the only assays needed routinely. Measurements of both drugs are used to ensure therapeutic and nontoxic levels. Table 1.28 summarizes the timing of the collection of specimens and the interpretation of the results for aminoglycoside and vancomycin assays.

Antibiograms

Antibiograms are compilations of antibiotic testing results over a defined period. In general, antibiograms list the percentage of bacteria susceptible to antimicrobial agents during an immediately preceding 1-year period. Antibiograms are used to assess the overall activity of antimicrobial agents against a pathogen. Every hospital or community has a different antibiogram. Commonly used antibiograms include those for gram-negative bacilli, *S. aureus*, and enterococci. Focused antibiograms, with data limited to specific microorganism–antimicrobial combinations, are useful in the management of emerging antimicrobial resistance. Antibiograms for vancomycin-resistant enterococci, Viridans group streptococci, coagulase-negative staphylococci, pneumococci, anaerobes, yeasts, and *M. tuberculosis* also can be useful. Antibiograms for groups of pathogens isolated from various anatomic sites (e.g., community-wide respiratory pathogens and stool pathogens, respectively) provide another way of representing antimicrobial susceptibility data. Table 1.29 is an example of a focused antibiogram for the viridans group streptococci.

REFERENCES

1. **Thomson RB, Peterson LR.** Role of the clinical microbiology laboratory in the diagnosis of infections. In Noskin GA (ed). *Management of Infectious Complications in Cancer Patients.* Boston: Kluwer Academic Publishers; 1998:143–65.

2. **Wilson ML.** General principles of specimen collection and transport. *Clin Infect Dis.* 1996;22:766–77.

3. **O'Grady NP, Barie PS, Bartlett J, et al.** Practice parameters for evaluating new fever in critically ill adult patients. *Crit Care Med.* 1998;26:392–408.

4. **College of American Pathologists.** *Compliance Guidelines for Pathologists.* Northfield, IL: College of American Pathologists; 1978:57–61.

5. **Morris AJ, Smith LK, Mirrett S, Reller LB.** Cost and time savings following introduction of rejection criteria for clinical specimens. *J Clin Microbiol.* 1996;34:355–7.

6. **Kiska DL, Jones MC, Mangum ME, et al.** Quality assurance study of bacterial antigen testing of cerebrospinal fluid. *J Clin Microbiol.* 1995;33:1141–4.

7. **Fredricks DN, Relman DA.** Applications of polymerase chain reaction to the diagnosis of infectious diseases. *Clin Infect Dis.* 1999;29:475–88.

8. **Forbes BA, Sahm DF, Weissfeld AS.** *Bailey and Scott's Diagnostic Microbiology,* 10th ed. St. Louis: Mosby; 1998:167–233.

9. **Miller JM, O'Hara CM.** Manual and automated systems for microbial identification. In Murray PR, Baron EJ, Pfaller MA, et al. (eds). *Manual of Clinical Microbiology,* 7th ed. Washington, DC: ASM Press; 1999:193–201.

10. **American Thoracic Society.** Diagnosis and treatment of disease caused by nontuberculous mycobacteria. *Am J Respir Care Med.* 1997;156:S1–25.

11. **McGinnis MR, Rinaldi, MG.** Some medically important fungi and their common synonyms and obsolete names. *Clin Infect Dis.* 1997;25:15–7.

12. **Garcia LS.** Classification of human parasites. *Clin Infect Dis.* 1997;25:21–3.

13. **Reisner BS, Woods GL, Thomson RB, et al.** Specimen processing. In Murray PR, Baron EJ, Pfaller MA, et al. (eds). *Manual of Clinical Microbiology,* 7th ed. Washington, DC: ASM Press; 1999:76–85.

14. **Weinstein AJ, Farkas S.** Serologic tests in infectious diseases. Clinical utility and interpretation. *Med Clin North Am* 1978; 62:1099–117.

15. **Woods GL, Walker DH.** Detection of infection or infectious agents by use of cytologic and histologic stains. *Clin Microbiol Rev* 1996;9:382–404.

16. **Jorgensen JH, Ferraro MJ.** Antimicrobial susceptibility testing: general principles and contemporary practices. *Clin Infect Dis* 1998; 26:973–80.

17. **Kiska, DL.** In vitro testing of antimicrobial agents. *Semin Pediatr Infect Dis* 1998;9:281–91.

2

Bacterial Meningitis

Carlos H. Ramirez-Ronda, MD

Carlos R. Ramirez-Ramirez, MD

Bacterial meningitis is a relatively infrequent disease with serious consequences. Central nervous system (CNS) infections account for approximately only 1% of hospital admissions, but even though bacterial meningitis is a rare disease, it requires prompt diagnosis and treatment. The morbidity and mortality from bacterial meningitis remain unacceptably high. A 1993 report observed that 61% of infants who survived gram-negative bacillary meningitis had developmental disabilities and neurologic sequelae (1). In 493 episodes of bacterial meningitis in adults, the overall case fatality rate was 25% (2). The increased frequency of isolates of *Streptococcus pneumonia* that are resistant to penicillin makes the prompt diagnosis and treatment of bacterial meningitis an urgent requirement (3–13).

Infection of the CNS can present in a great variety of forms, ranging from acute benign forms of viral meningitis to rapidly fatal bacterial meningitis; in other cases CNS infection can present with slow progressive mental deterioration that can be related to fungal, mycobacterial, or persistent viral infection (Fig. 2.1). The most common infectious diseases of the CNS are viral and bacterial meningitis, with the cumulative risk for CNS infection through age 80 years being 2.3% for men and 1.5% for women (14). Prompt treatment is usually effective for many of the severe presentations of CNS infections. The outcome is often determined by the efficacy and appropriateness of the treatment. Most deaths from bacterial infection occur at an early point, and usually within the first 48 hours of hospitalization. Because of its potential lethality, CNS infection must be recognized early and the probable infecting

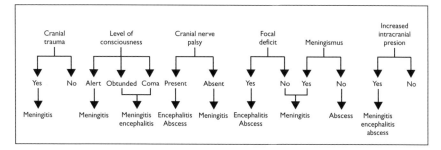

Figure 2.1   Algorithm for the evaluation and management of comminity-acquired or nosocomial meningitis. Clinical presentations are those seen in the acute clinic or emergency department or in hospitalized patients. The community-acquired diseases are divided into those that present with and without prior antibiotic treatment. In those with prior treatment, empirical therapy is started in patients with over 48 hours of pretreatment, irrespective of the CSF findings. If treatment was for less than 48 hours, empirical treatment is started only on those whose CSF examination shows a protein level of ≥150 mg/dL, a glucose level of ≤40 mg/dL, or a leukocyte count of ≥1200 cells/mL.

agent determined as rapidly as possible, either through laboratory examination or clinical diagnosis. Proper initial assessment of the patient requires a careful history, with attention to the evolution of the patient's disease, the history of exposures to infectious agents, and host factors that may result in increased susceptibility to certain infections. The physical examination is directed at localizing the neurologic disease and identifying evidence of systemic infection. These assessments are supplemented by examination of the cerebrospinal fluid (CSF) and imaging studies.

Epidemiology

The frequency of meningitis in children caused by *Hemophilus influenzae* has declined dramatically in the past 5 to 10 years because of widespread vaccination against *H. influenzae* type b. Specifically, from 1985 to 1991 there was an 82% reduction in the incidence of *H. influenzae* meningitis in children under 5 years of age (4,15). This reduction means that *S. pneumoniae* and *Neisscria meningitidis* have become the predominant causes of meningitis in non-neonates. Another important trend is the worldwide increase in infection with antibiotic-resistant strains of *S. pneumoniae*. Although penicillin-resistant strains of *S. pneumoniae* were first identified in the late 1960s, and meningitis caused by such strains was first diagnosed in 1974, the incidence of infection with *S. pneumoniae* resistant to penicillin and other beta-lactam antibiotics has increased worldwide in the past decade (4,16,17). The new findings are in contrast to the 1990 Centers for Disease Control and Prevention (CDC) report of a multistate surveillance study of bacterial meningitis based on data collected in 1986 (18). *H. influenzae* was the pathogen most commonly identified. The majority of cases were due to three species of bacteria: *H. influenzae* (45%), *S. peumoniae* (18%), and *N. meningitidis* (14%). The incidence rates of infection with specific pathogens were most influenced by age. Case fatality rates varied according both to type of bacteria and age group. For example, the overall case fatality rate for infection was higher for *S. pneumoniae* (19%) than for either *N. meningitidis* (13%) or *H. influenzae* (3%), but that for *S. pneumoniae* meningitis was much lower in children under 5 years old (3%) than in adults over the age of 60 years (31%) (18).

Antibiotic-resistant strains of *S. pneumoniae* have emerged as a major problem in the United States. For example, in metropolitan Atlanta, from January through October 1994, isolates from 25% of patients with invasive pneumococcal infection were resistant to penicillin (5% were highly resistant, with minimum inhibitory concentrations (MIC) ≥ 2 µg/mL), and isolates from 9% were resistant to cefotaxime (4% were highly resistant) (18).

Etiology

The most frequent bacterial pathogens of meningitis (*S. pneumoniae* , *N. meningitidis, H. influenzae*) have been responsible for about 80% of reported cases in the United States. Until the 1990s, *H. influenzae* had been the leading cause of bacterial meningitis, accounting for almost 50% of cases. The position of *H. influenzae* as the chief cause of bacterial meningitis in infants and young children has been changed by the widespread use of *H. influenzae* type b (Hib) conjugate vaccines. As a result, the relative frequencies of *S. pneumoniae* and *N. meningitidis* as agents of meningitis have increased among children (5,6, 8,10,11,13,19).

Other bacterial causes of meningitis are group B streptococci, *Listeria monocytogenes*, and enteric gram-negative bacilli. *L. monocytogenes* has become important in bacterial meningitis as the result of the increasing numbers of immunocompromised and otherwise vulnerable persons at risk (e.g., transplant recipients, patients undergoing hemodialysis, patients with liver disease). In New York City, cases of *Listeria* meningitis increased from 0.9% to 3.4% of all reported cases between 1972 and 1979. Similarly, gram-negative bacillary meningitis (excluding cases caused by *H. influenzae*) increased in New York City from 5.6% to 7.0% of reported cases between 1972 and 1979 (20).

The frequencies of the bacterial agents in meningitis are age related. In neonatal meningitis, *Escherichia coli* and group B streptococci predominate, but other streptococci and *L. monocytogenes* also have significant roles. After the neonatal period in children, the predominant position of *H. influenzae* as a cause of meningitis in the first few years of life declined dramatically since 1990 in the United States as a result of widespread immunization, with Hib-protein conjugate vaccines. *N. meningitidis* is the second most frequent cause of childhood bacterial meningitis. For adult meningitis, *S. pneumoniae* is the principal bacterial agent, causing about 40% of cases.

In adults with bacterial meningitis treated in tertiary care institutions, cases of nosocomial as well as community origin are seen. Among community acquired cases, *S. pneumoniae*, *N. meningitidis*, and *L. monocytogenes* are the leading causes, accounting for about 40%, 15%, and 10% of cases, respectively. Among nosocomial cases, gram-negative bacilli, various streptococcal species, *Staphylococcus aureus*, and coagulase-negative staphylococci are the principal infecting microorganisms, accounting for about 40%, 15%, and 10% of cases, respectively. Gram-negative bacillary meningitis is commonly a postneurosurgical (nosocomial) complication, but may be spontaneous (in hospitalized patients or in the community setting) (11,13,21).

S. aureus is the pathogen in 1% to 9% of cases of bacterial meningitis overall. Cases occur in several categories, based on predisposing circumstances: CNS disorders (usually involving prior neurosurgery) in about 50%, endocarditis in about 20%, and bacteremia from other sites of infection (often in the setting of diabetes, cancer, or alcoholism) in about 25% (22).

Obligate anaerobic bacteria rarely cause meningitis. About 1% of cases of bacterial meningitis are polymicrobial infections. The common predisposing factors for mixed bacterial meningitis have become cerebrospinal fluid (CSF) fistulae; neoplasms in proximity to the CNS, such as carcinoma of the rectosigmoid colon eroding through the sacrum to the subarachnoid space; and contiguous sites of infection (23).

Pathogens and Pathophysiology

A common feature among the bacterial meningeal pathogens are their polysaccharide capsules. These are present on *S. pneumoniae*, *H. influenzae*, *N. meningitidis*, *E. coli* K1, and *Streptococcus agalactiae* (group B streptococcus). Such encapsulation inhibits phagocytosis by neutrophils and antibody-independent, complement-mediated bactericidal activity in different ways. The capsular sialic acid of *N. meningitidis* appears to facilitate binding of complement factor H to C3b, and this interferes with binding of factor B and activation of the alternative pathway (24). In the case of *S. pneumoniae*, factor B binds poorly to C3b on the capsular surface of the organism, and the polyribosyl phosphate capsule of Hib cannot serve as an acceptor for covalent C3 deposition (24).

The initial site of entry of *H. influenzae* into the CNS is the vascular choroid plexus, which shows the earliest histophatologic evidence of inflammation. After exiting the inflamed plexus capillaries, the organisms enter the lateral ventricles and the subarachnoid space. Once infection is introduced into the CSF, bacteria multiply rapidly because of inadequate local defenses in the form of lack of complement-mediated lysis, opsonizing antibody, and neutrophil phagocytosis. A number of pathophysiologic changes develop as a consequence of bacterial meningitis, and involve the brain, its lining, cranial nerves, meningeal and other intracranial blood vessels, and the spinal cord (24). In experimental animal models, specific bacterial subcapsular components (in the case of *S. pneumoniae*, peptidoglycan or lipoteichoic acid; in the case of Hib, lipopolysaccharide) are the major inducers of the meningeal inflammation that follows bacterial entry and multiplication in the CSF. Ampicillin-induced lysis of pneumococci in the CSF results in a transient increase in polymorphonuclear cell pleocytosis, consistent with the release of cell-wall debris (24). This inflammatory response is caused by the release into the subarachnoid space of various proinflammatory cytokines, such as interleukin-1 (IL-1), IL-6, and tumor necrosis factor (TNF) from meningeal cells. By inducing the expression of several families of adhesion molecules on endothelium that interact with corresponding leukocytic receptors, these cytokines promote increased adherence and transendothelial movement of neutrophils (24).

A leukocyte adhesion of molecule (AM-1) belonging to the selectin family mediates adhesion to endothelium even under conditions of flow; its binding affinity for its endothelial receptor is increased by exposure to cytokines (TNF, granulocyte-macrophage colono-stimulating factor), thus furthering neutrophil trafficking into the subarachnoid space.

Once within the subarachnoid space, activated neutrophils release prostaglandins and toxic oxygen metabolites that increase vascular permeability and that may cause direct neurotoxicity. Early in the course of meningitis, as observed in animal models, changes take place in meningeal and cerebral capillaries. These vessels, by virtue of their tight intercellular endothelial junctions and their meager rate of pinocytosis, constitute the blood-brain barrier (BBB). They undergo morphologic changes (opening of tight junctions, enhanced pinocytosis) and become permeable to proteins. In experimental Hib meningitis, the increase in permeability in the BBB appears to correlate principally with the bacterial titer in the CSF, but is augmented by increasing pleocytosis.

A variety of mediators of the inflammatory response, such as IL-1, IL-6, TNF, complement components, and arachidonated metabolites probably contribute to the breakdown of the BBB and the cerebral manifestations of bacterial meningitis. The major physiologic consequence of altered vascular permeability is (vasogenic) cerebral edema (24). This edema may also have cytotoxic and interstitial components. Increased intracranial pressure (ICP) caused by cerebral edema and reduced reabsorption of CSF produces vomiting and obtundation (24).

Cerebral blood flow (CBF) appears to be enhanced in the early stages of bacterial meningitis, but it subsequently declines in accordance with the severity of the inflammatory process. Focal areas of marked hypoperfusion (attributable to local vasculitis or thrombosis) can occur in patients with normal overall CBF. In some patients, impaired autoregulation of CBF may contribute to the development of cerebral edema or ischemia or altering cerebral perfusion pressure (24).

With the spread of meningeal inflammation over the cerebral hemispheres and into the basal cisterns, superficial pial arteries and veins may be subject to thrombosis. Decreased CBF due to cerebral edema or vascular thrombosis, plus any element of hypoxia due to pneumonia or respiratory insufficiency, results in enhanced glucose metabolism via the anaerobic glycolytic pathway, with ensuing lactate accumulation in the brain and CSF. This central lactic acidosis may contribute considerably to the obtundation and coma of patients with severe meningitis (24).

Diagnosis

Clinical Evaluation

Figure 2.2 summarizes the steps in the diagnosis and management of bacterial meningitis.

General Manifestations

Headache or backache and fever are common, but not universal, indications of bacterial meningitis. Fever can accompany acute meningitis but may be absent. The initial physical evaluation should include evaluation for level of consciousness, cranial nerve palsy, focal deficits, meningismus, increased ICP and critical trauma (14).

Antecedent upper respiratory tract infection is common in bacterial meningitis (40% of cases), and another 10% to 15% of patients have an ill-defined prior illness (often diagnosed as otitis media). Between 25% and 75% of patients have a headache, lethargy, and confusion ("meningeal symptoms") of rapid onset (within 24 hours). Other patients have more prolonged (1 to 7 days) respiratory tract or otic symptoms, with meningeal symptoms that develop and progress more slowly. In patients with *L. monocytogenes* meningitis, the prodromal symptomatic period tends to be longer than in patients with other types of pyogenic meningitis (12, 25, 26).

Kerning and Brudzinski signs, along with fever, vomiting, irritability, lethargy, and headache, are features found on physical examination in most pa-

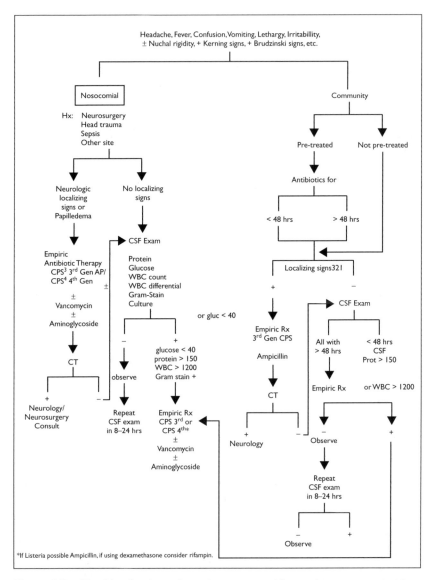

Figure 2.2   Algorithm for the patient who presents with granulomatous meningitis.

tients. Neck stiffness is a symptom in less than half of patients, but nuchal rigidity of some degree is noted as a sign in more than 80%. Myalgias (especially in meningococcal diseases) and backache occur less frequently. Reduced cognitive function is also seen. Photophobia is more often associated with viral meningitis.

A petechial or purpuric rash, predominantly on the extremities, in a patient with meningeal signs carries the high probability of a meningococcal cause, and requires immediate treatment because of the rapidity with which this type of infection can advance. About 50% of patients with meningococcal meningitis have such skin lesions. In more severe meningococcal infections, large purpuric areas develop, usually accompanying hypotension or shock and evidence of disseminated intravascular coagulation (DIC). Petechial and purpuric skin lesions sometimes occur in patients with acute *S. aureus* endocarditis who have meningeal signs and CSF pleocytosis (either from staphylococcal meningitis or cerebral embolic infarction). In this setting, one or two of the purpuric lesions often contain a purulent center, and aspirated material reveals gram-positive cocci in clusters (*Staphylococci*) on Gram-stain examination. Macular and petechial skin lesions accompanied by meningeal signs may occur with enteroviral aseptic meningitis in summer outbreaks (12).

Infections of the leptomeninges can present with signs and symptoms of meningeal irritation and altered mental status. Inflammation of the meninges causes reflex paraspinous muscle spasm, which is reflected in an opisthotonic posture as nuchal rigidity, inability to straighten a raised leg, and flexion of the leg when the neck is flexed, or opisthotonic posture. Most patients with acute bacterial meningitis after the neonatal period have signs of meningeal irritation at the time of presentation (14). Those without such signs are more likely to be elderly and to have gram-negative meningitis. Neonates usually exhibit listlessness but no clear CNS signs. Seizures are common.

Disease within the brain parenchyma may result in seizures, altered states of consciousness, acute changes in personality or behavior, or focal neurologic deficits. The hypothalamic–pituitary axis may be involved, causing severe hypothermia and diabetes insipidus.

The evidence of CNS infection in meningitis may be masked in elderly persons by other disease processes. Fever may be attributed to a recognized infection elsewhere, such as pneumonia, cellulitis, endocarditis, otitis, or sinusitis, and altered CNS function may be blamed on alcoholism, head trauma, stroke, brain tumor, subarachnoid hemorrhage, or metabolic abnormalities. Treatable CNS infection, particularly bacterial meningitis, must be ruled out in such patients. This is usually done by careful neurologic examination, including lumbar puncture.

Neurologic Manifestations

In adults the most frequent neurologic complications of bacterial meningitis are cerebrovascular, occurring in about 37% of patients with intracranial complications, followed in frequency by brain swelling, which is detected by computed tomography (CT) (in 34% of cases, and hydrocephalus in 29%) (27).

BRAIN SWELLING

As noted earlier, cerebral edema can occur in acute bacterial meningitis. Manifestations include obtundation and coma, palsies of cranial nerve VI, abnormal reflexes, hypertension, decerebrate posturing, an abnormal respiratory pattern, and bradycardia. Brain edema causes increased ICP, which in older infants has been shown to reduce cerebral blood flow velocity. The resulting decrease in cerebral perfusion is another potential cause of brain injury. Papilledema is rare because of the relatively brief duration of the meningeal process and increased CSF pressure.

A markedly increased ICP from meningitis may lead to herniation. Signs of herniation include 1) bradycardia and an abnormal respiratory patterns, 2) midposition, nonreactive pupils, 3) unequally sized or dilated, nonreactive pupils, 4) a skew deviation or dysconjugate movements of the eyes, and 5) decorticate or decerebrate posturing (12).

Marked hyperpnea sometimes occurs in patients with severe bacterial meningitis; in this condition, CSF acidosis, due mainly to increased lactic acid levels, provides much of the respiratory drive.

FOCAL CEREBRAL SIGNS

Focal cerebral signs (hemiparesis, quadriparesis, visual field defects, disorders of conjugate gaze, dysphasia) occur in 10% to 20% of patients with meningitis, more frequently with pneumococcal than with other types of meningitis. These signs may appear early in the course of meningitis, or, less frequently, later in the course of the disease as a result of cortical arteritis or phlebitis.

CRANIAL NERVE DYSFUNCTION

Cranial nerve dysfunction has been reported in 10% to 20% of patients with bacterial meningitis. Cranial nerves III, VI, and VIII are most often involved. The highest frequency of involvement is associated with *S. pneumoniae* meningitis. Vasculitis-induced infarction of cranial nerve VIII and necrosis of cells in the organ of Corti may be responsible for permanent deafness. Involvement of the inner ear is not a result of direct extension of infection from the middle ear to the inner ear, even when otitis media precedes meningitis (12, 28).

SEIZURES

Seizures in meningitis may be focal or generalized. Early seizures occur in 15% to 30% of cases of bacterial meningitis. In a study of adults with meningitis, *S. pneumoniae* was the cause of seizures in a greater percentage of those patients who had them, but alcoholism was a confounder. Seizures that occur early in hospitalization do not herald the onset of a permanent seizure disorder, but those that persist beyond the first few days or that develop later during hospitalization may do so (29).

Non-neurologic Complications

SEPTIC COMPLICATIONS

Because of the early treatment of acute bacterial endocarditis is an uncommon complication of the bacteremia associated with such meningitis. In the rare instance in which endocarditis develops, it usually involves the aortic valve. Pyogenic arthritis caused by the common agents of meningitis may complicate the presentation early in the course of CNS infection.

COAGULOPATHIES

In patients with meningitis, coagulation disorders (thrombocytopenia, DIC) may complicate bacteremia and hypotension. The coagulopathy may be mild and consist only of thrombocytopenia, but in patients with more profound bacteremia the clinical features and laboratory findings may be typically those of DIC.

SHOCK

Shock may develop early in the course of acute bacterial meningitis as a consequence of intense bacteremia, and this can also occur in meningococcemia-meningitis or in pneumococcal bacteremia in asplenic patients.

PROLONGED FEVER

Most patients with the common types of bacterial meningitis become afebrile within 2 to 5 days of initiation of appropriate antimicrobial therapy. Occasionally, fever persists for 8 to 10 days or longer, or recurs after initial defervescence. Such a febrile course, accompanied by persisting headache, a stiff neck, a depressed sensorium, and focal cerebral signs, suggests that antimicrobial therapy has been inadequate or that a neurologic complication (e.g., cortical vein thrombophlebitis and arteritis, ventriculitis, ventricular empyema, subdural effusion or empyema, sagittal sinus thrombosis) has supervened. Reevaluation of CSF findings, particularly Gram-stained smears and cultures, is of paramount importance; the appearance of new focal cerebral signs would be an indication for cranial CT. (Examination of CSF is described below, in the section "Laboratory Diagnosis.")

Drug fever or a serum sickness-like syndrome should be considered in a patient with persistent fever whose clinical course and CSF findings show continued improvement.

Laboratory Diagnosis

CSF Examination

Examination of CSF is the basis of the diagnostic approach to CNS infection. Normally, CSF is crystal clear, contains less than five mononuclear cells per cubic millimeter; has a protein content of less than 4.5 g/L, of which 14% or less is γ-globulin; has a glucose concentration about two thirds that of the blood; and is under a pressure of less that 180 mm H_2O (21).

CNS infection usually produces changes in the CSF. These may include an increased number of cells, increased protein concentration, and decreased glucose concentration. Total and differential cell counts should be made. Mononuclear cells usually predominate in nonbacterial (mycobacterial, fungal, rickettsial, and viral) infections; predominance of polymorphonuclear leukocytes (PMN) is typical of bacterial infections, but can also be seen in amebic infections and early in viral infections. One PMN or more than five mononuclear cells in an uncentrifuged CSF specimen are abnormal. Early in any of these diseases there may be no increase in the cell number. Repeated examination of the CSF after 8 to 24 hours in patients suspected of having a viral processes is often useful. A pleocytosis may be found in subacute bacterial endocarditis, after severe seizures, and during systemic viral infections such as measles. Large numbers of erythrocytes may be found in the CSF in herpes virus infection and in postinfectious and amebic encephalitis (12,19,30,31).

A CSF specimen should be stained and cultured for the possible infecting organism in meningitis. Because CNS infection is frequently a complication of systemic diseases, other body fluids (e.g., blood, stool, throat scrapings, sputum, and urine) should also be cultured. Short-term antibiotic treatment before hospital admission does not significantly alter the total or differential cell count or CSF protein or glucose values; however, it does reduce the frequency of positive cultures and diagnostic Gram stains (12). Some fungal and bacterial antigens (e.g., of *Cryptococcus*, *Haemophilus*, pneumococcus, and meningococcus) may be detected by immunodiagnostic techniques, providing a rapid clue to diagnosis and a potential mechanism for identifying the infecting organism in previously treated persons. The polymerase chain reaction (PCR) is increasingly useful for the diagnosis of viral infections of the CNS (32–35).

The CSF protein level increases with most infections, and in chronic infections an increased proportion of this protein may consist of locally synthesized immunoglobulin. The increase in protein concentration may be slight with viral infections, but is usually greater with bacterial, fungal, or tuberculous infections. An increased protein value may be the only CSF abnormality in brain abscess or parameningeal infection. The immunoglobulin present is often directed against the infecting agent.

The CSF glucose value is usually low in untreated bacterial meningitis, and is often also low in fungal, tuberculous, and amebic meningitis. The CSF glucose value can best be interpreted if a plasma glucose level is also available from a sample taken at approximately the same time. The CSF glucose value may be depressed in some encephalitides of viral meningitis (mumps, lymphocytic choriomeningitis viruses, herpes virus infection), and CNS sarcoid, tumors, and subarachnoid hemorrhage (36).

Infection at the site where the puncture will be performed is a contraindication to lumbar puncture. The major risk in performing a lumbar puncture occurs when there is evidence of increased ICP from a mass lesion in the brain. With removal of CSF, the ICP dynamics may be altered and the brain may shift and herniate through the tentorial notch or foramen magnum. If a mass lesion is suspected on the basis of the history or physical examination, or if increased ICP is evident on fundoscopic examination, an imaging technique such as OT or magnetic resonance imaging (MRI) should be used before lumbar puncture. If this occurs after culture, empiric antibiotic therapy should be begun. In other situations, lumbar puncture should not be delayed, because the information gained from examining the CSF is crucial for the differential diagnosis and early institution of treatment (19, 37).

Other Laboratory Studies

Blood cultures from patients with meningitis often reveal the pathogen, disclosing 90% of *H. influenzae*, 80% of *S. pneumoniae*, and 90% of *N. meningitidis* (34).

Bacteremic skin lesions associated with highly invasive organisms may reveal the agent on a Gram-stained smear. Thus, for example, aspiration of the whitish center of one of the purulent purpura associated with *S. aureus* bacteremia may reveal the pathogen. The purely petechial lesions of the skin in bacterial meningitis, however, are unlikely to be revealing on Gram stain examination.

Gram stain examination and culture of fluid aspirated from a middle-ear effusion may provide a clue to bacteriologic diagnosis when the findings of CSF smear examination are equivocal. The peripheral leukocyte count is commonly increased in patients with bacterial meningitis, ranging from 14,000 to 24,000 cells/mm^3, and is generally higher in pneumococcal and meningococcal than in *H. influenzae* disease (12).

Hyponatremia in the course of bacterial (or tuberculous or fungal) meningitis is commonly due either to the complicating syndrome of inappropriate antidiuretic hormone secretion (SIADH) or to inappropriate fluid administration.

Radiologic Studies

Chest radiographs should be made in cases of bacterial meningitis to discover any perdisposing pulmonary portal of infection. Films of the air sinuses and mastoids should be made at an appropriate time after commencing antimicrobial therapy if the history or findings suggest infection of these structures.

When the history, clinical setting, or physical signs (papilledema, focal cerebral findings) suggest a suppurative intracranial fluid collection, cranial CT should be done without delay, and before lumbar puncture (but after blood for cultures has been taken and therapy with appropriate antimicrobials for meningitis of unknown bacterial cause has been instituted) (12).

Patients with bacterial meningitis rarely have clinically significant CT findings without concomitant focal neurologic abnormalities. CT done during the second week of meningitis is most sensitive for cerebral infarction. In the course of meningitis in children, CT is most valuable when focal neurologic findings persist, when CSF cultures remain positive, or when meningitis is recurrent (38, 39).

In about 30% of adults with meningitis, CT shows abnormalities related to meningitis or its complications. Cerebral edema and dural enhancement are abnormalities seen on scans done within 72 hours of admission, whereas cerebral infarcts are seen on later scans. Ventriculomegaly is the most common CT abnormality in adult meningitis, occurring in 15% of all cases, of which 15% require a shunting procedure. In the study of adult meningitis in which this was found, 19 (49%) of the 39 patients who exhibited focal neurologic deficits or seizures had CT abnormalities related to meningitis. In contrast, of the 48 patients with nonfocal findings, only eight (17%) had CT abnormalities. Thus, CT in meningitis should not be routine, but should be employed as indicated by the clinical setting, neurologic findings, and clinical course (12,21).

Differential Diagnosis

The clinical manifestations of meningeal inflammation in bacterial meningitis (headache, fever, stiff neck, obtundation) are common to various other types of meningitis (viral, fungal mycobacterial, treponemal, borrelial, parasitic, hypersensitivity), as well as to acute pyogenic bacterial meningitis and to parameningeal infections. Analysis of CSF findings is central to development of the differential diagnosis.

Nonbacterial Meningitis

A retrospective analysis of the predictive value of initial clinical and laboratory observations was performed with 422 patients who had meningitis seen at one hospital between 1969 and 1980 (4). Five CSF values were found to be individual predictors of bacterial infection with 99% or greater certainty: 1) a CSF glucose level below 1.9 mmol/L (34 mg/dL), 2) a CSF/blood glucose ratio of less than 0.23, 3) a CSF protein level above 2.2 g/L, 4) more than $2000/mm^3$ CSF, or 5) more than 1180 CSF neutrophils per mm^3. Although any one of the foregoing tests could rule in bacterial meningitis with a high likelihood, none could exclude it. However, a logistic multiple regression model, utilizing the four parameters of 1) patient age, 2) month of onset, 3) total CSF neutrophil count, and 4) CSF/blood glucose ratio could be used to exclude acute bacterial meningitis with more than 95% confidence in patients whose CSF Gram stains were negative.

Aseptic enteroviral meningitis usually can be distinguished from bacterial meningitis by its epidemiology, more gradual onset, rare occurrence of outbreaks, accompanying macular or petechial rash, and lymphocytic pleocytosis without hypoglycorrhachia (9). Aseptic echovirus meningitis can present with an initial pleocytosis of up to 1000 cells per mm^3 and neutrophil predominance, which shifts in the next 12 to 36 hours to a predominance of lymphocytes. In nonbacterial meningitis, the CSF glucose level is usually above 40 mg/dL, but may be slightly reduced in occasional patients if the pathogen is the virus of lymphocytic choriomeningitis, mumps, or herpes simplex. Aseptic meningitis may be associated with the acute human immunodeficiency virus (HIV) mononucleosis-like syndrome. Acute aseptic herpes simplex virus type 2 (HSV-2) meningitis occurs in sexually active persons, and may be distinguished from bacterial meningitis by the presence of clustered vesicular lesions in the genital area or inguinal lymphadenopathy and by its lymphocytic pleocytosis.

The aseptic meningitis of neuroborreliosis can be distinguished from acute pyogenic meningitis by its more subacute onset, exposure of the patient to an area endemic for Lyme disease, positive serologic test result for Lyme disease, lymphocytic pleocytosis, and history of erythema chronicum migrans. Leptospiral meningitis might be suggested by a biphasic illness, conjunctivitis, and lymphocytic pleocytosis occurring in a person exposed to rodents, dogs, or cows. Diagnosis of this disease is usually made by serologic testing. Tuberculous meningitis occurs in a setting of either past tuberculous infection (breakdown of an old meningeal tuberculoma) or recently acquired infection with miliary dissemination to the meninges in an immunocompetent or immunocompromised (e.g., HIV-infected) patient. The onset of tuberculous meningitis tends to be less abrupt than that of acute pyogenic meningitis. The characteristic CSF changes are lymphocytic pleocytosis, hypoglycorrhachia, and an increased protein concentration. Bilateral palsies of cranial nerve VI suggest a basilar meningitis, and with the CSF algorithm described earlier, strongly suggest tuberculous meningitis.

Fungal meningitides are almost always more subacute in onset than is bacterial meningitis, produce a lymphocytic pleocytosis with hypoglycorrhachia, and are suggested by epidemiologic clues. Fungal meningitides most commonly present the clinical picture of chronic meningitis, and are diagnosed by culture and antigen detection (e.g., *Cryptococcus neoformans*) in the CSF, or by antibody determination in the CSF and serum. Rarely, chronic meningitis may be characterized by a predominantly neutrophilic CSF according to the algorithm previously described, for which any of several bacterial and mycotic agents may be responsible.

Parameningeal infections (particularly brain abscess, subdural empyema, and cranial and spinal epidural abscess) should be considered in the differential diagnosis of acute bacterial meningitis. These processes might be suspected in a patient with features of meningeal inflammation who also has a chronic ear, sinus, or lung infection. Focal cerebral signs and neurologic symptoms antedating the onset of the acute meningitis suggest a space-occupying intracranial infection, such as a brain abscess. In a patient with presumed bacterial meningitis whose CSF algorithm shows an atypical neutrophilic pleocytosis, a normal glucose level, and no demonstrable organisms on a Gram-stained smear, parameningeal infections warrant particular attention in the differential diagnosis. Isolation of anaerobic bacteria from CSF, especially in mixed culture, suggests parameningeal infection.

Naergleria fowleri can rarely produce a fulminant, acute, and usually fatal purulent meningitis. This diagnosis would be considered for a patient who had recently swum in warm freshwater. Early symptoms may include an altered sense of smell and taste. In addition to a neutrophilic pleocytosis with a low to normal glucose level, the CSF often contains numerous red blood cells. The diagnosis is made by finding motile amoebic trophozoites in fresh preparations of uncentrifuged CSF.

The clinical picture of acute meningitis may develop in bacterial endocarditis. It may represent true bacterial meningitis caused by a pyogenic organism (e.g., *S. pneumoniae*, *S. aureus*), or it may result from cerebral embolic infarction from endocarditis caused by a nonpyogenic organism. CSF findings of cerebral infarction in this latter situation include a pleocytosis of several hundred cells, with varying numbers of neutrophils, a normal glucose level, and absence of bacteria. In occasional patients with meningeal symptoms caused by small cerebral embolic infarctions from acute *S. aureus endocarditis*, the diagnosis may be made by examining Gram-stained smears of purulent cutaneous purpural lesions.

Chemical Meningitis

Chemical meningitis occasionally results from leakage into the subarachnoid space of debris from an intracranial tumor, commonly a craniopharyngioma or an epidermoid tumor of the posterior fossa. This may produce the picture of recurrent meningitis. CSF findings include an initial neutrophilic (or lymphocytic) pleocytosis, with or without hypoglycorrhachia. Birefringent material (keratinized debris) from an epidermoid tumor or a craniopharyngioma may be observed under polarized light microscopy (40).

Another rare, noninfectious cause of meningitis is systemic lupus erythromatosus. The CSF in such cases usually shows a lymphocytic pleocytosis with a normal glucose concentration, although rarely, numerous neutrophils and hypoglycorrhachia are features. Antinuclear antibodies are present in high titers. Rarely, unusual acute, recurrent episodes of nonbacterial meningitis of unknown cause are part of the course of Behçet's syndrome, Mollaret's meningitis (believed to be due to recurrent herpes meningitis), or familial Mediterranean fever. Hypopyon, orogenital lesions, and pathergic skin changes would be indicative of Behçet's syndrome.

Hypersensitivity Meningitis

Occasionally, meningitis is the principal manifestation of hypersensitivity to drugs such as sulfonamides and nonsteroidal antiinflammatory agents. The pleocytosis in such cases may be predominantly neutrophilic or lymphocytic, and some eosinophils may be present, but the glucose level in CSF is normal. Mollaret's meningitis, characterized by self-limited episodes of fever, meningeal findings, mononuclear pleocytosis (sometimes neutrophilic at inception), and the presence in the CSF of unusual cells variously described as "epithelial" or "endothelial," has been associated in some instances with underlying Herpes simplex virus type 1 (HSV-1) infections or with epidermoid cysts of the CNS (6,8,12,13,19,30,41–43).

Treatment

The efficacy of antimicrobial therapy in bacterial meningitis depends on a variety of factors, including the antimicrobial susceptibility of the organism, bactericidal activity of the antimicrobial agent, capacity of the antimicrobial agent to penetrate BBB, and effectiveness of various modes of antimicrobial drug administration in achieving desired concentrations of the drug in the CSF. Since there is a lack of intrinsic opsonic and antibacterial activity in the CSF early in bacterial meningitis, bactericidal rather than bacteriostatic agents are needed for treatment (44). The CSF concentration of β-lactam antibiotics or aminoglycosides must be 10 to 20 times higher than the minimal bactericidal concentration for the infecting organism if optimal bactericidal effects are to be achieved. The low pH and abundance of nucleic acids in purulent CSF inhibit rapid bacterial killing by aminoglycosides.

Most antimicrobial agents used in treating bacterial meningitis, with the exception of chloramphenicol, do not penetrate well through the normal BBB. β-Lactam antibiotics penetrate only to the extent of 0.5% to 2.0% of their peak serum concentrations, although higher concentrations are achieved when the meninges are inflamed. Clindamycin, erythromycin, and first- and second-generation cephalosporins should not be used to treat bacterial meningitis because effective bactericidal levels in the CSF cannot be obtained with these drugs. For antimicrobial drugs such as β-lactam drugs, aminoglycosides, and vancomycin, which poorly penetrate even inflamed meninges, intermittent bolus parenteral administration is preferred because higher peak levels are achieved (19).

Why Bactericidal Activity in CSF?

"Bacterial meningitis is an infection in an area of impaired host resistance" (19). Specific antibody and complement are frequently absent from the CSF in patients with this disease, resulting in inefficient phagocytosis and in rapid bacterial multiplication (to concentrations of 10 million or more colony-forming units per milliliter of CSF (45). Optimal antimicrobial treatment requires that the drug being used have a bactericidal effect in the CSF. Patients with pneumococcal and gram-negative bacillary meningitis who are treated with bacteriostatic antibiotics have poor clinical outcomes (12,19,46).

Factors Influencing Bactericidal Activity in Cerebrospinal Fluid

The major factors affecting the bactericidal activity of an antimicrobial drug in CSF are its relative degree of penetration into the fluid, its concentration there, and its intrinsic activity in infected CSF. The penetration of an antimicrobial drug into CSF is primarily influenced by the characteristics of the drug and the integrity of the BBB (Table 2.1). When the barrier is intact, penetration is limited because vesicular transport across cells is minimal and the junctions between the endothelial cells of the cerebral microvasculature are tight. However, during meningitis there is an increase in vesicular transport across cells in meningeal arterioles, and complete separation of the tight junctions between endothelial cells in meningeal venules. These changes result in increased permeability of the BBB, increasing the penetration of many microbial drugs (such as β-lactam drugs) into the CSF to 5% to 10% of their serum concentrations. For other antibiotics more highly soluble in lipids (such as chloramphenicol, rifampin, and trimethoprim), penetration into CSF is high (reaching 30% to 40% of their serum concentration) even when the meninges are not inflamed (1).

The CSF concentration of an antimicrobial agent needed for maximal bactericidal activity is unknown. In experimental meningitis, maximal bactericidal activity occurs when the concentration of drug is 10 to 30 times the minimal bactericidal concentration against the organism *in vitro* (47). One explanation for this difference is that infected CSF decreases the activity of an antimicrobial drug (19). Since the activity of a β-lactam drug (i.e., penicillin G) on bacterial cell-wall synthesis depends on bacterial cell division, fever may impair its bactericidal effect *in vivo* (48).

Hazards of Antimicrobial Therapy

Bactericidal therapy often results in bacteriolysis of the pathogen. As a result, treatment can promote the release of biologically active cell-wall products (e.g., the lipopolysaccharide of gram-negative bacteria and the teichoic acid and peptidoglycan of streptococci) into the CSF. This release of cell-wall fragments can increase the production of cytokines (IL-1, IL-6, and TNF-α) in CSF, exacer-

Table 2.1   Empiric Selection of Antibiotics for the Treatment of Suspected Bacterial Meningitis

Group of Patients	Likely Pathogen	Choice of Antibiotic
Neonate <1 month	S. agalactiae, E. coli, Group D Other enterobacteriae Listeria	Ampicillin plus cefotaxime or ceftriaxone
Infant 1–3 months	S. pneumoniae, N. meningitidis + neonatal pathogens or L. monocytogenes	Ampicillin plus cefotaxime, ceftriaxone; consider dexamethasone
Age, 3 mo to <7 years	N. meningitidis, S. pneumoniae, or H. influenaze (if DRSP)	Cefotaxime/ceftriaxone ± dexamethasone, if DRSP + vancomycin
Age, 7 to 50 years	S. pneumonia or N. meningitidis	Cefotaxime/ceftriaxone + Dexamethasone
	If DRSP	Vancomycin + cefotaxime/ceftriaxone
Age, >50 years	S. pneumoniae, L. monocytogenes, or gram-negative bacilli (rare)	Ampicillin plus cefotaxime or ceftriaxone
	If DRSP >2%	As above + vancomycin
With impaired cellular immunity (alcoholics, other, primary or secondary)	L. monocytogenes or gram-negative bacilli including P. aeruginosa	Ampicillin plus ceftazidime or cefepime
With head trauma, neuro-surgery, or cerebrospinal fluid shunt	Staphylococci, gram-negative bacilli, P. aeruginosa, or S. pneumoniae	Vancomycin plus ceftazidime
With recurrent episodes of meningitis	S. pneumoniae (most common)	Broad-spectrum cephalosporins Cefotaxime/ceftriaxone
	If DRSP	As above + vancomycin

bating inflammation and further damaging the BBB. Achieving a rapid bactericidal effect in CSF remains a primary goal of therapy for meningitis (19,30).

When Should Treatment Be Started?

It is important to promptly institute antibiotic therapy for bacterial meningitis, and the accusation of failure to promptly treat the disease is a common reason for malpractice litigation (19). The intuitive assumption is that a delay in therapy of even a few hours affects the prognosis adversely, although the clinical data on this are inconclusive (19).

One of the most important factors contributing to delayed diagnosis and treatment of bacterial meningitis is the decision to perform cranial CT imaging before lumbar puncture is done. If imaging is indicated, investigators have suggested obtaining blood cultures, instituting empirical antimicrobial therapy, and performing lumbar puncture immediately after imaging if it discloses no intracranial mass lesion (5,12,19). Instituting antimicrobial therapy 1 to 2 hours before lumbar puncture will not decrease the diagnostic sensitivity if the culture of CSF is done in conjunction with testing of CSF for bacterial antigens and with blood cultures (19,49).

Empiric Antimicrobial Therapy

When lumbar puncture is delayed or a Gram stain of CSF is nondiagnostic, empirical therapy is essential and should be directed at the most likely pathogens on the basis of the patient's age and underlying health status (Table 2.1; Fig. 2.3). For most patients, most authors recommend therapy with a broad-spectrum cephalosporin (cefotaxime or ceftriaxone), supplemented with ampicicllin in neonates (less than 1 month old) and in young infants (1 to 3 months old) as well as in immunocompromised patients and older adults (more than 50 years old), since in these groups infections with *S. agalactiae* and *L. monocytogenes* are more prevalent. These recommendations require modification under special circumstances (2,8,13,19,30). For immunocompromised patients, treatment should include ampicillin (for possible *Listeria*) and a broad-spectrum cephalosporin (such as ceftazidime or cefepime) that has more inclusive activity against gram-negative organisms, and specifically *P. aeruginosa*. Patients with recent head trauma or neurosurgery, and those with CSF shunts, should be given broad-spectrum antibiotics effective against both gram-positive and gram-negative organisms, such as a combination of vancomycin and ceftazidime. For patients with suspected *S. pneumoniae* infections and in practice environments in which drug-resistant *S. pneumoniae* is a problem, many clinicians consider adding vancomycin in a higher dose (15 mg/kg) until culture results are known (19).

For patients with identifiable bacteria on a Gram stain of CSF, microbial therapy should be directed toward the presumptive pathogen (Table 2.2). For all patients, therapy should be modified when the results of CSF culture and antibiotic susceptibility testing become available (12,19).

Empiric Glucocorticoid Therapy

Adjunctive glucocorticoid therapy was tested and found to ameliorate bacterial meningitis in laboratory animals, on the basis of evidence that inflammatory cytokines (e.g., IL-1, IL-6, and TNF-α) have a role in the pathophysiology of bacterial meningitis.

In a recent trial involving 56 children with *S. pneumoniae* meningitis, there were substantially fewer audiologic and neurologic sequelae in glucocorticoid-treated children 1 year later, but the difference was not statistically significant.

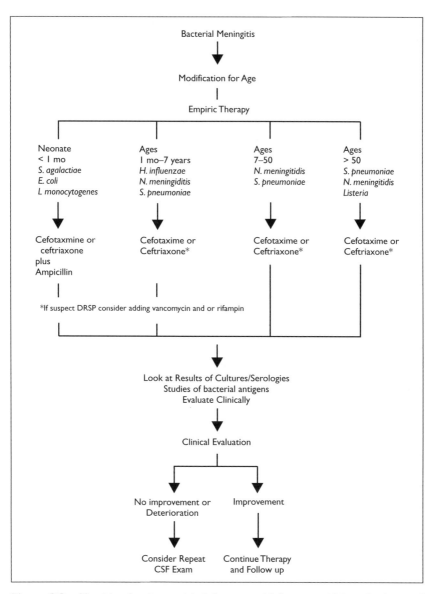

Figure 2.3   Algorithm for the empirical therapy and follow-up guidelines for bacterial meningitis based on the age of the patient.

The benefit of adjunctive glucorcoticoid therapy in adults is even less clear; in only one prospective, randomized trial (which was not placebo-controlled or double-blinded) was such therapy beneficial, and then only in the subgroup of patients infected with *S. pneumoniae* (50).

Table 2.2   Recommendations for Antibiotic Therapy in Patients with Bacterial Meningitis Who Have a Positive Gram Strain or Culture of Cerebrospinal Fluid*

Type of Bacteria	Choice of Antibiotic
By Gram stain	
Cocci	
Gram-positive	Vancomycin plus cefotaxime or ceftriaxone, consider dexamethasone
	If dexamethasone is used, add ceftriaxone + rifampin*
Gram-negative	Penicillin high dose (300,000 U/kg up to 24 million U)
Bacilli	
Gram-positive	Ampicillin 100 mg/kg every 18 hours in children and 12 g/day in adults (or penicillin G) plus gentamicin 1.5 mg/kg every 1.8 hours
Gram-negative	Cefotaxime/ceftriaxone/ceftazidime if *P. aeruginosa* likely/cefepime?
By culture	
S. pneumoniae	Vancomycin plus cefotaxime or ceftriaxone—see gram-positive cocci
H. influenzae	Ceftriaxone or cefotaxime
N. meningitidis	Penicillin G high dose
L. monocytogenes	Ampicillin plus gentamicin—see gram-negative bacilli
S. agalactiae	Penicillin G (some add gentamicin in neonates)
Enterobacteriaceae	Broad-spectrum cephalosporin plus aminoglycoside (intravenous gentamicin; may need intrathecal)
Pseudomonas aeruginosa, Acinetobacter	Ceftazidime with or without aminoglycoside

*Modified from Quagliarello VJ, Scheld WM. Treatment of bacterial meningitis. *N Engl J Med.* 1997;336:708-16.

Many authors recommend adjunctive dexamethasone therapy for children more than 2 months of age who have bacterial meningitis, particularly those not vaccinated against *H. influenzae* and thought to be infected with *H. influenzae*, and those with gram-negative coccobacilli and a Gram-stained preparation of CSF. Dexamethasone therapy should be started intravenously at the same time as, or slightly before, the first dose of antimicrobial drug, at a dose of 0.15 mg/kg body weight every 6 hours for 4 days (19,42,51). In adults with bacterial meningitis, the benefits of adjunctive glucocorticoid therapy are less convincing, and its use should be more limited (12,41,51). Some authors believe that the adults most likely to benefit are those with a high concentration of bacteria in their CSF (i.e., those with a positive Gram stain of CSF) and evidence of increased ICP; in such patients, they recommend the same regimen (0.15 mg of dexamethasone per kilogram of body weight given intravenously every 6 hours for 4 days) (19,51).

Treatment of Specific Infections

Common Pathogens

S. PNEUMONIAE

In treating meningitis caused by penicillin-susceptible strains of *S. pneumoniae*, penicillin G and ampicillin are similar in effectiveness and are the drugs of choice. For patients with suspected *S. pneumoniae* meningitis (for which the susceptibilities are unknown) and patients known to have antibiotic-resistant *S. pneumoniae*, the choices of drug are problematic. This is because the CSF concentrations of penicillin may not be bactericidal and second, because clinical failures have been reported with broad-spectrum cephalosporins (cefotaxime or ceftriaxone) even though they can be effective against penicillin-resistant strains. Almost all failures have occurred in children with strains of *S. pneumoniae* for which the MIC of cefotaxime or ceftriaxone is 2 μg/mL or higher, although some reports suggest that treatment may fail when the MICs of the two drugs are ≥ 1.0 μg per milliliter (52).

As the MIC of penicillin for *S. pneumoniae* increases, resistance increases to other antimicrobial agents, including cephalosporins, chloramphenicol, trimethoprim–sulfamethoxazole, and erythromycin, but not vancomycin. Therefore, vancomycin may be the most effective treatment agent for *S. pneumoniae* meningitis in the era of β-lactam resistance. However, concern about the penetration of vancomycin into the CSF in adults has promoted studies of combination regimens. In experimental *S. pneumoniae* meningitis, the combination of vancomycin and ceftriaxone was synergistic even against strains for which the MIC of ceftriaxone was above 4 μg/mL (53). However, in animals given dexamethasone concomitantly, the penetration of vancomycin into the CSF was reduced, and sterilization of the CSF was delayed (54). Only the combination of ceftriaxone and rifampin effectively sterilized the CSF with respect to highly resistant strains of *S. pneumoniae* when dexamethasone was given concomitantly (54). In children, vancomycin has been used in a dose of 15 mg/kg; the data for adults with higher double doses of vancomycin are not strong, but many clinicians recommend this practice, especially when suspected drug resistant *S. pneumoniae* are found or when the infection is documented.

Although these regimens have not yet been studied in humans, and recommendations for the management of bacterial meningitis are evolving, the increasing prevalence of antibiotic-resistant *S. pneumoniae* warrants the combination of ceftriaxone plus vancomycin in patients with a Gram stain of CSF that suggests the presence of *S. pneumoniae* (19). This regimen should be continued if the *S. pneumoniae* isolate is resistant to penicillin (MIC ≥ 0.1 μg/mL) and to ceftriaxone and cefotaxime (MIC > 0.5 μg/mL). In adults treated with adjunctive dexamethasone, ceftriaxone plus rifampin is the preferred combination regimen pending studies of susceptibility (19). Because the penetration of vancomycin into CSF is not reduced in children treated with dexamethasone, ceftriaxone plus vancomycin can still be given (55). Unless the isolate of *S. pneumoniae* is known to be susceptible to penicillin, many authors recommend a second lumbar puncture within 24 to 48 hours to document bacteriologic cure, because adjunctive dexamethasone therapy may prevent adequate clinical assessment of the response to therapy (54).

N. MENINGITIDIS

Penicillin and ampicillin are effective treatment agents for meningitis caused by *N. meningitidis*, although rare isolates of β-lactamase-producing strains have high-level resistance (MIC ≥ 250 µg/mL). Clinical isolates with altered penicillin-binding proteins and intermediate resistance to penicillin (MIC 0.1–1.0 µg/mL) have been identified in Europe and South Africa, and recently in North Carolina. The clinical importance of such resistance is unclear, because most patients with meningitis caused by these intermediately resistant strains can be treated effectively with penicillin. At present, penicillin is the drug of choice for meningitis caused by *N. meningitidis* the bacterial isolates from patients who do not have adequate responses should be formally tested, and the treatment should be changed to ceftriaxone (or cefotaxime) if the isolate is resistant to penicillin (MIC ≥ 0.1 µg/mL) (5,12,13,19).

Less Common Pathogens

LISTERIA

Ampicillin and penicillin are the treatments of choice for *L. monocytogenes* meningitis (13,19). However, neither drug is bactericidal against *Listeria in vitro*, and mortality rates as high as 30% have been reported with the use of these drugs in *Listeria*. These observations, and the enhanced bactericidal activity in experimental *Listeria* meningitis when penicillin (or ampicillin) is combined with gentamicin, have prompted many to recommend these latter combinations. Some authors recommend ampicillin (or penicillin) plus gentamicin for patients of all ages who have *Listeria* meningitis (12,13,19). Trimethroprim–sulfamethoxazole is bactericidal against *Listeria in vitro*, and has been a successful alternative agent in specific patients. Despite being effective *in vitro*, chloramphenicol and vancomycin have proved ineffective in patients with systemic *Listeria* infection. Meropenem is active *in vitro* and in laboratory animals with *Listeria* meningitis, but there are inadequate data to recommend its use in humans (19).

STREPTOCOCCUS AGALACTIAE

For neonates with meningitis caused by *S. agalactiae* (group B streptococcus), the combination of ampicillin and gentamicin is the regimen of choice because of the *in vitro* synergy of these drugs and reports of penicillin-tolerant strains of *S. agalactiae*. In adults with group B streptococcal meningitis, the benefit of the combination regimen over penicillin (or ampicillin) is unproved, and mortality is influenced primarily by the presence of underlying illness (12,13,19).

GRAM-NEGATIVE BACTERIAL MENINGITIS

With the advent of the broad-spectrum cephalosporins (cefotaxime, ceftriaxone, ceftazidime, and cefepime), clinical outcomes in bacterial meningitis have improved remarkably (success rate, 85%–90%) because of the high level of activity of these antibiotics against gram-negative pathogens, and their high degree of penetration into CSF. Ceftazidime in particular has enhanced activity against *Pseudomonas aeruginosa*, and has proved very effective (cure rate 70%–75%, with or without concomitant systemic aminoglycoside therapy). Other promising antimicrobial agents are aztreonam, trimethoprim–sultamethoxazole, ciprofloxacin, cefepime, and meropenem. Although no results are available from comparative trials, some authors (19) recommend ceftazidime combined with a parenterally administered aminoglycoside as first-line therapy for gram-negative bacillary meningitis. In patients who do not have a response, they recommend a repeat lumbar puncture with CSF culture and antibiotic susceptibility testing. If gram-negative bacilli continue to grow in cultures of CSF and resistance develops to cephalosporin during therapy, intrathecal (or intraventricular) therapy with aminoglycosides or alternative systemic antimicrobial agents can be given on the basis of the results of susceptibility studies.

Chloramphenicol has been found ineffective in gram-negative bacteria because its effect against gram-negative bacilli in CSF is only bacteriostatic. Although aminoglycosides are bactericidal *in vitro*, systemic therapy with gentamicin and amikacin was not highly effective because of inadequate penetration into CSF. Unfortunately, in neonates with gram-negative meningitis, the intrathecal administration of aminoglycosides was ineffective, and the mortality rate for patients given intraventricular aminoglycoside therapy was higher than for patients given intravenous aminoglycoside therapy. Subsequent smaller case series suggested that individualized dosing of aminoglycosides through an intraventricular reservoir may lead to better outcomes.

S. AUREUS

Treatment of *S. aureus* meningitis involves the use of intravenous nafcillin or oxacillin. For meningitis caused by methicillin-resistant *S. aureus*, or when such methicillin resistant organisms are likely, or for patients who are allergic to penicillin, vancomycin is the alternative drug of choice (12,13,19). Some investigators recommend the addition of rifampin to either nafcillin or vancomycin when the therapeutic response to these latter two drugs has been inadequate, or from the beginning when the infection is severe (13,19). Since coagulase-negative staphylococci are the most frequent causes of CSF shunt infections (and complicating meningitis), and because more than one third of such nosocomial strains of staphylococci are methicillin resistant, vancomycin is the initial drug of choice for treating shunt infections, although its penetration is limited in the absence of marked meningeal inflammation. If the response to treatment is unsatisfactory, rifampin (which readily penetrates the CSF) might be added.

Duration of Antibiotic Therapy

The optimal duration of antibiotic therapy for patients with bacterial meningitis is undefined (3,4,6–10,12,13,19,30,43,56). Most texts recommend a range of 7 to 10 days for meningococcal meningitis, and longer courses (10–21 days) for meningitis caused by other pathogens (Table 2.3). In a randomized trial of therapy with ceftriaxone in children with nonmeningococcal meningitis (primarily *H. influenzae* disease), 7 days of therapy was effective as 10 days of therapy (12,19,57). Clinical trials involving patients with meningococcal meningitis showed that 7-day treatment regimens (including penicillin, cefotaxime, ceftriaxone, and chloramphenicol) were very effective, and the vast majority of patients were cured in 4 or 5 days (12,19,58). No comparative studies have been done of the duration of treatment in patients with meningitis caused by *S. pneumoniae*, *L. monocytogenes*, *S. agalactiae*, or enteric gram-negative bacilli. We recommend that the duration of therapy be tailored to the individual patient on the basis of the clinical and microbiologic response.

Prevention

Meningococcal Diseases

The risk of meningococcal disease for household contacts of an initial case is 500 to 800 times greater than the endemic rate for meningococcal disease in the general population (12). Chemoprophylaxis is indicated for close contacts (e.g., household or day care center personnel, medical personnel in close direct contact with the patient) of patients with meningococcal disease. Rifampin is 80% to 90% effective in eliminating asymptomatic nasopharyngeal carriage of *N. meningitidis* and is the recommended drug for chemoprophylaxis of meningococcal meningitis. The dose is 600 mg orally every 12 hours for 2 days for adults, 10 mg/kg every 12 hours for children older than 1 month, and 5 mg/kg every 12 hours for children younger than 1 month. Because the carrier state may recur shortly after discontinuation of treatment with high doses of penicillin, rifampin should also be administered to patients with meningococcal disease before their discharge from the hospital.

Table 2.3   Guidelines for the Duration of Antibiotic Therapy

Pathogen	Suggested Duration of Thearpy (Days)
H. influenzae	7
N. meningitidis	7
S. pneumoniae	10–14
L. monocytogenes	14–21
Group B streptococci	14–21
Gram-negative bacilli (other than H. influenzae	21

*Modified from Quagliarello VJ, Scheld WM. Treatment of bacterial meningitis. N Engl J Med. 1997;336:708-16.

Minocycline has been almost as effective as rifampin in eliminating *N. meningitidis* from nasopharyngeal carriers, but is not commonly used because of reports of vestibular side effects. Oral ciprofloxacin reaches concentrations in nasal secretions that are above the MIC for *N. meningitidis*. Single-dose oral ciprofloxacin, 500 or 750 mg for adult patients, is about 90% effective in eradicating pharyngeal carriage of *N. meningitidis*.

Ceftriaxone (250 mg intramuscularly in adults and 125 mg in children) was reported to eliminate the carriage of serogroup A meningococci in more than 90% of patients for up to 2 weeks.

Immunoprophylaxis of meningococcal disease currently involves use of a quadrivalent (A/C/Y/W-135) polysaccharide vaccine. It is used in the military, in travelers to countries with hyperendemic or epidemic disease, in aborting outbreaks caused by meningococcal serogroups covered by the vaccine, and for persons at high risk, such as asplenic patients or those who have terminal complement-component deficiencies.

Meningococcal vaccines are important in quelling epidemics in developing countries where they are used as a componenet to prophylactic chemotherapy in neighborhood or school outbreaks.

H. influenzae Infection

The risk of secondary spread of invasive Hib infection from infected persons to nonimmunized household contacts younger than 4 years is 2% to 6% during the 30-day period after exposure (12). The highest rate occurs in contacts younger than 1 year. The majority of secondary cases occur within a week of onset of disease in the index case.

Rifampim is effective in eliminating nasopharyngeal carriage of Hib. If another child (whether previously given Hib vaccine or not) younger than 4 years resides in the household, rifampin prophylaxis is recommended for all household contacts, including adults (except pregnant women) of any index case. The dose is 20 mg/kg orally once daily for 4 days (maximal daily dose: 600 mg). Because nasopharyngeal carriage may reappear after discontinuation of antimicrobial thearpy for systemic Hib infection, the index patient should receive rifampin before hospital discharge.

Current recommendations of the American Academy of Pediatrics Committee on Infectious Diseases call for vaccination of all infants beginning at 2 months of age with one of three licensed Hib PRP (or PRP oligomer) protein-conjugate vaccines. There are 1) HbOC (HibTITER) (diphtheria CRM 197 protein conjugate), 2) PRP-OPM (PedvaxHIB), *N. meningitidis* serograoup B outer membrane protein complex conjugate, and 3) PRP-T (ActHIB, Omni-HIB), tetanus toxoid protein complex. A primary series of HbOC or PjRP-T consists of three doses given at 2, 4, and 6 months of age, whereas for PjR-OMP, only two doses, given at 2 and 4 months, are recommended. An additional booster dose of a conjugate vaccine should be given at 12 to 15 months of age. A fourth vaccine, PRP-D (ProHIBIT), a diphtheria toxoid-protein conjugate vaccine, is recommended only for use in children 12 months of age and older, and can be substituted at that time for one of the other vaccines as the booster dose.

REFERENCES

1. **Unhanand M, Mustaf MM, McCracken GH Jr, Nelson JD**. Gram-negative enteric bacillary meningitis: a twenty-one year experience. *J Pediatr* 1993;122:15–21.
2. **Durand ML, Calderwood SB, Weber DJ, et al**. Acute bacterial meningitis in adults: a review of 493 episodes. *N Engl J Med* 1993;328:21–8.
3. **Hosoglu S, Ozen A, Kokogly OF, et al**. Acute bacterial meningitis in adults: analysis of 218 episodes. *Indian J Med Sci* 1997;166:231–4.
4. **Schuchat A, Perkins BA, Lefkowitz L, et al**. Bacterial meningitis in the United States in 1995. Active Surveillance Team. *N Engl J Med* 1997;337:970–6.
5. **Andersen J Wandall JH, Skinhoj P, et al**. Acute meningococcal meningitis: analysis of features of the disease according to the age of 255 patients. *J Infect Dis* 1997; 34:227–35.
6. **Segreti J, Harris AA**. Acute bacterial meningitis. *Infect Dis Clin North Am* 1996; 10:797–809.
7. **Sigurdardottir B, Gudmundsson S, Erlendsdottir H, et al**. Acute bacterial overview. *Arch Intern Med* 1997;157:425–50.
8. **Tunkel AR, Scheld WM**. Acute bacterial meningitis in adults. *Curr Clin Top Infect Dis* 1996;16:215–39.
9. **Andersen J, Wandall JH, Voldsgaard P, et al**. Acute meningitis of unknown etiology: analysis of 219 cases admitted to the hospital between 1977 and 1990. *J Infect Dis* 1995;31:115–22.
10. **Towsend GC, Scheld WM**. Infections of the central nervous system. *Adv Intern Med*. 1998;43:403-7.

11. **Pruitt AA.** Infections of the nervous system. *Neurol Clin* 1998;16:419–47.

12. **Swartz M.** Acute bacterial meningitis. In Gourbach SL, Barlett JG, Blacklow NR, eds. *Infectious Diseases,* 2nd ed. Philadelphia: WB Saunders, 1998; 1377–81.

13. **Roos KL, Tunkel AR, Scheld WM.** Acute bacterial meningitis in children and adults. In Scheld WM, Whittey RJ, Durack DT, eds. *Infections of the Central Nervous System,* 2nd ed. Philadelphia: Lippincott-Raven, 1997; 297–312.

14. **Griffin DE.** Approach to the patient with infections of the central nervous system. In Gourback SI, Bartlett JG, Blacklow NR, eds. *Infectious Diseases,* 2nd ed. Philadelphia: WB Saunders, 1998; 1377–1381.

15. **Adams WG, Deaver KA, Cochi SL, et al.** Decline of childhood Haemophilus influenzae type b (Hib) disease in the Hib vaccine era. *JAMA* 1993;269:221–6.

16. **Naraqi S, Kirkpatrick GP, Kabin S.** Relapsing pneumococcal meningitis: isolation of an organism with decreased susceptibility to penicillin G. *J Pediatr* 1974;85:671–3.

17. **Fenoll A, Martin-Bourgon C, Munoz R, et al.** Serotype distribution and antimicrobial resistance of Streptococcus pneumoniae isolates causing systemic infections in Spain, 1979–1989. *Rev Infect Dis* 1991;13:56–60.

18. **Wenger JD, Hightower AW, Facklam RR, et al.** Bacterial Meningitis Study Group. Bacterial meningitis in the United States, 1986: report of a multistate surveillance study. *J Infect Dis* 1990;162:1316–23.

19. **Quagliarello VJ, Scheld WM.** Treatment of bacterial meningitis. *N Engl J Med* 1997;336:708–716.

20. **Cherubin CE, Marr JS, Sierra MF, et al.** Listeria and gram-negative bacillary meningitis in New York City, 1972–1979. *Am J Med* 1981;71:199.

21. **Durand MI, Calderwood SB, Weber DJ, et al.** Acute bacterial meningitis in adults: A review of 493 episodes. *N Engl J Med* 1993;328:21.

22. **Schlesinger LS, Ross SC, Schaberg DR.** *Staphylococcus aureus* meningitis: A broad-based epidemiologic study. *Medicine (Baltimore)* 1987;66:148.

23. **Swartz MN.** Central nervous system infection. In Finegold SM, George WL, eds. *Anaerobic Infections in Humans.* San Diego, CA: Academic Press, 1989; 155–212.

24. **Tunkel AR, Scheld WM.** Pathogenesis and pathology of bacterial infections of the central nervous system. In Scheld WM, Whitley RJ, Durack DT, eds. *Infections of the Central Nervous System.* Philadelphia: Lippincott-Raven, 1997; 297–312.

25. **Carpenter RR, Peterdorf RG.** The clinical spectrum of bacterial meningitis. *Am J Med* 1962;33:262.

26. **Salwen KM, Vikerfors T, Olcén P.** Increased incidence of childhood bacterial meningitis. *Scand J Infect Dis* 1987;19:1.

27. **Pfister H-W, Borasio GD, Diarnagl U, et al.** Cerebrovascular complications of bacterial meningitis in adults. *Neurology* 1992;42:1497.

28. **Eavey RD, Gao YZ, Schuknecht HF, et al.** Otologic features of bacterial meningitis of childhood. *J Pediatr* 1985;106:402.

29. **Bohr VA, Rasmussen N.** Neurologic sequelae and fatality as prognostic measures in 875 cases of bacterial meningitis. *Dan Med Bull* 1988;35:92.

30. **Tunkel AR, Scheld WM.** Issues in the management of bacterial meningitis. *Am Fam Physician* 1997;56:1355–62.

31. **Hoen B, Canton P, Gerard A, et al.** Multivariate approach to differential diagnosis of acute meningitis. *Eur J Clin Microbiol Infect Dis* 1996;15:252–4.

32. **Ferraro MJ.** Rapid immunologic diagnosis of meningitis–Is there a future? In Balows A, Tilton RC, Turano A, eds. *Rapid Methods and Automation in Microbiology and Immunology*, Italy, Brixia Academic Press, 1988, 481–7.

33. **Martin WJ.** Rapid and reliable techniques for the laboratory detection of bacterial meningitis. *Am J Med.* 1983;75:119.

34. **Bohr V, Rasmussen H, Hansen B, et al.** Eight hundred seventy-five cases of bacterial meningitis: Diagnostic procedures and the impact of preadmission antibiotic therapy. *J Infect* 1983;7:193.

35. **Wilson CB, Smith AL.** Rapid tests for the diagnosis of bacterial meningitis. *Curr Clin Top Infect Dis* 1986;7:134.

36. **Koskiniemi M, Vaheri A, Taskinen E.** Cerebrospinal fluid alterations in herpes simplex virus encephalitis. *Rev Infect Dis* 1984;6:608.

37. **Bryan CS, Reynolds KL, Crout L.** Promptness of antibiotic therapy in acute bacterial meningitis. *Ann Emerg Med* 1986;15:544.

38. **Packer RJ, Bilaniuk LT, Zimmerman RA.** CT parenchymal abnormalities in bacterial meningitis: Clinical significance. *J Comput Assist Tomogr* 1982;6:1064.

39. **Bodino J, Lylyk P, Del Volle M, et al.** Computed tomography in purulent meningitis. *Am J Dis Child* 1982;136:495.

40. **Crossly GH, Dismukes WE.** Central nervous system epidermoid cyst: A probable etiology of Mollaret's meningitis. *Am J Med* 1990;89:805.

41. **Prasad K, Haines T.** Dexamethasone treatment for acute bacterial meningitis: how strong is the evidence for routine use? *J Neurol Neurosurg Psychiatry* 1995;59:31–31.

42. **Wubbel L, McCracken GH Jr.** Management of bacterial meningitis: 1998. *Pediatr Rev* 1998;19:78–84.

43. **Rockowitz J, Tunkel AR.** Bacterial meningitis. Practical guidelines for management drugs. *Drugs.* 1995;50:838–53.

44. **Simberkoff M, Molover H, Rahal J Jr.** Absence of detectable bacterial and opsonic activities in normal and infected cerebrospinal fluids: A regional host defense deficiency. *J Lab Clin Med* 1980;95:362.

45. **Zwahlen A, Nydegger UE, Vaudeaux P, et al.** Complement-mediated opsonic activity in normal and infected human cerebrospinal fluid: early response during bacterial meningitis. *J Infect Dis* 1982;145:635–46.

46. **Crane LR, Lerner AM.** Nontraumatic gram-negative bacillary meningitis in the Detroit Medical Center, 1964–1974. *Medicine (Baltimore)* 1978;57:197.

47. **Strausbaugh LJ, Sande MA.** Factors influencing the therapy of experimental pneumococcal meningitis in rabbits. *Infect Dis* 1978;137:251–60.

48. **Small PM, Tauber MG, Hackbarth CJ, Sande MA.** Influence of body temperature on bacterial growth rates in experimental pneumococcal meningitis in rabbits. *Infect Immun* 1986;52:484–7.

49. **Coant PN, Korberg AE, Duffy LC, et al.** Blood culture results as determinants in the organism identification of bacterial meningitis. *Pediatr Emerg Care* 1992;8:200–5.

50. **Kanra GY, Ozen H, Secmeer G, et al.** Beneficial effects of dexamethasone in children with pneumococcal meningitis. *Pediatr Infect Dis J* 1995;14:490–4.

51. **Towsend GC, Scheld WM.** The use of corticosteroids in the management of bacterial meningitis. *J Antimicrob Chemother* 1996;37:1051–61.

52. **Friedland IR, Shelton S, Paris M, et al.** Dilemmas in diagnosis and management of cephalosporin-resistant Streptococcus pneumoniae meningitis. *Pediatr Infect Dis J* 1993; 12:196–200.

53. **Friedland IR, Paris MM, Ehrett S, et al.** Evaluation of antimicrobial regimens for treatment of experimental penicillin–and cephalosporin–resistant pneumococcal meningitis. *Antimicrob Agents Chemother* 1993;37:1630–6.

54. **Paris MM, Hickey SM, Uscher MI, et al.** Effect of dexamethasone on therapy of experimental penicillin and cephalosporin-resistant pneumococcal meningitis. *Antimicrob Agents Chemother* 1994;38:1320–4.

55. **Klugman KP, Friedland IR, Bradley JS.** Bactericidal activity against cephalosporin-resistant Streptococcus pneumoniae in cerebrospinal fluid of children with acute bacterial meningitis. *Antimicrob Agents Chemother* 1995;39:1988–92.

56. **Knockaert DL.** Bacterial meningitis: diagnostic and therapeutic considerations. *Eur J Emerg Med* 1994;1:92–103.

57. **Lin T-Y, Chrane DF, Nelson JD, McCracken GH Jr.** Seven days of ceftriaxone therapy is as effective as ten days treatment for bacterial meningitis. *JAMA* 1985;253: 3559–63.

58. **O'Neill P.** How long to treat bacterial meningitis. *Lancet* 1993;341:530 [Erratum, Lancet 1993;341:642.]

3

Viral Meningitis and Viral Encephalitis

K.V. Gopalakrishna, MD
James S. Tan, MD

Aseptic Meningitis

Aseptic meningitis syndrome is a self-limiting disease characterized by meningeal symptoms of acute onset, cerebrospinal fluid (CSF) pleocytosis (usually with a mononuclear cell predominance), and the inability to isolate a bacterial agent. At least 300,000 cases of this syndrome occur each year in the United States (1). Aseptic meningitis is commonly caused by an infectious agent but may be of noninfectious origin (2). Viruses are the most common identifiable agents of this syndrome, with enteroviruses being responsible for more than 80% of cases (3). Outbreaks of enteroviral meningitis are seasonal. Table 3.1 shows the common and uncommon causes of acute aseptic meningitis syndrome. The most commonly affected age groups are infants and children (4). The discussion in this chapter includes the clinical manifestations of aseptic meningitis syndrome in older children and adults. Acute meningitis caused by herpes virus is discussed in Chapter 38.

The clinical manifestations of acute bacterial meningitis and those of aseptic meningitis are difficult to distinguish from one another. In older children and adults, both conditions present with fever of acute onset (usually with a temperature of 38°–40°C), severe headache, and meningismus. Neck stiffness is of variable severity. Photophobia is a common accompanying sign of enteroviral meningitis. Nonspecific findings include vomiting, anorexia, rash, diarrhea, cough, and pharyngeal irritation. The course of aseptic meningitis is generally benign and self-limited. However, viral persistence, rheumatologic

Table 3.1   Causes of Acute Aseptic Meningitis Syndrome

More Common Infectious Causes

Viral
Enteroviruses (nonpolio)
HIV
Mumps virus
Herpes simplex virus type 2
Vector-borne viruses (e.g., mosquito- and tick-borne)
Lymphocytic choriomeningitis virus (arenavirus)

Spirochetes
Leptospira species
Borrelia burgdorferi

Mycobacteria
Mycobacterium tuberculosis

Less Common and Rare Infectious Causes

Viral
Adenovirus
Herpes simplex virus type 1
Varicella-zoster virus
Cytomegalovirus
Epstein–Barr virus
Influenza virus types A and B
Parainfluenza virus
Measles virus
Rubella virus
Poliovirus
Rotavirus
Encephalomyocarditis virus
Attenuated vaccine strains of poliovirus, mumps, measles, and vaccinia

Spirochetes
Treponema pallidum
Borrelia recurrentis
Bartonella henselae

Chlamydia
Chlamydia psittaci
Chlamydia trachomatis

Rickettsia
Rickettsia rickettsii
Coxiella burnetii
R. prowazekii
R. typhi
R. tsutsugamushi
Ehrlichia species

Mycoplasma
Mycoplasma pneumoniae
M. hominis
Ureaplasma urealyticum

Other Bacteria
Brucella species
Listeria monocytogenes
Nocardia species
Actinomycetes

Fungi
Cryptococcus neoformans
Coccidioides immitis
Histoplasma capsulatum
Blastomyces dermatidis
Sporothrix schenkii
Zygomycetes
Pseudoallescheria boydii
Cladosporium species

Parasites
Angiostrongylus cantonensis
Strongyloides stercoralis
Taenia solium
Schistosoma species
Trichenella spiralis
Paragonimus species
Echinococcus granulosus
Multiceps multiceps
Gnathostoma spinigerum
Toxoplasma gondii
Naegleria/Acanthomoeba species
Trypanosoma species

Other Infections
Partially treated bacterial meningitis
Parameningeal focus of infection
Endocarditis or bacteremia
Bacterial toxins
Viral postinfectious syndromes
Postvaccination for mumps, measles/mumps, poliovirus, pertussis, rabies, or vaccinia

Noninfectious Causes

Medications
NSAIDs (e.g., ibuprofen, naproxen, tolmetin, diclofenac, ketoprofen)
Antimicrobial agents (e.g., sulfisoxazole, isoniazid, ciprofloxacin, beta-lactam

agents, metronidazole, pyrazinamide)
Muromonab-CD3 (OKT-3)
Azathioprine
Carbamazepine
Phenazopyridine
Ranitidine
Immunoglobulin

Intracranial Tumor and Cysts
Craniopharyngioma
Dermoid/epidermoid cyst
Pituitary adenoma
Astrocytoma
Glioblastoma multiforme
Medulloblastoma
Pinealoma
Ependymoma
Teratoma

Lymphomatous Meningitis, Carcinomatous Meningitis, Leukemia

Neurosurgery-Related Illness
Intrathecal injections (e.g., air, isotopes, antimicrobial agents, antineoplastic agents, steroids, radiographic contrast media)
Chymopapain injection

Systemic Illness
Systemic lupus erythematosis
Sarcoidosis
Behçet's disease
Sjögren's syndrome
Mixed connective tissue disease
Rheumatoid arthritis
Polymyositis
Wegener's granulomatosis
Lymphomatoid granulomatosis
Polyarteritis nodosa
Granulomatous angiitis
Cerebral vasculitis
Familial Mediterranean fever
Kawasaki's disease
Multiple sclerosis
Vogt–Koyanagi–Harada syndrome
Serum sickness
Heavy-metal poisoning (e.g., lead, mercury)
Procedure-related complications (e.g. spinal anesthesia)

NSAIDs = nonsteroidal anti-inflammatory drugs; TMP-SMX = trimethoprim–sulfamethoxazole.
Modified from Hasbun R. The acute aseptic meningitis syndrome. *Curr Infect Dis Rep.* 2000;3:345–51; and Connolly KJ, Hammer SM. The acute septic meningitis syndrome. *Infect Dis Clin North Am.* 1990;4:599–622.

manifestations, and even death may occur in patients with immunoglobulin deficiency (5). Because of the difficulty in differentiating acute bacterial meningitis from the nonbacterial type, examining the CSF is usually helpful but not conclusive. Table 3.2 shows the differential findings in the CSF. The CSF in a patient with acute bacterial meningitis usually contains more than 1000 cells/mm^3 with a predominance of neutrophils, whereas in viral meningitis the CSF has fewer than 1000 cells/mm^3 with a predominance of mononuclear cells. In the early stage of the disease, neutrophils may predominate for a few hours. A mild increase in the CSF protein concentration and a mild decrease in the CSF glucose concentration are typical. After lumbar puncture, CSF specimens should be tested for bacterial agents and subjected to rapid viral diagnostic techniques. Use of the polymerase chain reaction (PCR) test for enteroviruses has been shown to reduce the duration of hospitalization of patients with enterovirus meningitis (3).

From findings in a large enterovirus meningitis outbreak in Rhode Island in the summer of 1991, Rice and coworkers (6) recommended that lumbar puncture be performed routinely to differentiate bacterial from viral meningitis. They recommended that if the CSF is suggestive of viral meningitis during an outbreak, patient observation alone is sufficient. Empirical antibacterial therapy and hospitalization are indicated only for patients who present with atypical clinical and laboratory features. The clinical features of viral meningitides not caused by enterovirus infection are listed in Table 3.3.

Currently, there is no antiviral agent effective for treating viral meningitis. Use of antienteroviral agents (e.g., pleconaril) is being investigated for treating enteroviral meningitis but has not been approved (2). Most patients with aseptic meningitis do not need hospitalization; treatment is largely supportive once bacterial meningitis has been ruled out.

Table 3.2 Cerebrospinal Fluid Findings in Patients Who Present with Meningeal Signs

Diagnosis	Pressure (cm H$_2$0)	Leukocytes ($\lozenge$10^5/L)	PMNLs (per mm^3)	Glucose (CSF:blood ratio)	Protein (g/L)	Lactate (mmol/L)
Normal	<20	1–2	<1	>0.5	<0.45	<2
Acute bacterial meningitis	>20	>1000	>50	<0.4	>1.00	>4
Chronic meningitis	Variable	>1000	Variable	<0.4	>0.45	>2
Aseptic (viral)	<20	<1000	<50	>0.4	Variable	<2

CSF = cerebrospinal fluid; PMNLs = polymorphonuclear leukocytes.
Republished with permission from Leib SL, Tauber MG. Acute and chronic meningitis. In Armstrong D, Cohen J (eds). *Infectious Diseases*. London: Mosby; 1997.

Table 3.3 Clinical Features of the Common Viral Causes of Meningitis

Viral Agent	Season	Age	Exposure History	CSF Profile	Diagnostic Tests
Enteroviruses	Summer, early fall	Children, young adults	Known outbreak of enteroviral disease in community	Early (first 48 hours) neutrophilic pleocytosis with a shift to mononuclear cells	Culture of CSF, blood, stool, throat; PCR
HSV-2	No seasonal pattern	Young adults	Sexually active, new partner	<500 cells with lymphocyte predominance	HSV-2 culture from CSF and genital lesions; seroconversion
HIV	No seasonal pattern	Any age (peak in young adults)	Sexual history, IV drug use, transfusion, specific exposure (needle stick)	<200 cells with lymphocyte predominance	HIV testing
Mumps virus	Late winter to spring	Classically peaks in children aged 5–9 years*	Known community outbreaks	Low CSF glucose in 25% of patients; CSF pleocytosis <500 cells	CSF culture and serology
LCMV	Late fall to early winter	Young adults	Contact with pet rodents (e.g., hamsters, mice) or their excreta	Low CSF glucose in 25% of patients. Pleocytosis usually <750 cells†	Culture of CSF, blood, urine; serology

CSF = cerebrospinal fluid; HSV-2 = herpes simplex virus type 2; IV = intravenous; LCMV = lymphocytic choriomeningitis virus; PCR = polymerase chain reaction test.
* In the vaccine era, adolescents now comprise a more significant proportion of those infected.
† Counts over several thousands have been found.
Hammer SM, Connolly KJ. Viral aseptic meningitis in the United States: Clinical features, viral etiologies, and differential diagnosis. In Remington JS, Swartz MN (eds). *Current Clinical Topics in Infectious Disease*, vol 12. Boston: Blackwell Scientific; 1992.

Viral Encephalitis

The term *encephalitis* means inflammation of the substance of the brain. Because inflammation of the brain and the meninges often accompany each other, terms such as *meningoencephalitis* are also used to describe such conditions. Acute encephalitis associated with a viral infection has two distinct types. In the first type, the virus invades neuronal tissues directly and causes perivascular inflammation and tissue necrosis. In the second type, called *postinfectious encephalomyelitis*, demyelination is localized to the white matter, without infection of the neuronal cells themselves.

The incidence of viral encephalitis varies greatly with the specific causative virus, geographical location, and season. The reported incidence of acute encephalitis is between 3.5 and 7.4 cases per 100,000 patient-years (7).

Etiology

Many viruses have been associated with encephalitis; however, even with the help of sophisticated techniques, a definitive cause is identified in only approximately half of all cases (8). Although enteroviruses are the most common causes of acute viral meningitis, these viruses account for less than 3% of the cases of acute viral encephalitis (9). Enterovirus infections occur primarily in late summer and fall. Arbovirus infections vary widely in occurrence throughout the world. Because arboviruses are arthropod-borne, the incidence of arbovirus encephalitis increases when the viruses' insect vectors are active. Mosquito-borne encephalitis peaks in late summer in regions of temperate climate. Tick-borne diseases occur most often in spring and early summer (10). In the United States, viruses of the California serogroup (LaCrosse strain) and St. Louis encephalitis, western equine encephalitis, and eastern equine encephalitis viruses are the most common arboviruses (Table 3.4). A first-known outbreak of West Nile virus encephalitis was reported in the New York City metropolitan area in 1999 (11).

Herpes simplex virus (HSV) type 1 is the most common cause of the localized, sporadic form of encephalitis seen in the United States. This disease has no seasonal preference. Approximately 1000 cases are reported annually.

In addition to arboviruses and HSV, many other viruses can cause encephalitis. These encephalitides usually present with milder disease and have fewer sequelae and a lower mortality than does arbovirus or HSV encephalitis (12). The ease of world travel, urbanization, and encroachment on natural environments have led to the spread of viruses and disease vectors from the developing world to the developed world. An example of this scenario is the importation of the Asian tiger mosquito (*Aedes albopictus*, the vector for both

Table 3.4   Characteristics of Viral Encephalitis

Virus	Transmission	Diagnostic Studies	Comments
Enteroviruses	Person to person	Culture of throat, stool, and CSF; PCR test of CSF	Rare fatal encephalitis in neonates
Arboviruses*	Mosquitoes	CSF viral specific IgM; acute and convalescent sera	Japanese encephalitis is the most widespread around the world; West Nile encephalitis emerged in New York City area in 1999
HSV	Person to person	PCR test of CSF; MRI and EEG	Only viral encephalitis with effective antiviral therapy
EBV	Person to person	PCR test of CSF	Lymphadenopathy
CMV	Person to person, bloodborne	Culture and PCR test of CSF	Immunosuppressed host
HIV	Person to person, bloodborne	Serum ELISA Western blot	Encephalitis found at the time of primary infection is rare
Mumps virus	Person to person	Culture of CSF and saliva; serology	Associated parotitis or orchitis
Rabies virus	Animal to person	Culture of CSF and saliva; PCR test of CSF and skin	Disease can be fatal

CMV = cytomegalovirus; CSF = cerebrospinal fluid; EBV = Epstein–Barr virus; EEG = electroencephalography; ELISA = enzyme-linked immunosorbent assay; HSV = herpes simplex virus; IgM = immunoglobulin M; MRI = magnetic resonance imaging; PCR = polymerase chain reaction test.
* Including Japanese encephalitis, St. Louis encephalitis, California serogroup (LaCrosse) encephalitis, Eastern and Western equine encephalitis, and West Nile encephalitis.

dengue and yellow fever) to the southern United States in a shipment of used tires from Japan (13).

Pathogenesis and Pathology

Infectious agents can invade the central nervous system via the blood (e.g., arbovirus, mumps virus, measles virus) or the peripheral nerves (e.g., HSV, herpesvirus B from monkeys, rabies virus). HSV encephalitis is thought to result either from reinfection or from reactivation of the latent virus in the trigeminal and other cranial ganglia. More than 90% of adults have antibody to HSV type 1, and approximately 25% of patients with encephalitis have a history of cold sores.

Clinical Findings

Patients with viral encephalitis often present with headache, fever, nuchal rigidity, and alteration of consciousness. The degree of this latter alteration may vary from mild lethargy to stupor and coma. Various focal features (e.g., motor weakness, accentuated deep tendon reflexes, abnormal movements, tremors, seizures) have been described. Increased intracranial pressure can lead to papilledema, and cranial nerve palsies may develop.

Encephalitis caused by HSV may have an insidious or abrupt onset. Affected patients often present with bizarre behaviors or hallucinations. These findings suggest temporal lobe localization of the disease (14).

Laboratory Findings

Examining the CSF is essential for the diagnosis of viral encephalitis. Pleocytosis is variable (10–1000 cells/mm^3), with a predominance of mononuclear cells; however, considerable numbers of polymorphonuclear cells may be present at an early stage of infection. Erythrocytes are frequently present in HSV encephalitis. The CSF protein is usually increased, and the CSF glucose is typically normal or slightly below normal.

Although CSF can be cultured for arboviruses and enteroviruses, attempts to culture CSF for HSV have been unsuccessful. Rapid diagnosis of arbovirus encephalitis is possible with an enzyme-linked immunosorbent assay for virus-specific IgM antibodies in the CSF. Serum antibody measurements made in the acute and convalescent phases sometimes help in establishing the diagnosis of arbovirus encephalitis. Because identifying the cause in arbovirus encephalitis outbreaks is so important, certain State agencies offer laboratory assistance in making the laboratory diagnosis.

In HSV encephalitis, cerebral tissue biopsy with virus isolation has been the gold standard of diagnosis. PCR analysis of the CSF for HSV recently has become available in reference laboratories. In laboratories that are experienced in performing this test, the specificity of PCR approaches 100%, and the sensitivity is between 75% and 98% (7).

In viral encephalitis, electroencephalography often reveals a diffuse slowing of brain waves. Slow-wave complexes, at regular intervals of two to three per second in the temporal lobe, are characteristic of HSV encephalitis.

Computed tomography of the brain in HSV encephalitis reveals low-density lesions in one or both temporal lobes; however, this finding tends to appear late in the disease. Magnetic resonance imaging of the brain may show the abnormality at an early stage of disease and is superior to computed tomography in sensitivity and in localizing lesions in the temporoparietal region.

Treatment

The only form of viral encephalitis for which effective treatment exists is that caused by HSV. Treatment with acyclovir therapy has proven superior to that with vidarabine in reducing morbidity and mortality in HSV encephalitis (15). Untreated HSV encephalitis carries a 70% mortality rate. Acyclovir reduces the mortality to less than 19% (16). Usually, intravenous acyclovir 10 mg/kg is given every 8 hours for 14 days. The patient's age and level of consciousness at the beginning of therapy are important prognostic factors. Younger age and a Glasgow Coma Scale score of greater than 6 favor recovery.

The management of other viral encephalitides is usually supportive and is intended to avoid nosocomial complications. Cerebral edema may be treated with mannitol or corticosteroids. Seizures should be controlled with anticonvulsants.

Summary

Acute viral infections of the CNS produce illnesses that range from mild to serious. Acute viral meningitis is usually mild and self-limiting. Acute viral encephalitis may result in serious brain injury and even death. Treatment is available for HSV encephalitis, and its prognosis depends on early recognition and treatment with acyclovir.

REFERENCES

1. **Parasuraman TV, Deverka PA, Toscani MR.** Estimating the economic impact of viral meningitis in the United States. *Infect Med.* 2000;17:417–27.
2. **Hasbun R.** The acute aseptic meningitis syndrome. *Curr Infect Dis Rep.* 2000;3:345–51.
3. **Ramers C, Billman G, Hartin M, et al.** Impact of a diagnostic cerebrospinal fluid enterovirus polymerase chain reaction test on patient management. *JAMA.* 2000;283:2680–5.
4. **Rotbart HA, Brennan PJ, Fife KH, et al.** Enterovirus meningitis in adults. *Clin Infect Dis.* 1998;27:896–8.
5. **Rotbart HA.** Viral meningitis and the aseptic meningitis syndrome. In Scheld WM, Whitley RJ, Durak DT (eds). *Infections of the Central Nervous System.* New York: Raven Press; 1991:19–40.
6. **Rice SK, Heinl RE, Thornton LL, Opal SM.** Clinical characteristics, management strategies, and cost implications of a statewide outbreak of enterovirus meningitis. *Clin Infect Dis.* 1995;20:931–7.
7. **Johnson RT.** Acute encephalitis. *Clin Infect Dis.* 1996; 23:219–226.
8. **Bergstrom SM, Hagberg L.** Acute viral encephalitis in adults: a prospective study. *Scand J Infect Dis.* 1998;30:215–20.

9. **Meyer HM Jr, Johnson RT, Crawford IP, et al.** Central nervous system syndromes of "viral" etiology: a study of 713 cases. *Am J Med.* 1960;29:334–7.

10. **Montalbano MA, Knowles CM, Adams DA, et al.** Summary of notifiable diseases–United States, 1996. *MMWR Morbid Mortal Weekly Rep.* 1997;45:1-87.

11. **Anonymous.** Update: West Nile virus encephalitis–New York 1999. *MMWR Morbid Mortal Weekly Rep.* 1999;48:944–6.

12. **Griffin DE.** Encephalitis, myelitis, and neuritis. In Mandell GL, Bennett JE, Dolin R (eds). *Principles and Practice of Infectious Diseases,* 4th ed. New York: Churchill Livingstone; 1995:874–81.

13. **Rogers DJ, Parker MJ.** Vector-borne diseases, models, and global change. *Lancet.* 1993;342:1282–4.

14. **Whitley RJ, Soong S-J, Linneman C, et al.** Herpes simplex encephalitis: clinical assessment. *JAMA.* 1982;247:317–20.

15. **Whitley RJ.** Herpes simplex virus infections of the central nervous system: therapeutic and diagnostic considerations. *Clin Infect Dis.* 1995;20:414.

16. **Whitley RJ.** Viral encephalitis. *N Engl J Med.* 1990;323:242.

4

Brain Abscess

Scott A. Fulton, MD

Robert A. Salata, MD

Brain abscess is a relatively rare diagnosis, with 1500–2500 cases occurring annually in the United States (1). Its prevalence has not increased significantly, despite increases in patients who are chronically immunosuppressed by medical therapy (e.g., corticosteroids, cytotoxic chemotherapy), systemic inflammatory diseases (e.g., sarcoidosis, systemic lupus erythematosis), and HIV infection. Brain abscess occurs with a striking male predominance (from 2–3:1) and generally occurs in patients 20 to 40 years of age (2–6). However, children with congenital heart disease represent most brain abscess patients under 20 years of age (6–8). Not all patients with a space-occupying lesion of the central nervous system have a pyogenic brain abscess. The differential diagnosis is relatively limited to infectious and neoplastic causes. Knowledge of a patient's medical, surgical, travel, and HIV-exposure histories is important during the initial evaluation and treatment of brain abscess. This chapter provides a concise review of the pathogenesis and approaches to the diagnosis and management of cerebral brain abscesses and focuses primarily on bacterial abscesses in immunocompetent patients. A more extensive discussion of brain abscesses in immunocompromised patients can be found in several excellent reviews (9–11).

Definition and Differential Diagnosis

A brain abscess is a focal collection of purulent material within the brain parenchyma. Involvement of the overlying pia and arachnoid meninges usually occurs only in the setting of concomitant meningitis or after an intraventricular rupture. By definition, *cerebral brain abscess* does not comprise subdural, epidural, or spinal abscesses, which vary in pathogenesis and etiology. *Brain abscess* is a term reserved for an encapsulated (matured), nonneoplastic, space-occupying mass seen with contrast-enhanced computed tomography (CT) or magnetic resonance imaging (MRI) either as a finely nodular or ring-enhancing lesion (12–14). The ring enhancement represents the vascularized capsule that surrounds a central area of necrosis. Abscess formation begins as a focal inflammatory reaction or cerebritis that allows diffusion of contrast medium centrally within the lesion. The cerebritis stage of abscess formation can present a diagnostic difficulty, because there is no collection of material for diagnostic aspiration. In addition, the early inflammatory changes seen in cases of brain abscess are not specific to this condition and also may arise from encephalitis, vasculitis, and in some cases from a tumor or the early stage of an infarct (12,13).

The differential diagnosis of a brain abscess takes into consideration the cause of ring-enhancing lesions. The typical pathogens involved in brain abscesses include a broad range of microorganisms, including aerobic, microaerophilic, and anaerobic bacteria. Fungi, mycobacteria, and parasites also may cause brain abscesses. However, opportunistic pathogens such as *Nocardia asteroides*, *Aspergillus*, and *Toxoplasma gondii* are identified almost exclusively in patients who have an underlying immunodeficiency that results from corticosteroid treatment, cancer chemotherapy, transplantation, or HIV infection (15–19). The differential diagnosis can be prioritized on the basis of comorbid conditions and the patient's immunocompetence. Additionally, travel history or point of origin may identify patients who are at risk for brain abscesses caused by mycobacteria, *Brucella*, or *Coccidioides* (20–22).

Pathogenesis

Anatomical Considerations

The brain parenchyma is covered by the pia mater, arachnoid, and dura mater, which are penetrated by emissary and diploic (valveless) veins that drain into the cerebral venous sinuses. Additionally, venous drainage of the soft tissues of the head converges within cerebral venous sinuses (9). Because these valveless conduits allow retrograde blood flow directly to the brain, brain abscesses can result from infections in the periorbital and facial soft tissues, paranasal sinuses, ears, and dentition. Brain abscesses that arise hematogenously from distant infectious foci also have been described in cases of endocarditis, lung abscess, hepatic abscess, and inflammatory bowel disease; however, many "cryptic" abscesses arise without an obvious distant focus (2,10,23–25). Brain abscesses that arise from direct extension from adjacent bony structures (e.g., the frontal, sphenoid, and mastoid sinuses, but not usually the maxillary sinuses) and from direct inoculation during surgery or after a penetrating trauma also are well described (11,26–28). Thus, the seeding of the brain with pathogenic microorganisms may occur hematogenously, by direct implantation, or by contiguous inoculation.

Brain Abscess Formation and Radiographic Correlates

The classic studies of Britt and Enzmann (13) correlated neuropathologic and CT findings in experimental streptococcal brain abscesses induced in dogs. In subsequent studies, 14 human cases of brain abscess were analyzed pathologically and radiographically, yielding findings that paralleled those in the animal model (12). In brief, a focal area of inflammation (cerebritis) that is caused largely by small-vessel thrombosis and perivascular inflammation, marks early abscess formation. Microscopically, these lesions contain neutrophils, lymphocytes, and plasma cells. CT shows variable central diffusion of contrast medium and, because neovascularization is minimal, absence of or scant ring enhancement. Delayed images show continued diffusion and minimal decay of contrast medium during the early cerebritis stage of abscess formation. The late cerebritis stage is characterized by more prominent diffusion centrally and by ring enhancement that may be finely nodular, thick, or thin. The decay of ring enhancement in delayed images remains minimal. Pathologically, central necrosis begins and is associated with increased edema and maximal cerebritis. Although the time course for abscess formation is variable, the cerebritis stage evolves over a period of 3 to 10 days.

Capsule formation around an abscess results from organization of collagen by fibroblasts and from neovascularization that is accompanied by reduced inflammation. CT at this stage of abscess development shows less central enhancement and a marked decay in capsular enhancement because of maximal neovascularization and capsular blood flow. The time to encapsulation also varies but is generally within 10 to 14 days. Matured abscesses tend to have well-defined capsules; however, because neovascularization is more rapid at the cortical aspect of an abscess, the abscess walls adjacent to the ventricle tend to be thinner and more prone to rupture. Depending on anatomical location and the degree of edema, abscesses may remain undetected for days or even weeks. However, most patients present within 10 to 14 days of their initial symptoms (3,4,6).

Location of Brain Abscesses

Abscesses that involve the basal ganglia, cerebellum, all lobes of the cerebrum, and rarely the brain stem have been described. However, most abscesses are located in the cerebrum, where the frontal and temporal lobes represent the major sites of involvement (50%) that are reported in most series (2–4,6,18). Table 4.1 shows the distribution of abscesses in the central nervous system in six large studies. This comprehensive summary illustrates the location of abscesses in six patient populations that varied in demographics and comorbid medical conditions, illustrating some changes in epidemiology and abscess location over time. In early studies (4), a large percentage of abscesses involved the temporal lobes, which has been attributed to the greater incidence of otogenic infections (e.g., chronic otitis) in both children and adults before 1967. In other series (4,6,28,29) in which the incidence of otogenic and rhinogenic infection was also high, the temporal lobe was involved in approximately 42% of cases. Apparently, the spread of otogenic infections to the temporal lobe occurs primarily through contiguous spread or direct extension.

More recent studies from the United States (3) and Singapore (5) suggest a decline (from 25%–42% to 14%–22% of all brain abscesses) in temporal lobe abscesses, presumably from the expedient antibiotic treatment of otitis media. Frontal lobe abscesses are the most common; however, the temporal and parietal lobes are involved at a similar rate (*see* Table 4.1). In other reports, the percentages of frontal and temporal lobe abscesses have been similar (11). Furthermore, although the populations reported in major studies were heterogeneous with respect to age, sex, and comorbid conditions, the distribution of

Table 4.1   Percent Distribution of Brain Abscesses by Anatomical Location

Anatomical Location	UK 1957 (4)*	UK 1967 (4)*	USA 1986 (3)	Singapore 1993 (5)	Japan 1997 (8)[†‡]	USA 1994 (18)[†§]	Mean
Cerebellum							
Frontal lobe	31	35	33	33	30	30	32
Temporal lobe	42	25	14	22	24	21	25
Parietal lobe	22	34	24	19	25	37	26
Occipital lobe	NR	NR	8	6	15	27	14
Cerebellum	NR	NR	6	18	15	17	16
Other[¶]	NR	NR	15	NR	4	24	—

NR = not reported.
* Percentages adjusted to exclude 18% subdural abscess included in original set.
[†] Total >100% because some patients had more than two abscesses.
[‡] All patients had congenital cyanotic heart disease.
[§] All patients were bone marrow transplant recipients.
[¶] Brain stem and basal ganglia.

abscesses among the frontal, parietal, and temporal lobes was remarkably similar among the individual studies (*see* Table 4.1).

It is important to note that in pediatric and adolescent patients with congenital cyanotic heart disease (CCHD), the distribution of abscesses in the cerebrum did not differ significantly when the mechanism of inoculation was considered to be strictly hematogenous (8). However, the incidence of cerebellar and occipital brain abscesses was greater and seemed to correlate with the percentage of multiple abscesses occurring hematogenously. Similarly, a higher incidence of occipital lobe and cerebellar abscesses was reported in bone marrow-transplant patients who had disseminated fungal infections (18). Thus, one might predict that recurrent occult bacteremia or fungemia might increase the distribution of lesions to the occipital lobes and cerebellum, which are served by the posterior circulation. However, no cerebral or cerebellar lobe shows a unique proclivity for abscess formation except when inoculated by direct extension (e.g., chronic otitis media that affects the temporal lobe, mastoiditis that affects the cerebellum).

Epidemiology

The risk of brain abscess formation through direct inoculation or extension from rhinogenic or otogenic foci has been recognized for many years; however, such cases represent only half the reported cases in the literature (2,3,5,7,30,31). Table 4.2 summarizes five studies that represent four different countries and shows the percentage of patients with brain abscess and the following risk factors: CCHD, otogenic, rhinogenic, dental, pulmonary, and cryptogenic infections. Although the distribution of associated factors varies among studies, rhinogenic and otogenic infections were identified in 15% to 40% of the 192 adult and pediatric patients reported. In a review only of pediatric patients from 1960–1989 (7), 38% of 535 patients with brain abscesses had concomitant rhinogenic and otogenic infections. Although the percentage of abscesses that involved the temporal lobes has declined somewhat with time (*see* Table 4.1), the overall prevalence of brain abscess caused by rhinogenic and otogenic infections has not changed markedly in the past 30 to 40 years (*see* Table 4.2). Additionally, approximately 5% to 20% of brain abscesses occurred in the setting of CCHD, dental, or pulmonary disease. In studies that involved a greater number of children, the association of brain abscess with CCHD ranged from 18% to 20% (5,31). No associated infection was identified in 22% to 45% of the patients reported (*see* Table 4.2); however, the general distribution of attributable causes of brain abscess is remarkably similar in early and recent series.

It is important to note that most series reported single abscesses in 70% or more of patients. There are fewer data for patients with multiple brain ab-

Table 4.2   Percentage of Patients with Attributable Risk Factors for Brain Abscess Formation

Brain Abscess Risk Factors	USA 1970–83 (3)	USA 1961–73 (2)	Canada 1986–93 (30)	Switzerland 1982–92 (5)	Singapore 1989–93 (5)*
Cases[†]	40	60	28	34	30
CCHD	None	8.3	None	8	20
Otogenic infection	16	20	15	None	33
Rhinogenic infection	20	‡	None	13	7
Odontogenic infection	13	7	10	13	None
Pulmonary infection	16	13	5	21	None
Cryptogenic infection	22	25	45	29	40

CCHD = cyanotic congenital heart disease.
* Excluding trauma and postsurgical patients.
† 70% to 87% solitary abscesses.
‡ Rhinogenic percentage included in the otogenic percentage for this study.

scesses, which presumably arise hematogenously. However, Sharma et al. (31) reported multiple abscesses in 25% and 26% of patients with CCHD and otogenic infections, respectively. Thus, otogenic infections also may inoculate the brain hematogenously to yield multiple abscesses. In contrast, another study found multiple abscesses in only 11% of CCHD patients with brain abscesses (8), suggesting that hematogenous inoculation does not necessarily result in multiple abscesses. Moreover, another study found that 44% of patients with two or more abscesses had no identifiable comorbid infection (1). Thus, no clear association can be drawn between a specific medical condition and abscess multiplicity.

Data in Table 4.2 also show a large percentage of patients with brain abscess that do not have an identifiable source. Many case reports implicate several clinical conditions in brain abscess formation (Table 4.3). In this regard, CCHD represents a prototypical risk factor for hematogenous brain abscess formation and accounts for 75% of cases of brain abscess in patients under 20 years of age. Right-to-left shunts within the cardiopulmonary vasculature increase the opportunity for microorganisms to bypass pulmonary host defenses and gain access to the brain. It is not known how chronic hypoxemia

Table 4.3   Medical Conditions Associated with Brain Abscess

Diabetes mellitus	Inflammatory bowel disease
Portal hypertension	Pelvic inflammatory disease
Cirrhosis	Systemic lupus erythematosus
Infective endocarditis	Intravenous drug use
Postdental care	Cyanotic congenital heart disease
Transplantation	Hemolytic uremic syndrome
Pneumonia	Chronic mastoiditis, otitis, or sinusitis
Periodontal disease	Premature birth
HIV disease	Trauma and neurosurgery
Liver abscess	Congenital pulmonary arteriovenous fistula
Sarcoidosis	Cystic fibrosis

or secondary polycythemia contributes to the pathogenesis of brain abscess in patients with CCHD (10). Arteriovenous shunting also occurs in advanced cirrhosis with portal hypertension, hereditary hemorrhagic telangiectasia, and congenital pulmonary arteriovenous fistula, which also have been described as conditions predisposing to brain abscess formation (32,33). Interestingly, bacteremia associated with intravenous narcotic abuse has not been reported to cause a disproportionately large number of brain abscesses, a finding that underscores the complexity of brain abscess formation via hematogenous mechanisms (2,3,6). It is interesting to hypothesize that intermittent or sporadic bacteremia would be less likely to cause brain abscesses than would chronic conditions (e.g., pulmonary arteriovenous fistulas, CCHD), in which bacteremia may be more frequent, continuous, and profound. Other medical conditions associated with brain abscesses have included infective endocarditis, hemolytic uremic syndrome, cystic fibrosis, premature birth, and pelvic inflammatory disease (7,23,34).

The principal pathophysiologic mechanisms for brain abscess formation in normal and immunosuppressed patients are not well understood. For example, in patients with inflammatory bowel disease, brain abscess formation may result from an impaired mucosal barrier or as a consequence of corticosteroid treatment. When opportunistic pathogens such as *Nocardia asteroides* are identified within a brain abscess, an underlying immunologic defect must be considered. However, even in conditions with relatively normal immune function (e.g., pregnancy), opportunistic pathogens have been identified in brain abscesses (35). Nevertheless, brain abscess formation has typically been associated with a definitive array of clinical conditions, which should help physicians maintain a high clinical suspicion of its existence when accompanied by the appropriate epidemiologic, clinical, and radiographic findings.

Clinical Manifestations

Signs and symptoms of brain abscess are extremely variable and often are masked by comorbidities. The classic triad of fever, headache, and neurological deficit is present in less than 50% of patients (3,8,18,31). Fever and headache, however, have been present in from 40% to 75% of patients in most series for which data are available (9,36). Table 4.4 summarizes the signs and symptoms associated with brain abscess from four studies in which abscess multiplicity was also known. In a comprehensive description reported by Chun et al. (3), fever and headache were present in 40% to 72% of patients. Other signs associated with increased intracranial pressure (e.g., nausea, vomiting, confusion) were present in 20% to 35% of patients. Multiple abscesses were present in 27% of patients. In the study by Sharma et al. (31), in which all patients had two or more abscesses, the presence of headache, fever, and seizures were similar to those in other reports. However, patients with multiple brain abscesses presented more often with hemiparesis and cranial nerve deficits. In bone marrow-transplant patients (48% with multiple abscesses), 26% and 31% of the patients presented with hemiparesis and cranial nerve deficits, respectively (18). Notably, only 7% of bone marrow-transplant patients with brain abscesses complained of headache. In patients with CCHD, 52% presented with hemiparesis, even though only 20% of the patients had

Table 4.4   Percentage of Patients with Signs and Symptoms Associated with Brain Abscesses at Presentation

Signs and Symptoms	USA (3)	India (31)*	Japan (8)†	USA (18)‡
Headache	72	76	60	7
Fever or chills	42	65	65	83
Seizure	35	39	47	22
Nausea or vomiting	35	—	42	2
Confusion	26	7.9	—	50
Motor weakness	21	—	—	—
Visual disturbances	21	13	7	—
Hemiparesis	9	26	52	26
Speech disturbances	9	—	3	—
Dizziness	7	—	—	—
Syncope	7	—	—	—
Stiff neck	5	26	—	—
Cranial nerve abnormality	—	34	—	31

* All patients had two or more abscesses.
† All patients had congenital cyanotic heart disease.
‡ All patients were bone marrow transplant recipients only.
Data from references 3, 8, 18, and 31.

two or more abscesses (8). Thus, abscess multiplicity does not consistently predict the presenting signs and symptoms of brain abscess. Interestingly, seizures were reported in 22% to 47% of patients and also did not distinguish patients with a single abscess from those with multiple abscesses (8,18).

Patients with brain abscess come to clinical attention at different times. Most often, signs and symptoms of the abscess evolve insidiously. Patients with minimal symptoms may not seek attention for weeks, by which time the abscess has matured. However, delayed presentation (1–2 weeks) is not generally associated with an increased mortality (14). In other cases, abscess location and associated edema cause severe symptoms, usually headache or seizure (30%), forcing the patient to seek medical attention at an early stage (2–5 days). Symptom duration is highly variable, with patients tending to present within 10 to 14 days of the their initial symptoms (3,6,35). Early presentation with abrupt neurological changes (e.g., seizure, blindness, hemiparesis) or coma portends a poor prognosis (because there may be a rupture of an intraventricular abscess or associated meningitis) and is observed more often at the extremes of age. Furthermore, patients with multiple abscesses do not seem to present earlier than patients with single lesions (31).

Despite the variable presentation of brain abscesses, only the grading of mental status at evaluation is predictive of mortality (37). Essentially, the more obtunded the patient is at the time of presentation, the higher the mortality. Although the diagnosis and treatment are more rapid today than in the past, patients with a neurological status of grade C (i.e., responding to painful stimuli only) or grade D (coma) have the highest predicted mortality rates. Overall, mortality rates have decreased from 17% to 83% in the pre-CT era to less than 20% with the aid of modern imaging techniques, including MRI (1,4,6,29). Although the variability in mortality among reported series is extensive, overall mortality averaged 30% when 2825 patients who presented in the pre- and post-CT eras (1950–1993) were evaluated (38). Mortality rates that exceeded 80% were reported in cases of brain abscess complicated by meningitis and of ruptured intraventricular brain abscesses (38). Generally, most patients (>80%) present with grade A or B neurological status, which accounts for the relatively low mortality from brain abscess (3,39). Interestingly, patients with multiple abscesses do not seem to present more often with neurological status of grades C and D (1,5,23). Thus, abscess multiplicity does not correlate well with mental status at the time of diagnosis.

Diagnosis

The data in Table 4.4 illustrate the clinical findings associated with brain abscess. However, because less than 50% of patients present with "hard" neurological findings (e.g., cranial nerve deficit, focal weakness, seizure), a high index of suspicion is necessary for initiating a diagnostic evaluation. Altered mental status, particularly headache, often prompts a CT or MRI of the brain. In the past, cerebral angiography and radionuclide scanning were used as adjuncts in the diagnosis of brain abscess. The modern imaging era began with the availability of CT (c. 1974), which has been regarded as a revolutionary advance in the diagnosis of cerebral brain abscess. CT and MRI also have been important in evaluating brain lesions in HIV-infected and other immunosuppressed patients (12,14,40).

Britt and Enzmann (12, 13) have provided crucial histopathologic and radiographic data about the evolution of brain abscess. Although imaging characteristics consistent with brain abscess are variable, patients typically have lesions that demonstrate ring enhancement when injected with iodinated contrast medium or gadolinium. Figure 4.1A shows a CT scan (with contrast) of two abscesses with surrounding hypodense edema in the left parietal lobe. Multiple ring-enhancing lesions also are shown in Figure 4.1B, in which the left frontal and right occipital lobes are involved. Figure 4.2 shows a T_1-weighted MRI scan of a typical mature abscess with gadolinium enhancement of the peripheral capsule. T_2-weighting generally produces a hyperintense signal within the abscess and the surrounding edematous tissue. Because the etiology of ring-enhancing lesions tends to be infectious or neoplastic, a major concern in the diagnosis of brain abscess is ruling out malignancy. Rare instances have been cited in which both an abscess and a tumor coexisted

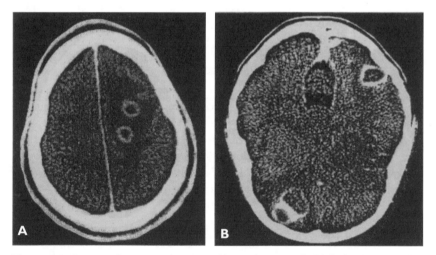

Figure 4.1 Computed tomography scans of brain abscesses. **A,** Multiple abscesses that involve the left frontoparietal region. **B,** Multiple abscesses that involve the left frontal and right occipital lobe.

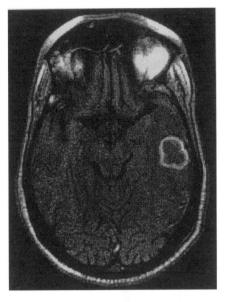

Figure 4.2 Magnetic resonance imaging scan of a brain abscess. This T_1-weighted image shows a mature (encapsulated) abscess that involves the left temporal lobe.

(41,42). If there is high suspicion for malignancy, biopsy is essential; a search for a primary malignancy (especially in the lung) may be necessary. Radionuclide scanning with either ^{99m}Tc- or ^{111}In-labeled white blood cells may help differentiate tumor from infection (41). However, biopsy remains the "gold standard" and is often feasible with modern stereotactic techniques. Some lesions that are small, immature, or located within the brainstem may not be amenable to stereotactic aspiration or biopsy. Therefore, close consultation with both a neurosurgeon and a neuroradiologist is essential.

Although identification and localization of the lesion are key elements of imaging in brain abscess cases, diagnostic aspiration and/or biopsy are critical in establishing a microbiological diagnosis. Because 20% to 40% of abscesses are cryptogenic (*see* Table 4.2), an effort should be made to obtain abscess material (e.g., aerobic, anaerobic, fungal) for cultivation in the microbiology laboratory. Results of abscess cultures reveal organisms in 60% to 80% of cases (3,5,6,31), unless the patients have been given antibiotics previously (37,43). Obtaining cultures of abscess fluid allows more directed antibiotic therapy and may suggest an anatomical source of infection. Clinicians should be prompted to evaluate patients for extraneural sources of infection that may reveal the offending pathogens, especially when diagnostic aspiration is not possible or when cultures are negative. There are no strict guidelines for this, and results are often negative. CT or MRI may help identify rhinogenic or otogenic disease. Additionally, cultures of sputum, pleural fluid, and blood may be helpful in cases of pneumonia, pleural empyema, and endocarditis. Positive blood cultures have been noted in 60% to 70% of brain abscess patients with active endocarditis and are of help in directing the appropriate antibiotic therapy. In one series, candidemia was present in 21% of bone marrow-transplant patients with candidal brain abscesses (18). In contrast, other studies have reported positive blood cultures in only 10% to 12% patients (3,37). Thus, obtaining blood cultures during the initial evaluation may have some use, especially if diagnostic aspiration is delayed or not performed (3).

On the basis of associated risk factors, empirical therapy for brain abscess can be governed by a knowledge of the microbiological flora that are typical for this condition. Table 4.5 summarizes some expected pathogens associated with brain abscess. With regard to the usual risk factors (*see* Table 4.2), aerobic and anaerobic streptococci predominate (40%–80% of cases) when the source is considered to be rhinogenic, otogenic, odontogenic, pulmonary, or cardiac. Enteric bacilli also may arise from chronic otogenic infection. Staphylococci, including methicillin-resistant *Staphylococcus aureus*, and Enterobacteriaceae predominate in neurosurgical and trauma patients. Additionally, penetrating trauma to the head should alert the physician to such organisms as *Bacillus* (26). Even in immunocompromised patients, typical streptococci (aerobic and microaerophilic), including *Streptococcus pneumoniae* (44), must be considered in cases of brain abscess, along with opportunistic pathogens. In most cases for which aspirates are available for cultivation in the laboratory, positive results are obtained in well over 80% of the samples evaluated in many series (2,3,45). Importantly, 10% to 40% of positive cultures in cases of brain abscess yield polymicrobial results; therefore, antibiotic therapy must be tailored appropriately.

Ancillary laboratory evaluation is generally of little value in the diagnosis of brain abscess. Many patients have a modestly increased leukocyte count (>10,000 cells/mm^3). Although an increased erythrocyte sedimentation rate is likely in brain abscess, few data have evaluated this indicator. Interestingly, some studies have monitored levels of C-reactive protein. Jamjoom et al. (46) reported 18 of 24 patients with C-reactive protein levels above 20 mg/dL. However, C-reactive protein probably has little diagnostic use beyond being a helpful correlate or in monitoring the response to treatment. Presently, the treatment of brain abscess is monitored clinically along with repeat CT or MRI.

The use of cerebrospinal fluid analysis in the diagnosis of brain abscess dates back to studies done in the pre-CT era. Cerebrospinal fluid analysis may reveal pleocytosis and increased protein levels. However, cultures are usually negative. The high mortality rates associated with lumbar puncture in patients with brain abscess were determined before the availability of modern imaging (4,29). Lumbar puncture is best avoided until a space-occupying lesion or severe edema has been ruled out. If necessary, cerebrospinal fluid sampling is performed most optimally in consultation with a neurologist or neurosurgeon.

Table 4.5   Brain Abscess in Adults: Microbiology and Antimicrobial Therapy

Source of Abscess	Site of Abscess	Microbial Flora	Antimicrobial Therapy*†
Paranasal sinus	Frontal lobe	Aerobic streptococci (usually *Streptococcus milleri* group) Anaerobic streptococci *Haemophilus* species *Bacteroides* species *Fusobacterium* species	Penicillin + metronidazole or cefotaxime or ceftriaxone + metronidazole‡
Otogenic infection	Temporal lobe, cerebellum	*Streptococcus* species Enterobacteriaceae *Bacteroides* species (including *B. fragilis*) *Pseudomonas aeruginosa*	Penicillin + metronidazole + ceftazidime or ceftriaxone
Metastatic spread	Multiple cerebral lesions are common, especially in the middle cerebral artery; however, any lobe can be involved	Depends on source Endocarditis: *Staphylococcus aureus, Streptococcus viridans* Urinary tract: Enterobacteriaceae, Pseudomonadaceae Intra-abdominal: *Streptococcus* species, Enterobacteriaceae, anaerobic organisms Lung abscess: *Streptococcus* species, *Actinomyces* species, *Fusobacterium* species	Nafcillin + metronidazole + cefotaxime
Penetrating trauma	Depends on wound site	*Staphylococcus aureus* *Clostridium* species Enterobacteriaceae *Staphylococcus epidermidis*	Nafcillin + cefotaxime or ceftriaxone
Postoperative		*Staphylococcus aureus* Enterobacteriaceae Pseudomonadaceae	Vancomycin + ceftazidime

*These are the suggested antimicrobial therapies for empirical treatment. The antibiotic selection varies depending on the clinical situation and culture results.

†The recommended antibiotic dosages for a 70-kg patient are as follows: penicillin, 2–4 million units IV q4h; metronidazole, 500 mg IV q6h; cefotaxime, 1–2 g IV q4–8h (maximum 12 g/d); ceftriaxone, 2 g IV q12h; ceftazidime, 1–2 g IV q4–8h (maximum 12 g/d); nafcillin, 2 g IV q4h; and vancomycin, 1 g IV q12h. Dosages may need to be adjusted in patients with underlying renal or liver disease. Ceftriaxone and cefotaxime can be used interchangeably.

‡ Cefotaxime plus metronidazole has been demonstrated to have efficacy in two studies with limited numbers of patients.

Republished with permission from Mathisen GE, Johnson JP. Brain abscess. *Clin Infect Dis.* 1997;25:763–81.

Management

The treatment of patients with brain abscess is complicated and necessitates the close interaction of the primary physician, a neurosurgeon, and an infectious disease specialist. Two key elements are critical in the initial evaluation and treatment of the patient with a brain abscess. First, as discussed previously, a regimen of antibiotics must be chosen on the basis of an assessment of attributable risk factors and the infection site (*see* Table 4.5). If no obvious focus of infection is present, a search for other infection sites is necessary, even though 30% to 40% of patients have no identifiable source of brain abscess. In these patients, a thorough medical history may help identify other clues. For example, a history of drug abuse indicates a need for either a semisynthetic penicillin (e.g., nafcillin) or vancomycin, depending on corroborative cultures, allergy history, and the prevalence of methicillin-resistant staphylococci. Additionally, risk factors for HIV should be discussed. If HIV infection is a possibility, consent should be obtained and testing should be performed. This is especially important because the therapy for a common cause of brain abscess in these patients (*T. gondii*) is different (e.g., sulfadiazine, pyrimethamine).

The second crucial element in the initial management of patients with brain abscess is the decision to evacuate or aspirate the lesion surgically or stereotactically. The approach is affected by the location, size, and number of lesions. Perhaps most critical is the patient's mental status at the time of diagnosis, because mortality is high for patients who present acutely or with grade C or D neurological status. This following section briefly considers these issues, with treatment guidelines that must be individualized to each patient.

Antibiotic Penetration of Brain Abscess Cavities

Ideally, antibiotic choice in the therapy of brain abscess is guided by data that demonstrates penetration into the abscess cavities. Unfortunately, these data are limited. Penicillin G has considerable efficacy and has been measured in abscesses at concentrations ranging from two to 380 times the minimal inhibitory concentration of typical offending streptococci (47,48). Chloramphenicol and nafcillin penetration into abscess cavities was more erratic, producing concentrations up to 4 times the minimal inhibitory concentration. Nonetheless, chloramphenicol and nafcillin have been used with excellent success in treating brain abscesses (3,10,23,48). Other important antibiotics that reach measurable levels within abscess cavities include metronidazole, vancomycin, cefotetan, ceftriaxone, cefotaxime, ceftazidime, and fluoroquinolones (47,49–53). Of these, metronidazole has been a pivotal agent against anaerobic streptococci, which are frequently present (40%–50%) and often tolerant or resistant to penicillin. The clinical evaluation of antibiotic combinations in treating brain abscess has not been systematic or well controlled.

It should be emphasized that first- and second-generation cephalosporins and aminoglycosides are not recommended for treating brain abscesses. In cases of ventricular rupture that involve Enterobacteriaceae, the intraventricular instillation of an aminoglycoside may have benefit. Although the efficacies of newer antimicrobial agents have not been well studied, a recent neonatal case of brain abscess caused by resistant *Enterobacter cloacae* was successfully treated with meropenem (54).

Treatment Strategies

Antibiotic Treatment: General Guidelines

All patients with cerebral brain abscesses require antibiotic treatment (see Table 4.5). The antibiotics used must have activity against suspected pathogens or those related to an identified source of infection. For example, if there is a history of intravenous drug abuse, coverage must include an antistaphylococcal antibiotic such as nafcillin. If there is reason to suspect methicillin-resistant staphylococci as the source of infection, vancomycin should be used. Antibiotic selection is even more critical when attributable risk factors are absent. Because brain abscesses that arise from rhinogenic, otogenic, odontogenic, pulmonary, and cryptogenic sources are often infected with anaerobic bacteria, combination therapy must ensure adequate coverage of anaerobes. This has been accomplished classically with combinations of penicillin G and chloramphenicol, with the latter drug having been replaced successfully by metronidazole in the past 20 years. When an otogenic source is implicated or suspected, a third-generation cephalosporin (e.g., ceftriaxone, ceftazidime, ceftizoxime, cefotaxime) should be included in the treatment regimen, because Enterobacteriaceae and Pseudomonas may be present. When comorbid immunosuppressive conditions are known to exist (e.g., chronic renal failure, corticosteroid therapy, or diabetes), the physicians treating the case must, in consultation with an infectious diseases physician, either rule out or empirically direct antimicrobial therapy against Listeria, Nocardia, Aspergillus, and Candida. This is especially true in the setting of functional or absolute neutropenia (18). Abscesses that arise from trauma or neurosurgery are empirically treated with nafcillin or vancomycin in combination with a third-generation cephalosporin; however, ceftazidime, which has better antipseudomonal activity, is often reserved for treating postoperative abscesses. Despite extensive, successful experience with empirical treatment of brain abscesses, the identification of organisms within the abscess cavity should be sought. Mathisen and Johnson (10) and Tunkel et al. (11) have summarized empirical treatment guidelines for brain abscesses, which have been modified in Table 4.5. Definitive or empirical treatment of nocardial, fungal, and my-cobacterial brain abscesses is discussed in detail in other sources (10,11,55).

Surgical Treatment and Aspiration

Although antibiotics are critical in the treatment of brain abscesses, surgical intervention is usually necessary. For this reason, prompt neurosurgical consultation and evaluation are essential. Before modern imaging techniques were available, open craniotomy and the excision of an abscess provided contents for definitive culture. This approach was successful for most patients, especially when the abscess was solitary and located peripherally (5). Today, most authors suggest an open procedure for patients with either grade C (obtunded) or grade D (comatose) neurological status, both of which have been associated with mortality rates that range from 20% to 100% (2,3,4,6,29,38). Similarly, a poor neurological status has been associated with a 30% mortality rate in children and infants with brain abscess (7). Indeed, rapidity of disease progression and the patient's mental status on admission are predictive of high mortality (37). Additionally, old age or a pulmonary source for a brain abscess seems to increase mortality (3). Certainly, the decision to perform open craniotomy must take into consideration any comorbid conditions that may increase operative mortality (56).

Less invasive, CT-guided aspiration of single peripheral abscesses has been successful (39,45,57). Precise stereotactic aspiration has been used with success for peripheral lesions but is reserved more often for deep lesions of the brain stem or cerebellum in stable patients with either grade A (normal) or grade B (lethargic) neurological status (1,10,45). It should be stressed that, regardless of the surgical technique chosen, abscess contents or tissue must be obtained and sent promptly to the laboratory for Gram and fungal stains and for aerobic, anaerobic, and fungal cultures. Additional cultures for my-cobacteria also should be considered in consultation with an infectious diseases specialist.

The availability of modern CT and MRI techniques has revolutionized the surgical treatment of brain abscesses (43,45). Mampalam and Rosenblum (45) reported a reduction in mortality from 41% in the pre-CT era (before 1970–1974) to 4% in the post-CT era. In a prospective study of multiple abscesses from 1976 to 1992, Mamelak et al. (1) compared stereotactic aspiration with craniotomy. Stereotactic aspiration was the treatment of choice for patients after 1984 except for lesions that were located in the posterior fossa or those that were superficial, well matured, and excisable. In seven patients evaluated and treated with aspiration alone, no difference in outcome was found for stereotactic aspiration versus open craniotomy (1). However, this is not the case for the treatment of nocardial brain abscesses, which may require evacuation through a craniotomy (55). Other studies have advocated placement of catheters for repeated aspiration and instillation of antibiotics (39); however, this approach has not been used widely. The literature supports the efficacy of stereotactic aspiration (when available) for brain abscesses, and a recent review reported that only 14 of 102 patients treated in this manner had moderate neurological disability after the procedure (45). This outcome is similar to that for patients undergoing craniotomy and emphasizes the failure of any study to have demonstrated a surgical procedure of choice for brain abscess. When resources for advanced neuroradiographic intervention have been unavailable, open procedures (e.g., craniotomy, the classic free-hand burr-hole approach) have been used with success (4,29).

Antibiotics Alone

Although abscesses are traditionally thought to require drainage for cure, some clinicians have noted successful treatment of these lesions with antibiotics alone. Antibiotics alone can be considered for the treatment of an abscess if the patient is of grade A or B neurological status at the time of clinical suspicion or diagnosis. The efficacy of antibiotic treatment alone may rely on improved antibiotic penetration during the cerebritis stage of an abscess, emphasizing the importance of early diagnosis. Additionally, most studies show that the success of antibiotic therapy is dictated by abscess size: Small abscesses (<2.0–2.5 cm), even when numerous, have been treated successfully with antibiotics alone (23,48). The success of this approach, however, depends on careful antibiotic selection and close clinical monitoring. Boom and Tuazon (23) reported successful treatment of multiple mature brain abscesses with antibiotics alone. The duration of therapy was individualized , varying from 2.5 to 48.0 months, with the longest period required for a patient with *Nocardia asteroides*. Rosenblum et al. (56) reported similar results, with antibiotics alone being curative in six of eight patients considered as candidates for nonsurgical treatment; however, failures of antibiotic therapy also have been reported (30,37). The success of antibiotic therapy alone as the primary modality for treating a brain abscess rests on close clinical monitoring of the patient and repeat CT or MRI scans at weekly or biweekly intervals until a definitive response is seen (1,43,45).

Because abscesses tend to shrink in size by the second or third week of treatment, patients with lesions that do not improve should be considered for prompt surgical treatment (30,45,56). Patients who develop new lesions or show declining mental status with antibiotic therapy alone also should be treated surgically. A change in these patients' antibiotic regimens should be considered in close consultation with an infectious diseases specialist. The duration of antibiotic therapy is dictated primarily by clinical improvement, but most studies support at least 6 weeks of parenteral therapy, followed by oral therapy for an additional 2 to 4 weeks (9,10,40). Some authors suggest that antibiotic treatment alone requires a prolonged course of at least 12 weeks, but such choices must be individualized to each patient on the basis of clinical and radiographic findings. Despite extensive experience with empirical treatment, identifying organisms within the abscess cavity or from distant sites should be pursued diligently, and therapy should be directed toward the most likely pathogens (*see* Table 4.5), especially in immunocompromised patients. Definitive or empirical treatment of nocardial, listerial, fungal, and mycobacterial brain abscesses is discussed in detail in other sources (10,11,55).

Supportive Therapy and Outcome

Corticosteroids have been used to reduce cerebral edema associated with brain abscess. However, there is some controversy about whether corticosteroids impair immune defenses and antibiotic efficacy. Although the role of corticosteroids has not been studied systematically, most authors recommend weaning the patient from steroids when his or her edema has resolved.

As prophylaxis against seizure in patients with brain abscesses, most clinicians administer anticonvulsants during the treatment phase and wean the patient from the drugs when the abscess has resolved completely (10). These decisions are best made in consultation with a neurologist or neurosurgeon. A variety of neurological deficits have been reported in cases of brain abscess, encompassing a spectrum of disabilities including hemiparesis, aphasia, blindness, and weakness. In most series that we have studied, the incidence of neurological deficits has been highly variable, has borne no relationship to abscess multiplicity, and has ranged from 0% to 20% among the patients reported.

Summary

Although pyogenic brain abscesses are relatively infrequent, the clinician should maintain a high index of suspicion for their existence when confronted with suggestive clinical signs and symptoms. With advances in stereotactic aspiration and surgery, craniotomy may be avoided without increasing mortality, even in cases of multiple abscesses. However, craniotomy remains a time-honored surgical modality that should be considered particularly for large, single, peripheral abscesses (e.g., cortical lesions). In all cases, efforts to identify pathogens should be diligent even in the face of culture-negative aspirates (15%–20%), and antibiotic therapy should be tailored appropriately to the findings. Duration of therapy is highly variable and is dictated by the patient's clinical status, the etiologic organism's antibiotic sensitivity, adverse antibiotic effects, and resolution of lesions on radiographic images. Therapy generally requires at least 8 to 12 weeks for best outcomes. The treatment of patients with pyogenic brain abscess is highly individualized and critically dependent on dialogue among the primary care physician, neurosurgeon, radiologist, and infectious disease specialist.

REFERENCES

1. **Mamelak AN, Mampalam TJ, Obana WG, Rosenblum ML.** Improved management of multiple brain abscesses: a combined surgical and medical approach. *Neurosurgery*. 1995;36:76–86.

2. **Brewer NS, MacCarty CS, Wellman WE.** Brain abscess: a review of recent experience. *Ann Intern Med.* 1975;82:571–6.

3. **Chun C-H, Johnson JD, Hofstetter M, Raff RJ.** Brain abscess: a study of 45 consecutive cases. *Medicine.* 1986;65:415–31.

4. **Garfield J.** Management of supratentorial intracranial abscess: a review of 200 cases. *BMJ.* 1969;2:7–11.

5. **Ng PY, Seow WT, Ong PL.** Brain abscesses: review of 30 cases treated with surgery. *Aust NZ J Surg.* 1995;65:664–6.

6. **Yang S, Zhao C.** Review of 140 patients with brain abscess. *Surg Neurol.* 1993; 39:290–6.

7. **Saez-Llorens XJ, Umana MA, Odio CM, et al.** Brain abscess in infants and children. *Pediatr Infect Dis.* 1989;8:449–58.

8. **Takeshita M, Kagawa M, Yato S, et al.** Current treatment of brain abscess in patients with congenital cyanotic heart disease. *Neurosurgery.* 1997;412:1270–9.

9. **Heilpern KL, Lorber B.** Focal intracranial infections. *Infect Dis Clin North Am.* 1996;10:879–898.

10. **Mathisen GE, Johnson JP.** Brain abscess. *Clin Infect Dis.* 1997;25:763–81.

11. **Tunkel AR, Wispelwey B, Scheld WM.** Brain abscess. In Mandell GL, Bennett, Dolin R (eds). *Mandell, Douglas, and Bennett's Principles and Practice of Infectious Diseases, 5th Ed.* New York: Churchill Livingstone; 1999:1014–23.

12. **Britt RH, Enzmann DR.** Clinical stages of human brain abscesses on serial CT scans after contrast infusion. *J Neurosurg.* 1983;59:972–89.

13. **Britt RH, Enzmann DR, Yeager AS.** Neuropathological and computerized tomographic findings in experimental brain abscess. *J Neurosurg.* 1981;55:590–603.

14. **Haimes AB, Zimmerman, RD, Morgello S, et al.** MR imaging of brain abscesses. *Am J Roentgenol.* 1989;152:1073–85.

15. **Cheng Y-T, Huang C-T, Leu HS, et al.** Central nervous system infection due to *Clostridium septicum*: a case report and review of the literature. *Infection.* 1997;25:171–4.

16. **Green M, Wald ER, Tzakis A, et al.** Aspergillosis of the CNS in a pediatric liver transplant recipient: case report and review. *Rev Infect Dis.* 1991;13:653–7.

17. **Gupta SK, Manjunath-Prasad KS, Sharma BS, et al.** Brain abscess in renal transplant recipients: report of three cases. *Surg Neurol.* 1997;48:284–7.

18. **Hagensee ME, Bauwens JE, Kjos B, Bowden RA.** Brain abscess following marrow transplantation: experience at the Fred Hutchinson Cancer Research Center, 1984–1992. *Clin Infect Dis.* 1994;19:402–8.

19. **Maniglia RJ, Roth T, Blumberg EA.** Polymicrobial brain abscess in a patient infected with human immunodeficiency virus. *Clin Infect Dis.* 1997;24:449–51.

20. **Banuelos AF, Williams PL, Johnson RH, et al.** Central nervous system abscesses due to *Coccidioides* species. *Clin Infect Dis.* 1996;22:240–50.

21. **Guvenc H, Kocabay K, Okten A, Bektas S.** Brucellosis in a child complicated with multiple brain abscesses. *Scand J Infect Dis.* 1989;21:333–6.

22. **Monno L, Carbonara S, Costa D, et al.** Cerebral lesions in two patients with AIDS: the possible role of *Mycobacterium kansasii. Clin Infect Dis.* 1996;22:1130–1.

23. **Boom WH, Tuazon CU.** Successful treatment of multiple brain abscesses with antibiotics alone. *Rev Infect Dis.* 1985;7:189–99.

24. **Dykhuizen RS, Douglas G, Weir J, Gould IM.** *Corynebacterium afermentans* subsp. *lipophilum:* multiple abscess formation in brain and liver. *Scand J Infect Dis.* 1995;27:637–9.

25. **Vohra P, Burroughs MH, Hodes DS, et al.** Disseminated nocardiosis complicating medical therapy in Crohn's disease. *J Pediatr Gastroenterol Nutr.* 1997;25:233–5.

26. **Bert F, Ouahes O, Lambert-Zechovsky N.** Brain abscess due to *Bacillus macerans* following a penetrating periorbital injury. *J Clin Microbiol.* 1995;33:1950–3.

27. **Wohl TA, Kattah JC, Kolsky MP, et al.** Hemianopsia from occipital lobe abscess after dental care. *Am J Ophthalmol.* 1991;112:689–94.

28. **Yen P-T, Chan S-T, Huang T-S.** Brain abscess: with special reference to otolaryngologic sources of infection. *Otolaryngol Head Neck Surg.* 1995;113:15–22.

29. **Jefferson AA, Keogh AJ.** Intracranial abscesses: a review of treated patients over 20 years. *Q J Med.* 1977;46:389–400.

30. **Shahzadi S, Lozano AM, Bernstein M, et al.** Stereotactic management of bacterial brain abscesses. *Can J Neurol Sci.* 1996;23:34–9.

31. **Sharma BS, Khosla VK, Kak VK, et al.** Multiple pyogenic brain abscesses. *Acta Neurochir.* 1995;133:36–43.

32. **Kubaska SM, Chew FS.** Brain abscess in hereditary hemorrhagic telangiectasia. *Am J Roentgenol.* 1997;169:240–4.

33. **Momma F, Ohara S, Ohyama T, et al.** Brain abscess associated with congenital pulmonary arteriovenous fistula. *Surg Neurol.* 1990;34:439–41.

34. **Kum N, Charles D.** Cerebral abscess associated with an intrauterine contraceptive device. *Obstet Gynecol.* 1979;52:375–8.

35. **Braun TI, Kerson LA, Eisenberg FP.** Nocardial brain abscess in a pregnant woman. *Rev Infect Dis.* 1991;13:630–2.

36. **Powers JH, Scheld WM.** Fever in neurologic diseases. *Infect Dis Clin North Am.* 1996;10:45–66.

37. **Seydoux, C, Francioli P.** Bacterial brain abscesses: factors influencing mortality and sequelae. *Clin Infect Dis.* 1992;15:394–401.

38. **Zeidman SM, Geisler FH, Olivi A.** Intraventricular rupture of a purulent brain abscess: case report. *Neurosurgery.* 1995;36:189–93.

39. **Hasdemir MG, Ebeling U.** CT-guided stereotactic aspiration and treatment of brain abscesses: an experience with 24 cases. *Acta Neurochir.* 1993;125:58–63.

40. **Walot I, Miller BL, Chang L, Mehringer CM.** Neuroimaging findings in patients with AIDS. *Clin Infect Dis.* 1996;22:906–19.

41. **Nassar SI, Haddad FS, Hanbali FS, Kanaan NV.** Abscess superimposed on brain tumor: two case reports and review of the literature. *Surg Neurol.* 1997;47:484–8.

42. **Ng WP, Lozano A.** Abscess within a brain metastasis. *Can J Neurol Sci.* 1996;23: 300–2.

43. **Dyste GN, Hitchon PW, Menezes AH, et al.** Stereotaxic surgery in the treatment of multiple brain abscesses. *J Neurosurg.* 1988;69:188–94.

44. **Grigoriadis E, Gold WL.** Pyogenic brain abscess caused by *Streptococcus pneumoniae*: case report and review. *Clin Infect Dis.* 1997;25:1108–12.

45. **Mampalam TJ, Rosenblum ML.** Trends in the management of bacterial brain abscesses: a review of 102 cases of 17 years. *Neurosurgery.* 1988;23:451–8.

46. **Jamjoom AB.** Short course of antimicrobial therapy in intracranial abscess. *Acta Neurochir.* 1996;138:835–9.

47. **Black P, Graybill JR, Charache P.** Penetration of brain abscess by systemically administered antibiotics. *J Neurosurg.* 1973;38:705–9.

48. **De Louvois J, Gortvai P, Hurley R.** Antibiotic treatment of abscesses of the central nervous system. *BMJ.* 1977;2:985–7.

49. **Green HT, O'Donoghue MAT, Shaw MDM, Dowling C.** Penetration of ceftazidime into intracranial abscess. *J Antimicrob Chemother.* 1989;24:431–6.

50. **Levy RM, Gutin PH, Baskin DS, Pons VG.** Vancomycin penetration of a brain abscess: case report and review of the literature. *Neurosurgery.* 1986;18:632–6.

51. **Sjolin J, Eriksson N, Arneborn P, Cars O.** Penetration of cefotaxime and desacetyl-cefotaxime into brain abscesses in humans. *Antimicrob Agents Chemother.* 1991;35: 2606–10.

52. **Sjolin J, Lilja A, Eriksson N, et al.** Treatment of brain abscesses with cefotaxime and metronidazole: prospective study of 15 consecutive patients. *Clin Infect Dis.* 1993;17: 857–63.

53. **Yamamoto M, Jimbo M, Ide M, et al.** Penetration of intravenous antibiotics into brain abscesses. *Neurosurgery.* 1993;33:44–9.

54. **Meis JFGM, Groot-Loonen J, Hoogkamp-Korstsanje JAA.** A brain abscess due to multiply-resistant *Enterobacter cloacae* successfully treated with meropenem. *Clin Infect Dis.* 1995;20:1567.

55. **Mamelak AN, Obana WG, Flaherty JF, Rosenblum ML.** Nocardial brain abscess: treatment strategies and factors influencing outcome. *Neurosurgery.* 1994;35:622–34.

56. **Rosenblum ML, Hoff JT, Norman D, et al.** Nonoperative treatment of brain abscesses in selected high-risk patients. *J Neurosurg.* 1980;52:217–25.

57. **Chacko AG, Chandy MJ.** Diagnostic and staged stereotactic aspiration of multiple bihemispheric pyogenic brain abscesses. *Surg Neurol.* 1997;48:278–83.

5

Endocarditis

Chatrchai Watanakunakorn, MD†

Definition

Infective endocarditis is a disease that results from infection primarily of the valvular endocardium and occasionally of the mural endocardium. This disease may have clinical manifestations in all organ systems and may vary clinically from an indolent chronic illness to an acute, rapidly fatal, catastrophic event. A high degree of clinical suspicion is needed for diagnosis (1–8).

Epidemiology

The prevalence of endocarditis is approximately 1.7 to 4.2 cases per 100,000 population or 0.32 to 1.30 per 1000 hospital admissions in the United States (1,9). Although it can occur at any age, endocarditis tends to occur more frequently in older individuals (1,2). This may be due in part to the large population of older individuals who have underlying conditions. However, endocarditis is prevalent among young people who habitually use nonsterile intravenous drugs (i.e., those who practice "mainlining") (10). Endocarditis is also increasingly a disease of medical progress (11). It occurs in patients with prosthetic heart valves or indwelling intravascular catheters during hospitalization and in those who have received parenteral nutrition or have undergone invasive cardiac procedures (1–3,5,7,8,10,12).

†Deceased.

Pathogenesis

Trauma to the endocardial endothelium is probably the most common pathogenic mechanism for infective endocarditis. Three hemodynamic characteristics have been implicated as predisposing to endothelial trauma: regurgitant blood flow, the presence of high-pressure gradients, and a narrow orifice (13). Cardiac abnormalities marked by these characteristics, such as aortic stenosis or ventricular septal defect, are associated with a high incidence of infective endocarditis. In contrast, structural abnormalities that lack these characteristics, such as an ostium secundum atrial septal defect, do not predispose to endocarditis. Except among the population of intravenous drug abusers, the prevalence of endocarditis of the right side of the heart (where there is low pressure) is very low.

Trauma to the endothelium triggers the local deposition of platelets and fibrin, forming a sterile thrombotic endocardial lesion or vegetation. If bacteremia or fungemia occurs even transiently at the time of the formation of this sterile vegetation, the involved microorganisms may adhere to the surface of the vegetation. Because of the absence of a local host-defense mechanism at the vegetation site, the microorganisms multiply and more platelets and fibrin deposit onto the vegetation. In the absence of therapeutic intervention, this cycle continues, resulting in an ever-larger vegetation that consists of platelets, fibrin, and colonies of microorganisms.

Certain microorganisms adhere to the altered valvular surface better than others. The best-characterized mechanism of adherence of microorganisms to a sterile thrombotic endocardial lesion is through the extracellular polysaccharides synthesized by certain bacteria, such as the dextran produced by *Streptococcus mutans*. There is also experimental evidence that the *in vitro* binding of *Staphylococcus aureus*, group A streptococci, and *S. viridans* to epithelial cells is augmented by the presence of fibronectin, a plasma glycoprotein that is also a major surface constituent of mammalian cells. However, certain host-defense mechanisms, such as the bactericidal activity of serum complement, protect against endocardial infection. It is known that gram-negative enteric bacilli such as *Escherichia coli*, which are usually serum sensitive, seldom cause infective endocarditis. In one of the rare instances of *E. coli* endocarditis, it was determined that the infective strain of the organism was serum resistant (14).

The pathogenetic mechanism by which organisms such as *S. aureus* cause acute bacterial endocarditis that affects a previously normal heart valve remains unknown. It has been postulated that the endothelial cells of the cardiac valves have specific receptors for *S. aureus* (15). The reason for the high prevalence of tricuspid valve endocarditis among intravenous drug abusers remains speculative. Trauma to the endothelium, by repeated insult with impure substances injected intravenously, may be one mechanism responsible for such disease.

Pathophysiology

Infective endocarditis is a systemic disease. Emboli from the infective vegetation may circulate to every organ system in the body (especially the lungs when the vegetations are at the right side of the heart), resulting in septic infarcts or abscesses. Large arterial emboli are known to occur with certain organisms, such as *Candida, Aspergillus, Haemophilus,* and group B streptococci (16).

With progression of the infective vegetations of endocarditis, the host produces an IgM antibody directed against IgG commonly known as *rheumatoid factor*. Immune complexes that involve the two antibodies are then formed and deposited in certain organ systems, creating an autoimmune phenomenon that can clinically manifest as a variety of disorders, including glomerulonephritis, arthritis, or arthralgia.

Infecting Organisms

Staphylococci, streptococci, and enterococci are the major microorganisms responsible for infective endocarditis; however, many other microorganisms may cause the disease under the appropriate circumstances. Table 5.1 lists the important microorganisms that cause endocarditis in different clinical settings.

The major infecting organisms in subacute bacterial endocarditis (SBE) are non–beta-hemolytic streptococci (also known as *viridans* groups of streptococci), which include many species (e.g., *Streptococcus sanguis, S. mitis, S. salivarius, S. intermedius*) (1,17,18). *S. bovis* is an important cause of endocarditis and is known to be associated with colonic pathologies such as carcinoma or villous adenoma (19,20). Enterococci (especially *Enterococcus faecalis*, a well-known cause of endocarditis in elderly men and women of childbearing age) have now been associated with hospital-acquired endocarditis (1,7,21,22). The HACEK microorganisms (*Haemophilus aphrophilus, Actinobacillus actinomycetamcomitans, Cardiobacterium hominis, Eikenella corrodens,* and *Kingella kingae*, a group of fastidious gram-negative bacilli that are part of the normal flora of the oral cavity) are also capable of causing endocarditis (1,23). Prolonged incubation is usually required for growth of these microorganisms in blood culture. Occasionally, endocarditis caused by *Staphylococcus aureus* may run an indolent course. *S. epidermidis* may cause SBE of a native valve (24).

S. aureus is the most important cause of acute endocarditis, and the prevalence of endocarditis caused by this organism has increased markedly in recent years (1,2,8). *S. aureus* is a major cause of hospital-acquired endocarditis, especially in cases associated with infected intravascular catheters (1–3,5,7,8,25). Additionally, beta-hemolytic streptococci of groups A, B, C,

Table 5.1 Microorganisms That Cause Endocarditis in Different Clinical Settings

Subacute Endocarditis (Indolent Course)

Viridans streptococci (*S. mitis, S. salivarius, S. sanguis, S. intermedius*, etc.)*
Group D streptococcus (*Streptococcus bovis*)*
Enterococcus (*E. faecalis, E. faecium, E. durans, E. avium*)*
Haemophilus (*H. aphrophilus, H. paraphrophilus*)
Actinobacillus actinomycetamcomitans
Cardiobacterium hominis
Eikenella corrodens
Kingella kingae
Staphylococcus epidermidis
Staphylococcus aureus

Acute Endocarditis (Aggressive Course)

Staphylococcus aureus*
Group A, B, C, G streptococci
Haemophilus (*H. parainfluenzae, H. influenzae*)
Streptococcus pneumoniae
Staphylococcus lugdunensis
Enterococcus (*E. faecalis, E. faecium, E. avium, E. durans*)
Neisseria (*N. gonorrhea, N. mucosa*)

Endocarditis in Intravenous Drug Abusers

Staphylococcus aureus*
Streptococcus group A
Pseudomonas aeruginosa
Enterococcus faecalis
Burkholderia cepacia
Candida species
Polymicrobial

Prosthetic Valve Endocarditis

Staphylococcus epidermidis*
Staphylococcus aureus
Candida species
Gram-negative bacilli
Viridans streptococci
Enterococcus faecalis
Aspergillus species

Some Unusual Causes of Native Valve Endocarditis

Bartonella (*B. quintana, B. henselae*)
Gram-negative bacilli
Brucella species
Coxiella burnetii
Chlamydia species
Legionella pneumophila
Mycobacterium species
Opportunistic fungi

* Most common microorganism(s).

and G increasingly have been reported as causes of acute endocarditis (1,16,26–29). Recently, *S. lugdunensis*, a coagulase-negative species, has been reported to cause endocarditis with an acute destructive clinical course (25,30). *Bartonella* species have been reported to be the etiologic agents in some cases of culture-negative endocarditis, with *Bartonella henselae* found in individuals who own kittens and *B. quintana* found in homeless people (31–33). *Streptococcus pneumoniae* and *Neisseria* species are rare causes of endocarditis. Enterococcal endocarditis occasionally presents with an acute clinical course.

Staphylococcus aureus is by far the most common cause of endocarditis in intravenous drug abusers, in whom it often infects the tricuspid valve (10). Group A streptococci, *Pseudomonas aeruginosa*, *Candida* species, and other microorganisms also can cause endocarditis in this population.

Prosthetic valve endocarditis (PVE) traditionally is divided into early and late disease based on its occurrence before or after 60 postoperative days, respectively. All bacteria, fungi, and other microorganisms are capable of causing PVE; however, coagulase-negative staphylococci are the most important causes of both early and late PVE, *S. aureus* causes more cases of early PVE, and streptococci cause more cases of late PVE (12). *Candida* species and various gram-negative bacilli are also important causes of PVE.

Beyond those discussed here, some of the many other microorganisms that can cause endocarditis of native valves are listed in Table 5.1.

Clinical Manifestations

Although the terms *acute endocarditis* and *subacute endocarditis* have fallen into disfavor in recent years (some physicians have instead used the terms *endocarditis of aggressive course* and *endocarditis of indolent course*), these remain useful in describing the clinical presentation of patients with infective endocarditis. The onset of illness in acute endocarditis is usually within 1 week of infection. High fever is a common feature but, in older patients, confusion with or without fever may be the presenting symptom. These patients often appear acutely ill. The cause of their endocarditis is usually a more virulent organism (*see* Table 5.1). On the other hand, patients with subacute endocarditis typically have been ill for a longer period; they often appear chronically ill and may not recall the exact onset of their illness. Malaise, low-grade fever, and night sweats may continue for weeks or even months before the patient seeks medical attention. The infecting organism in such cases is usually less virulent than in acute endocarditis (*see* Table 5.1).

Fever is an important symptom of infective endocarditis, but the patient may not notice a low-grade fever. There is no characteristic fever pattern in infective endocarditis, although fever usually occurs in the evening or at night. In some cases, and especially in patients with PVE, fever may be the only symptom of infective endocarditis. There may be a chilly sensation and perspiration, especially at night. Polyarthralgia is not uncommon, and acute rheumatic fever must be part of the differential diagnosis. Pyarthrosis may be the presenting event in acute endocarditis. Other presenting complaints of endocarditis include musculoskeletal symptoms, such as joint pain, back pain, and shoulder pain from diffuse or localized myalgia. Severe back pain is an important symptom at clinical presentation (1,2). Some patients may recall transient pain at the tip of a finger or toe, representing the expression of an Osler's node (i.e., a transient, painful erythematous nodule that may occur on the tip of a finger or toe or on the foot) (34).

Infective endocarditis is a systemic disease, and affected individuals may present with diverse clinical manifestations.

- **Headache and stiff neck:** may be due to metastatic infection to the brain, meninges, or both.
- **Cerebral emboli or a ruptured mycotic aneurysm:** may account for the clinical presentation of a cerebrovascular accident.
- **Complaints of a cold extremity:** from embolization to a major artery
- **Numbness:** from nerve compression by an adjacent mycotic aneurysm or embolization to vasonervorum
- **Gross hematuria from emboli to the kidneys or immune complex disease:** may be a presenting symptom
- **Acute chest pain:** from myocardial infarction caused by coronary embolization
- **Symptoms of congestive heart failure (CHF):** from a severely damaged heart valve
- **Fever, pleuritic chest pain, cough, and dyspnea resulting from septic pulmonary infarction:** prominent presenting symptoms of tricuspid valve endocarditis in intravenous drug abusers

Physical findings

Patients with subacute endocarditis may exhibit pallor. Petechiae, especially on the palpebral conjunctiva, buccal mucosa, or on the skin of the trunk may be a useful clue to the disease. Rarely, the skin may show purpura caused by disseminated intravascular coagulation. Osler's nodes (34), Janeway lesions (painless erythematous lesions, usually of the palms of hands or soles of the feet), or Roth's spots (round or oval, white-centered hemorrhagic spots in the retina) may be present in some patients. Clubbing of fingers is now a rare finding in endocarditis, and splinter hemorrhages of the nails are a nonspecific finding.

Signs of CHF may be found in patients with severe valvular regurgitation caused by a vegetation or by the acute rupture of valve cusps, valve leaflets, chordae tendineae, or papillary muscles; if so, murmurs of valvular regurgitation should be obvious. Other types of cardiac murmur also may be present. Patients who have acute endocarditis that affects a previously normal valve, mural endocarditis, or right-sided endocarditis may not have a murmur. The murmur of tricuspid valve endocarditis is usually a systolic ejection murmur when it first develops. The typical holosystolic murmur of tricuspid regurgitation does not appear until late in the course of the illness. A change in the quality of a preexisting murmur is infrequent. In older patients who have arteriosclerotic heart disease, there is often no change in an existing systolic ejection murmur when a valve first becomes infected. Cardiac arrhythmia may occur in patients with myocardial infarction resulting from coronary embolization, abscesses involving the conduction system, or severe CHF. A pericardial friction rub is uncommon in infective endocarditis and may be indicate purulent pericarditis caused by the rupture of a myocardial abscess or a valvering abscess into the epicardium.

A palpable spleen may occur in subacute endocarditis but is not encountered in patients with acute endocarditis. In subacute endocarditis, the spleen is usually firm and nontender and seldom extends more than two finger-breadths below the costal margin. Patients with acute or subacute endocarditis also may present with acute left upper quadrant pain from a splenic infarct (1). Spleen tenderness may result from a splenic abscess caused by a septic infarct. Muscle tenderness in the lumbar region is present in patients with severe back pain.

Laboratory Findings

The leukocyte count in subacute endocarditis is normal, whereas acute endocarditis usually is accompanied by polymorphonuclear leukocytosis. A moderate normocytic anemia is common in subacute endocarditis, with the hemoglobin level usually not less than 9 g/dL. If severe anemia is present, an alternate diagnosis should be considered. Anemia is rare in acute endocarditis. The erythrocyte sedimentation rate is always increased and may remain so for several weeks after successful therapy of endocarditis.

Urinalysis may reveal erythrocytes in patients with endocarditis, and occasionally there may be gross hematuria. Mild proteinuria is a common finding. Rheumatoid factor may be present in subacute endocarditis, especially in patients who have had symptoms for more than 6 weeks. Hyperbilirubinemia may occur in patients who are acutely ill with acute staphylococcal endocarditis (35).

Both two-dimensional transthoracic and transesophageal echocardiography—the latter being the preferred method—have been used as adjuncts in the diagnosis of infective endocarditis. A positive finding in either examination may be helpful, but a negative finding does not exclude endocarditis.

Table 5.2 Duke Criteria for Diagnosis of Infective Endocarditis*

Major Criteria

A. Positive blood culture for infective endocarditis

1. Typical microorganism for infective endocarditis from two separate blood cultures:

a. Viridans streptococci[†], *Streptococcus bovis*, or HACEK group, *or*

b. Community-acquired *Staphylococcus aureus* or enterococci in the absence of a primary focus, *or*

2. Persistently positive blood culture—defined as recovery of a microorganism consistent with infective endocarditis from:

a. Blood cultures drawn more than 12 hours apart, *or*

b. All of three or a majority of four or more separate blood cultures, with the first and last ones drawn at least 1 hour apart

B. Evidence of endocardial involvement

1. Positive echocardiogram for infective endocarditis

a. Oscillating intracardiac mass on valve, on supporting structures, in the path of regurgitant jets, on implanted material, or in the absence of an alternative anatomic explanation, *or*

b. Abscess, *or*

c. New or partial dehiscence of prosthetic valve, *or*

2. New valvular regurgitation (an increase or change in preexisting murmur is not sufficient)

Minor criteria

A. Predisposition: predisposing heart condition or intravenous drug use

B. Fever ≥38.0°C (100.4°F)

C. Vascular phenomena: major arterial emboli, septic pulmonary infarcts, mycotic aneurysm, intracranial hemorrhage, conjunctival hemorrhage, or Janeway lesions

D. Immunologic phenomena: glomerulonephritis, Osler's nodes, Roth's spots, or rheumatoid factor

E. Microbiological evidence: positive blood culture, but not meeting major criterion as noted previously[‡] or serologic evidence of active infection with organism consistent with infective endocarditis

F. Echocardiogram: consistent with infective endocarditis, but not meeting major criterion as previous noted

HACEK = *Haemophilus* species, *Actinobacillus actinomycetamcomitans*, *Cardiobacterium hominis*, *Eikenella* species, *Kingella kingae*

* Requirements for the diagnosis of infective endocarditis: two major criteria, one major and three minor criteria, or five minor criteria.

† Including nutritional variant strains

‡ Excluding single positive cultures for coagulase-negative staphylococci and organisms that do not cause endocarditis

Adapted from Durack DT, Lukes AS, Bright DK, and the Duke Endocarditis Service. New criteria for diagnosis of infective endocarditis: utilization of specific echocardiographic findings. *Am J Med.* 1994;96:200-9.

Blood Culture

Blood culture is the most important laboratory procedure in the diagnosis of infective endocarditis. The hallmark of bacterial endocarditis is the constant shed-

Table 5.3 Treatment Regimens for Infective Endocarditis

Infecting Organism	Regimen	Comments
Viridans groups of streptococci, *Streptococcus bovis*	1. Penicillin 2–3 MU IV q4h for 2 wk + gentamicin 1 mg/kg IV q8h for 2 wk 2. Same as regimen 1 except that penicillin is given for 4 wk (6 wk for PVE endocarditis) 3. Penicillin 2–3 MU IV q4h for 4 wk 4. Ceftriaxone 2 g IV qd for 4 wk 5. Vancomycin 15 mg/kg (max 1 g) IV q12h for 4 wk	1. For patients aged ≥65 years without renal dysfunction, CN VIII defects, or serious complications 2. For patients with complicated disease (e.g. shock, CNS involvement, penicillin MIC > 0.1 µg/mL, PVE) 3. For patients aged ≥65 years with renal dysfunction or CN VIII defects 4. For patients with non–IgE-mediated penicillin allergy or on outpatient therapy 5. For patients with IgE-mediated penicillin allergy
Enterococcus species	1. Penicillin 3–5 MU IV q4h for 4–6 wk + gentamicin 1 mg/kg IV q8h for 4–6 wk 2. Penicillin as in regimen 1 + streptomycin 7.5 mg/kg (max 500 mg) IM q12h for 4–6 wk 3. Vancomycin 15 mg/kg (max 1 g) IV q12h for 4–6 wk + gentamicin as in regimen 1 4. Vancomycin as in regimen 3 + streptomycin as in regimen 2	1. Monitor renal function and gentamicin serum levels (peak = 3 µg/mL, trough < 1 µg/mL); gentamicin MIC < 2000 µg/mL 2. Only if gentamicin MIC ≥ 2000 µg/mL and streptomycin MIC < 2000 µg/mL 3. Same as for regimen 1; for patients with penicillin allergy 4. Same as for regimen 2; for patients with penicillin allergy
Group A, B, C, and G streptococci and *Streptococcus pneumoniae*	1. Penicillin 2–3 MU IV q4h for 4 wk 2. Ceftriaxone 2 g IV qd for 4 wk 3. Vancomycin 15 mg/kg (max 1g) IV q12h for 4 wk	1. May add gentamicin 1 mg/kg IV q8h for 2 wk in seriously ill patients infected with group B streptococci 2. For patients with non–IgE-mediated penicillin allergy or on outpatient therapy 3. For patients with IgE-mediated penicillin allergy

Staphylococcus species	1. Nafcillin or oxacillin 2 g IV q4h for 6 wk	1. May add gentamicin 1 mg/kg IV q8h for 3 d in seriously ill patients
	2. Penicillin 3 MU IV every 4 h for 6 wk	2. When penicillin MIC $\leq$ 0.1 μg/mL and beta-lactamase negative; may add gentamicin as in regimen 1
	3. Vancomycin 15 mg/kg (max 1 g) IV q12h for 6 wk	3. For patients with IgE-mediated penicillin allergy or those infected with methicillin-resistant *Staphylococcus* species; may add gentamicin as in regimen 1
	4. Cefazolin 2 g IV q8h for 6 wk	4. For patients with non-IgE-mediated penicillin allergy; may add gentamicin as in regimen 1
	5. Nafcillin or oxacillin 2 g IV q4h + gentamicin 1 mg/kg IV q8h for 2 wk	5. For intravenous drug abusers with right-sided endocarditis
Staphylococcal prosthetic valve	1. Vancomycin 15 mg/kg (max 1 g) IV q12h for $\geq$6 wk + rifampin 300 mg PO q8h for $\geq$6 wk + gentamicin 1 mg/kg IV q8h for 2 wk	1. For patients with penicillin allergy or those infected with methicillin-resistant *Staphylococcus* species
	2. Nafcillin or oxacillin 2 gm IV q4h for $\geq$6 wk + rifampin and gentamicin as in regimen 1.	2. For patients infected with methicillin-susceptible *Staphylococcus* species
HACEK microorganisms	1. Ceftriaxone 2 g IV qd for 4 wk	1. Administer for 6 wk in patients with prosthetic valve endocarditis
Culture-negative endocarditis	1. Use the treatment regimens for infection with *Enterococcus* species above	1. If there is no clinical response, consider alternate diagnosis; obtain fungal blood cultures; order serology for *Chlamydia, Bartonella, Brucella,* and *Coxiella burnetii*

CN VIII = eighth cranial nerve; HACEK = *Haemophilus* species, *Actinobacillus actinomycetamcomitans, Cardiobacterium hominis, Eikenella* species, *Kingella kingae*; IgE = immunoglobulin E; IM = intramuscularly; IV = intravenously; max = maximum dose; MIC = minimum inhibitory concentration; MU = million units; PO = orally; PVE = prosthetic valve endocarditis.

Table 5.4 Indications for Surgical Intervention in Infective Endocarditis

Refractory congestive heart failure

More than one serious systemic embolic episode

Uncontrolled infection (e.g., *Pseudomonas endocarditis*)

Valve dysfunction as demonstrated by fluoroscopy or two-dimensional echocardiography

Ineffective antimicrobial therapy (e.g., fungal endocarditis)

Resection of mycotic aneurysms

Most cases of prosthetic valve endocarditis (especially in the presence of dehiscence or relapse)

Local suppurative complications, including perivalvular or myocardial abscesses with conduction system abnormalities, heart block, etc.

ding of bacteria from an infected vegetation into the systemic circulation, resulting in persistent bacteremia. Three to six blood cultures should be taken to document persistent bacteremia. In patients with clinically indolent disease, blood cultures can be taken over a period of 2 to 3 days. In patients who are acutely ill, blood cultures should be taken over a period of 2 to 3 hours before empirical antibiotic therapy is instituted. In bacterial endocarditis, the infecting organism should grow in all or most blood cultures. By contrast, blood cultures in cases of fungal endocarditis may not be positive with routine blood culture media, and special culture techniques may be needed to grow the causative organism.

Occasionally, a patient has a clinical picture that is compatible with bacterial endocarditis but also has multiple blood cultures in which there is no growth. The true incidence of such so-called *culture-negative endocarditis* is unknown but may vary from 0% to 40%. The most common reason for negative blood cultures is the administration of antibiotics before specimens for blood cultures are taken. Positive blood cultures can be obtained for most patients when antibiotics are discontinued. Fastidious organisms or organisms that require special growth factors, such as *Brucella* species, may give negative blood cultures if inadequate methods are used. Prolonged incubation may be required for fastidious organisms such as the HACEK group. In rare instances, endocarditis may be caused by *Coxiella burnetii*, *Bartonella* species, and *Chlamydia* species. These organisms do not grow in blood culture, and their identification as the source of endocarditis in such cases usually is made serologically. As mentioned earlier, fungal organisms (e.g., *Candida*, *Aspergillus*, and *Histoplasma* species) should be considered in patients with culture-negative endocarditis.

Diagnostic Criteria

The diagnosis of infective endocarditis is based on clinical and laboratory findings. A group of researchers at Duke University has proposed criteria (major and minor) for the diagnosis of infective endocarditis (Table 5.2) (36).

The typical echocardiographic finding of vegetation (preferably by trans-esophageal echocardiography) is considered a major criterion. Further experience with the Duke criteria is needed, and there probably will be refinement of these criteria (37). The Duke criteria should be considered only as a guide to the diagnosis of infective endocarditis; clinical judgment is still the most important element in making the diagnosis.

Management

In most cases, infective endocarditis is potentially curable. It is important to make the clinical diagnosis early and to identify the causative pathogen correctly so that a proper antibiotic treatment regimen can be prescribed. The antimicrobial susceptibility of clinical isolates should be determined. In general, treatment involves giving high doses of bactericidal antibiotics over a prolonged period. Usually, an antibiotic that inhibits bacterial cell wall synthesis is used and, in certain situations, an aminoglycoside is added for synergistic effect (38–42). Table 5.3 lists recommended antibiotic regimens for infective endocarditis on the basis of the infecting organisms (43).

Monitoring of Antibiotic Treatment

Blood cultures for most of the bacterial pathogens responsible for infective endocarditis show no growth after antibiotic therapy is begun. However, for some pathogens (e.g., *S. aureus*), the patient may have positive blood cultures for up to 1 week of therapy (2). In the case of endocarditis caused by *P. aeruginosa*, persistent bacteremia during therapy may necessitate surgical excision of infected vegetations.

The serum bactericidal titer is a test of the ability of the patient's serum, during antibiotic therapy, to kill a certain number of infecting organisms *in vitro*. Traditionally, it has been recommended that for optimal therapy of bacterial endocarditis, the peak serum bactericidal titer should be at least 1:8, preferably 1:16. However, no good clinical data have confirmed the validity of this recommendation. Until convincing data become available in the future, the determination of the serum bactericidal titer in patients with endocarditis is not routinely recommended (43).

Surgical Intervention

Cardiac surgery is an important adjunct in the management of infective endocarditis. When there is an indication, the infected valve should be re-

Table 5.5 Prophylaxis Recommendations for Conditions and Procedures Associated with Endocarditis

Cardiac Conditions Associated with Endocarditis

Endocarditis Prophylaxis Recommended

High-Risk Category

> Prosthetic cardiac valves, including bioprosthetic and homograft valves
>
> Previous bacterial endocarditis
>
> Complex cyanotic congenital heart disease (e.g., single-ventricle states, transposition of the great arteries, tetralogy of Fallot)
>
> Surgically constructed systemic pulmonary shunts or conduits

Moderate-Risk Category

> Most other congenital cardiac malformations (other than those mentioned in the high-risk category above and the negligible-risk category below)
>
> Acquired valvar dysfunction (e.g., rheumatic heart disease)
>
> Hypertrophic cardiomyopathy
>
> Mitral valve prolapse with valvar regurgitation and/or thickened leaflets

Endocarditis Prophylaxis Not Recommended

*Negligible-Risk Category**

> Isolated secundum atrial septal defect
>
> Surgical repair of atrial septal defect, ventricular septal defect, or patent ductus arteriosus (without residua beyond 6 mo)
>
> Previous coronary artery bypass graft surgery
>
> Mitral valve prolapse without valvar regurgitation
>
> Physiologic, functional, or innocent heart murmurs
>
> Previous Kawasaki disease without valvar dysfunction
>
> Previous rheumatic fever without valvar dysfunction
>
> Cardiac pacemakers (intravascular and epicardial) and implanted defibrillators

Dental Procedures and Endocarditis Prophylaxis

Endocarditis Prophylaxis Recommended[†]

> Dental extractions
>
> Periodontal procedures, including surgery, scaling and root planing, probing, and recall maintenance
>
> Dental implant placement and reimplantation of avulsed teeth
>
> Endodontic (root canal) instrumentation or surgery only beyond the apex
>
> Subgingival placement of antibiotic fibers or strips
>
> Initial placement of orthodontic bands (but not brackets)
>
> Intraligamentary local anesthetic injections
>
> Prophylactic cleaning of teeth or implants where bleeding is anticipated

Endocarditis Prophylaxis Not Recommended

> Restorative dentistry[‡] (operative and prosthodontic) with or without retraction cord[§]
>
> Local anesthetic injections (nonintraligamentary)
>
> Intracanal endodontic treatment (after placement and buildup)
>
> Placement of rubber dams
>
> Postoperative suture removal
>
> Placement of removable prosthodontic or orthodontic appliances
>
> Taking of oral impressions
>
> Fluoride treatments

Taking of oral radiographs
Orthodontic appliance adjustment
Shedding of primary teeth

Other Procedures and Endocarditis Prophylaxis

Endocarditis Prophylaxis Recommended

Respiratory Tract

Tonsillectomy and/or adenoidectomy
Surgical operations that involve respiratory mucosa
Bronchoscopy with a rigid bronchoscope

Gastrointestinal Tract¶

Sclerotherapy for esophageal varices
Esophageal stricture dilation
Endoscopic retrograde cholangiography with biliary obstruction
Biliary tract surgery
Surgical operations that involve intestinal mucosa

Genitourinary Tract

Prostatic surgery
Cystoscopy
Urethral dilation

Endocarditis Prophylaxis Not Recommended

Respiratory Tract

Endotracheal intubation
Bronchoscopy with a flexible bronchoscope, with or without biopsy**
Tympanostomy-tube insertion

Gastrointestinal Tract

Transesophageal echocardiography**
Endoscopy with or without gastrointestinal biopsy**

Genitourinary Tract

Vaginal hysterectomy**
Vaginal delivery**
Cesarean section
In uninfected tissue:

Urethral catheterization
Uterine dilatation and curettage
Therapeutic abortion
Sterilization procedures
Insertion or removal of intrauterine devices

Other

Cardiac catheterization, including balloon angioplasty
Implanted cardiac pacemakers, implanted defibrillators, and coronary stents
Incision or biopsy of surgically scrubbed skin
Circumcision

---

* No greater risk than the general population.
† Prophylaxis is recommended for patients with high- and moderate-risk cardiac conditions.
‡ This includes restoration of decayed teeth (filling cavities) and replacement of missing teeth.
§ Clinical judgment may indicate antibiotic use in selected circumstances that may create significant bleeding.
¶ Prophylaxis is recommended for high-risk patients; it is optional for medium-risk patients.
** Prophylaxis is optional for high-risk patients.
Adapted from Dajani AS, Taubert KA, Wilson W, et al. Prevention of bacterial endocarditis: recommendation by the American Heart Association. *JAMA.* 1997;277:1794–801.

Table 5.6 Prophylactic Regimens for Dental, Oral, Respiratory Tract, and Esophageal Procedures

Situation	Agent	Regimen
Standard general prophylaxis	Amoxicillin	2.0 g PO 1 hour before procedure
Patient unable to take oral medications	Ampicillin	2.0 g IM or IV within 30 minutes before procedure
Patient allergic to penicillin	Clindamycin	600 mg PO 1 hour before procedure
Patient allergic to penicillin and unable to take oral medications	Clindamycin	600 mg IV within 30 minutes before procedure

IM = intramuscularly; IV = intravenously; PO = orally.
Adapted from Dajani AS, Taubert KA, Wilson W, et al. Prevention of bacterial endocarditis: recommendation by the American Heart Association. *JAMA.* 1997;277:1794–801.

placed regardless of the duration for which the patient has received antibiotic therapy. It has been shown that the risk of infection of a newly implanted prosthetic valve is very low, even if there is active valvular infection at the time of surgery (provided that antibiotic therapy is continued postoperatively). Table 5.4 lists the indications for cardiac surgery in infective endocarditis (44).

Follow-Up

Relapse of endocarditis is uncommon if the patient is treated with an appropriate antibiotic regimen. However, relapse may occur, especially in medically treated PVE. After cessation of antibiotic therapy, the patient should be seen every 2 weeks for the first month and monthly for 2 more months. Blood cultures should be taken if the patient's temperature rises above 100.4°F more than once and there is no obvious reason for fever. Relapse is unlikely after 3 months.

Antimicrobial Prophylaxis

Although there is no conclusive proof that the prophylactic use of antibiotics in humans can prevent bacterial endocarditis, it is justified on theoretical and experimental grounds. The aim is to provide high serum concentrations of effective antibiotics during procedures that are associated with a high incidence of transient bacteremia in patients with cardiac and intravascular defects that are known to predispose to infection. Only one dose of appropriate antibiotics, given shortly before the performance of a high-risk procedure, is

Table 5.7 Prophylactic Regimens for Genitourinary and Gastrointestinal Procedures*

Situation	Agents	Regimen[†]
High-risk patient	Ampicillin + gentamicin	Ampicillin 2.0 g IM or IV + gentamicin 1.5 mg/kg (max 120 mg) within 30 minutes of starting procedure; 6 hours later, amoxicillin 1 g PO or ampicillin 1 g IM or IV
High-risk patient allergic to penicillin	Vancomycin + gentamicin	Vancomycin 1.0 g IV over 1–2 hours + gentamicin 1.5 mg/kg IV or IM (not to exceed 120 mg); complete injection or infusion within 30 minutes of starting procedure
Moderate-risk patient	Amoxicillin or ampicillin	Amoxicillin 2.0 g PO 1 hour before procedure or ampicillin 2.0 g IM or IV within 30 minutes of starting procedure
Moderate-risk patient allergic to penicillin	Vancomycin	Vancomycin 1.0 g IV over 1–2 hours complete infusion within 30 minutes of starting procedure

IM = intramuscularly; IV = intravenously; max = maximum dose; PO = orally.
* Excluding esophageal procedures (see Table 5.6).
† No second dose of vancomycin or gentamicin is recommended.
Adapted from Dajani AS, Taubert KA, Wilson W, et al. Prevention of bacterial endocarditis: recommendation by the American Heart Association. *JAMA*. 1997;277:1794–801.

needed. The guidelines listed in Tables 5.5, 5.6, and 5.7 are recommended by the American Heart Association (45).

REFERENCES

1. **Watanakunakorn C, Burkert T.** Infective endocarditis at a large community teaching hospital, 1980–1990: a review of 210 episodes. Medicine. 1993;72:90–102.

2. **Watanakunakorn C.** *Staphylococcus aureus* endocarditis at a community teaching hospital, 1980–1991: an analysis of 106 cases. *Arch Intern Med.* 1994;154:2330–5.

3. **Watanakunakorn C, Tan JS, Phair JP.** Some salient features of *Staphylococcus aureus* endocarditis. *Am J Med.* 1973;54:473–81.

4. **Watanakunakorn C, Tan JS.** Diagnostic difficulties of staphylococcal endocarditis in geriatric patients. *Geriatrics.* 1973;28;168–73.

5. **Watanakunakorn C, Baird IM.** *Staphylococcus aureus* bacteremia and endocarditis associated with a removable infected intravenous device. *Am J Med.* 1977;63:253–6.

6. **Espersen F, Frimodt-Moller N.** *Staphylococcus aureus* endocarditis: a review of 119 cases. *Arch Intern Med.* 1986;146:118–21.

7. **Fernandez-Guerrero ML, Verdijo C, Azofra J, et al.** Hospital-acquired infectious endocarditis not associated with cardiac surgery: an emerging problem. *Clin Infect Dis.* 1995;20:16–23.

8. **Fowler VG Jr, Li J, Corey GR, et al.** Role of echocardiography in evaluation of patients with *Staphylococcus aureus* bacteremia: experience in 103 patients. *J Am Coll Cardiol.* 1997;30:1072–8.

9. **Watanakunakorn C.** Endocarditis, infective. In Dambro MR (ed). *Griffith's 5-Minute Clinical Consult.* Baltimore: Williams & Wilkins; 1998:356–9.

10. **Watanakunakorn C.** Changing epidemiology and newer aspects of infective endocarditis. *Adv Intern Med.* 1976;22:21–47.

11. **Watanakunakorn C.** Infective endocarditis as a result of medical progress. *Am J Med.* 1978;64:917–19.

12. **Watanakunakorn C.** Prosthetic valve infective endocarditis. *Prog Cardiovasc Dis.* 1979;22:181–92.

13. **Weinstein L, Schlesinger JJ.** Pathoanatomic, pathophysiologic, and clinical correlations in endocarditis (Part 1). *N Engl J Med.* 1974;291:832–7.

14. **Watanakunakorn C, Kim J.** Mitral valve endocarditis caused by a strain of serum-resistant *Escherichia coli. Clin Infect Dis.* 1992;14:501–5.

15. **Johnson CM, Hancock GA, Goulin GD.** Specific binding of *Staphylococcus aureus* to cultured porcine cardiac valvular endothelial cells. *J Lab Clin Med* 1988;112:16–22.

16. **Gallagher PG, Watanakunakorn C.** Group B streptococcal endocarditis: report of seven cases and review of the literature, 1962–1985. *Rev Infect Dis.* 1986;8:175–88.

17. **Tan JS, Watanakunakorn C, Phair JP.** *Streptococcus viridans* endocarditis: favorable prognosis in geriatric patients. *Geriatrics.* 1973;28:68–73.

18. **Watanakunakorn C, Pantelakis J.** Alpha-hemolytic streptococcal bacteremia: a review of 203 episodes during 1980–1991. *Scand J Infect Dis.* 1993;25:403–8.

19. **Watanakunakorn C.** *Streptococcus bovis* endocarditis. *Am J Med.* 1974;56:256–60.

20. **Watanakunakorn C.** *Streptococcus bovis* endocarditis associated with villous adenoma following colonoscopy. *Am Heart J.* 1988;116:1115–16.

21. **Malone DA, Wagner RA, Myers JP, et al.** Enterococcal bacteremia in two large community teaching hospitals. *Am J Med.* 1986;81:601–6.

22. **Watanakunakorn C, Patel R.** Comparison of patients with enterococcal bacteremia due to strains with and without high-level resistance to gentamicin. *Clin Infect Dis.* 1993;17:74–8.

23. **Wilson WR, Karchmer AW, Dajani AS, et al.** Antibiotic treatment of adults with infective endocarditis due to streptococci, enterococci, staphylococci, and HACEK microorganisms. *JAMA.* 1995;274:1706–13.

24. **Whitener C, Caputo GM, Weitekamp MR, et al.** Endocarditis due to coagulase-negative staphylococci: microbiologic, epidemiologic, and clinical considerations. *Infect Dis Clin North Am.* 1993;7:81–96.

25. **Watanakunakorn C.** Staphylococcal endocarditis. *Curr Opin Infect Dis.* 1996;9:105–108.

26. **Watanakunakorn C, Habte-Gabr E.** Group B streptococcal endocarditis of tricuspid valve: report of three cases and review of the literature. *Chest.* 1991;100:569–71.

27. **Burkert T, Watanakunakorn C.** Group A streptococcus endocarditis: report of 5 cases and review of the literature. *J Infect* 1991;23:307–16.

28. **Watanakunakorn C.** Endocarditis due to beta-hemolytic streptococci. *Chest.* 1992;102:333–4.

29. **Baddonr LM.** Infectious Diseases Society of America's Emerging Infectious Network: infective endocarditis caused by beta-hemolytic streptococci. *Clin Infect Dis.* 1998; 26:66–71.

30. **Vandenesch F, Etienne J, Reverdy ME, et al.** Endocarditis due to *Staphylococcus lugdunensis*: report of 11 cases and review. *Clin Infect Dis.* 1993;17:871–6.

31. **Drancourt M, Mainardi JL, Bronqui P, et al.** *Bartonella (Rochalimaea) quintana* endocarditis in three homeless men. *N Engl J Med.* 1995;332:419–23.

32. **Holmes AH, Greenough TC, Balady GJ, et al.** *Bartonella henselae* endocarditis in an immunocompetent adult. *Clin Infect Dis.* 1995;21:1004–7.

33. **Hadfield TL, Warren R, Kass M, et al.** Endocarditis caused by *Rochalimaea henselae.* *Hum Pathol.* 1993;24:1140–1.

34. **Watanakunakorn C.** Osler's nodes on the dorsum of the foot. *Chest.* 1988;94: 1088–90.

35. **Watanakunakorn C, Chan SJ, Demarco DG, et al.** *Staphylococcus aureus* bacteremia: significance of hyperbilirubinemia. *Scand J Infect Dis.* 1987;19:195–203.

36. **Durack DT, Lukes AS, Bright DK, and the Duke Endocarditis Service.** New criteria for diagnosis of infective endocarditis: utilization of specific echocardiographic findings. *Am J Med.* 1994;96:200–9.

37. **Bayer AS.** Diagnostic criteria for identifying cases of endocarditis: revisiting the Duke criteria two years later. *Clin Infect Dis.* 1996;23:303–4.

38. **Watanakunakorn C.** Penicillin combined with gentamicin or streptomycin: synergism against enterococci. *J Infect Dis.* 1971;124:581–6.

39. **Watanakunakorn C, Bakie C.** Synergism of vancomycin–gentamicin and vancomycin–streptomycin against enterococci. *Antimicrob Agents Chemother.* 1973;4:120–4.

40. **Watanakunakorn C, Glotzbecker C.** Enhancement of the effects of antistaphylococcal antibiotics by aminoglycosides. *Antimicrob Agents Chemother.* 1974;6:802–6.

41. **Watanakunakorn C, Glotzbecker C.** Synergism with aminoglycosides of penicillin, ampicillin, and vancomycin against enterococcal group D streptococci and viridans streptococci. *J Med Microbiol.* 1977;10:133–8.

42. **Watanakunakorn C, Tisone JC.** Synergism between vancomycin and gentamicin or tobramycin for methicillin-susceptible and methicillin-resistant *Staphylococcus aureus* strains. *Antimicrob Agents Chemother.* 1982;22:903–5.

43. **Wilson WR, Karchmer AW, Dajani AS, et al.** Antibiotic treatment of adults with infective endocarditis due to streptococci, enterococci, staphylococci, and HACEK microorganisms. *JAMA.* 1995;274:1706–13.

44. **Scheld WM, Sande MA.** Endocarditis and intravascular infections. In Mandell GL, Bennett JE, Dolin R, (eds). *Principles and Practice of Infectious Diseases,* 4th ed. New York: Churchill Livingstone; 1995:740–83.

45. **Dajani AS, Taubert KA, Wilson W, et al.** Prevention of bacterial endocarditis: recommendation by the American Heart Association. *JAMA.* 1997;277:1794–801.

6

Vascular Infections

Louis D. Saravolatz, MD

Vascular infections are uncommon but serious infections that may arise from the deposition of bacteria circulating in the bloodstream onto the vascular endothelial surface, or from contiguous spread of bacteria to a vessel wall. This chapter will address mycotic aneurysms, infected pseudoaneurysms, and septic thrombophlebitis.

Mycotic Aneurysms

Mycotic aneurysms were described in 1885 by Sir William Osler in association with bacterial endocarditis arising in a patient with multiple aneurysms of the aorta (1). Osler described the bacterial nature of endocarditis and its association with an aneurysm as a consequence of hematogenous seeding of of an organism through the vascular supply to the large blood vessels. However, mycotic aneurysms had in fact originally been noted as many as three decades earlier by Edward Koch, who described a superior mesenteric artery aneurysm associated with "rheumatism" (2). Mycotic aneurysms were traditionally described as primary and secondary. Primary aneurysms were those that were considered "cryptogenic." These arise from a primary intravascular focus of infection, without any evidence of an inflammatory process in the surrounding tissue. A primary mycotic aneurysm may be suspected when the patient presents clinically with evidence of infection as the result of bacteremia from an obscure focus of infection. The clinician's suspicion of this diagnosis would be increased if the bacteremia were antedated by an illness caused by the same bacterial agent. Primary infections basically arise from bacterial embolic seeding from the vasa vasorum to the media of arterial walls. Secondary mycotic aneurysms are associated with another focus of infection and sometimes with an inflammatory process in the adjacent tissue. These latter forms of aneurysm are often referred to as pseudoaneurysms, and will be addressed separately.

Clinical Manifestations

The clinical manifestations of mycotic aneurysms can vary substantially according to the virulence of the organism. Often characterized by a long, febrile course that eludes the diagnostic acumen of the clinician, a mycotic aneurysm becomes clinically apparent when the affected blood vessel ruptures. In 75% of cases, rupture is the initial presentation. If the site is intracranial, the presentation is headache and rapid neurologic deterioration. If the site is intrathoracic, a catastrophic aortic rupture is the presentation, and in the case of an intra-abdominal site, retroperitoneal hemorrhage is commonly found. Leukocytosis occurs in the majority of patients, but blood cultures are positive in only approximately half of patients. Primary mycotic aneurysms are associated with atherosclerosis, cystic medial necrosis, or syphilitic aortitis. The underlying disease process generally involves the intima of the vessel wall. The microbial etiology of mycotic aneurysms has included *Streptococcus viridans* and *Staphylococcus aureus*, and to a lesser extent *Salmonella species* and enterococci.

In a series of 330 patients, bacterial endocarditis was the disease most commonly associated with infectious aneurysms, and occurred in 294 cases.[2] Coarctation of the aorta occurred in approximately 15% of cases. Pneumonia, osteomyelitis, lung abscess, primary bacteremia, otitis media, urinary sepsis, and meningitis each occurred in less than 5% of cases. The average age at presentation was 33 years. Blood vessels involved were most commonly the aorta, followed by superior mesenteric, cerebral, femoral, hepatic, pulmonary, splenic and even coronary arteries.

Diagnosis

The diagnosis of a mycotic aneurysm requires a high index of suspicion in unexplained bacteremias associated with systemic signs of sepsis, or in the case of systemic sepsis in the abacteremic patient. The existence of infective endocarditis in the year before presentation, or of other recent serious bacterial infections, should heighten suspicion of the possibility of a mycotic aneurysm. Laboratory findings are generally nonspecific and are those associated with sepsis. Radiographic evaluations may help. A palpable aneurysm is rarely seen, and unfortunately a diagnosis is established before rupture in only slightly more than half of cases. Angiography of the site of suspected involvement is the definitive test before surgical exploration. For intracranial mycotic aneurysms, magnetic resonance angiography and intravenous digital subtraction angiography are promising techniques (3,4). During the operative procedure, affected tissue should be collected for both histology and culture.

Treatment

Optimal treatment of mycotic aneurysms requires surgical excision and concomitant antimicrobial therapy (5). In the case of rupture of aneurysms of large vessels such as the abdominal aorta, survival is infrequent even for patients who undergo emergency surgery. Even in the case of elective surgery, excision of an aneurysm and revascularization may be associated with severe perioperative morbidity and mortality. Adequate excision of all infected material and establishment of adequate drainage is essential. Unfortunately, this is extremely difficult to do when a large vessel is involved, and particularly if there is pre-existing prosthetic material that cannot be removed. Several investigators have shown that placing arterial homografts or plastic prosthesis through contaminated tissues, even in the face of systemic antibiotic coverage, may result in persistent infection and frequent disruption of the graft anastomoses. In contrast, arterial bypass reconstruction through clean tissue planes has produced healing with favorable results. In the surgical approach to the peripheral vessels, a bypass is created with an uninvolved vessel. In such cases, a vein graft may also be employed. In these cases, there has been greater success in eradicating infection even in the face of persistent infection in the adjacent tissue (6,7).

Optimal antimicrobial therapy for infectious aneurysms requires selection of bactericidal antimicrobial agents that can be given in high doses for prolonged periods. These requirements are general, and there are no controlled studies that provide objective evidence for an optimal duration of therapy. The dose, selection, and duration of antimicrobial therapy are similar to those for infective endocarditis. Some clinicians utilize an even longer duration because of the potential contamination of prosthetic material that may be implanted into an infected surgical site. In such cases it would be prudent to administer antimicrobial therapy for a minimum of 6 weeks via a parenteral route, and a combination therapy should be considered for more resistant organisms, as in the case of infective endocarditis. Moreover, even though the infection may appear to have been brought under control, the patient's clinical course may deteriorate rapidly and terminate in early disruption of the arterial suture line with associated hemorrage. In such cases, the patient develops evidence of the hemorragic shock and death is to be expected. Such complications may occur at anytime from 1 to 2 months after surgery, thus necessitating careful long-term follow-up to permit intervention on an emergent basis.

Prognosis and Prevention

Today, the overall prognosis in the case of a mycotic aneurysm is generally poor. The onset is often abrupt, making the diagnosis difficult at best. There are no noninvasive diagnostic procedures available for making rapid diagnosis. Utilization of magnetic resonance angiography should be considered in place of traditional angiography. After the diagnosis is made, the challenge is to excise the infected tissue and destroy any organisms that may be in the vascular suture line or that may be clinically inapparent on areas of the blood vessel wall. Some organisms are more virulent than others, making it even more difficult to eradicate them and necessitating prolonged antibiotic therapy. However, the penetration of these antimicrobials to atherosclerotic plaques and thrombi is poor. These areas tend to be avascular, and this may result in subtherapeutic levels of antimicrobial agent. Thus, antimicrobial therapy for indefinite periods may be given consideration in some infections because of the fear of relapse and its devastating consequences. Prevention of such infections is best achieved by eradicating the primary focus of infection, which will be either infective endocarditis or bacterial infection at another site. With available therapy and the high cure rate in infective endocarditis, most cases of infectious aneurysm can be prevented. The clinician should monitor patients for evidence of relapse of these infections and promptly treat them.

The evidence for primary prophylaxis for infectious aneurysms is limited. If a prosthetic graft is placed, patients may be treated like patients with a cardiac valve graft in place, and given antimicrobial prophylaxis for high-risk procedures such as dental and genitourinary procedures.

Infected False Aneurysms ("Pseudoaneurysms")

A variety of terms have been associated with infected "mycotic aneurysms" involving the major or peripheral vessels and resulting in destruction of the vessel wall, aneurysm formation, and aneurysm rupture (8). False aneurysms, in contrast to true mycotic aneurysms, involve a blood vessel that was normal before the infection. Thus, there is no intimal involvement, and the lesion does not result in embolomycotic event. These false or pseudoaneurysms are usually triggered by an unsuccessful attempt at femoral vein access, often for use of illicit injectable drugs. Failure to use aseptic technique establishes a perivascular infection. There is inadvertent trauma to the arterial wall resulting in a vascular or perivascular hematoma, which in turn leads to the formation of a false aneurysm. As the infection continues to spread, there is a destructive process involving the blood vessel wall, and eventual rupture leading to rapid clinical deterioration and demise within a relatively short ensuing period.

Etiology

Infected false aneurysms are most often associated with parenteral drug abuse as a risk factor, although other techniques, such as intravascular catheter placement and angiography, may be associated with mycotic aneurysms. However, because aseptic technique is generally used during these procedures, the risk for such for such complications is extremely low. Nonetheless, there are reports of hematoma with local infection resulting in contiguous spread and infected aneurysm formation in association with cardiac catheterization. Thus, the evolution of a false aneurysm involves trauma to the outer layer of the arterial wall, or externa, resulting in perivascular hematoma and infection leading to aneurysm formation with intimal sparing.

Clinical Manifestations

The history and physical findings made by McIlroy et al. in a series of 60 patients with infected false aneurysms of the femoral artery included groin swelling and/or a mass in the femoral artery area in more than 90% with pain and tenderness in 80% (8). Fever and chills were found in 62%; other symptoms were nonspecific and included nausea, vomiting, paresthesias, and purulent drainage in less than 15% of patients. A pulsatile mass in the groin or femoral artery area was found in only 63% of the patients in this series, but its presence should alert the clinician to the high probability of an infected aneurysm. Fever and/or groin tenderness were present in only slightly more than half of the patients on admission. Other findings, such as an audible bruit over the palpable mass, were made in only 27% of the cases. Associated cellulitis, erythema, and purulent drainage were found in less than 25% of the patients. Absence of a pulse distal from the involved artery was present in less than 10% of the patients, and distal emboli were found in only 1 of the 60 patients. The history of groin swelling, pain, and tenderness with the finding on physical examination of a mass in cases of mycotic aneurysm of the femoral artery make the clinical presentation indistinguishable from that of a groin abscess or phlegmon evolving into an abscess. The findings that one would like to make, such as bruit, diminished pulses, distal emboli, and even a pulsatile mass, are often absent, thus making the diagnosis extremely difficult to establish.

Diagnosis

As in the case of mycotic aneurysms, laboratory findings in cases of infected false aneurysm are nonspecific. Leukocytosis is present in many cases, but is not always found. Blood cultures should be done, but were positive in only 60% of the 60 patients in McIlroy and colleagues series. Nonetheless, the organisms were discovered in the blood vessels at the time of surgery in more than 90% of these patients. The most common isolated pathogen was *Staphylococcus aureus*, in 80% of the latter patients; other organisms that were noted, which included *Streptococcus pyogenes* other streptococci, and anaerobes, were each found in 20% of the patients. The anaerobes included *Bacteroides, Fusobacterium, and Peptococcus*. Gram-negative aerobic bacilli occurred in 15% of the patients, with no single predominant organism, but included *Pseudomonas aeruginosa, Proteus mirabilis, Escherichia coli, Klebsiella pneumoniae, Serratia marcescens*, and *Citrobacter freundii*.

The procedures used to diagnose false aneurysms have included digital subtraction angiography (DSA), conventional arteriography, ultrasonography (US), and computed tomography (CT). In addition small numbers of patients have false aneurysms diagnosed at the time of surgical intervention for drainage of an abscess when the surgeon discovers that he is inadvertently dissecting into the blood vessel wall. In the case of DSA and arteriography, the sensitivity is 90% to 96% (9). US is considerably less effective, with a diagnostic sensitivity of only 24%. The value of US is that it may quite accurately reveal the presence of a perivascular abscess, which, if detected might arouse suspicion of contiguous spread of infection leading to a mycotic aneurysm.

Treatment

Treatment of infected false aneurysms requires a combined medical and surgical approach (8,10,11). The empiric treatment used before organisms are identified should include vancomycin, gentamicin, and metronidazole for beta-lactam-resistant *S. aureus*, gram-negative bacilli, and anaerobes. Once the organisms are identified and appropriate susceptibility testing has been performed, a specific antimicrobial regimen can be prescribed. In a large published series, the mean duration of effective antibiotic therapy for infected false aneurysms was 24 days for patients who were successfully cured (8).

Bacteriologic treatment failure was accompanied by a recurrence rate of 10% (six of 60 patients) for cellulitis and/or wound infection at the site of the aneurysm. However, these six patients had initially received short-term (less than 15 days) parenteral antibiotic therapy, versus the other patients who were cured with more than 16 days of therapy (p=0.002, Fisher's exact test). In this series, in contrast to in findings with mycotic aneurysms, all treatment failures occurred within the first month after discharge from the hospital. There was no one predominant organism among the cases of treatment failure, with *S. aureus* being most common both in cases of treatment failure and treatment success. Interestingly, none of the patients who experienced bacteriologic treatment failure required amputation, and all were subsequently cured with the second course of antimicrobial treatment. We may therefore conclude that prolonged antimicrobial therapy of at least three weeks and even as long as six weeks will provide a reasonable margin of safety. For false aneurysms that manifest as swelling in the groin and with evidence of overlying infection, management requires a combined medical surgical approach. Initial antimicrobial therapy should be broad spectrum, to treat beta-lactam-resistant *S. aureus*, anaerobes, and gram-negative bacilli. Thus, combination therapy with vancomycin, gentamicin, and metronidazole should be considered. In cases in which the groin is not involved, anaerobes are less relevant and metronidazole may be deleted.

Perivascular abscesses and infected hematomas should be appropriately excised. Interestingly, in the large published series mentioned above (8), a variety of surgical approaches were taken, including grafting and/or reanastomotic procedures involving saphenous vein grafts and prosthetic grafts (Dacron). Graft failures did occur, and in the case of femoral mycotic aneurisms, 10% of the patients required above-knee amputation. Interestingly there were no deaths in this series of 60 aneurysms with the current availability of optimal antimicrobial therapy and vascular surgical techniques. Infected false aneurysms need to be ligated and removed, with the wound left open, and adequate surgical debridement of the infected perivascular tissue. Surgical management is an area for future investigation in terms of defining the extent of debridement, optimal graft material, and revascularzation procedures (11,12). State-of-the-art vascular surgery and advances in this discipline with prosthetic or homologous graft procedures will determine the surgical management.

Prevention

Among the 169 cases of infected false aneurysm reported in the United States literature between 1966 and 1988, the overwhelming majority occurred in intravenous drug users, and the main mechanism for preventing these lesions is therefore dealing with socioeconomic considerations of illicit drug use, which is not within the scope of this chapter (8). To prevent infected false aneurysms associated with cardiac catheterizations, optimal aseptic technique should be used during the catheterization procedures. Antimicrobial therapy for infected hematomas and consideration of pressure decompression for noninfected pseudoaneurysms should be given before surgical intervention is needed.

Septic Thrombophlebitis

Septic thrombophlebitis evolves from an infected venous thrombosis that becomes associated with venous obstruction, septic emboli, and high-grade bacteremia.

Etiology

Septic thrombophlebitis has changed with time from chiefly involving intracranial veins and the dural sinus, both of which are now rarely involved, to mainly consist of suppurative phlebitis of cannulated and great veins as a complication of intravenous therapy (13–15). Other sites at which the condition may occur, but again relatively rarely, include pylephlebitis and septic thrombophlebitis. Local infection is the major factor predisposing to septic thrombophlebitis.

Most cases of septic thrombophlebitis arise from bland phlebitis that develops because of stasis, hypercoagulability, and endothelial injury. These risk factors are all increased when there is adjacent inflammation. If the inflammatory process is associated with microorganisms, the latter migrate via lymphatics or the vascular supply to the wall of the vein. The associated infection may be anywhere in the body, including intracranial veins, neck veins, great veins of the thorax, abdominal veins, pelvic veins, and peripheral veins. In addition to the periphlebitic method of acquisition, a more common current route for the development of septic thrombophlebitis is the endovascular route, via an intravenous cannula, especially if the latter is left in place for more than 48 hours. However, cannula-associated infections usually have both perivascular and endovascular components, and it is often unclear which route initiated the infection in such cases. A third possible route is hematogenous seeding from a distant site. Certain pathogens, such as streptococci, *Bacteroides fragilis*, and *Campylobacter fetus* have a higher rate of occurrence in septic phlebitis than do other pathogens that are isolated more frequently from the primary source of infection. There is evidence that these organisms may release substances that inhibit the coagulation cascade.

Clinical Manifestations

The clinical manifestations of septic thrombophlebitis are local inflammation and infection, sepsis, and embolic manifestations. The latter include fever, hyperthermia, rigors, diaphoresis, confusion, tachycardia, tachypnea, hypotension, abdominal pain, and ecchymoses. The local process varies with the site of involvement. Patients with thrombophlebitis generally present with fever (70%–90%). The signs and symptoms are described in Table 6.1 on the basis of the site of involvement. Understanding the anatomy of the site of involvement in the case of intracranial veins and dural sinuses may assist the clinician in understanding what to expect in terms of clinical manifestations.

Diagnosis

The laboratory findings in cases of septic thrombophlebitis are those of sepsis. An increased white blood cell (WBC) count with a left shift and laboratory evidence of disseminated intravascular infection are common.

Blood cultures are essential in the diagnosis of septic thrombophlebitis. Two sets of culture results should be obtained initially, and two additional after 24 to 48 hours. If bacteremia persists despite appropriate empiric antimicrobial therapy, it may point to the need for surgical intervention.

Careful examination of initial and subsequent chest radiographs may disclose evidence of septic pulmonary emboli. Irregularly defined pulmonary infiltrates progressing to cavitation suggest this complication. Ventilation perfusion scanning may be more sensitive than plain radiography, and can be performed if the diagnosis is strongly considered in the face of a negative chest radiograph.

The diagnosis of septic phlebitis is definitively established by venotomy with histologic and microbiologic examination of the thrombus. When this is done, the laboratory must be asked to perform aerobic, anaerobic, and fungal cultures.

In seeking a specific site of infection as the source of septic thrombophlebitis, the clinician should order cultures appropriate for probable sites. If, for example, an intracranial focus is suspected, cerebrospinal fluid should be obtained, culture of which will reflect either meningitis or a parameningeal inflammatory process (increased WBC count with both polymorphonuclear leukocytes and mononuclear cells, a normal glucose, a slightly elevated protein concentration and culture negativity).

Radiographic assessment with CT or magnetic resonance imaging (MRI) may be helpful. If utilized, contrast-enhanced CT or MRI with gadolinium can be very sensitive modalities in demonstrating filling defects consistent with thrombus caused by septic phlebitis (16,17).

Table 6.1   Clinical Manifestations of Intracranial Septic Thrombophlebitis

Vein	Predisposing Illness	Symptoms/Signs
Cavernous sinus	Chronic sinusitis, diabetes mellitus, facial cellulitis	Headache (ophthalmic and maxillary branch CN.V), periorbital edema, unilateral progressing to bilateral eye findings, diplopia, photophobia, tearing, ptosis, and mental status changes. Hemiparesis, and seizures are less common. Sinus tenderness to palpation, exophthalmus, chemosis, ophthalmoplegia CN. III, IV, and VI), papilledema, V I and V2 defecit.
Lateral sinus	Usually absent other than chronic otitis media	Subacute onset with headache (fronto–occipital and temporal occipital), nausea vomiting, vertigo, signs of ear infection, ruptured tympanic membranes (40%), posterior auricular swelling (Cresinger's sign; 50%), papilledema (15%), CN.VI palsy (33%), nuchal rigidity (33%).
Superior sagittal sinus	Bacterial meningitis, extension from cavernous or lateral sinus septic phlebitis, sinusitis (ethmoid and maxillary), scalp infection. Less common: pulmonary or odontogenic infections.	Similar to those of bacterial meningitis: headache, nausea, vomiting, seizure, coma, hemiparesis, brain stem compression, and papilledema
Cortical	Bacterial meningitis and sinusitis	Seizures, focal deficits and signs and symptoms of meningitis

CN = cranial nerve.

Treatment

Antimicrobial therapy with high-dose intravenous antibiotics should be initiated empirically for septic thrombophlebitis on basis of the site of the lesion and most likely pathogens (Table 6.2). The optimal duration of therapy has not been established, but 2 weeks of therapy would be a minimum, with at least 4 weeks if *S. aureus* is the pathogen (18).

Table 6.2 Microbial Etiology and Treatment Considerations for Septic Phlebitis

Site	Microbial Etiology	Empiric Treatment Options*
Cavenous sinus	Staphylococcus aureus (70%), group A streptococci, Streptococcus pneumoniae, gram (-) bacilli, anaerobes	Penicillinase-resistant penicillins[†] (or vancomycin), ceftriaxone (or cefotaxime) + metronidazole
Lateral sinus	Group A streptococcus, S. aureus, Bacteroides, gram (-) (Proteus mirabilis and Escherichia coli)	Penicillinase-resistant penicillins +, ceftriaxone (or cefotaxime) plus metronidazole.
Sagittal sinus	S. aureus, Group A streptococci	Penicillinase resistant penicillin's
Cortical	S. pneumoniae, Hemophilus influenzae, Neisseria meningitis	Vancomycin plus ceftriaxone (or vancomycin and aminoglycosides. If brain abscess or sinus source add metronidazole
Internal jugular vein	S. aureus, gram (-) bacilli, candida	Penicillinase resistant penicillins[†] (or vancomycin) and aminoglycosides
	If candida is suspected	Add amphotericin
Great vein	S. aureus, gram (-) bacilli	As in internal jugular sources
Pelvic veins	Anaerobes (Bacteroides fragilis), microaerophilic, streptococci	Metronidazole plus aminoglycosides or carbapenems or Beta lactam/Beta lactamase inhibitors plus an aminoglycoside
Pylephlebitis	Anaerobes (Clostridium), gram (-) bacilli	As in pelvic veins
Peripheral	S. aureus, Group A streptococci	Penicillinase resistant penicillins[†] or vancomycin.
		Add an aminoglycoside if patient had had prolonged hospitalization or prior antimicrobial agents.

*Dosing with normal renal and hepatic function: penicillinase-resistant penicillin (nafcillin 1.5–2.0 g every 4 hours); ceftriaxone 2g IV every 12 hours; cefotaxime 2 g IV every 4–6 hours; aminoglyosides (gentamicin/tobramycin 1.5 mg/kg IV every 8 hours; amphotericin 0.6–1.0 mg/kg every 24 hours; beta-lactam/beta-lactamase inhibitors (ticarcillin/CA 3.1 g every 4 hours; ampicillin–sulbactam 3.0 g every 6 hours; piperacillin–tazobactam 3.375 g every 6 hours.
[†]Penicillinase resistant penicillins (nafcillin or oxacillin).

If the vein is accessible and the patient demonstrates persistent bacteremia or perivascular infection, surgical excision of the infected clot should be considered (19).

Other ancillary measures include drainage of any primary focus of infection such as a contagious abscess. The involved area should be elevated to a 45-degree angle to enhance venous drainage. The use of anticoagulation remains controversial. There is some anecdotal evidence for a benefit of anticoagulation in the case of internal jugular vein involvement and pelvic septic phlebitis. In cases involving other sites, the risk of hemorrhage and complications of therapy must be carefully weighed before anticoagulation is instituted, in the view of the lack of convincing evidence to support such therapy.

Prevention and Future Developments

Prompt and appropriate treatment of bacterial infections of the skin, ear, dentition, sinuses, and pelvis is the main measure that can be effective in preventing septic thrombophlebitis. In case a venous cannula is in place, its removal should occur within 48 to 72 hours whenever possible, and more promptly when there is development of local infection or sepsis of unknown source. A detailed discussion of strategies for preventing infected emboli from vascular catheters has been recently published by the Centers for Disease Control and Prevention (20).

As for further research, the role of anticoagulants should be critically evaluated in a randomized, placebo-controlled trial. Unfortunately, the difficulty in agreeing on a diagnostic criteria, and the low rate of septic thrombophlebitis at most sites, may make such a trial difficult if not impossible to perform.

REFERENCES

1. **Osler W.** The Gustonian Lecture on Malignant Endocarditis. *Br Med J* 1885; 1:467–70.

2. **Goadby HK, McSwiney RR, Rob CG.** Mycotic aneurysm. *St. Thomas Hospital Report* 1949; 5:44–52.

3. **Tunkel AR, Kaye D.** Neurologic complications of infective endocarditis, *Neurol Clin* 1993:11:419.

4. **Kimura I, Okmura R, Yamashita K, et al.** Mycotic aneurysm. *Radiat Med* 1989;7:121.

5. **Meridith ED, Darling RC, Alvarado RU, et al.** Surgical management of mycotic aneurysms and the complications of infections or vascular reconstructive surgery. *Am J Surg* 1969; 117:460–70.

6. **Johansen K, Devin J.** Mycotic aortic aneurysms. A reappraisal. *Arch Surg* 1983: 118:583.

7. **Bitseff EJ, Edwards WH, Mulheim JL Jr, et al.** Infected abdominal aortic aneurysms. *South Med J* 1987;80:309–12.

8. **McIlroy MA, Reddy D, Markowitz N, Saravolatz LD,** Infected false aneurysms of the femoral artery in intravenous drug addicts. *Rev Infect Dis* 1989; 11:578–85.

9. **Shetty PC, Kasicky GA, Sharma RP, et al.** Mycotic aneurysms in IVDA: the utility of intravenous digital substraction angiography. *Radiology* 1985; 155:319–21.

10. **Johnson JR, Ledgerwood AM, Lucas CE.** Mycotic aneurysm: new concepts in therapy. *Arch Surg* 1983; 118:577–87.

11. **Reddy DJ, Smith RF, Elliot JP Jr, et al.** Infected femoral artery false aneurysms in drug addicts: evolution of selective vascular reconstruction. *J Vasc Surg* 1986;3:718–25.

12. **Johnson JR, Ledgerwood AM, Lucas CE.** Mycotic aneurysm: new concepts in therapy. *Arch Surg* 1983; 118:577–82.

13. **Maki DG.** Septic thrombophlebitis. *Hosp Med* 1976:36–49.

14. **Southwick IS.** Septic thrombophlebitis of major dual venous sinuses. *Curr Clin Infect Dis* 1995; 15:179–203.

15. **Rupp ME.** Infections of intravascular catheters and vascular devices. In Crossley KB, Archer GL, eds. *The Staphylococci in Human Disease.* New York: Churchill Livingstone; 1997;379–399.

16. **Ellie E, Houang B, Louail C, et al.** CT and highfield MRI in septic thrombosis of the cavernous sinuses. *Neuroradiology* 1992; 34:22–4.

17. **Komiyama M.** Magnetic resonance imaging of the cavernous sinus. *Radiat Med* 1990; 8:136–44.

18. **Raad I, Narro J, Khan, et al.** Serious complications of the vascular catheter-related *Staphylococcus aureus* bacteremia in cancer patients. *Eur J Clin Microbiol Infect Dis.* 1992; 11–675.

19. **Verghese A, Winrich WC, Arbeit RD.** Central venous septic thrombophlebitis—the role of medical therapy. Medicine. 1985; 64 (6) 394–400.

20. **Centers for Disease Control and Prevention.** Part 1. Intravascular device-related infection: An overview: Part 2. Recommendations for prevention of intravascular device-related infections. *Fed Regist* 1995;60:49978.

7

Infectious Diarrhea and Gastroenteritis

Keith B. Armitage, MD

Robert A. Salata, MD

Infectious gastroenteritis is one of the most common infections throughout the world and is a leading worldwide cause of infant mortality, with 4 million to 6 million deaths per year. In the United States, most cases of infectious gastroenteritis are self-limited, a sharp contrast to the situation in the developing world where cases are more often chronic and debilitating. Diarrhea may be the most common symptom experienced by travelers, immigrants, and refugees. The pathogens that cause diarrhea range from viruses that cause self-limited illness in adults and more serious syndromes in children to bacterial and protozoan pathogens that may cause significant morbidity and mortality in healthy and immunocompromised adults and children alike. New and emerging pathogens (e.g., *Escherichia coli* serotype 0157:H7, *Cryptosporidium*) have received much attention from the lay press and the medical community. In this chapter, a general approach to the adult patient with acute diarrhea is followed by a discussion of selected pathogens that cause diarrhea. Chronic diarrhea, food poisoning, and traveler's diarrhea are discussed separately. The discussion generally excludes infectious diarrhea in patients with AIDS and/or HIV infection.

Epidemiology

In the United States, most cases of infectious gastroenteritis go unreported, and the incidence of the disease is based on estimates. On average, adults in the United States and Europe have approximately one episode per year of infectious gastroenteritis (1). In the United States, infectious diarrhea accounts for approximately 8 million visits to physicians, 250,000 hospitalizations, and 10,000 deaths annually (2). Together, gastroenteritis and acute diarrhea account for 1.5% of hospitalizations for inpatients under 20 years of age. In the developed world, most of the morbidity and mortality from infectious gastroenteritis occurs in the elderly. Exceptions to this rule occur with infection by *E. coli* 0157:H7 (which produces hemolytic uremic syndrome [HUS] in children) and by rotavirus (which causes diarrhea leading to dehydration in young children).

Although the United States has an average of one case of infectious gastroenteritis per adult, these cases are not evenly distributed in the population. Groups at special risk include adults who have small children in daycare centers, international travelers, homosexual men, immunosuppressed patients, and individuals living in poor hygienic conditions. These risk groups account for a disproportionate number of cases of infectious gastroenteritis. Animal populations are the primary reservoir for most bacterial enteropathogens in the United States. *Salmonella*, *Campylobacter*, and pathogenic strains of *E. coli* usually enter humans from poultry, bovine, or porcine sources, and the route of illness is usually via undercooked or contaminated food. Infectious agents that rely on a human reservoir and are spread directly from one person to another or by human fecal contamination and include *Salmonella typhi*, *Shigella*, and *Vibrio cholerae* are much less common in the United States than in the developing world.

Pathogenesis

The vast majority of microorganisms found in the human intestine are not pathogenic, but those that are rely on a variety of virulence factors to produce disease. Microbial virulence factors include enterotoxins that alter intestinal salt and water transport mechanisms, adherence (and colonization) factors, and invasive and penetrability properties.

Enterotoxins usually act in the upper small intestine to provoke fluid and electrolyte secretion and either cause no significant alteration in mucosal histology (e.g., cholera toxin) or are cytotoxins that can alter mucosal histology to the point of epithelial cell death (e.g., clostridial and staphylococcal enterotoxins). Adherence to the intestinal surface is required for many enteropathogens and involves specific cell-surface determinants. Invasive bacteria primarily colonize the colon and have the ability to invade and survive in host cells and to bring about cell death. Gross mucosal ulceration can occur, particularly in shigellosis, and is responsible for dysenteric stools in that disease. In the case of systemic pathogens such as *S. typhi*, virulence factors include the ability to infect and persist in host immune cells, which permits access to the circulation and leads to extraintestinal disease.

The role of host factors in the susceptibility to infectious gastroenteritis is discussed below.

Etiology

Infectious diarrhea can be classified as inflammatory or noninflammatory (Table 7.1) (2). This classification has practical application for the clinician, because examining the stool for fecal leukocytes (Fig. 7.1) can help distinguish the two conditions, and this distinction can alter the diagnostic and therapeutic approach. Noninflammatory diarrhea most often results from interference with absorption of fluid and electrolytes and does not involve pathogenic invasion of the intestinal mucosa. Virtually all viral and most protozoan pathogens give rise to a noninflammatory diarrhea. In most cases, these pathogens cause disease by interfering with the absorptive functions of entero-

Table 7.1 Characteristics and Causes of Inflammatory and Noninflammatory Diarrhea

	Noninflammatory	Inflammatory
Location	Small intestine	Large intestine
Diarrhea	Watery, large volume	Small volume, loose stools, blood, pus
Stool examination	No fecal leukocytes	Fecal leukocytes
Cause (infectious organism)	Norwalk-like viruses	*Shigella* species
	Rotavirus	*Salmonella enteritidis*
	Giardia lamblia	*Campylobacter* species
	Enterotoxigenic *Escherichia coli*	Enteroinvasive *E. coli*
	Vibrio cholerae	*V. parahaemolyticus*
	Clostridium perfringens	*C. difficile*
	Bacillus cereus	*Entamoeba histolytica***
	Staphylococcus aureus	*Yersinia enterocolitica*
	Cryptosporidium	
	Cyclospora	
	Microsporidium	
	Enterohemorrhagic *E. coli*	

* Toxins produced by *E. histolytica* that destroy leukocytes may lead to the absence of fecal leukocytes in patients with colitis due to *E. histolytica*. Patients with risk factors for acquiring bacterial or protozoan pathogens or intestinal parasites and their ova should have their stool examined for fecal leukocytes. The presence of fecal leukocytes should prompt a stool culture, which may lead to the initiation of specific therapy (see Table 7.2).

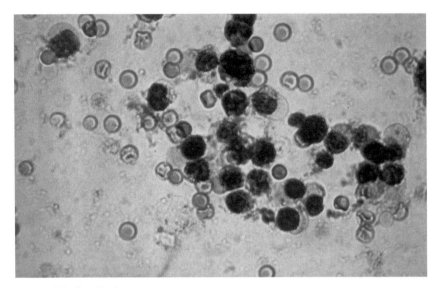

Figure 7.1 Fecal leukocytes.

cytes in the small intestine through the production of toxins that alter the handling of fluids and electrolytes (e.g., as in cholera [which is discussed in a later section]) or cause villous damage. These processes result in the delivery of excess fluid and electrolytes to the large intestine. Once the absorptive capacity of the large intestine is exceeded, a high-volume, watery diarrhea results.

In contrast with the aforementioned viruses and protozoans, many bacterial pathogens invade the intestinal mucosa (usually the colon), provoking an inflammatory response that results in colonic malabsorption and the presence of leukocytes and blood in the stool. This diarrhea is characterized by mucus and blood and by a smaller volume of stool than is seen with noninflammatory diarrhea. *E. coli* can produce either syndrome, depending on the strain of the infecting organism (which is discussed in a later section). Other bacterial pathogens also cause noninflammatory diarrhea by producing preformed toxins that are ingested in contaminated food (*see* section on Food Poisoning Syndromes below).

Diagnosis

The risk of acquiring a gastrointestinal infection varies with the host and the potential for exposures to infectious agents. Host factors that influence susceptibility to infection include age, intestinal dysmotility, integrity of the normal intestinal flora, gastric acidity, and intestinal mucosal immunity. Potential for exposure to infectious agents varies with socioeconomic conditions and sanitation, travel to areas endemic to intestinal pathogens to which the host lacks immunity, and the occurrence of food- or water-borne outbreaks of disease caused by these agents. When evaluating a patient with diarrhea, it is impossible to overemphasize the importance of a careful history that focuses on issues such as travel, antibiotic use, illness in close contacts, exposure to potentially contaminated food or water, and the presence of decreased gastric acidity or gastrointestinal motility.

A careful history also helps differentiate patients who are likely to have a self-limited viral process that requires only symptomatic therapy from those who have a bacterial or protozoan pathogen that might necessitate further testing and specific therapy. In adults, viral gastroenteritis typically lasts 24 to 36 hours and no longer than 72 hours. The illness usually is not associated with significant abdominal pain, and there is no (or only a low-grade) fever. Viral gastroenteritis is associated with watery stools without blood or pus. In infants and small children, some viral pathogens (rotavirus, most notably) may produce a prolonged illness.

Risk factors for infection by bacterial or protozoan pathogens also can be determined from a history of potential exposures. In tropical countries, acute diarrhea occurs endemically and epidemically, and any recent travel in a tropical country increases the likelihood of infection by a nonviral pathogen. In the United States, camping and hiking may be associated with exposure to *Giardia*. Exposure to imported fruits and undercooked meats or poultry products may be associated with infection by bacterial pathogens or *Cyclospora*. Antibiotic use, achlorhydria, or an immunocompromised state may influence the risk of infection by a bacterial pathogen. Patients whose history suggests either a bacterial process or risk factors for the acquisition of bacterial pathogens should have their stool examined for fecal leukocytes (*see* Fig. 7.1); patients at risk for acquiring protozoan or other intestinal parasites should have a fresh stool specimen examined for ova and parasites. The presence of fecal leukocytes should prompt a stool culture and may lead to the initiation of specific therapy (*see* section on Treatment below). This approach is illustrated in Figure 7.2.

Treatment

When treating patients with diarrhea, be aware that an otherwise healthy subject with a history that suggests a self-limited viral process and no risk factors for acquiring other pathogens does not require any further workup and should be treated with oral rehydration and symptomatic support.

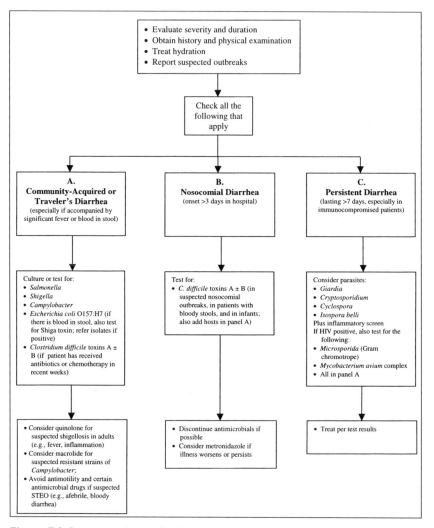

Figure 7.2 Recommendations for the diagnosis and management of diarrheal illnesses. (Republished with permission from Guerrant RL, Van Gilder T, Steiner TS, et al. Practice guidelines for the management of infectious diarrhea. *Clin Infect Dis.* 2001;32: 331.

For patients with acute inflammatory diarrhea or those from whom a pathogen has been isolated, the decision to institute specific antimicrobial therapy is based on host factors and the specific pathogen. For most healthy adults, antimicrobial therapy has a limited role in the management of acute diarrhea. For many enteropathogens (e.g., *Salmonella*) and enterohemorrhagic *E. coli*, antimicrobial therapy has not been proven to have a benefit and may prolong the carrier state in *Salmonella* infection. Furthermore, antimicrobial resistance is a growing problem with some enteropathogens, such as *Shigella* and *Salmonella*. In contrast, antimicrobial therapy is indicated for dysentery caused by *Shigella* or *Entamoeba histolytica*; in cholera, antimicrobial therapy can decrease the volume of fluid lost and shorten the clinical syndrome. However, patients who are at high risk for bacteremia and other complications of bacterial gastroenteritis (e.g., the elderly, immunocompromised patients, patients with vascular grafts, patients with sickle cell disease) benefit from antibiotic therapy. In these patients, empirical therapy is warranted in the setting of acute inflammatory diarrhea. In crowded conditions (e.g., refugee camps, areas of poor hygiene), epidemics of acute diarrhea caused by enteropathogens are common. In such settings, steps should be taken to ensure the safety of the water supply, to improve hygienic conditions, and to decrease the interpersonal spread of disease.

As with noninflammatory diarrhea, patients with inflammatory diarrhea require adequate hydration. In the past quarter century, oral rehydration therapy has revolutionized the treatment of a variety of acute diarrheal illnesses. Oral rehydration formulas in which the addition of glucose increases the efficiency of absorption of fluid and electrolytes have decreased the need for intravenous hydration. Antimotility agents should be used with caution in patients with inflammatory diarrhea, particularly in children. In a very small minority of patients with severe colitis, especially in the setting of infection with *Shigella* or *E. histolytica*, antimotility agents have been associated with complications such as colonic perforation and death. Most experts advise caution in the use of antimotility agents in patients with fever and bloody diarrhea and do not recommend their use without concomitant antimicrobial therapy.

The use of biotherapeutic agents in preventing and treating intestinal infections has been studied but not widely applied (3). *Lactobacillus* and *Saccharomyces* species have been shown in placebo-controlled studies to be effective in preventing or treating antibiotic-associated colitis, acute infantile diarrhea, recurrent *Clostridium difficile* diarrhea, and other diarrheal illnesses (4). These agents have not gained widespread use, but they have potential benefit in selected patients.

Specific Pathogens

Viruses

Norwalk-Like Viruses

A family of viral pathogens known as small round-structured viruses (SRSVs) or Norwalk-like viruses are the major cause of viral gastroenteritis in adults worldwide (5,6). These human enteric viral pathogens belong to the family

Caliciviridae. They can be distinguished both clinically and epidemiologically from rotavirus (which is discussed in the following section). SRSVs cause illness in adults and children and usually produce a mild clinical syndrome characterized by nausea, vomiting, and diarrhea that lasts no more than 24 to 36 hours. The diarrhea is watery and noninflammatory, and abdominal pain and fever are usually mild or absent. There have been large, well-documented outbreaks of such illness caused by interpersonal transmission of SRSVs as well as common-source outbreaks caused by food handlers. SRSV-associated illness in schools, hospitals, and cruise ships and a multistate outbreak caused by contaminated oysters are testimony to the highly contagious and ubiquitous nature of these enteric viral pathogens (6). Illness caused by SRSVs has a higher incidence in the winter and is often referred to as "winter-vomiting disease." Treatment consists of rehydration and symptomatic relief with antimotility agents.

Rotavirus

Rotavirus infection is much more common in children than is infection by Norwalk-like agents and produces a longer and more severe illness. Most studies show rotavirus to be the most common cause of pediatric diarrhea. An estimated 75 to 125 deaths and 65,000 to 75,000 hospitalizations for rotavirus infection occur each year in the United States. By the age of 2 years, most children are immune to rotavirus (7). Unlike the large, antigenically heterogeneous Norwalk virus family, only a few strains of rotavirus are antigenically heterogenous; thus, infection leads to protective immunity. Trials of a rotavirus vaccine seem promising (8). In addition to infecting children, rotavirus has been associated with illness in parents of infected children and travelers, and water-borne and nosocomial outbreaks of rotavirus disease have been reported. Treatment consists of hydration and supportive care.

Bacteria

Salmonella

In the developed world, salmonellosis is primarily a food-borne gastrointestinal disease. Outside the developed world, systemic illness caused by *S. typhi* and *S. paratyphi* is unusual (and is discussed briefly later). Approximately 40,000 culture-proven cases of *Salmonella* gastroenteritis are reported to the Centers for Diseases Control and Prevention each year (9). However, this is believed to represent only a small fraction of cases, because for each reported case 10 to 100 cases go unreported. Gastroenteritis related to different *Salmonella* species can be differentiated by a serotyping system; approximately 10 of these serotypes are responsible for most cases in the United States. The vast majority of *Salmonella* infections in the United States arise from an animal reservoir, and specific species of *Salmonella* are associated with particular food types and animals. Poultry, beef, and pork frequently have been associated with *Salmonella*. Undercooking meat products and inoculating food-preparation surfaces, which leads to cross-contamination, are common sources of *Salmonella* gastroenteritis. Although such gastroenteritis is associated most often with meat products and eggs, two recent large outbreaks were described in connection with ice cream and dry oat cereal, and there are case reports of other food products and animals having been contaminated with *Salmonella* (9). Interpersonal spread plays a small role in the transmission of *Salmonella* gastroenteritis.

Clinically, *Salmonella* gastroenteritis is characterized by inflammatory diarrhea that may be accompanied by abdominal pain and fever. The illness may be more severe in the very young, the elderly, and the immunosuppressed (10). Clinically significant bacteremia associated with *Salmonella* gastroenteritis is unusual in healthy adults but is seen in elderly and, most significantly, in immunosuppressed persons. Severe and prolonged illness, including bacteremia, has been well described in patients with AIDS (11). Most cases of *Salmonella* gastroenteritis in otherwise normal hosts do not require antibiotic treatment. Antibiotic therapy has not been shown to have a significant benefit in such cases and has been associated with relapses and prolonged carriage of *Salmonella*. Very young, elderly, and immunosuppressed persons and those with underlying illnesses (e.g., severe vascular disease, sickle cell disease) are at risk for complications or prolonged illness in *Salmonella* gastroenteritis and benefit from antibiotic therapy (Table 7.2). Antimicrobial resistance is an increasing issue, but the fluoroquinolones (e.g., ciprofloxacin) and third-generation cephalosporins usually are reliable (12).

S. typhi and related species produce a prolonged systemic illness characterized by invasion of the reticuloendothelial system and bacteremia. Patients may not have diarrhea during the illness, or it may be present only at the outset and may be mild. In contrast to nontyphoidal species of *Salmonella*, *S. typhi* and related species are highly adapted human pathogens and have no animal reservoir. Infection is based on human-to-human spread through direct contact or, more often, through fecal contamination of food and water. Typhoid fever is unusual in the United States, with fewer than 500 cases reported per year (70% or more of which occur in travelers or immigrants) (11). In addition to having fever, patients with typhoid fever can present with hepatosplenomegaly and a rash. The diagnosis is made by serology or by culturing *S. typhi* from the blood, stool, urine, or bone marrow. Antimicrobial therapy with quinolones or other agents improves survival and shortens the duration of illness (13). Most patients respond clinically to antimicrobial therapy within a week.

Antimicrobial resistance is increasing worldwide, and knowledge of local resistance patterns should be used in selecting therapy for typhoid fever. From

Table 7.2 Recommended Antimicrobial Therapies for the Infectious Organisms That Cause Diarrhea

Diseases	Infectious Organism	Recommended Antimicrobial Therapy
Bacterial		
Shigellosis	*Shigella* species	Adults: SXT 160–800 mg q12h for 3 days
		Fluoroquinolone: Ofloxacin 300 mg, norfloxacin 400 mg, or ciprofloxacin 500 mg q12h for 3 days
		Children: SXT 5–25 mg/kg/d in 2 divided doses for 3–5 days
Salmonellosis	*Salmonella enteritidis*	Adults*: SXT 160–800 mg q12h for 3 days (if susceptible); norfloxacin 400 mg, ciprofloxacin 500 mg, or ofloxacin 200 mg q12h for 5–7 days
		Children*: If ≤3 months of age, ceftriaxone 50 mg/kg/d; if >3 months and healthy, no treatment necessary; if >3 months with underlying illness, ceftriaxone <2 g/d
Campylobacteriosis	*Campylobacter jejuni*	Adults: Azierythromycin 500 mg/d for 5 days; fluoroquinolones as for shigellosis above
		Children: Azierythromycin 10 mg/kg/d for 5 days
ETEC, EPEC, EIEC	*Escherichia coli*	Same as for shigellosis above
EHEC	*E. coli* O157:H7 and other enteric bacteria that produce Shiga-like toxins	Role of antimicrobial therapy unclear
Aeromonas *Plesiomonas* diarrhea	*Aeromonas* *Plesiomonas shigelloides*	Same as for shigellosis above
Antibiotic-associated diarrhea†	*Clostridium difficile*	Metronidazole 500 mg tid for 10 days; vancomycin 125 mg qid for 10 days; bacitracin also has been used
Yersiniosis	*Yersinia enterocolitica*	Antimicrobial therapy usually is not required except for severe infections or associated bacteremia
		Adults: combination of two of the following: doxycycline, aminoglycoside, SXT, fluoroquinolones
		Children: ceftriaxone 50 mg/kg/d q24h for 5 days
Cholera	*Vibrio cholerae*	Doxycycline 300 mg PO in a single dose; tetracycline 500 mg qid for 3 days; SXT 160 mg/800 mg bid for 3 days
		A fluoroquinolone in a single dose
Parasitic		
Giardiasis	*Giardia lamblia*	Metronidazole 250–750 mg q8h for 7–10 days
		Infants: furazolidone 7 mg/kg/d in 4 divided doses for 7 days
		Older children: metronidazole 20 mg/kg/d in 3 divided doses for 7 days
Amebiasis	*Entamoeba histolytica*	Metronidazole 750 mg q8h for 5–10 days + diiodohydroxyquin 650 mg q8h for 20 days
		or
		paromomycin 500 mg tid for 10d
		For children: Metronidazole 50 mg/kg/d IV in 3 divided doses + diiodohydroxyquin 40 mg/kg/d in 3 divided doses for 20 days
Cryptosporidiosis	*Cryptosporidium* species	No treatment necessary except in severe cases or in patients with AIDS
		Severe cases: Paromomycin 500 mg q8h for 7 days
		AIDS patients: give 14–28 days then q12h indefinitely
Isosporiasis	*Isospora* species	SXT 160–800 mg q12h for 7–10 days
		AIDS patients: SXT 320–1600 mg q12h for 2–4 weeks, then 160–800 mg/d indefinitely
		Children: SXT 10–50 mg/kg/d in 2 divided doses for 7 days
Microsporidiosis	*Microsporidium* species	Albendazole 400 mg q12h for 3 weeks
Cyclosporiasis	*Cyclospora* species	SXT 160–800 mg q6h for 10 days
		AIDS patients: SXT 320–1600 mg q12h for 2–4 weeks, then 160–800 mg/d indefinitely
		Children: SXT 10–50 mg/kg/d in 2 divided doses for 7 days

*Treatment for salmonellosis is recommended only for severe cases, for patients aged <6 months or >50 years or for those with prostheses, valvular heart disease, severe atherosclerosis, malignancy, or uremia.
† Discontinue the offending agent
EHEC = Enterohemorrhagic *E. coli*; EIEC = Enteroinvasive *E. coli*; EPEC = Enteropathogenic *E. coli*; ETEC= Enterotoxigenic *E. coli*; SXT = sulfamethoxazole–trimethoprim.

1% to 3% of patients may become chronic fecal carriers of *S. typhi*. The fluoro-quinolones or ampicillin (for ampicillin-sensitive strains) may be used to attempt eradication of the chronic carrier state in selected individuals (e.g., health care workers, food preparers). Avoiding contaminated food and water supplies can prevent typhoid fever. Several vaccines for typhoid fever are available, and have an efficacy of approximately 70% to 80%. In the United States, vaccination is given most often to travelers to areas in which *S. typhi* is endemic, which includes most tropical destinations.

Campylobacter

Before the 1970s, when selective culture media simplified the isolation of several enteropathogens, infection with *Campylobacter* was thought to be unusual. It is now recognized as the most common cause of bacterial gastroenteritis in the developed world. An estimated 2 million to 4 million cases occur every year in the United States, with a summer–fall seasonality (14). *Campylobacter* is by far the most common cause of bacterial gastroenteritis in young adults, causing gastroenteritis 10 times more often than does *Salmonella*. The primary animal reservoir of *Campylobacter* is the chicken, and most cases of infection with the organism are associated with undercooked poultry or cross-contamination of other foodstuffs. Contact with animals other than chickens, including kittens, also has been associated with *Campylobacter* infection. Most cases are sporadic, and large outbreaks and interpersonal spread are unusual.

Campylobacter causes an acute inflammatory colitis that is indistinguishable from that caused by *Salmonella* or other bacterial enteropathogens. Diarrhea, abdominal pain, and fever are present in most patients. The illness usually lasts from 4 to 7 days. Severe prolonged colitis that mimics inflammatory bowel disease has been reported. *Campylobacter* also has been associated with pseudoappendicitis, and in rare instances has been believed to cause appendicitis. Hepatitis and pancreatitis also have been reported infrequently in association with campylobacteriosis. Bacteremia occurs in approximately 2% of culture-confirmed cases, and immunocompromised patients are at increased risk. Additionally, *Campylobacter* is associated with the Guillain–Barré syndrome and is by far the most common identified infection preceding this syndrome, with evidence of antecedent *Campylobacter* infection found in 20% to 40% of Guillain–Barré cases (14a,14b). The overall incidence of Guillain–Barré syndrome is much lower than that of campylobacteriosis, and the individual risk of acquiring the syndrome after this enteric infection is low.

Most patients with *Campylobacter* enteritis require only supportive therapy with rehydration. In clinical trails, antimicrobial therapy has not been shown to be of benefit when given after several days of illness. However, when given at the onset of illness, antimicrobial therapy shortens the duration of illness and is clearly beneficial for patients with severe or prolonged disease, which can occur in immunosuppressed patients. *Campylobacter* is resistant to trimethoprim and most cephalosporins. Fluoroquinolones showed early promise as therapeutic agents against *Campylobacter*; however, resistance has developed during therapy and is spreading in fields in which quinolones are heavily used (e.g., animal husbandry). Azierythromycin remains the antimicrobial agent of choice for the treatment of *Campylobacter* enteritis.

Escherichia coli

E. coli is the predominant nonpathogenic bacterial species in the human intestinal flora, but some strains have developed the ability to cause gastrointestinal disease. Diarrheagenic strains of *E. coli* cause disease through a variety of mechanisms and produce varying clinical syndromes, including traveler's diarrhea, hemorrhagic colitis, HUS, persistent watery diarrhea in infants, and persistent diarrhea (15). The genetic information responsible for the pathogenesis is often carried by plasmids or phages. During the past decade, the detailed pathogenic mechanisms associated with specific stains of *E. coli* have been perceived, but their details are beyond the scope of this chapter (15). We focus on the most common and clinically significant diarrheal syndromes caused by *E. coli*.

Enterotoxigenic *E. coli* strains are responsible for more than one third of cases of traveler's diarrhea. They produce diarrhea by the elaboration of a toxin that induces secretion of fluid and electrolytes by the small bowel. The strains are noninvasive and noninflammatory and are acquired by ingesting contaminated food and water. The illness that they cause is characterized by watery diarrhea (mild or severe) that usually lasts approximately 5 days but can be prolonged (rare). The illness is usually self-limited, but antimicrobial therapy (e.g., trimethoprim–sulfamethoxazole, quinolones) has been shown to significantly shorten the duration of illness. Antimotility agents used with antibiotics also have been shown to decrease the frequency of stools. (For treatment of traveler's diarrhea, see section on Diarrhea in Travelers below.)

E. coli 0157:H7 and other enterohemorrhagic *E. coli* strains have gained prominence in the past 15 years by producing a severe syndrome in children that is characterized by bloody diarrhea and subsequent HUS (16). These strains also produce a nonbloody diarrhea and a hemorrhagic colitis (which may be severe, particularly in the elderly) without HUS. *E. coli* 0157:H7 and related stains produce two toxins that account for the intestinal and systemic pathogenesis of disease. Cattle are the primary reservoir for *E. coli* 0157:H7, and most cases of illness caused by the organism can be traced to the consumption of contaminated beef or of food products contaminated with bovine fecal matter. Interpersonal spread of the organism also has been documented. Diagnosis of *E. coli* 0157:H7 gastroenteritis is made by isolating the organism from stool.

Managing the illness caused by *E. coli* 0157:H7 and related strains consists of supportive care. Antimicrobial therapy has not been shown to shorten the duration of illness, and there are inconclusive reports that suggest that antimicrobial therapy may increase the risk for HUS. Pending large clinical trails, no rational recommendation can be made for or against antimicrobial therapy. However, dialysis instituted early in the course of *E. coli* 0157:H7–related HUS may provide a survival advantage, increasing the importance of early recognition of the syndrome. Recent reports have indicated that the type of grain given to cattle in feedlots may dramatically increase the amount of *E. coli* 0157:H7 in the animals' intestines, and many efforts are underway to prevent or minimize this. Preventing *E. coli* 0157:H7–related illness by thoroughly cooking meat and avoiding contamination of beef or other food products is also critical and is receiving increasing government attention.

Two other types of pathogenic *E. coli* deserve brief mention. Enteroinvasive *E. coli* strains are pathogenically related to *Shigella* (*see* section below) and produce a similar colitis/dysentery syndrome. Enteropathogenic *E. coli* strains are a heterogeneous subset of pathogenic *E. coli* strains. They have been shown to be responsible for large outbreaks of diarrhea in both the developed and developing world. Management of diarrhea caused by either of these types is similar to that for diarrhea caused by other bacterial enteropathogens. Decisions about the use of antimicrobial therapy for disease caused by these types of *E. coli* are based on the severity of illness at presentation and the characteristics of the host.

Vibrio cholerae

Cholera is a scourge of antiquity and an infection of immense historical significance that remains a major public health issue today. The seventh cholera pandemic, caused by the 01 El Tor strain of *V. cholerae*, began in 1961 and continues today. The World Health Organization (WHO) estimates that more than 3 million cases have occurred in the past 40 years (17). The Western Hemisphere was free of cholera for almost 100 years, but the disease has gained a foothold in the past decade, spreading from the coast of Peru to other areas of South and Central America (18). In the United States, cases have been seen in travelers and in consumers of raw food imported from South America. Cholera causes an acute and explosive diarrhea that can lead rapidly to loss of up to 10% of the body's fluids and electrolytes. *V. cholerae* produces a toxin that acts on the enterocytes of the small bowel, causing derangement of the normal handling of solute and water, leading to hypersecretion of fluid and electrolytes. The resultant voluminous "rice water" diarrhea can lead to dehydration and death. The diagnosis is made by isolating the organism from the stool. The use of oral rehydration solutions, which contain glucose and electrolytes, has been associated with a marked decrease in morbidity and mortality from cholera. Intravenous or oral rehydration is the mainstay of therapy, along with use of antibiotics (particularly fluoroquinolones).

V. parahemolyticus is a worldwide cause of food-borne illness, and is the most common pathogen associated with food in Japan (19). *V. parahemolyticus* is a salt water–loving organism, and the illness it causes is associated with the consumption of seafood and exposure to salt water. In addition to producing gastrointestinal illness, *V. parahemolyticus* causes the infection of wounds exposed to salt water and can produce a severe sepsis syndrome, particularly in patients with liver disease or other impaired host defenses.

Shigella

Shigella species differ from other common bacterial enteropathogens because it lacks an animal reservoir and relies instead on human-to-human contact or human fecal contamination for spread of the infection. As a result, *Shigella* infection is more common in areas of the world where living conditions are poor and where the infrastructures for handling human waste and delivering safe drinking water are insufficient. In the United States, children who attend daycare facilities and homosexual men are identified as risk groups for shigellosis. There are four species of *Shigella*—*Shigella dysenteriae*, *S. flexneri*, *S. boydii*, and *S. sonnei*)—all of which vary in their epidemiology and pathogenicity. *S. sonnei* is the major species that causes illness in the developed world.

Shigella causes a spectrum of enteritis that ranges from mild self-limited disease to fulminant dysentery. *Shigella* requires the smallest inoculum size (102 organisms) to cause infection of any of the major bacterial enteropathogens. In addition to severe dysentery, HUS, and bacteremia, obtundation and seizures are known complications of shigellosis. The diagnosis can be made by isolating the organism in stool culture. Empirical therapy should be considered when patients have dysentery. The other common infectious cause of dysentery syndrome in travelers and immigrants is amebiasis, which should be ruled out, particularly in adults. Resistance to antibiotics (e.g., ampicillin, trimethoprim–sulfamethoxazole, fluoroquinolones [less common]) among *Shigella* species is increasing around the world (20). If determining the antimicrobial resistance of an isolate is not possible, patients who fail to respond to antibiotic treatment within 48 hours should be switched to another antibiotic. There is no effective vaccine for *Shigella*.

Yersinia enterocolitica

Infection with *Yersinia enterocolitica* most often leads to inflammatory diarrhea but also can produce septicemia, arthritis, and abdominal pain that mimics appendicitis (21). In the United States, infection with *Y. enterocolitica* is less common than infection with the bacterial enteropathogens discussed previously and accounts for approximately 1% of bacterial gastroenteritis cases. Swine are an important animal reservoir for *Y. enterocolitica*, and the consumption of undercooked pork or chitterlings (raw pork intestines) is an important epidemiologic clue to the presence of *Y. enterocolitica*. Cows and other animals are also hosts for the organism, and its spread from dogs to humans and from humans to humans have been documented.

The diarrheal illness caused by *Y. enterocolitica* is similar to that caused by *Salmonella* or *Campylobacter*. Pseudoappendicitis is more common in older children and in adults. In clinical trials, antimicrobial therapy was not helpful in self-limited cases of *Y. enterocolitica* infection in otherwise healthy individuals; however, in most studies, antibiotic therapy was not begun until several days into the illness. Antibiotic therapy is indicated for severe presentations, patients with medical complications, or cases of septicemia. *Y. enterocolitica* is resistant to ampicillin and first-generation cephalosporins and is sensitive to doxycycline, aminoglycosides, fluoroquinolones, and trimethoprim–sulfamethoxazole. Another species of *Yersinia*, *Y. pseudotuberculosis*, is an animal pathogen that occasionally produces diarrheal illness in humans similar to that caused by *Y. enterocolitica*.

Clostridium difficile

Clostridium difficile is harmless under normal environmental conditions in the colon, its growth suppressed by the normal colonic flora. Disruption of the normal colonic flora permits *C. difficile* to proliferate and produce cytopathic toxins that cause mild to severe diarrhea. Asymptomatic carriage of *C. difficile* is found in 7% of all patients admitted to hospitals (22). The carriage rate increases to more than 20% after hospitalization, with the organism being spread from one patient to another by the hands of health care workers. Therefore, *C. difficile* is both a community-acquired and a nosocomially acquired organism. Broad-spectrum antimicrobial agents, particularly those that are active against anaerobes, are the most common causes of alterations in the ecology of the colon that lead to *C. difficile* disease. The illness can develop after a single dose of antibiotics or at any time up to 2 months after cessation of therapy. Chemotherapeutic agents that alter the intestinal flora also have been implicated in *C. difficile* disease. Not all patients who carry *C. difficile* and receive antibiotics develop diarrhea, and most mild cases of antibiotic-associated diarrhea (75%) are not due to *C. difficile* but instead result from alterations in the flora or other effects of the antibiotics that are given.

Clinically, *C. difficile* diarrhea ranges from a mild, self-limited illness to the severe but less frequent syndrome of pseudomembranous colitis (Fig. 7.3). The latter condition is characterized by the development of whitish yellow plaques in the colon that can become confluent (23), and it can lead to colonic perforation, necrosis, and death. Patients with this syndrome are often febrile

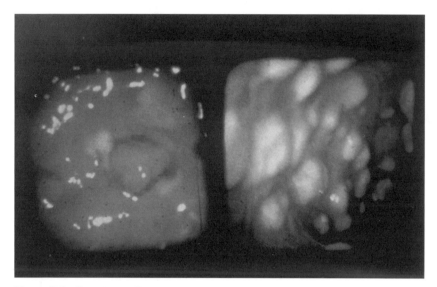

Figure 7.3 *Clostridium difficile* colitis.

and appear ill. Although occurring in a minority of patients, extreme leukocytosis (with peripheral white blood cell counts over 40,000 cells/mm^3) can be an important clue to the presence of pseudomembranous colitis, particularly in elderly patients. The diagnosis of *C. difficile* diarrhea is made by the demonstration of toxin in a patient's stools; several different assays exist for this purpose. Isolating the organism from the stool of symptomatic patients is considered presumptive but not definitive evidence of infection, because carriage of *C. difficile* is not always associated with illness. Fecal leukocytes may or may not be present (sensitivity 30%–60%). Endoscopic examination can be used to establish a diagnosis of pseudomembranous colitis, and the findings in computed axial tomographic scans of the abdomen are often characteristic.

Treatment for mild cases of *C. difficile* diarrhea can consist of simply stopping the infecting organism, if possible. In more severe cases, antibiotic therapy with oral vancomycin or oral or intravenous metronidazole should be used. Oral vancomycin is not absorbed and is effective in inhibiting the growth of *C. difficile*. An oral dose of 125 mg given four times daily is recommended except for the most severe cases. Oral vancomycin therapy is expensive compared with metronidazole and has been linked to colonization of vancomycin-resistant enterococcus. Intravenous vancomycin does not reach measurable levels in the bowel and is not an effective treatment agent for colitis caused by *C. difficile*. Metronidazole is also active against *C. difficile* and has the advantages of lower cost and availability for intravenous delivery in patients who cannot take anything by mouth and/or have ileus. Clinical trials of vancomycin and metronidazole in severe cases of *C. difficile* diarrhea have been inconclusive; many experts favor oral vancomycin for the sickest patients; combinations of oral vancomycin and intravenous metronidazole have been used in severe cases. Oral vancomycin has not been shown to provide any advantage in less severe cases of *C. difficile* diarrhea, and most authorities recommend metronidazole as a cheaper alternative. Probiotic therapy with *Saccharomyces boulardii* or *Lactobacillus* has shown promise in clinical trials but has not gained widespread popularity. Many experts recommend against anti-motility agents because they may prolong exposure to *C. difficile* toxin.

Relapsing *C. difficile* diarrhea occurs in 10% to 20% of patients (22). Neither vancomycin nor metronidazole is active against *C. difficile* spores. If the colonic milieu remains altered after successful therapy, *C. difficile* diarrhea may recur after sporulation and the production of metabolically active toxin-producing bacteria. Multiple relapses are a particular problem in the elderly, perhaps because of the tendency for spores to persist in diverticula and to resist being removed from the bowel through normal peristalsis. Therapeutic approaches to relapsing *C. difficile* diarrhea have included long tapering courses of oral van-comycin and probiotic therapy (*see* Table 7.2) (24).

Protozoa

Entamoeba histolytica

Entamoeba histolytica is an enteric protozoan parasite that causes amebiasis, the third most deadly parasitic disease worldwide (after malaria and schistosomiasis). Infection with *E. histolytica* is highly endemic in Africa, South America, Mexico, and southern Asia. The infection is transmitted through contaminated food and water, and less frequently by direct fecal–oral contact with the cyst form of the organism. Although most infected individuals are asymptomatic, *E. histolytica* causes a variety of intestinal and extraintestinal syndromes. The most common clinical presentation is a noninvasive colitis that is characterized by nonspecific abdominal pain and loose stools. Amebic colitis, which is caused when *E. histolytica* trophozoites invade intestinal epithelial cells, is characterized by abdominal pain and tenderness, with bloody stools and without fecal leukocytes. Fulminant amebic colitis, which may lead to toxic megacolon, is infrequent but can be seen in malnourished patients, in children, and in patients taking corticosteroids. This syndrome is characterized by fever, an outward appearance of toxicity, profuse diarrhea, and occasionally intestinal perforation. Intestinal amebiasis can be diagnosed by identifying amebic trophozoites and/or cysts in the stool; several stool specimens are often required for this and at least three stool specimens should be examined before amebiasis is ruled out. Additionally, *E. histolytica* must be differentiated from nonpathogenic intestinal protozoans. The colitis caused by *E. histolytica* is inflammatory, but fecal leukocytes may be few or absent because the amebic form of *E. histolytica* can lyse host inflammatory cells.

The most common extraintestinal site of amebiasis is a liver abscess. Amebic liver abscess can present acutely, with fever, abdominal pain, and weight loss, or can have a more insidious course. Amebic liver abscesses most often occur from 2 to 6 months after exposure to *E. histolytica* and can be seen in refugees and immigrants with relatively remote exposures. Other extraintestinal sites of infection are rare and include brain abscesses, pleural and pericardial abscesses, and sites of cutaneous and genitourinary infection. Only a minority of patients with extraintestinal amebiasis have *E. histolytica* in their stool, in which cases the diagnosis of amebiasis is based on clinical suspicion, serologic findings (positive in >85% of patients with invasive infection), and imaging studies (e.g., computed tomography, ultrasound).

Treatment of amebiasis depends on the site of infection and other factors. Treatment of asymptomatic persons who pass cysts of *E. histolytica* in their stools is given only to patients who live in nonendemic areas or to those who are at high risk for colitis. A variety of luminal agents are available for treating asymptomatic persons who pass cysts of the organism, including diloxanide, paromomycin, and diiodohydroxyquin. Colitis is usually treated with a nitroimidazole (e.g., metronidazole) followed by a luminal agent to eradicate the cyst state. Metronidazole is the treatment of choice for extraintestinal amebiasis (*see* Table 7.2).

Preventing amebiasis is an important consideration in situations of crowding and poor sanitation. The simple act of boiling water eliminates cysts of *E. histolytica*; however, treating drinking water with chlorine or iodine is ineffective.

Giardia lamblia

Giardia lamblia is the most common parasitic cause of diarrhea in the developed world (25). Because most states in the United States do not mandate that giardiasis be reported, data on the incidence of the disease in this country are not highly reliable. The annual incidence is estimated to be 50 cases per 100,000 population, with toddlers and young adults the major groups at risk. Infection is passed from person to person and by ingesting contaminated water or food. Outbreaks of waterborne *G. lamblia* infection have been well described and usually involve the ingestion of untreated river, lake, well, and occasionally municipal water. Giardiasis occurs in travelers, accounting for approximately 5% of cases of traveler's diarrhea. *G. lamblia* is resistant to chlorine and can be reliably removed from water only by ultrafiltration. Person-to-person transmission of the organism has been demonstrated most often in daycare centers. *G. lamblia* can be found in many large mammals; however, because the organism is difficult to subtype, the role of these animal reservoirs is unknown.

G. lamblia causes a noninflammatory diarrhea characterized by watery stools, cramping, flatulence, and little or no fever. The illness usually lasts approximately 1 week but can persist in immunocompromised patients, including those with IgA deficiency who may otherwise not show manifestations of immunodeficiency. The diagnosis is made by demonstrating the organism in a wet mount of a fresh stool specimen (Fig. 7.4). Some symptomatic patients may shed few organisms, and empirical therapy is warranted for patients in whom there is a high index of suspicion of giardiasis but who have negative stool specimens. Standard therapy consists of metronidazole in a dose of 250 to 750 mg orally thrice daily for 7 to 10 days. Lower doses are associated with treatment failure, and higher doses are associated with increased side effects. Other treatment options include quinacrine hydrochloride, furazolidone, and tinidazole (which is not available in the United States).

Microsporidia

Microsporidia are an order of small, obligate, intracellular protozoal parasites found widely in animals and in the environment. In the past decade, they have been recognized as having a role in human disease, particularly in immunocompromised patients, including those with HIV infection and/or AIDS. At least four genera are known to cause human disease: *Encephalitozoon, Enterocytozoon, Nosema,* and *Pleistophora* (26). Cases of infection are most often recognized in residents of tropical countries and in travelers. The most common symptoms are chronic diarrhea and wasting. Infection also has been rec-

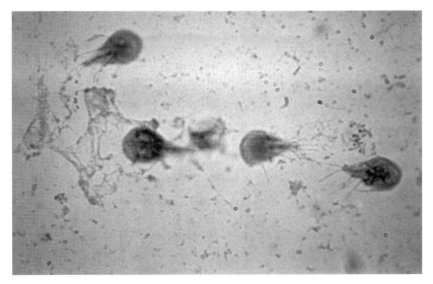

Figure 7.4 *Giardia lamblia* trophozoites in the stool.

ognized at extraintestinal sites. Diagnosis requires electron microscopy of biopsy specimens. Clearly defined therapies are lacking; albendazole has been used successfully in some cases of infection with *Enterocytozoon*.

Cryptosporidia

Cryptosporidium parvum is a protozoan parasite found throughout the world but was not known as a human pathogen until the early 1980s. It is now recognized as a cause of sporadic cases of self-limited diarrhea in healthy individuals and of intractable diarrhea in immunocompromised patients (27). Groups at risk for acquiring the organism include travelers, animal handlers, and day-care center personnel. In 1994, an outbreak of cryptosporidiosis in Milwaukee that was associated with contamination of the city's water supply affected several hundred thousand residents.

Illness caused by *C. parvum* follows the ingestion of spores and the infection of small-bowel enterocytes, leading to disruption of intestinal absorption and producing a watery, noninflammatory diarrhea. The duration of the illness is usually 10 to 14 days but can be chronic in immunocompromised patients; chronic cryptosporidial diarrhea has been well described in patients with HIV infection and/or AIDS. Cholecystitis has been reported in immunocompromised patients. Diagnosis is made by identifying oocysts in stool with a modified acid-fast stain. Treatment consists of hydration and supportive care. A variety of antimicrobial agents have been used in chronic, severe cases of cryptosporidiosis, with no consistent response.

Cyclospora

Cyclospora cayetanensis is a coccidian parasite recently recognized as a cause of acute and chronic diarrhea (28,29). Originally described in travelers and ex-patriates in Kathmandu who presented with prolonged diarrhea, *Cyclospora* has been linked to outbreaks of diarrhea in the United States associated with imported fruit, particularly berries. The clinical illness caused by *Cyclospora* is characterized by diarrhea, nausea, and weight loss that can persist for months or weeks if left untreated. Treatment with trimethoprim–sulfamethoxazole has been successful. An alternative therapy for patients with sulfa allergy has not been established (30).

Food-Poisoning Syndromes

Food poisoning can result from the ingestion of a variety of infectious agents, preformed bacterial toxins, and noninfectious substances, and it encompasses many clinical presentations. For the purposes of this section, food poisoning is defined as any illness occurring within 48 hours of food ingestion. Not all food poisoning syndromes produce gastrointestinal symptoms, and many (e.g., scombroid, ciguatera, shellfish, botulism) present with primarily neurological syndromes that are beyond the scope of this chapter.

Bacteria cause 92% of food-borne illnesses for which a cause is identified (31). In the United States, most cases of food-borne illness go unreported, and the incidence of food-borne gastroenteritis is based on estimates. In 1996, the Centers for Disease Control and Prevention began active surveillance for *Campylobacter*, *E. coli* 0157:H7, *Listeria*, *Salmonella*, *Shigella*, *Vibrio*, *Yersinia*, *Cyclospora*, and *Cryptosporidium* in specific regions of the United States (the data include illnesses with onset after 48 hours). The incidence of illness was highest for *Campylobacter* (24.7 cases per 100,000 population), followed by salmonellosis (13.7) and shigellosis (7.8) (32). The major risk factors for food-borne disease are improper food storage and preparation, most often related to the temperature at which the food is stored before preparation or the temperature at which it is held before consumption after being prepared. Poor personal hygiene of the food preparer, inadequate cooking, and contaminated equipment (including cross-contamination of food-preparation surfaces) are also important risk factors. Food poisoning syndromes are often suspected by patients who present with gastrointestinal illness. The presence of similar symptoms in two or more people who have consumed the same food should raise suspicion for food poisoning.

Food poisoning syndromes can be categorized by incubation time and symptoms, such as the presence or absence of vomiting. Gastrointestinal symptoms that occur within 6 hours of food ingestion suggest the presence of a preformed bacterial toxin, such as those produced by *Staphylococcus aureus* or *Bacillus cereus*, or a chemical substance. Both *S. aureus* and *B. cereus* proliferate and produce toxins under conditions of improper food storage. Syndromes of food poisoning from both *S. aureus* and *B. cereus* present with prominent nausea and vomiting. *S. aureus* food poisoning occurs when food is contaminated with enterotoxin-producing strains of staphylococci under conditions favoring growth of the bacteria and with time for accumulation of enough toxin to produce illness. Because *S. aureus* enterotoxins are relatively heat stable, proper cooking is not protective against disease. Vomiting is the predominant symptom, but diarrhea and fever also can occur. The diagnosis is suggested by the history and time frame of illness occurrence and can be confirmed by isolating a toxin-producing strain of *S. aureus* from the suspected food. Large outbreaks of illness caused by *S. aureus* food poisoning have been well documented. Custards, other egg products, and potato salads are among the foods most commonly associated with staphylococcal food poisoning. *B. cereus* poisoning is similar to that caused by *S. aureus* and is frequently associated with the consumption of fried rice.

The differential diagnosis of short-incubation food poisoning also includes Norwalk-like viral gastroenteritis (discussed previously). The incubation period for this illness is usually longer than that for food poisoning caused by *S.*

aureus or *B. cereus* (usually >8 hours), and diarrhea is usually a prominent feature of the illness. Heavy-metal ingestion can produce upper intestinal symptoms within an hour of ingestion. Zinc ingestion caused by improper storage of acidic beverages in galvanized containers has been reported. Faulty fluoridation that results in high fluoride levels also has been shown to produce nausea and vomiting. Ingestion of poisonous mushrooms and raw fish containing helminths are also included in the differential diagnosis.

The onset of nausea, vomiting, and abdominal pain within 8 to 16 hours after ingestion of food suggests illness caused by the ingestion of preformed toxins from *Clostridium perfringens* or *B. cereus*. The longer incubation time results from the production of toxins after the ingestion of food. Food poisoning caused by *C. perfringens* typically presents with abdominal cramping and non-inflammatory diarrhea with little or no vomiting. The diagnosis of *C. perfringens* food poisoning is difficult to make because the organism is normally present in the intestinal flora. The diagnosis is based on the isolation of the toxin from stool. Food poisoning caused by *C. perfringens* resembles *B. cereus* food poisoning of long incubation.

Diarrhea related to food-borne infection that occurs with an incubation period of more than 16 hours is usually due to the bacterial enteropathogens discussed above, including *Salmonella, Campylobacter, E. coli, Yersinia,* and *V. parahemolyticus.*

The management of food-borne gastroenteritis consists primarily of rehydration and supportive care. Treatment issues for bacterial pathogens have been discussed previously. Food-borne illnesses are largely preventable through proper handling, storage, and preparation of food.

Diarrhea in Travelers

A wide variety of enteropathogens cause diarrhea in travelers, including *Salmonella, Shigella, E. coli, Campylobacter,* rotavirus, and protozoan parasites. In the developing world, these enteric pathogens circulate in the community and, at times, are isolated from both symptomatic and asymptomatic subjects. Travelers are at increased risk for developing infectious gastroenteritis because they typically lack immunity to the local enteropathogens and are often exposed to infection via contaminated food or water. The increased incidence of bacteria and parasites in travelers should prompt a more aggressive approach should diarrhea or other gastrointestinal symptoms develop, especially if these are severe or chronic.

Enterotoxigenic *E. coli* is the most common cause of diarrhea in travelers, followed by *Salmonella, Shigella,* and viral pathogens (33). *G. lamblia* is responsible for approximately 5% of cases of traveler's diarrhea, and should be suspected in patients who develop diarrhea after returning from short-term travel, have an illness characterized by bloating and flatulence, and have prolonged symptoms (>3 weeks).

In counseling travelers about diarrhea, it is important to give advice that helps them to avoid acquiring enteropathogens and to develop a strategy in case they do develop illness. Travelers should be advised to drink only bottled or boiled water (and to use such water when brushing their teeth), to eat fruits and vegetables only if they have been cooked or if they are peeled by the travelers themselves, and to avoid ice cubes. These precautions should be maintained even on the way home, because the food and water on the airplane or on other transportation may be prepared locally. Travelers also should be advised that handheld filtration systems and purification tablets do not always work and should not be considered reliable protection against diarrhea.

Experts in travel medicine advise presumptive therapy in the event of diarrhea. The traveler is given a prescription for an antibiotic (usually a quinolone, trimethoprim–sulfamethoxazole, or doxycycline) and is instructed to begin taking the antibiotic together with an antimotility agent if diarrhea develops. This strategy is effective for diarrhea caused by enterotoxigenic *E. coli*, the most common pathogen responsible for traveler's diarrhea. Persistent fever or bloody stools should prompt the traveler to seek medical attention. Use of antibiotics to prevent diarrhea may be associated with side effects, may contribute to the pool of resistant pathogens worldwide, may put the traveler at increased risk for some pathogens owing to the disturbance of the normal flora, and is generally not recommended.

Bismuth sulfates (e.g., Pepto-Bismol) work by coating the intestine, preventing bacterial adherence and colonization, and inhibiting production of bacterial toxin. They are effective only if taken at least four or five times per day, which most travelers find inconvenient.

Chronic Diarrhea

A large number of conditions, both infectious and noninfectious, can lead to chronic diarrhea, which is defined as diarrhea that persists for more than 4 weeks. Patients with chronic diarrhea can be subclassified further according to whether or not they have malnutrition and/or blood in their stool. Patients with chronic diarrhea who do not have malnutrition but who do have blood in their stool should be evaluated for a colonic neoplasm or parasite-associated conditions, such as ameboma, whipworm colitis, chronic campylobacteriosis, and schistosomiasis. Inflammatory bowel disease also should be considered.

Patients without blood in the stool but with signs or symptoms of malnutrition usually have an underlying malabsorption syndrome, which may stem from a variety of conditions. Among the infectious causes of malabsorption syndromes are tropical sprue, bacterial overgrowth syndrome, and several parasites, including *G. lamblia, Strongyloides stercoralis, Capillaria,* and *Cryptosporidium.* Some cases of filariasis and intestinal psuedo-obstruction from Chagas' disease can cause lymphatic obstruction that can lead to chronic diarrhea. The term *tropical enteropathy* (or *sprue*) has been used to describe a syndrome of malabsorption and minor intestinal mucosal abnormalities seen in otherwise healthy subjects from tropical countries. Tropical enteropathy is thought to be an adaptation to frequent enteric infections. The wide variety of noninfectious causes of malabsorption is beyond the scope of this chapter.

Chronic diarrhea, malnutrition, and wasting are common manifestations of HIV infection in tropical countries. Referred to as *slim disease* in many parts of Africa, this syndrome has not been linked to a single specific pathogen. It may be related to exposure to multiple enteric pathogens or to the involvement of the bowel mucosa by HIV infection. Many enteric pathogens cause diseases of more severe and prolonged course in patients with AIDS (*see* Chapter 36).

Nosocomial Diarrhea

Diarrhea that occurs after 3 days of hospitalization is by definition considered to be nosocomial diarrhea. Patients with nosocomial diarrhea are not likely to have the standard enteric pathogens, such as *Campylobacter, Salmonella,* and *Shigella.* The yield for ova and parasites is similarly low. In 15% to 20% of these patients, *C. difficile* toxin may be detected in the stool. Among hospitalized patients, it is recommended that stool cultures be made for the following groups:

- Patients who have diarrhea within 72 hours after admission
- Patients whose onset of diarrhea occurs more than 72 hours after admission and who are 65 years or older, have preexisting disease that causes alteration of organ function, have HIV infection, or have a neutropenia of 500 cells/mm^3 or less or when an outbreak of nosocomial infection is suspected
- Patients with a suspected nondiarrheal manifestation of enteric infection, such as erythema nodosum, mesenteric lymphadenitis, polyarthritis, or fever of unknown origin (34).

Additionally, testing for *C. difficile* toxin is an important part of the work-up for diarrhea (35).

Summary

In the United States, most cases of gastroenteritis and diarrhea in adults are self-limited. A careful history helps identify patients at risk for complications of bacterial or protozoal infection. Specific antimicrobial therapy is indicated for some pathogens, and a subset of patients may benefit from therapy for bacterial pathogens that cause self-limited disease in normal healthy adults.

REFERENCES

1. **Cook GC.** Diarrhoeal disease: a world-wide problem. *J R Soc Med.* 1998;91:192–4.

2. **DuPont HL.** Guidelines on acute infectious diarrhea in adults: the Practice Parameters Committee of the American College of Gastroenterology. *Am J Gastroenterol.* 1997;92: 1962–75.

3. **Elmer GW, Surawicz CM, McFarland LV.** Biotherapeutic agents: a neglected modality for the treatment and prevention of selected intestinal and vaginal infections [See comments]. *JAMA.* 1996;275:870–6.

4. **Roffe C.** Biotherapy for antibiotic-associated and other diarrhoeas. *J Infect.* 1996; 32:1–10.

5. **Caul EO.** Viral gastroenteritis: small round structured viruses, caliciviruses and astroviruses. Part II: The epidemiological perspective. *J Clin Pathol.* 1996;49:959–64.

6. **Kapikian A.** Overview of viral gastroenteritis. *Arch Virology.* 1996;12:7–19.

7. **Jin S, Kilgore PE, Holman RC, et al.** Trends in hospitalizations for diarrhea in United States children from 1979 through 1992: estimates of the morbidity associated with rotavirus. *Pediatr Infect Dis J.* 1996;15:397–404.

8. **Vesikari T.** Rotavirus vaccines against diarrhoeal disease. *Lancet.* 1997;350:1538–41.

9. **Vought KJ, Tatini SR.** *Salmonella enteritidis* contamination of ice cream associated with a 1994 multistate outbreak. *J Food Prot.* 1998;61:5–10.

10. **Bruce-Jones PN, Allen SC.** Variations of invasive *Salmonella* infection in elderly people. *Br J Clin Pract.* 1996;50:470–1.

11. **Aliaga L, Mediavilla JD, Lopez de la Osa A, et al.** Nontyphoidal *Salmonella* intracranial infections in HIV-infected patients. *Clin Infect Dis.* 1997;25: 1118–20.

12. **Rankin SC, Coyne MJ.** Multiple antibiotic resistance in *Salmonella enterica* serotype enteritidis [Letter]. *Lancet.* 1998;351:1740.

13. **Waiz A.** The new quinolones in the treatment of diarrhoea and typhoid fever. *Drugs.* 1995;49(Suppl 2):132–5.

14. **Stutman HR.** *Salmonella, Shigella,* and *Campylobacter:* Common bacterial causes of infectious diarrhea. *Pediatr Ann.* 1994;23:538–43.

14a. **McCarthy N, Giesecke J.** Incidence of Guillain-Barre syndrome following infection with *Campylobacter jejuni. Am J Epidemiol.* 2001;153:610–4.

14b. **Mishu B, Blaser MJ.** Role of infection due to the *Campylobacter jejuni* in the initiation of Guillain-Barre syndrome. *Clin Infect Dis.* 1993;17:104–8.

15. **Nataro JP, Kaper JB.** Diarrheagenic *Escherichia coli* [Published erratum appears in *Clin Microbiol Rev.* 1998 Apr;11(2):403]. *Clin Microbiol Rev.* 1998;11:142–201.

16. **Slutsker L, Ries AA, Greene KD, et al.** *Escherichia coli* O157:H7 diarrhea in the United States: clinical and epidemiologic features. *Ann Intern Med.* 1997;126: 505–13.

17. **Kuruvilla A, Jesudason MV, Mathai D, et al.** The clinical pattern of diarrhoeal illness caused by the new epidemic variant of non-O1 *Vibrio cholerae. Trans R Soc Trop Med Hyg.* 1994;88:438.

18. **Begue R, Castellares G, Hayashi K, et al.** Diarrheal disease in Peru after the introduction of cholera. *Am J Trop Med Hyg.* 1994;51:585–9.

19. **Akeda Y, Nagayama K, Yamamoto K, Honda T.** Invasive phenotype of *Vibrio parahaemolyticus. J Infect Dis.* 1997;176:822–4.

20. **Materu SF, Lema OE, Mukunza HM, et al.** Antibiotic resistance pattern of *Vibrio cholerae* and *Shigella* causing diarrhoea outbreaks in the eastern Africa region: 1994–1996 [see comments]. *East Afr Med J.* 1997;74:193–7.

21. **Currie B.** *Yersinia enterocolitica. Pediatr Rev.* 1998;19:250.

22. **Johnson S, Gerding DN.** *Clostridium difficile*-associated diarrhea. *Clin Infect Dis.* 1998; 26:1027–34.

23. **Brazier JS.** The diagnosis of *Clostridium difficile*-associated disease. *J Antimicrob Chemother.* 1998;41(Suppl C):29–40.

24. **Wilcox MH.** Treatment of *Clostridium difficile* infection. *J Antimicrob Chemother.* 1998; 41(Suppl C):41–6.

25. **Heresi G, Cleary TG.** *Giardia. Pediatr Rev.* 1997;18:243–7.

26. **Wanke CA, DeGirolami P, Federman M.** *Enterocytozoon bieneusi* infection and diarrheal disease in patients who were not infected with human immunodeficiency virus: case report and review [See comments]. *Clin Infect Dis.* 1996;23:816–8.

27. **Tzipori S, Griffiths JK.** Natural history and biology of *Cryptosporidium parvum. Adv Parasitol.* 1998;40: 5–36.

28. **Gumbo T, Gordon SM, Adal KA.** *Cyclospora*: update on an emerging pathogen. *Cleve Clin J Med.* 1997;64: 299–301.

29. **Brennan MK, MacPherson DW, Palmer J, Keystone JS.** Cyclosporiasis: a new cause of diarrhea. *CMAJ.* 1996;155:1293–6.

30. **Connor BA.** *Cyclospora* infection: a review. *Ann Acad Med Singapore.* 1997;26:632–6.

31. **Humphrey T.** Food-and milk-borne zoonotic infections. *J Med Microbiol.* 1997;46: 28–33.

32. **Hogue A, White P, Guard-Petter J, et al.** Epidemiology and control of egg-associated *Salmonella enteritidis* in the United States of America. *Rev Sci Tech.* 1997;16:542–53.

33. **Castelli F, Carosi G.** Epidemiology of traveler's diarrhea. *Chemotherapy.* 1995; 41(Suppl 1):20–32.

34. **Wood M.** When stool cultures from adult inpatients are appropriate. *Lancet.* 2001; 357:901–2.

35. **Guerrant RL, Van Gilder T, Steiner TS, et al.** Practice guidelines for the management of infectious diarrhea. *Clin Infect Dis.* 2001;32:331–50.

8

Biliary Tract Infections

Curtis J. Donskey, MD
Louis B. Rice, MD

Biliary tract infections are common causes of morbidity and mortality throughout the world. Although most of these infections are complications of gallstone disease, biliary infections in the absence of gallstones are increasingly recognized in immunocompromised and critically ill patients and as complications of biliary tract instrumentation. The clinician must distinguish infection of the biliary system from other illnesses that may have a similar presentation. Additionally, clinicians must determine whether urgent surgical or endoscopic drainage of such infections is indicated. New imaging, endoscopic, and surgical drainage techniques have improved the diagnosis and management of biliary tract infections; however, they have also increased the complexity of decision making with regard to these conditions.

Overview

The biliary system includes the gallbladder and bile ducts. In the healthy biliary system, bile is sterile. In the presence of biliary tract pathology, however, bactibilia (the presence of bacteria in the biliary system) is common. Bacteria may reach the biliary tract from the portal circulation or by ascending from the small intestine through the ampulla of Vater. Bactibilia has been demonstrated in 12% of patients who have undergone elective cholecystectomy for gallstones (i.e., *chronic cholecystitis*) (1), in approximately one third of patients with common bile duct obstruction caused by malignancy, and in up to 80%

to 90% of patients with common bile duct stones or strictures (2). Additional factors associated with bactibilia include diabetes mellitus, jaundice, advanced age, and instrumentation of the biliary tree. Bactibilia most often represents colonization rather than infection. The development of biliary tract infection generally requires obstruction of bile ducts, and the most common cause of this obstruction is gallstones.

Cholelithiasis (gallstone disease) is present in 10% to 15% of adults in the Western industrialized countries (3). Cholelithiasis increases in frequency with age and is more common in women than in men. By 75 years of age, approximately 35% of women and 20% of men in the United States have developed gallstones. Seventy-five percent of these stones are cholesterol stones and 25% are pigment stones. Risk factors for cholesterol gallstones include female gender, obesity, pregnancy, rapid weight loss, total parenteral nutrition, and certain medications (e.g., estrogens, clofibrate). Risk factors for pigment stones include chronic hemolysis, cirrhosis, and pancreatitis.

The clinical manifestations of gallstones are illustrated in Figure 8.1. Seventy-five percent of individuals with gallstones remain asymptomatic. The most common presenting symptom of cholelithiasis is biliary pain or colic, a visceral pain caused by transient or partial obstruction of the bile ducts that is not associated with inflammation or secondary infection. In a study of people with asymptomatic gallstones, the annual risk of new biliary pain was 2% within the first 5 years after gallstone diagnosis, falling to approximately 0.5% annually thereafter (4). Once biliary pain develops, the likelihood of infection and other complications of gallstone disease increases (3). Obstruction of the cystic duct results in acute cholecystitis, whereas obstruction of the common bile duct may result in cholangitis. Approximately 10% of gallstone patients have stones in the common bile duct. Although these may be asymptomatic, the incidence of serious complications (e.g., obstructive jaundice, pancreatitis, cholangitis) ranges from approximately 25% to 50%.

Acute Calculous Cholecystitis

Pathogenesis and Bacteriology

Cholecystitis refers to inflammation of the gallbladder, which may or may not be secondarily infected. In more than 90% of patients with acute cholecystitis, a gallstone obstructs the cystic duct (acute calculous cholecystitis). This obstruction leads to bile stasis and to increased intraductal pressures, with subsequent gallbladder distension, a compromised blood supply, and impaired lymphatic drainage. Damage to the gallbladder mucosa from ischemia and bile stasis promotes further inflammation through the production of inflammatory me-

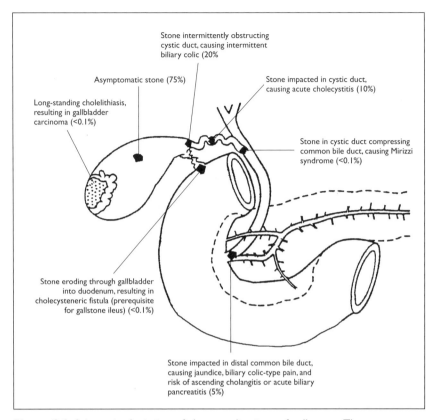

Figure 8.1 Schematic depiction of the complications of gallstones. The percentages, based on natural history data, approximate the frequency of gallstones occurring in untreated patients. As shown, the most frequent outcome is for gallstones to remain asymptomatic throughout life. Biliary colic, acute cholecystitis, and cholangitis are the most common complications; Mirizzi's syndrome, cholecystenteric fistula, and gallbladder cancer are relatively rare. (Republished with permission from Bilhartz LE, Horton JD. Gallstone disease and its complications. In *Sleisenger and Fordtran's Gastrointestinal and Liver Disease: Pathophysiology, Diagnosis, Management,* vol 2, 6th ed. Philadelphia: WB Saunders; 1998.)

diators, such as prostaglandins and lysolecithin. The pathologic changes in cholecystitis range from initial edema and congestion to neutrophilic infiltration and perforation or gangrene.

Although bacteria do not play a direct role in initiating cholecystitis, they can be cultured from approximately 50% of patients with acute cholecystitis. Early reports suggested that bacterial infection was often a late complication of cholecystitis, but a recent study found that 81% of patients who underwent cholecystectomy within 2 days of symptom onset had positive gallbladder cultures, whereas patients from whom cultures were made after symptoms of a longer duration had lower rates of positive cultures (5). The organisms isolated from bile in acute cholecystitis are usually members of the normal intestinal flora. Approximately half are aerobic gram-negative rods, approximately 30% are enterococci or streptococci, and 15% are anaerobes (5). In 70% of cases, the infection is polymicrobial. When polymicrobial infection is present, aerobic gram-negative rods are the organisms most likely to be cultured from the blood. Fungal organisms, predominantly *Candida* species, are isolated occasionally. When *Candida* species are isolated from the gallbladder of a nonneutropenic patient without evidence of candidemia or of candidiasis outside the biliary tract, cholecystectomy without antifungal therapy has been reported to be adequate therapy (6). However, severe cases of acalculous cholecystitis caused by *Candida* species have been reported (7). Consultation with an infectious diseases specialist is recommended when *Candida* species are isolated from bile cultures.

Clinical Manifestations

Most patients who present with acute calculous cholecystitis have had previous episodes of biliary pain. Biliary pain is constant, poorly localized (although usually in the epigastrium or right upper quadrant [RUQ]), and typically lasts from 1 to 6 hours. Pain that lasts longer than 6 hours suggests acute cholecystitis. As inflammation of the gallbladder develops, the pain localizes to the RUQ and becomes more severe. It is often associated with nausea and mild vomiting.

Physical examination commonly reveals fever in patients with acute calculous cholecystitis, but the temperature rarely exceeds 102°F unless complications, such as gangrene or perforation, are present. Mild jaundice is seen in 20% of patients. RUQ tenderness is detected on abdominal examination, and a palpable gallbladder is detected in one third of patients. In patients who have had multiple attacks of cholecystitis, the gallbladder is often not palpable because it has become fibrotic and unable to distend. Murphy's sign refers to pain and inspiratory arrest during palpation of the right subcostal region and is relatively specific for acute cholecystitis.

Elderly patients or debilitated patients with acute cholecystitis often present with minimal localizing signs or symptoms, and the diagnosis is often delayed. Compared with younger populations, the elderly population has a greater incidence of complications, such as perforation, gangrene, and empyema. As a result, the mortality rate from acute cholecystitis in the elderly is approximately 7% compared with 1.6% in younger persons (8).

Complications

Perforation of the gallbladder occurs in approximately 5% to 10% of acute cholecystitis cases. A small percentage of these cases involve free perforation with diffuse peritonitis. More often, a localized pericholecystic abscess occurs. Persistent fever and abdominal pain may be noted in these cases, but the signs and symptoms are not distinctive. Many cases are diagnosed late or are missed, which accounts for the 30% to 50% mortality rate among patients with free perforation.

Empyema or suppurative cholecystitis occurs when gross pus is present in the gallbladder. The reported frequency of this condition varies from 1% to 9%. Fever, leukocytosis, and a tender mass are typical; however, as with perforation, minimal signs and symptoms may be present, especially in elderly patients.

Emphysematous cholecystitis occurs when gas-forming bacteria infect the gallbladder wall and produce pockets of gas that are visible by plain radiography, ultrasonography, or computed tomography (CT) (9). Approximately two thirds of patients affected with this condition have poorly controlled diabetes. Bacteria associated with emphysematous cholecystitis include *Clostridium perfringens*, anaerobic streptococci, and *Escherichia coli*. Early cholecystectomy is indicated because of the high risk of perforation. All three of the aforementioned complications occur most commonly in the elderly, in patients with diabetes mellitus, and in patients with acalculous cholecystitis.

A cholecystenteric fistula develops when a gallstone erodes through the wall of the gallbladder and into the intestinal tract, usually at the duodenum. The presentation is similar to that of acute cholecystitis. The presence of air in the biliary tree (pneumobilia) suggests the diagnosis. Obstruction of the small bowel may occur when a large gallstone fills the lumen of the bowel, usually at the ileocecal valve.

Biliary tract infections are the most common source of liver abscess in the United States. In patients with cholecystitis, contiguous spread of infection may result in liver abscess. In patients with cholangitis, infection ascends through the biliary tree. Liver abscesses that result from a biliary source are commonly multiple.

Differential Diagnosis

Clinicians who evaluate patients with pain in the RUQ and fever must consider many conditions in addition to acute cholecystitis (Table 8.1). In one prospective study of 100 patients who had suspected acute cholecystitis, the diagnosis was correct in only two thirds of cases (4). Cholangitis must always

Table 8.1   Differential Diagnosis of Right Upper Quadrant Pain and Fever

Acute cholecystitis
Cholangitis
Myocardial infarction or ischemia
Right lower lobe pneumonia
Pulmonary embolism or infarction
Intestinal obstruction
Hepatitis
Perihepatitis (Fitz-Hugh–Curtis syndrome)
Liver abscess
Pancreatitis
Right-sided nephrolithiasis or pyelonephritis
Appendicitis
Peptic ulcer disease

be considered in the differential diagnosis because the spectrum of clinical and laboratory findings for this condition overlaps that of acute cholecystitis (Table 8.2). High fever or frank jaundice, stones in the common bile duct or a dilated common bile duct (as seen with ultrasound), and bilirubin concentration that exceeds 4 mg/dL should suggest cholangitis. Appendicitis may cause pain in the RUQ if the appendix is retrocecal or if the cecum is positioned in the subhepatic area. Acute pancreatitis is difficult to distinguish from cholecystitis because the two conditions may present similarly and the serum amylase and lipase concentrations may be nonspecifically increased in cholecystitis. However, an amylase level above 1000 U/dL should suggest pancreatitis as a concurrent or alternative diagnosis. Renal colic and acute pyelonephritis that involves the right kidney are usually easily excluded by urinalysis. Small bowel obstruction usually causes more prominent nausea and vomiting than does cholecystitis and may be excluded by plain abdominal radiography. Myocardial infarction, pulmonary embolism, and Fitz-Hugh–Curtis syndrome (perihepatitis caused by infection with *Neisseria gonorrhoeae* or *Chlamydia trachomatis*) should be considered if risk factors for these conditions are present.

Diagnosis

In a patient with suspected acute cholecystitis, judicious laboratory testing and imaging are needed to confirm the diagnosis and to exclude complications and other conditions that are part of the differential diagnosis. Initial laboratory testing for all patients with RUQ pain should consist of a complete blood count with differential; measurement of transaminase, alkaline phos-

Table 8.2   Clinical Features, Diagnosis, and Treatment of Acute Calculous Cholecystitis, Acalculous Cholecystitis, and Cholangitis

	Acute Calculous Cholecystitis	Acalculous Cholecystitis	Cholangitis
Patient demographics	Women > men; middle-age to elderly	Critically ill or postoperative setting; elderly outpatients with vascular disease; patients with AIDS	No female predominance; middle-age to elderly
Pathophysiology	Gallstone obstructing a cystic duct; ischemia and/or bile stasis caused by inflammation; secondary bacterial infection in ~50%	Ischemia and/or bile stasis caused by hypoperfusion and fasting state; secondary bacterial infection	Gallstone obstruction common; bile duct in 80%–90% (strictures, malignancy, and instrumentation cause most other cases); bile cultures positive in 80%–100%
Symptoms	Previous episodes of biliary pain in most patients; poorly localized epigastric pain initially, then moderate to severe localized right upper quadrant pain; nausea commonly present; pain lasting >6 hours suggests cholecystitis rather than uncomplicated biliary pain	Presentation similar to calculous cholecystitis but often subtle depending on patient population	Charcot's triad of fever, jaundice, and abdominal pain present in 70%–85%; abdominal pain may be mild, transient, or poorly localized; elderly patients may present with only fever or altered mental status
Physical examination	Febrile but usually <102°F unless complicated by perforation or gangrene; right subcostal tenderness with inspiratory arrest (Murphy's sign); palpable gallbladder in ~1/3; mild jaundice in 20%	Unexplained fever may be the only sign; right upper quadrant tenderness is present in only ~25%	Fever in >90%; right upper quadrant tenderness in 90%; jaundice in 60%–80%
Laboratory	Leukocytosis plus bandemia common; mild elevation of bilirubin (2–4 mg/dL), transaminases, alkaline phosphatase, and amylase common; if bilirubin >4 or amylase >1000, suspect common bile duct stone and/or cholangitis	Laboratory findings similar to those seen in acute calculous cholecystitis	Leukocytosis in most patients; bilirubin >2 in 80%; alkaline phosphatase elevated in most patients; blood cultures positive in ~50%
Diagnostic imaging	Ultrasound, cholescintigraphy (HIDA, DISIDA scans); CT in select cases	Ultrasound, CT; cholescintigraphy is of limited utility because of the high incidence of false-positive results in the critically ill	CT, transhepatic cholangiogram; ERCP is the "gold standard"; ultrasound shows common duct stones in 50% and a dilated duct in 75% (normal ultrasound does not exclude cholangitis)
Management	Cholecystectomy with intraoperative cholangiography (if common bile duct stones are present, explore or use ERCP for stone removal); give antibiotics perioperatively to all patients and on initial presentation for selected patients	Cholecystectomy; surgical or percutaneous cholecystotomy for selected patients with high surgical risk; give antibiotics in all cases	Surgical decompression, ERCP (emergent decompression for severely ill patients or those with progression on antibiotics); antibiotics in all cases

Adapted from Bilhartz LE, Horton JD. Gallstone disease and its complications. In *Sleisenger and Fordtran's Gastrointestinal and Liver Disease: Pathophysiology, Diagnosis, Management*, vol 2, 6th ed. Philadelphia: WB Saunders; 1998.

phatase, gamma-glutamyltransferase, and serum amylase activities; serum bilirubin concentration; urinalysis; and blood culture. Ultrasound or radionuclide imaging of the RUQ should be performed on all patients (*see* discussion later in this section). On the basis of the previously described findings in the differential diagnosis and of the history and findings on physical examination, selected patients should undergo cardiac isoenzyme assays, electrocardiography, abdominal plain radiography, chest radiography, pelvic examination with cervical cultures, and total abdominal ultrasonography or CT.

Laboratory findings seen in acute cholecystitis are shown in Table 8.2. Mild leukocytosis with a left shift and mild increases in alkaline phosphatase, transaminase, and amylase activities are common. The bilirubin level is increased in 20% of patients, usually into the 2- to 4-mg/dL range. Plain abdominal radiography is rarely useful in the diagnosis of acute cholecystitis. In Western countries only 10% to 25% of gallstones are visible on plain radiography; however, it may help in the diagnosis of bowel obstruction, emphysematous cholecystitis, and cholecystenteric fistula.

Ultrasonography is the most useful imaging study in the initial evaluation of patients who present with acute RUQ pain and fever (10). It is the best modality for detecting gallstones within the gallbladder, with sensitivity and specificity both exceeding 90%. Because gallstones are highly prevalent and usually asymptomatic, abdominal pain in a patient with gallstones should not be attributed to acute cholecystitis without other supportive evidence. Thickening of the gallbladder wall to more than 4 mm and collections of pericholecystic fluid seen on ultrasound examination lend support to the diagnosis of acute cholecystitis; however, these findings also may be seen in patients with ascites or hypoalbuminemia. A sonographic Murphy's sign is a much more specific sign of acute cholecystitis. This consists of focal gallbladder tenderness with the patient beneath the transducer and has a positive predictive value of more than 90% if gallstones are present. Advantages of ultrasonography include the absence of radioactivity, portability of the equipment, and the ability to evaluate for other causes of abdominal pain.

Radionuclide imaging of the biliary system (cholescintigraphy) may be used as an initial diagnostic technique for acute cholecystitis, but is most useful as an adjunct to ultrasonography (10). The technique involves intravenous administration of technetium-99m-labeled iminodiacetic acid derivatives (HIDA, DISIDA) that are rapidly excreted into the bile and on serial scans show radioactivity in the gallbladder, common bile duct, and small bowel within 30 to 60 minutes. If the diagnosis of acute cholecystitis remains uncertain (e.g., in a patient in whom gallstones are seen by ultrasonography but who has features that suggest the possibility of nonbiliary causes of pain), a normal scan essentially excludes acute calculous cholecystitis. An abnormal or positive scan may be caused by an obstruction of the cystic duct by a stone that prevents visualization of the gallbladder in the presence of excretion of imaging agent into the common bile duct and small bowel. However, false-positive results (i.e., a failure to visualize the gallbladder of a patient who does not have acute cholecystitis) often occur in severely ill patients who receive parenteral nutrition. The sensitivity of a positive radionuclide imaging test is 95% and the specificity is approximately 90%. Jaundiced patients with serum bilirubin levels as high as 20 mg/dL may be imaged with this technique only if DISIDA is used (4).

Abdominal CT is not indicated in the management of most cases of acute calculous cholecystitis. When the diagnosis is in doubt, CT scanning is useful for excluding other intra-abdominal pathology that may have a similar presentation to acute cholecystitis. CT scanning is also useful in severe cases of acute cholecystitis when complications are suspected.

Treatment

The management of acute calculous cholecystitis requires a combined medical and surgical approach. Initial medical management of all patients should include administration of intravenous fluids and pain medication. Nasogastric suctioning may be used if persistent vomiting occurs. Early surgical consultation is recommended.

Antibiotic Therapy

Antibiotic therapy is recommended in complicated or severe cases of acute cholecystitis and for perioperative prophylaxis of all patients (Table 8.3). The role of antibiotics in the initial management of uncomplicated acute cholecystitis is not clear. One retrospective study of a series of patients with acute cholecystitis suggested that preoperative administration of antibiotics did not affect the incidence of local complications (e.g., pericholecystic abscess, empyema) but did decrease the incidence of postoperative wound infections and sepsis in elderly, debilitated patients and in those with local septic complications (11). The inability of antibiotics to reach significant concentrations within the gallbladder when the cystic duct is obstructed may explain these findings. For uncomplicated acute cholecystitis, our practice is to prescribe antibiotics to all elderly patients and those with underlying chronic medical conditions. Among younger patients without chronic medical conditions, we give antibiotics to those with high fever, leukocytosis, or progression of symptoms during hospitalization. However, it is not unreasonable to give antibiotics to all patients with acute cholecystitis, because positive bile cultures are common soon after symptoms begin (5). For cases of uncomplicated disease, treatment

Table 8.3   Common Bacterial Pathogens Isolated from Biliary Tract Infections and Recommended Empirical Antimicrobial Therapy*

Infections
Cholecystitis
Cholangitis

Bacterial Isolates
Enterobacteriaceae (50%)
Enterococci (30%)
Anaerobes (15%)
Polymicrobial (70%)

Suggested Regimens
Ampicillin–sulbactam 3 g IV q6h
Piperacillin–tazobactam 3.375 g IV q6h
Ampicillin 2g IV q4–6h + gentamicin
Ampicillin 5 mg/kg IV q24h + metronidazole
Ampicillin 500 mg IV q8h
Imipenem 0.5–1.0 g IV q8h
Ciprofloxacin 200–400 mg IV q12h ± metronidazole 500 mg IV q8h
Clindamycin 600 mg q6–8h ± ampicillin 2g IV q4–6h
Cefotaxime 1–2 g IV q8h

* All empirical antimicrobial regimens should provide coverage for Enterobacteriaceae. For severely ill patients with cholecystitis or cholangitis, the initial antimicrobial regimen includes coverage of anaerobes and enterococci. The antimicrobial regimen should be adjusted appropriately based on information gained from cultures of blood and bile. The dosages listed are for healthy adults and may require adjustment for patients with abnormal renal or hepatic function. The recommended duration of antimicrobial therapy for uncomplicated cases of cholangitis is 7–10 days. Antimicrobial therapy for uncomplicated cases of cholecystitis should not be continued for more than 3–5 days postoperatively.

with a variety of antibiotics with activity against aerobic gram-negative rods has been shown to be effective. Antimicrobial activity against anaerobic intestinal flora and enterococci is not essential for the treatment of uncomplicated acute cholecystitis. Acceptable antibiotic choices for treating uncomplicated cases include piperacillin, piperacillin–tazobactam, ampicillin–sulbactam, ampicillin plus gentamicin, ciprofloxacin, and cefoxitin.

Severely ill patients and those with infectious complications such as perforation should be given antimicrobial therapy with activity against gram-negative aerobes and anaerobes, including *Bacteroides fragilis*. We also routinely include coverage of enterococci in these patients' regimens; an inhibitor combination, such as piperacillin–tazobactam, or a carbapenem, is an ideal choice. Bacterial cultures should be obtained at the time of surgery, and antimicrobial therapy may be adjusted on the basis of the results.

Surgical Therapy

Cholecystectomy is the definitive therapy for acute cholecystitis. In cases of severe and complicated disease, cholecystectomy should be performed at an early point if possible. The timing of cholecystectomy in cases of uncomplicated disease is controversial. Randomized controlled trials of early (within days following presentation) compared with delayed (>6–8 weeks) cholecystectomy for acute cholecystitis have shown that early operation is preferred in most cases because it prevents morbidity and mortality from progressive acute cholecystitis and reduces total hospitalization time and costs (12–14). Laparoscopic cholecystectomy is an acceptable alternative to open surgery in most patients with uncomplicated acute cholecystitis (4). In patients with severe concurrent medical conditions that significantly increase the risks of morbidity and mortality of surgery, percutaneous tube cholecystotomy may be an appropriate temporizing measure (15).

Acute Acalculous Cholecystitis

Acute acalculous cholecystitis refers to acute inflammation of the gallbladder in the absence of gallstones and accounts for 5% to 10% of all cases of acute cholecystitis (3). In Western industrialized countries, most cases of acalculous cholecystitis are seen in critically ill patients and after any surgery. Acalculous cholecystitis sometimes also occurs in outpatients, particularly in elderly patients with underlying vascular disease (16). Additionally, patients with AIDS may develop acalculous cholecystitis as a result of infection with a number of organisms, including cytomegalovirus, *Cryptosporidium* species, and microsporida (17). Other individuals in which acalculous cholecystitis may occur include children, those with vasculitis, and AIDS patients.

Pathogenesis and Bacteriology

In most cases of acalculous cholecystitis, the gallbladder mucosa is injured by ischemia in combination with bile stasis. Ischemia may be caused by hypoperfusion in critically ill patients or by vascular insufficiency in patients with vasculitis or atherosclerosis. Bile stasis occurs in fasting patients because the gallbladder does not receive a cholecystokinin stimulus to empty itself. As in calculous cholecystitis, inflammatory mediators such as prostaglandins promote further injury in acalculous cholecystitis. The bacteria that secondarily infect the gallbladder in this condition are similar to those seen in calculous cholecystitis, but anaerobic flora are more commonly seen. As noted previously, *Candida* species have been associated with occasional cases of acalculous cholecystitis (7). Rare cases of acalculous cholecystitis have been associated with a variety of illnesses, including typhoid fever and leptospirosis.

Clinical Manifestations

Although acute acalculous cholecystitis may have a presentation similar to that of calculous cholecystitis, the presentation is more often subtle, owing to the preponderant occurrence of the disease in elderly and postoperative or critically ill patients. RUQ tenderness is initially absent in three fourths of cases (4). Acalculous cholecystitis should always be considered when unexplained fever or leukocytosis occurs in a critically ill or postoperative patient. Delays in diagnosis contribute to the much higher rates of gangrene and perforation seen in acalculous cholecystitis compared with calculous cholecystitis; mortality rates are also higher in the former disease (10%–50% vs. 1%).

Diagnosis

Because clinical signs of acalculous cholecystitis may be subtle, a high index of suspicion for this illness is needed in patients at risk for it. Mildly increased amylase, alkaline phosphatase, or transaminase activities may be seen but are nonspecific. Ultrasonographic findings are similar to those in calculous cholecystitis (i.e., a gallbladder wall thickened to >4 mm in the absence of ascites or hypoalbuminemia, pericholecystic fluid collection, and a sonographic Murphy's sign). The sensitivity of ultrasonography for detection of acute acalculous cholecystitis ranges from 67% to 92%, and its specificity is greater than 90% (18). CT scanning is also useful for detecting acalculous cholecystitis. Radionuclide scintigraphy is of limited use in most cases owing to the high incidence of false-positive tests in fasting, critically ill patients.

Management

Antibiotic coverage for patients with acalculous cholecystitis should include aerobic gram-negative organisms and anaerobes. Urgent surgical intervention is needed because of the high risk of progression to gangrene or perforation. Open cholecystectomy is the preferred procedure in most cases. Surgical or percutaneous cholecystotomy has been used successfully in patients considered to be too unstable to undergo urgent surgical therapy.

Prevention

In patients who receive total parenteral nutrition, the use of intravenous cholecystokinin to promote gallbladder contraction has been shown to reduce the formation of gallbladder sludge, which is a risk factor for acalculous cholecystitis (19). Daily cholecystokinin administration in critically ill patients has been proposed as a means of preventing acalculous cholecystitis. The effectiveness of this measure has not been established.

Cholangitis

The term *cholangitis* refers to inflammation of the biliary ducts, which may be caused by infection or mediated immunologically (e.g., primary sclerosing cholangitis). A wide variety of infectious agents have been associated with cholangitis, including bacteria, parasites, viruses, and fungi. This chapter focuses primarily on acute bacterial cholangitis.

Pathogenesis and Bacteriology

As in acute cholecystitis, bile duct obstruction plays an essential role in the development of bacterial cholangitis, and most cases are associated with gallstones. In 80% to 90% of cases, a gallstone obstructs the common bile duct (3). In most of the remaining cases, obstruction of the common bile duct is caused by malignancy, biliary strictures, or instrumentation. Rare cases are caused by congenital abnormalities of the bile ducts, parasites, or sclerosing cholangitis. Cholangitis occurs much more commonly in patients with biliary obstruction from gallstones or strictures than in patients with malignant obstruction. Obstruction results in increased bile stasis, which promotes growth of the bacteria that colonize the bile ducts, and intraluminal pressure, which promotes entry of these organisms into the bloodstream.

The bacteria isolated from the bile of patients with acute cholangitis are similar to those associated with bacterial colonization of the biliary tree and that seen with acute cholecystitis. Infections are often polymicrobial. Gram-negative aerobic bacteria are the most common organisms isolated, with *E. coli* and *Klebsiella* species accounting for most isolates. *Enterococcus* species are commonly isolated from bile cultures; however, they are not commonly recovered from blood cultures. Anaerobic bacteria are cultured from bile in up to 40% of cases of cholangitis, usually as part of a polymicrobial infection. Positive blood cultures are seen in approximately 50% of cases of cholangitis; in most such cases, gram-negative rods are isolated. In hospitalized patients or in those who have undergone instrumentation of the biliary tract, infection with more resistant organisms is common. As in cholecystitis, *Candida* species are occasionally associated with cholangitis.

Endoscopic retrograde cholangiopancreatography (ERCP) is used more commonly in the management of biliary tract diseases such as gallstones and obstruction than in cholangitis. This intervention may introduce intestinal flora into the biliary tract and promote the dissemination of bile bacteria through the blood (20). Postprocedural biliary tract sepsis is a serious complication associated with ERCP; enteric flora and *Pseudomonas aeruginosa* are the organisms commonly found.

Clinical Manifestations

Acute cholangitis has a wide range of clinical presentations, from a mild illness that may be self-limiting to a fulminant illness with septic shock (4,21). The classic clinical presentation of cholangitis includes Charcot's triad of fever and chills, jaundice, and RUQ pain; however, the complete triad is seen in only 70% to 85% of patients (*see* Table 8.2). Fever occurs in more than 90% of cases. Jaundice is seen in 60% to 80% of cases. Abdominal pain is described by approximately 70% of patients but may be mild and is not always localized to the RUQ. Elderly or debilitated patients may present only with fever or altered mental status as an indication of illness. In contrast with acute cholecystitis, cholangitis is seen as often in men as in women.

Differential Diagnosis

The differential diagnosis of cholangitis includes the same previously discussed entities in the differential diagnosis of cholecystitis (*see* Table 8.1) as well as other illnesses associated with fever and jaundice. The abdominal pain associated with cholangitis is often less severe than that of acute cholecystitis, whereas fever and other signs of systemic illness are often more pronounced. Liver abscess must be considered in the differential diagnosis of cholangitis but also may occur concurrently as a complication of cholangitis. Jaundice associated with sepsis caused by gram-negative or -positive bacteria (the *hepatopathy of sepsis*) also must be considered in the differential diagnosis. In cholangitis, systemic infection results in increased serum levels of conjugated bilirubin caused by a defect in the excretion of conjugated bilirubin from hepatocytes (22). Other infectious diseases associated with fever and jaundice (e.g., viral hepatitis, malaria, babesiosis, leptospirosis, typhoid fever) must be considered if relevant risk factors are present.

Diagnosis

Initial laboratory testing of patients with suspected cholangitis should include assays of alkaline phosphatase, transaminase enzymes, bilirubin, and amylase; urinalysis; a complete blood count with differential; and blood cultures. As in cholecystitis, other selected tests should be ordered on the basis of other illnesses suspected in the differential diagnosis. Typical laboratory findings in cholangitis are shown in Table 8.2. The bilirubin level is increased in more than 80% of patients. A bilirubin level above 4 mg/dL suggests cholangitis rather than cholecystitis as a cause of fever and RUQ pain. Leukocytosis and an increased serum alkaline phosphatase are present in most patients.

In cholangitis, the sensitivity of ultrasonography for the detection of common bile duct stones is 50%, whereas it is 75% for the detection of dilated common bile ducts (4). The bile ducts may not be significantly dilated early in the illness and may never become dilated in patients with chronic inflammation related to sclerosing cholangitis or recurrent infection. CT is approximately 75% sensitive for the detection of common bile duct stones and is superior to ultrasound for the detection of obstructing malignancy and abscesses. ERCP is the "gold standard" procedure for the diagnosis of common bile duct stones, with both sensitivity and specificity of 95% (4). Additionally, this technique allows therapeutic drainage at the time of diagnosis. Percutaneous transhepatic cholangiography is an alternative diagnostic technique to ERCP if the latter is unavailable or cannot be performed. Recently, magnetic resonance imaging cholangiography has been shown to be a useful method for detecting choledocholithiasis, with a sensitivity that exceeds 90% (23).

Treatment

The management of acute cholangitis usually includes both decompression of the obstructed common bile duct and antibiotic therapy. Patients with mild illness may respond to supportive measures and antibiotic therapy, allowing a delay of definitive surgical or radiologic procedures to relieve the obstruction until the acute illness is resolved. However, if the patient's clinical condition does not improve after 6 to 12 hours of antibiotic therapy, emergent decompression of the common bile duct is recommended. In recent years, endoscopic drainage techniques have become the initial procedure of choice in managing acute cholangitis. In a prospective randomized trial, initial endoscopic drainage for severe cholangitis caused by choledocholithiasis was associated with significantly lower morbidity and mortality than was initial surgical decompression (24).

When cholangitis is suspected, antibiotic therapy should be started promptly after blood specimens are drawn for culture. Initial antibiotic therapy should include an agent that is active against aerobic gram-negative rods, including *E. coli* and *Klebsiella* species. It is unclear whether antimicrobial activity directed against *Enterococcus* species and anaerobes is necessary in the initial management of patients with cholangitis. Antibiotic agents with little or no activity against these organisms (e.g., cefoperazone) have been shown to be effective in managing cholangitis. No studies have shown that a particular antibiotic regimen is superior to others in the management of cholangitis (2). Our practice is to include coverage for *Enterococcus* species and anaerobes for most patients with moderate to severe illness. Appropriate antibiotic choices for covering these organisms in addition to gram-negative rods would include piperacillin–tazobactam, imipenem, ampicillin–sulbactam, and ampicillin in combination with metronidazole and an aminoglycoside or quinolone. Antibiotic therapy usually can be directed at specific organisms when the results of blood and biliary cultures are available. Antibiotic therapy for 7 to 10 days is usually recommended, but the duration of therapy may be adjusted on the basis of the patient's clinical course and adequacy of drainage.

REFERENCES

1. **Chetlin SH, Elliott DW.** Biliary bacteremia. *Arch Surg.* 1971;102:303–7.

2. **van den Hazel SJ, Speelman GNJ, Dankert J, van Leeuwen DJ.** Role of antibiotics in the treatment and prevention of acute and recurrent cholangitis. *CID.* 1994;19: 279–86.

3. **Bilhartz LE, Horton JD.** Gallstone disease and its complications. In Feldman M, Scharschmidt BF, Sleisenger MH, eds. *Sleisenger and Fordtran's Gastrointestinal and Liver Disease: Pathophysiology, Diagnosis, and Management,* vol 2, 6th ed. Philadelphia: WB Saunders; 1998:948–72.

4. **Gracie WA, Ransohoff DF.** The natural history of silent gallstones: the innocent gallstone is not a myth. *N Engl J Med.* 1982;307:798.

5. **Claessonn BEB, Holmlund DEW, Matzsch TW.** Microflora of the gallbladder related to duration of acute cholecystitis. *Surg Gynecol Obstet.* 1986;162:531–5.

6. **Morris AB, Sands ML, Shiraki M, et al.** Gallbladder and biliary tract candidiasis: nine cases and review. *Rev Infect Dis.* 1990;12:483–9.

7. **Diebel LN, Raafat AM, Dulchavsky SA, Brown WJ.** Gallbladder and biliary tract candidiasis. *Surgery.* 1996;120:760–5.

8. **Morrow DJ, Thompson J, Wilson SE.** Acute cholecystitis in the elderly: a surgical emergency. *Arch Surg.* 1978;113:1149–52.

9. **Mentzer RM, Golden CT, Chandler JG, et al.** A comparative appraisal of emphysematous cholecystitis. *Am J Surg.* 1975;125:10–5.

10. **Saini S.** Imaging of the hepatobiliary tract. *N Engl J Med.* 1997;336(26):1889–94.

11. **Kune GA, Burdon JGW.** Are antibiotics necessary in acute cholecystitis? *Med J Aust.* 1975;2:627–30.

12. **Linden W, Sunzel H.** Early versus delayed operation for acute cholecystitis: a controlled clinical trial. *Am J Surg.* 1970;120:7–13.

13. **McArthur P, Cuschieri A, Sells RA Shields R.** Controlled clinical trial comparing early with interval cholecystectomy for acute cholecystitis. *Br J Surg.* 1975;62:850–2.

14. **Jarvinen HJ, Hastbacka J.** Early cholecystectomy for acute cholecystitis: a prospective randomized study. *Ann Surg.* 1980;191:501–5.

15. **Melin MM, Sarr MG, Bender CE, van Heerden J.** Percutaneous cholecystostomy: a valuable technique in high-risk patients with presumed acute cholecystitis. *Br J Surg.* 1995;82:1274–7.

16. **Savoca PE, Longo WE, Zucker KA, et al.** The increasing prevalence of acalculous cholecystitis in outpatients: results of a 7-year study. *Ann Surg.* 1990;211:433–7.

17. **French AL, Beaudet LM, Benator DA, et al.** Cholecystectomy in patients with AIDS: clinicopathologic correlations in 107 cases. *CID.* 1995;21:852–8.

18. **Mirvis SE, Vainright JR, Nelson AW.** The diagnosis of acute acalculous cholecystitis: a comparison of sonography, scintigraphy, and CT. *AJR.* 1986;147:1171–7.

19. **Sitzmann J, Pitt HA, Steinborn P, Pasha ZR, Sanders RC.** Cholecystokinin prevents parenteral nutrition induced biliary sludge in humans. *Surg Gynecol Obstet.* 1990;170:25–31.

20. **Westphal J-F, Brogard J-M.** Biliary tract infections: a guide to drug treatment. *Drugs.* 1999;57:81–91.

21. **Hanau LH, Steigbigel NH.** Cholangitis: pathogenesis, diagnosis, and treatment. *Curr Clin Trop Infect Dis.* 1995;25:153–78.

22. **Miller DJ, Keeton GR, Webber BL, Saunders SJ.** Jaundice in severe bacterial infection. *Gastroenterology.* 1976;71:94–7.

23. **Van DJ.** Magnetic resonance cholangiography: a field with attraction. *Gastroenterology.* 1995;108:1948–52.

24. **Lai ECS, Mok FPT, Tan ESY, et al.** Endoscopic biliary drainage for severe acute cholangitis. *N Engl J Med.* 1992;326:1582–6.

9

Hepatitis A–E

Ian Woolley, MD, MB

Arjun Venkataramani, MD, MPH

W. Henry Boom, MD

Although many viruses, including cytomegalovirus and Epstein–Barr virus, are associated with inflammation of the liver, this chapter discusses the various syndromes associated with the heterogeneous, alphabetized group of viruses A through E (Table 9.1), which are most directly associated with hepatitis. Other alphabetized viruses, such as GBV-C, TT virus, and the SEN virus seem to be agents that might be said to be "in search of a human disease" (1) and are not discussed here.

The public health consequences of viral hepatitis are evident in the burgeoning morbidity and mortality rates, the diminished quality of life, and the high health care costs associated with it. Almost 4 million Americans are positive for hepatitis C, and more than a million have hepatitis B. Furthermore, 700,000 new cases of hepatitis are reported annually, chronic liver disease claims at least 15,000 lives per year, and acute liver disease is respoonsible for approximately 300 deaths annually. Chronic viral liver disease is now the leading cause of cirrhosis, hepatocellular carcinoma, and liver transplantation.

Hepatitis A

Virology

The hepatitis A virus (HAV) is a single-stranded, nonenveloped RNA virus of the Picornaviridae family. Its lack of an envelope may make the virus more stable in bile and, hence, may enable it to be transmitted via the fecal–oral route.

Epidemiology

The HAV is excreted in human feces for up to 2 weeks before any clinical illness becomes apparent and for the same period after the onset of jaundice (2). HAV may survive and remain infectious for 3 to 10 months in water. It may be found in blood and saliva; however, this seems to be far less epidemiologically significant. Thirty-eight percent of Americans have antibody evidence of past HAV infection. Approximately 6% of cases of hepatitis A in the United States are due to travel abroad. The risk of acquiring the disease ranges from approximately 3 to 5 per 1000 population per month of stay in a country with endemic infection. Approximately 100 deaths from fulminant HAV infection occur annually. The risk of death increases with age and with coexistent liver disease. Vertical transmission does not occur.

Clinical Manifestations

The course of acute HAV is highly variable in terms of onset, associated prodrome, and associated jaundice (3). A critical determinant of the pattern of disease is age, with most affected individuals under 5 years of age having asymptomatic infection. The number of symptomatic infections increases with the age of the involved group, as does the ratio of jaundiced to nonjaundiced cases. The usual incubation period is 30 days (range 15–60 days). Prodromal symptoms (fever, fatigue, myalgias, anorexia, and headache) may occur 1 week before the onset of jaundice. Atypical symptoms, especially diarrhea, are more often seen in children than in adults. Subsequently, specific signs and symptoms of a hepatic illness (dark-colored urine, clay-colored stools, pruritus, and jaundice) develop. These may last 1 or more weeks and rarely follow a relapsing pattern. Rare (but frequently fatal) fulminant hepatitis occurs in less than 0.1% of cases. Preexisting liver disease, including chronic viral hepatitis, may be associated with more severe disease. Extrahepatic manifestations of HAV are rare, and the virus does not cause chronic hepatitis or cirrhosis.

Diagnosis

Serum transaminase enzyme activities rise rapidly during the prodromal period of HAV, with bilirubin levels peaking later. Serology is diagnostic (3). An HAV-positive IgM is almost always found at clinical presentation and may remain so for up to 1 year. There seems to be only one serotype of HAV, and the presence of antibody leads to lifelong protection against reinfection by the virus. Production of the antibody also leads to the abatement of clinical illness and infectivity. HAV-specific IgG can be used to test for past exposure and on-going protection against the virus.

Prevention

Recommendations for prophylaxis with immunoglobulin after exposure of at-risk groups to HAV apply to all close personal or household contacts of in-dex cases (2). Apart from daycare centers, there is no general indication for immunoglobulin prophylaxis in the workplace unless an outbreak with a common source, such as a food handler, is identified. Preexposure prophy-laxis for travelers should be accomplished by vaccination, except when travel is undertaken at short notice or when vaccination is contraindicated. Two in-activated (formalin-killed) vaccines (Havrix and Vaqta) are available for pre-venting hepatitis A. Both have excellent efficacy and safety profiles. They are recommended for international travelers who visit areas endemic to hepatitis A, sexually active homosexual men, injection-drug users, people with preex-isting liver disease, and children who live in communities at high risk for in-fection. Good responses to the vaccine have been documented in people with chronic liver disease and HIV infection. Two doses of vaccine given 6 months apart seems to provide adequate antibody levels for a minimum of 10 years.

Treatment

No specific therapy has been shown to be of benefit for hepatitis A.

Hepatitis B

Virology

The hepatitis B virus (HBV) is a member of the Hepadnaviridae family. These viruses are double-stranded DNA viruses with lipid envelopes.

Epidemiology

The United States has 1.25 million carriers of HBV (a prevalence of 5%), with 300,000 new infections occurring annually (4). HBV is responsible for approximately 300 deaths per year. On a worldwide basis, the pattern of disease varies. In areas endemic for hepatitis B (e.g., parts of East Asia and Africa), well over 10% of the population may be chronic carriers and most have an acute infection during their lifetime. Transmission of HBV occurs parenterally, via sexual contact, or perinatally. Those at high risk include injection-drug users, sexual partners of infected people, children of infected mothers, those who receive tattoos or body-piercings, unvaccinated health care workers, and dialysis patients.

Clinical Manifestations

The HBV may cause both an acute and a chronic infection (5). The acute illness may be asymptomatic. The classic features of malaise, fatigue, hepatic discomfort, anorexia, and nausea, followed by jaundice, dark urine, and pale stools occur after an incubation period of 45 to 160 days. A serum sickness–like illness (maculopapular rash, arthralgias, and fever) precedes clinical hepatitis in a minority of patients. Findings on examination may include jaundice, hepatomegaly with tenderness of the liver, splenomegaly, and lymphadenopathy. Abnormalities in liver function test results are similar to those seen with acute HAV infection. The clinical illness in hepatitis B typically lasts from 1 to 2 months but may last longer. Children usually have asymptomatic infection or a milder illness. Occasionally, the acute hepatitis may be prolonged or may take a relapsing course. Rarely, a fulminant, fatal hepatitis occurs.

Chronic HBV infection occurs as a consequence of 1% to 20% of cases of acute infection. Infection early in life is a clear risk factor for chronic infection; neonatal transmission seems to lead to chronic infection in most cases. Immunosupressed states also are associated with a milder initial disease and persistence of virus. Patients with chronic HBV infection can be classified broadly into two groups: 1) healthy carriers, who are usually asymptomatic, have undetectable viral replication, and have histologically inactive disease; and 2) people with detectable, high-frequency viral replication, increased transaminase enzyme activities, and histologically active disease. In the latter group, hepatitis B is likely to cause serious ensuing diseases, such as cirrhosis and hepatocellular carcinoma. The proportion of people who develop cirrhosis varies with the population studied, the duration of the infection, and possibly other factors, including coinfection with the hepatitis D virus (see section below). Extrahepatic manifestations of chronic HBV infection include glomerulonephritis and vasculitis. HBV is strongly linked with polyarteritis nodosa, and people with this disease should be routinely tested for HBV.

Diagnosis

The key to comprehending the serology of hepatitis B (Table 9.2) lies in understanding the structure of the HBV (6). The HBV has a double-shelled structure, which includes an inner core surrounded by a nucleocapsid containing the viral DNA (HBV DNA) and an outer membrane containing the hepatitis B surface antigen (HBsAg). HBsAg is produced after a successful immune response to infection or vaccination. It is the first marker of acute infection and is detected before transaminase enzyme activity increases. HBsAg usually disappears between 4 to 8 weeks after the development of jaundice, and a period of time (or "window") may elapse between the disappearance of HBsAg and the appearance of HBsAb. The major protein of the nucleocapsid is the core antigen (HBcAg), which does not circulate in the blood; however, in the development of immunity, it appears at an earlier point than does HBsAg. Therefore, IgM antibody to HBcAg may be an early marker of response to infection and may be the only detectable marker of infection during the previously mentioned "window" between the disappearance of HBsAg and appearance of HBsAb. The antibody to HBcAg is not protective against HBV; the HBV early antigen (HBeAg) is a protein cotranslated with the core antigen of the virus, and its presence in the blood is a qualitative marker of viral replication and infectivity. Serum HBV DNA is the best quantitative marker of replication of the virus.

The interpretation of serologic tests for hepatitis B has been made more complex by the discovery of a number of variant hepatitis B viruses. Several mutations have been described in different parts of the HBV genome. These include mutations in the S or pre-S regions of the genome. Those in the S region have been shown to be associated with vaccine escape by production of a mutant that is immunologically distinguishable from the antigen used in the vaccine. As a consequence, the antibodies elicited by the vaccine are not protective against the mutant virus; therefore, it is also possible that such viruses may escape the effect of passive immunization or even detection with an antibody-based detection method. The clinical significance of pre-S mutants is less clear. Pre-C or core mutations in the HBV genome affect HBeAg expression. The clinical significance of this is unclear, but patients may as a consequence have persistent HBV DNA expression despite having antibodies against HBeAg.

Prevention

The best form of prophylaxis against hepatitis B is immunization (7). According to current guidelines, candidates for vaccination include all infants, all children under 11 years of age, and individuals at increased risk for the disease.

They include people with multiple sexual partners, injection-drug users, patients who undergo hemodialysis, household and sexual contacts of infected people, health care workers, and travelers to endemic areas. Because the list of those at increased risk for HBV infection is not exclusive, there has been a trend toward universal coverage. Among immunocompetent people, a routine course of three injections (scheduled at 0, 1, and 6 months) provides immunity in 90% to 95% of cases. Instituting appropriate measures for those who do not seroconvert with vaccination but who are at high risk for hepatitis B is controversial. Alternatives to vaccination include giving a course of one of two commercially available vaccines (Recombivax and Engerix-B) or giving further or larger doses of the same vaccine. Postvaccination testing of people at high risk for HBV infection (e.g., health care workers) is worthwhile to determine appropriate prophylaxis if an exposure occurs. Revaccination in people who seroconvert after a first vaccination is not currently recommended.

Decreased exposure to a known risk factor for HBV is also important in preventing the disease and may take many forms. HBsAg-positive health care workers should be informed about the following:

• Their potential infectivity
• The need for vaccination of household or sexual contacts
• The danger of donating their organs, tissue, blood, or semen
• The need to cover wounds to prevent the transmission of HBV
• The risk of vertical or nosocomial transfer of the virus

Actively viremic health care workers should not perform invasive procedures.

The two most commonly encountered clinical situations in which passive immunization against hepatitis B is indicated are vertical transmission and needlestick injury. In the case of vertical transmission, the combination of active and passive immunization provides approximately 95% protection against the transmission of HBV. This is an important measure because of the development of chronic HBV infection in more than 90% of infected neonates. HBV-specific immunoglobulin (HBIG) in a dose of 0.5 mL should be given in the delivery room, and active vaccination with the hepatitis B vaccine should begin within a week of delivery. A similar protocol should be followed in cases of known nosocomial exposure of unimmunized or nonimmune people. In these cases, the recommended dose of HBIG is 0.06 mL/kg, which should be given as early as possible and always within the first 48 hours after exposure; however, it can still provide some benefit at least 1 week later and possibly even after. Again, active immunization should be given concurrently.

Prophylactic measures also may be taken for those with chronic hepatitis or cirrhosis. Consideration should be given to vaccinating such patients against HAV. They should be discouraged from consuming alcohol and should not be given hepatotoxic drugs if possible. Those with chronic HBV infections should be monitored for the development of cirrhosis or hepatocellular carcinoma. Screening for hepatocellular carcinoma is by annual ultrasound examination and testing for alpha-fetoprotein.

Treatment

The development of treatment options has been a relatively recent phenomenon in the management of viral hepatitis (8). The first available option was a synthetic version of a cytokine (interferon) produced in response to infection. Patients who benefit most from interferon therapy are typically HBeAg positive and have an increased alanine-aminotransferase level, low HBV DNA level, minimal fibrosis on biopsy, and have had the illness for a relatively short time. Even in such a restricted subgroup of patients, success (in terms of long-term clearance of virus and seroconversion) occurs only in 14% to 45%. Interferon therapy has multiple physical, psychological, and hematologic side effects. Other agents, such as nucleoside analogues (e.g., lamivudine, famciclovir), also have been used to treat chronic HBV infection. Because prolonged nucleoside analogue monotherapy induces drug-resistant strains of HBV, such agents should ideally be used in consultation with a hepatologist. Results of clinical trials with newer nucleoside analogues alone or in combination are awaited.

The ultimate treatment for HBV-related cirrhosis is liver transplantation; however, the rate of posttransplant infection of the donor liver is quite high without prophylaxis or preemptive treatment at the time of transplantation. Nevertheless, in approximately half of cases, recurrence of infection has no major effect on the patient's quality of life. Regimens used to decrease the risk of reinfection include the use of HBIG and nucleoside analogues. Successful transplantation in the context of fulminant HBV infection carries less of a risk of recurrence than that of transplantation for chronic hepatitis.

Hepatitis C

Virology

The hepatitis C virus (HCV) is an enveloped, single-stranded RNA virus of the Flaviviridae family. Interestingly, its molecular structure has been elucidated despite the failure to grow it in cell cultures (8). There are multiple subtypes of HCV, which are divided broadly into six families or genotypes. Additionally, variants referred to as quasispecies develop in individual patients (9). It is hypothesized that the development of quasispecies creates chronic infection and resistance to therapy.

Epidemiology

Hepatitis C is a significant human health problem, affecting 3% of the world's population (10). Rates of infection vary from 0.1% in Scandinavia and Britain to 1% to 5% in other Western European countries and the United States; higher rates (20%) occur in Egypt and other parts of the Middle East. Because well over 80% of patients infected with HCV develop chronic infection (which may lead to cirrhosis in 20% and hepatocellular carcinoma in up to 5% of those with cirrhosis), the mortality and morbidity rates that are associated with such infection are significant. However, because the natural history of hepatitis C has yet to be determined prospectively; it may take two or three decades for HCV infection to become clinically apparent.

Approximately 3.9 million U.S. citizens are infected with HCV. Additionally, the virus is responsible for 16% of cases of acute hepatitis in the United States, killing 8000 to 10,000 people annually. Although the availability of HCV testing and its use since mid-1992 have significantly reduced transmission of the virus via blood products, many people had been infected in this way before that time. The current risk of transmission of HVC is estimated to range from 0.001% to 0.010% per unit of blood. The main risk factors for HCV infection include blood (or blood factor concentrate) transfusion before testing is begun, injection-drug use, and sexual and/or household contact with an infected person. The risk of sexual transmission of HCV, even within a monogamous relationship, is estimated at 5% over a 10- to 20-year period. The risk of vertical transmission of the virus is estimated at 5%. The rate of HCV transmission by needlestick injury seems to be lower (~3%) compared with the frequency associated with HBV (up to 33%). Breastfeeding does not seem to be a risk factor for HCV transmission.

Clinical Manifestations

The HCV usually causes an insidious illness, with more than half of infected people remaining asymptomatic (10). The incubation period may vary from 2 weeks to 6 months but is typically 6 to 7 weeks. Up to 40% of infected individuals report some illness, often a mild hepatitis. The transition to chronic hepatitis is the usual pattern. Chronic hepatitis caused by HCV may be asymptomatic or associated with nonspecific symptoms, such as fatigue. Cirrhosis and hepatocellular carcinoma are common complications. Extrahepatic syndromes that are strongly associated with HCV infection include porphyria cutanea tarda, membranous glomerulonephritis, and mixed cryoglobulinemia.

Diagnosis

Serologic tests for hepatitis C include enzyme-linked immunosorbent assays
(ELISAs) and radioimmunoassays for antibodies to antigens of the virus
rather than for the virus itself (12). These serologic tests do not distinguish
acute from chronic or active from resolved disease and must be interpreted in
the context of the overall clinical picture. Newer ELISAs and radioimmunoassays for antibodies to HCV have become more sensitive and specific than
their precursors; however, false-negative and -positive results still occur. To
clarify the results of serologic testing, all positive ELISAs should be repeated;
if the repeat test is positive, then viremia should be confirmed with the HCV
RNA polymerase chain reaction (PCR) test, which provides a direct measure
of viral replication. As with all PCR testing, the HCV RNA PCR is operator
dependent; thus, for reliable results, a regional laboratory with expertise
should be used. The viral load (i.e., the number of copies of viral RNA per
milliliter of blood as estimated by the HCV RNA PCR) is of value in determining response to therapy.

The HCV genotype has been shown to predict the response to therapy;
genotyping is now an integral part of the work-up that should be performed
before instituting anti-HCV therapy. Notwithstanding, the finding of an HCV
genotype that is less responsive to therapy is not a contraindication to therapy,
although the genotype may affect the duration of therapy. Pretreatment testing—in the absence of decompensated cirrhosis—also includes a liver biopsy.
Increased activities of liver transaminase enzymes can raise the suspicion of
chronic hepatitis. However, they have little further use in the diagnosis and
management of chronic viral hepatitis because 1) they can be normal in the
presence of active liver disease, especially in immunocompromised individuals; 2) the degree of increase in enzyme activity does not correspond to activity of disease; and 3) normalization of enzyme activity with therapy does not
necessarily correlate with viral clearance.

Prevention

The great difference between preventive management for hepatitis B and C is
the absence of effective passive or active immunization for the latter, necessitating even greater emphasis on behavioral intervention (12). Counseling patients about their possible infectivity is mandatory and should include 1)
advice about sharing toothbrushes, razors, and nail clippers (hypodermic nee-
dles should never be shared); 2) the risk of sexually transmitting HCV (which
is negligible in a monogamous relationship); and 3) the possible infectivity of
blood. Alcohol consumption in any quantity should not be condoned. In
cases of needle-stick injury, a successful strategy has been to use interferon if

there is evidence of seroconversion for HCV; however, management in this situation is not standardized.

Treatment

Combination therapy with interferon and ribavirin is the standard of care for patients with chronic HCV infection (13). Newer, long-acting formulations of interferon are expected to become standard in caring for the disease in the near future. Predictors of a positive response include a younger age at the time of infection, a short duration of disease, a lower hepatitis C viral load, female gender, low body weight, the absence of significant fibrosis on liver biopsy, a low serum ferritin or hepatic iron content, and an HCV genotype other than type 1. Patients with a persistently increased ALT level and evidence of chronic hepatitis on biopsy are suitable for such therapy. At the end of a treatment course of 12 months, approximately 50% of such patients have a sustained virologic response to therapy (i.e., an absence of viremia 6 months after the cessation of therapy).

The only treatment for HCV-infected patients with decompensated cirrhosis is transplantation; however, recurrence of viral disease in the graft is universal. The consequences of such recurrence range from minimal to transplant failure. Strategies for reducing the rate of recurrence are currently being investigated and include treatment with a combination of interferon and ribavirin. Patients with chronic HCV should have regular monitoring of their disease activity, and those with cirrhosis should undergo annual screening for hepatocellular carcinoma, with ultrasound and testing for alpha-fetoprotein.

Hepatitis D

Virology

The hepatitis D virus (HDV), or delta hepatitis virus, is a small RNA-containing satellite virus or subviral agent that requires circulating HBsAg to infect hepatocytes (14). The infection may occur as a superinfection (in which HBV infection predates that of the delta virus) or as a coinfection (in which the two viruses are transmitted together). Once it is within the liver cell, HDV requires cellular RNA polymerase and a small hepatitis delta antigen (HDAg) for replication. There is no evidence of delta virus replication outside the liver.

Epidemiology

The HDV causes chronic infection in approximately 10 million people worldwide (15). The geographic distribution of such infection varies and includes foci in the Mediterranean area, South America, Africa, and the Middle East. In the United States, 6000 to 13,000 new HDV infections occur annually, including 35 that are fatal. Additionally, approximately 1000 U.S. citizens die each year from chronic HDV infection. The groups affected are primarily those at risk for parenteral infection, most notably injection-drug users. The sexual spread of disease is less efficient than that of hepatitis B, and vertical transmission is extremely rare.

Clinical Manifestations

The critical determinant of the clinical picture in HDV infection is whether superinfection or coinfection occurs; however, both may be associated with clinical disease more often than with HBV infection that is unaccompanied by HDV infection (16). If coinfection occurs, it is more likely to be self-limited and to proceed to chronic disease in only 5% of cases (as normally occurs with HBV infection). However, coinfection may be associated with acute disease of greater severity and a higher risk of fulminant hepatitis and liver failure than with HBV infection alone. This is particularly true with the HbeAg-negative strains of HBV. Superinfection, which is more common, is more likely to lead to chronic HDV infection, owing to the persistence of HBsAg. In such patients, cirrhosis seems to be more likely to develop than in isolated chronic hepatitis B. The clinical manifestations of hepatitis, cirrhosis, and hepatocellular carcinoma do not differ from those seen with other types of viral hepatitis.

Diagnosis

The ELISA for the antibody to HDAg is positive in cases of both recent and remote infection; a positive IgM antibody result for HDV indicates recent infection (14). Such serology is relevant only in the context of HBV serology. If the patient is HBsAb positive, active HDV infection is impossible unless a rare HBV mutant is present or the HBV infection has been cleared recently and the HDV is replicating within already-infected cells. PCR for hepatitis D RNA in serum (where available) is probably the most sensitive test for HDV infection; however, immunostaining and detection of HDAg in liver biopsy specimens is more practical.

Prevention

The principles of prophylaxis for HDV infection are similar to those for HBV infection, which is essential for the transmission of HDV (7). The most important goal is to prevent superinfection of patients already infected with HBV. Some vaccine development for HDV has been performed in animal models, but no immunization against the disease is currently available.

Treatment

Interferon is the only nonexperimental therapy available for chronic HDV infection, but the results are even more disappointing than those for the treatment of chronic HBV infection alone (14). Again, transplantation is the ultimate treatment for acute or chronic liver failure. In such cases, graft reinfection seems to be relatively infrequent, especially when HBV-specific immunoglobulin is used as prophylaxis.

Hepatitis E

Virology

The hepatitis E virus (HEV) is an unenveloped RNA virus that belongs to the Caliciviridae family.

Epidemiology

The HEV is most commonly seen in the Indian subcontinent, the Middle East, and Africa (17). It is spread via the fecal–oral route and is associated with contaminated food and water and with point-source outbreaks of disease.

Clinical Manifestations

The incubation period of hepatitis E ranges from 15 to 60 days. Symptoms are similar to those of hepatitis A and include fever, abdominal discomfort, dark urine, and pale stools (18). Less commonly, diarrhea, arthralgia, and urticarial rash may occur. The disease is usually self-limited but is associated with severe illness in pregnant women. It is not associated with chronic hepatitis. Preexisting liver disease, including chronic viral hepatitis, may be associated with more severe HEV disease.

Diagnosis

The diagnosis of hepatitis E can be made in travelers from endemic areas on the basis of a specific IgM to HEV in serum or by testing stool for viral antigen

(18); PCR for HEV also may be available in some centers. In the United States, testing is undertaken most optimally on returned travelers with acute viral hepatitis who are serologically negative for HAV, HBV, or HCV infection.

Prevention

Research is being done on the development of vaccines for hepatitis E. The best current form of prophylaxis is appropriate advice to travelers with respect to food and water (e.g., avoidance of uncooked and unpeeled foods, ice, and tap water for drinking or teeth cleaning) before they visit an area endemic for HEV.

Treatment

No specific therapy has been shown to be of benefit for hepatitis E.

REFERENCES

1. **Menon KVN, Zein NN.** What do we need to know about non-A-to-E viral hepatitis? *Curr Gastroenterol Rep.* 2000;2:33–9.

2. **Feinstone SM.** Hepatitis A: epidemiology and prevention. *Eur J Gastroenterol Hepatol.* 1996;8:300–5.

3. **Koff RS.** Clinical manifestations and diagnosis of hepatitis A virus infection. *Vaccine.* 1992;10(Suppl 1):S15-S17.

4. **Kaur S, Rybicki L, Bacon BR, et al.** Performance characteristics and results of a large-scale screening program for viral hepatitis and risk factors associated with exposure to viral hepatitis B and C: results of the National Hepatitis Screening Survey. National Hepatitis Surveillance Group. *Hepatology.* 1996;24:979–86.

5. **Lee WM.** Hepatitis B virus infection. *N Engl J Med.* 1997;337:1733–45.

6. **Davis GL.** Hepatis B: diagnosis and treatment. *South Med J.* 1997;90:866–70.

7. **From the Centers for Disease Control and Prevention.** Update: recommendations to prevent hepatitis B virus transmission–United States. *JAMA.* 1999;281:790.

8. **Malik AH, Lee WM.** Chronic hepatitis B virus infection: treatment strategies for the next millennium. *Ann Intern Med.* 2000;132:723–31.

9. **Davis GL.** Hepatitis C virus genotypes and quasispecies. *Am J Med.* 1999;107:21S-6S.

10. **Williams I.** Epidemiology of hepatitis C in the United States. *Am J Med.* 1999; 107:2–9S.

11. **Sarbah SA, Younossi ZM.** Hepatitis C: an update on the silent epidemic. *J Clin Gastroenterol.* 2000;30:125–43.

12. **Schafer D, Sorrell MF.** Conquering Hepatitis C, step by step. *N Engl J Med.* 2000;343:1723–4.

13. **Hadziyannis SJ.** Review: hepatitis delta. *Eur J Gastroenterol Hepatol.* 1997;12:289–298.

14. **Navascues CA, Rodriguez M, Sotorrio NG, et al.** Epidemiology of hepatitis D virus infection: changes in the last 14 years. *Am J Gastroenterol.* 1995;90:1981–4.

15. **Liaw YF, Tsai SL, Sheen IS, et al.** Clinical and virological course of chronic hepatitis B virus infection with hepatitis C and D virus markers. *Am J Gastroenterol.* 1998; 93:354–9.

16. **Aggarwal R, Naik SR.** Epidemiology of hepatitis E: past, present, and future. *Trop Gastroenterol.* 1997;18:49–56.

17. **Aggarwal R, Krawczynski K.** Hepatitis E: an overview and recent advances in clinical and laboratory research. *Eur J Gastroenterol Hepatol.* 2000;15:9–20.

10

Peritonitis

Jennifer A. Hanrahan, DO
Robert A. Bonomo, MD

Definition

Peritonitis is the condition of acute or chronic inflammation of the abdominal cavity from any cause. It may result from diffuse or localized infection or from chemical irritation and may be associated with an intra-abdominal infection such as an abscess. Infectious organisms can reach the peritoneum to cause peritonitis in a variety of ways, including direct seeding through the bloodstream, rupture of a hollow viscus, entry through pelvic organs in women, seeding through the diaphragm, and entry through an abdominal wound.

Generally, peritonitis can be divided into the three main categories of primary, secondary, and tertiary peritonitis. *Primary peritonitis* is a diffuse bacterial peritonitis that occurs in the absence of disruption of hollow viscera. There is no apparent source of infection in primary peritonitis. Examples of primary peritonitis include spontaneous bacterial peritonitis (SBP) in patients with liver disease, spontaneous peritonitis in children, and tuberculous peritonitis (TBP). In contrast, secondary peritonitis results from intra-abdominal infection, usually as a result of rupture of hollow viscera. *Secondary peritonitis* can be localized with abscess formation, or it may be diffuse. This type of peritonitis can result from a number of conditions, including a ruptured appendix, perforated gastric ulcer, intestinal ischemia, ruptured diverticuli, perinephric abscess, anastomotic leak, and trauma. *Tertiary peritonitis* is a fairly recent term used to describe a syndrome in which peritonitis results from inadequate host defenses. This usually occurs in the setting of chronic illness or prolonged hospitalization and may involve fungi or highly resistant nosocomial pathogens. The classification of peritonitis is summarized in Table 10.1.

Anatomy of the Peritoneal Cavity

Understanding anatomical relationships is important in appreciating the manner in which infection spreads in the abdomen. The peritoneal cavity expands from the base of the diaphragm to the floor of the pelvis and is divided into multiple compartments (Fig. 10.1). The upper and lower peritoneal cavities are separated by the transverse mesocolon. The greater omentum extends from the transverse mesocolon to the lower pole of the stomach to line the lower peritoneal cavity. The pancreas, duodenum, and ascending and descending colon are located in the anterior retroperitoneal space. The kidneys, ureters, and adrenal glands are located in the posterior retroperitoneal space. The liver, stomach, gallbladder, spleen, jejunum, ileum, transverse and sigmoid colon, cecum, and appendix are found within the peritoneal cavity itself. The peritoneal cavity is a closed space in men, whereas the fallopian tubes provide an opening from it in women. The peritoneal cavity is lined with a highly permeable serous membrane that provides lubrication. This is normally present through a small amount of fluid that permits movement of the

Table 10.1   Classification and Microbiology of Peritonitis

Type	Microbiology

Primary peritonitis
  Diffuse bacterial peritonitis with no
    disruption of hollow viscera (e.g., SBP,
    TBP, fungal peritonitis)
	SBP: *Escherichia coli, Klebsiella pneumoniae,*
	    streptococci, enterococci, anaerobes, and
	    Staphylococcus aureus (rare)
	TBP: *Mycobacterium tuberculosis*
	Fungal peritonitis: blastomycosis,
	    coccidioidomycosis, histoplasmosis

Secondary peritonitis
  Localized (abscess) or diffuse peritonitis
    from rupture of hollow viscus (e.g.,
    ruptured appendix, ischemic bowel,
    perforated gastric ulcer)
	E. coli and anaerobes, including *Bacteroides*
	    species, streptococci, *Clostridium* species,
	    and enterococci

Tertiary peritonitis
  Persistent peritonitis not responding to
    therapy or peritonitis in patients with
    multiple organ failure (e.g., peritonitis
    with low-grade pathogens, fungal
    peritonitis)
	Staphylococcus epidermidis, Candida species,
	    enterococci (including VRE), *Pseudomonas
	    aeruginosa, Stenotrophomonas maltophilia,
	    Aspergillus* species

SBP = spontaneous bacterial peritonitis; TBP = tuberculous peritonitis; VRE = vancomycin-resistant enterococcus.

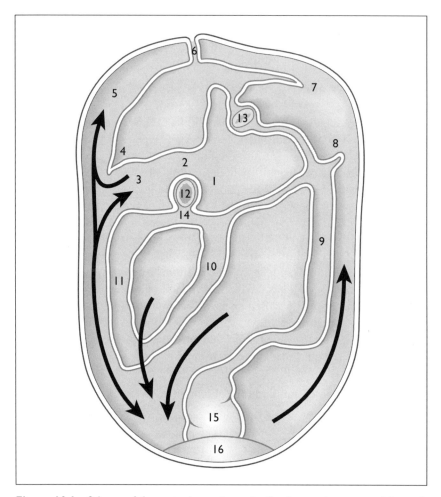

Figure 10.1   Schema of the posterior peritoneal reflections and recesses of the peritoneal cavity. 1 = lesser sac; 2 = foramen of Winslow; 3 = Morison's pouch; 4 = right triangular ligament; 5 = right subphrenic space; 6 = falciform ligament; 7 = left subphrenic space; 8 = phrenicolic ligament; 9 = bare area of ascending colon; 10 = root of the small bowel mesentery; 11 = bare area of ascending colon; 12 = duodenum; 13 = esophagus; 14 = root of the transverse mesocolon; 15 = bare area of rectum; 16 = bladder. Adapted with permission from Mandell, Douglas, and Benetté Principles and Practice of Infectious Diseases, 5th ed. Churchill Livingstone; 2000:821.

internal organs without hindrance. The protein content of normal peritoneal fluid (which consists mostly of albumin) is less than 30 mg/mL, and the fluid contains fewer than 250 white blood cells per milliliter.

The presence of separate spacing compartments and recesses in the peritoneal cavity helps sequester infection. These compartments include the pelvis in the lowest portion of the peritoneal cavity, the subphrenic spaces on the right and left sides of the peritoneal cavity, and Morison's pouch. Morison's pouch is the posterior superior extension of the subhepatic space and, when a patient is recumbent, is in the lowest part of the paravertebral groove. The falciform ligament separates the right and left subphrenic spaces and acts as a barrier to the spread of infection. The pouch of Douglas rests between the rectum and the body of the uterus.

Primary Peritonitis

Primary peritonitis is a diffuse infection in the peritoneal cavity that occurs in the absence of another source of infection. Examples of primary peritonitis include primary peritonitis in children, fungal peritonitis, TBP, and SBP. SBP is currently the most commonly encountered type of primary peritonitis and involves the infection of ascitic fluid in patients with ascites. This condition most commonly occurs with ascites from liver disease but also can occur with ascites caused by a number of other diseases, including nephrotic syndrome, congestive heart failure (especially chronic constrictive pericarditis), systemic lupus erythematosus, rheumatoid arthritis, and Budd-Chiari syndrome (Table 10.2). SBP also has been described in patients with chronic active hepatitis, acute viral hepatitis, and lymphedema (1).

The prevalence of SBP in patients hospitalized with ascites ranges from 7% to 27%, and mortality from this condition ranges from 44% to 95% (2–4).

Pathogenesis

A variety of mechanisms have been proposed for the pathogenesis of SBP. When SBP was initially described, the infection was presumed to result from transient enteric bacteremia followed by sepsis (4). More recently, it has been maintained that the existence of portal hypertension increases the translocation of bacteria to the lymphatic system and portal vein, with subsequent bacteremia. Direct translocation of bacteria from the gut is thought to be less likely given that SBP is usually monomicrobial. If direct translocation from the gut were responsible, polymicrobial infection would be expected to occur and anaerobes would be expected to play a greater role in SBP. Another likely factor in the development of SBP is delayed clearance of bacteria from the hepatic reticuloendothelial system in individuals with portal hypertension.

Table 10.2   Conditions Associated with Spontaneous Bacterial Peritonitis

Hepatic cirrhosis (from any cause)	Rheumatoid arthritis
Nephrotic syndrome	Budd–Chiari syndrome
Congestive heart failure (especially from constrictive pericarditis)	Viral hepatitis
	Lymphedema
Systemic lupus erythematosus	Malignancy

Risk Factors

A number of risk factors that predispose to the development of SBP have been identified (Table 10.3) (5). Patients with a serum bilirubin concentration above 2.5 mg/dL were found to have a threefold greater incidence of SBP than those with a bilirubin below 2.5 mg/dL. As would be expected, patients with a prothrombin time exceeding 1.6 times normal also were found to be at substantially greater risk for SBP than those with a normal prothrombin time. In addition, patients with a serum sodium concentration below 130 mmol/L, thrombocytopenia with a platelet count below 116,000 cells/mm^3, and an ascitic fluid protein content of 1 g/dL or less also were found to be at increased risk of SBP. Patients who developed SBP in one series were found to have a 69% recurrence rate at 1 year and a 1-year survival probability of only 38% (3). Patients who survive an initial episode of SBP often die later of liver failure and complications of portal hypertension.

Clinical Manifestations

The diagnosis of SBP should be considered in any patient with ascites who exhibits clinical deterioration, and diagnostic paracentesis should be performed in such cases. The clinical findings in SBP can be quite subtle. As many as one third of patients may be asymptomatic. Furthermore, although all patients with SBP have ascites, it may not be evident on physical examination. If a small amount of ascites is present, ultrasonography can be helpful in localizing fluid for paracentesis. Approximately 50% to 80% of patients with SBP have fever, and approximately half have abdominal pain. Hypotension and hypothermia can occur but are uncommon. Hepatic encephalopathy is often present, and worsening encephalopathy can occur in the absence of other signs. Because the presentation of SBP is variable and can have subtle manifestations, a high index of suspicion is required.

Table 10.3   Risk Factors for Development of Spontaneous Bacterial Peritonitis

Total bilirubin ≥2.5 mg/dL	Hyponatremia (Na⁺ ≤130 mEq/L)
Prolonged prothrombin time (≥1.6 times normal)	Thrombocytopenia (≤116,000 cells)
	Ascites fluid protein content ≤1 g/dL

Microbiology

Organisms usually recovered in SBP include normal enteric flora. As noted previously, SBP is generally a monomicrobial infection. Aerobic gram-negative bacilli are responsible for most cases, with *Escherichia coli* and *Klebsiella pneumoniae* causing more than 70% of cases (*see* Table 10.1) (2,6). Gram-positive organisms (e.g., enterococci, streptococci [including pneumococcus]) account for an additional 25% of cases of SBP. Anaerobes are rare and account for less than 5% of cases. Additionally, polymicrobial infection is unusual, and secondary peritonitis should be considered when this is found. *Staphylococcus aureus* is rarely isolated from patients with SBP, accounting for only 2% to 4% of all cases (2), and has been found in patients with erosion of an umbilical hernia. Other sites of infection should be sought when this organism is recovered.

Culture-Negative Neutrocytic Ascites and Bacterascites

In 1984, Runyon and Hoefs (7) originally described a variant of SBP called *culture-negative neutrocytic ascites* (CNNA). This entity was described as existing when a neutrophil count of more than 500 cells/mm³ is present in the absence of positive ascites fluid cultures. Negative ascites fluid cultures were found in up to 35% of suspected cases of SBP that were otherwise clinically indistinguishable from diagnosed SBP. The diagnosis of CNNA should be made only when patients have not received antibiotics in the recent past and when no alternate explanation exists for an increased neutrophil count. The clinical presentation, laboratory findings, mortality, and response to treatment are similar in patients with SBP and CNNA. Despite yielding negative cultures, CNNA is thought to be caused by bacterial infection. Repeat paracentesis usually shows improvement after initiation of antibiotic therapy. It is possible that the number of organisms present in CNNA is below the threshold of detection for culture. Although the original case series defined CNNA in patients with a neutrophil count of more than 500 cells/mm³, a neutrophil count of more than 250 cells/mm³ is used as a cutoff (2,7a).

The converse of CNNA, in which ascites fluid culture is positive but the neutrophil count is less than 250 cells/mm³, also can occur. This clinical situation is called *bacterascites*, which may be caused by transient passage of bacteria into ascitic fluid. Although CNNA should be treated with antibiotics, BA may not require treatment (2). In the setting of bacterascites, symptoms of peritonitis correlate with progression to SBP, whereas asymptomatic patients often do not experience this progression (6). Careful monitoring with repeat paracentesis when SBP is suspected may obviate the need for antibiotic therapy.

Diagnosis

The diagnosis of SBP is made by performing a diagnostic paracentesis. This procedure is safe, and although a coagulopathy may be present, most patients do not require correction of the coagulopathy before paracentesis (8). The commonly ordered tests for analyzing peritoneal fluid are summarized in Table 10.4. The neutrophil count is the single best predictor of infection, and one above 250-500 cells/mm^3 is indicative of infection, even in the absence of positive cultures (Table 10.5). The peritoneal fluid neutrophil count has a sensitivity of 80%, a specificity of 97%, and a diagnostic accuracy of 92%. Although a Gram stain is usually negative, it is a simple and useful diagnostic test and can help guide empirical antibiotic administration and identify bowel perforation.

Cultures should be obtained by directly inoculating from 10 to 15 mL of ascites fluid into blood culture bottles. Runyon and coworkers (9) found that the diagnostic yield for positive cultures increased from 42% to 91% when blood culture bottles were inoculated at the bedside as opposed to using conventional plating methods. The pH of ascitic fluid pH is also helpful in making the diagnosis; however, this generally reflects the size of the neutrophil population and is therefore lower with a larger neutrophil population. The ascites fluid albumin and total protein concentrations should be obtained, because they help establish both the diagnosis of portal hypertension and the risk of recurrence of SBP. Although peritoneal fluid cytology is rarely diag-

Table 10.4   Evaluation of Ascites Fluid

Recommended Tests	Optional Tests
Cell count and differential	Glucose
Albumin (serum and ascites fluid)	Amylase
Total protein	Lactate dehydrogenase
Gram stain	pH
Bacterial culture	Ziehl–Neelsen stain
	Mycobacterial and fungal culture
	Cytology
	Bilirubin (ascites fluid and serum)

Table 10.5   Characteristics of Ascites Fluid in Various Disease States

Condition	Appearance	Cell Count (WBCs/mL)
SBP	Turbid or purulent	≥250 PMNLs
Secondary peritonitis	Turbid or purulent	>1000 (mostly PMNLs)
Malignancy	Straw colored, bloody, chylous	>1000 (variable)
Cirrhosis, nephrotic syndrome	Clear	<250
TBP	Turbid, bloody	>1000 (mostly lymphocytes)

PMNLs = polymorphonuclear leukocytes; SBP = spontaneous bacterial peritonitis; TBP = tuberculous peritonitis; WBC = white blood cells

Table 10.6   Other Laboratory Tests for Evaluating Peritonitis

Complete blood count	Chest radiography
Serum electrolytes, glucose, blood urea nitrogen, and creatinine	Abdominal series (supine, left lateral decubitus, and upright films)
Liver function tests, including albumin	Abdominal ultrasound
Prothrombin time	Abdominal computed tomography
Blood cultures	

nostic of SBP, it can be performed in a search for tumor cells. The amylase concentration can help establish the diagnosis of pancreatic ascites and bowel perforation. Other optional tests that should be performed when TBP is suspected include smears for acid-fast bacilli and mycobacterial cultures.

Blood culture may be positive in one third to one half of cases of SBP (*see* Table 10.3 for further steps in the work-up of patients with SBP) and may be particularly helpful in patients whose ascites fluid cultures are negative. Urine culture is not usually helpful in the diagnosis of SBP because the organism it yields rarely coincides with the organism isolated from ascites fluid. Despite this, it is probably worthwhile to perform both blood and urine cultures on patients with suspected SBP (Table 10.6).

Differentiating Spontaneous Bacterial Peritonitis from Secondary Peritonitis

Although most patients who present with infected ascites fluid are found to have primary peritonitis, approximately 15% have secondary peritonitis (10).

Because the management of primary peritonitis differs from that of secondary peritonitis, it is important to distinguish them from each other. A history and physical examination are insufficient for differentiating primary from secondary peritonitis; however, a number of ascites-fluid parameters have been found to be helpful in this regard. Ascites fluid in peritonitis associated with bowel perforation usually has two of the following parameters: 1) a total protein concentration above 1 g/dL, 2) a glucose concentration below 50 mg/dL, and/or 3) an ascites-fluid lactate dehydrogenase concentration above the upper limit of normal. Additionally, if the ascites fluid is deeply bile stained with a bilirubin concentration above 6 mg/dL and if the ascites fluid-to-serum bilirubin ratio is greater than 1, then biliary perforation should be suspected. As previously stated, more than one organism in a Gram stain or a polymicrobial culture also suggests bowel perforation. Patients who meet these criteria should undergo evaluation to rule out perforation of a hollow viscus. Plain radiographs of the abdomen can be obtained to look for free air under the diaphragm. If these are unrevealing, a computed tomographic scan of the abdomen should be performed on patients with suspected secondary peritonitis.

Secondary peritonitis also may have other causes than those named above, which may not be as readily distinguishable. Repeat paracentesis is helpful in these situations. Akriviadis and Runyon (10) performed many repeat paracenteses on patients with SBP and found that all patients with the disease had a decrease in their peritoneal fluid neutrophil count at 48 hours. Furthermore, all patients who had positive ascites fluid cultures with organisms susceptible to the initially given antibiotic had negative cultures at 48 hours. All patients who were found to have secondary peritonitis had persistently positive ascites fluid cultures at 48 and 96 hours despite antibiotic therapy, and more than half had multiple organisms.

The clinical presentations of SBP and secondary peritonitis can be similar in patients with ascites. However, because secondary peritonitis often requires surgical intervention, it is critical to differentiate these two entities (*see* section on Treatment of Secondary Peritonitis below). It is recommended that repeat paracentesis be performed at 48 hours in patients being treated for SBP. If the neutrophil count fails to decline or if the ascites fluid culture remains positive, then further evaluation is indicated.

Treatment of Spontaneous Bacterial Peritonitis

Initial treatment of SBP should include the administration of antibiotics with activity against enteric flora. After the infecting organism has been identified by culture and susceptibility testing, treatment should be pinpointed to the specific pathogen (Table 10.7). Empirical therapy of SBP should include consideration of the following antibiotics: ampicillin-sulbactam, piperacillin-tazobactam, and a third-generation cephalosporin. In our institution, aminoglycosides are generally avoided because of the potential for nephrotoxicity, particularly in patients with cirrhosis. Cefotaxime, which has activity against

Table 10.7   Empirical Antibiotics for Primary, Secondary, and Tertiary Peritonitis

Type	Dosage*	Microbiology
Primary peritonitis		Enterobacteriaceae,
Cefotaxime	2 g IV q8h	*Streptococcus pneumoniae,*
Piperacillin–tazobactam	3.375 g IV q6h or 4.5 g q8h	*Enterococcus* species, anaerobes (<1%–2%)
Secondary peritonitis		Enterobacteriaceae,
Ampicillin–sulbactam + gentamicin	3 g IV q6h + 1.7 mg/kg IV q8h	*Bacteroides* species, *Pseudomonas aeruginosa,*
Piperacillin–tazobactam + gentamicin	3.375 g IV q6h + 1.7 mg/kg IV q8h or 4.5 g q8h	*Enterococcus* species
Ciprofloxacin + metronidazole	400 mg IV q12h + 500 mg q8h	
Tertiary peritonitis		*Staphylococcus epidermidis,*
Meropenem	1 g IV q8h	*Stenotrophomonas*
Imipenem	500 mg IV q6h	*maltophilia, P. aeruginosa,*
Cefepime + vancomycin	2 g IV q12h + 1 g IV q12h	*Candida* species, fungi
Fluconazole	200–400 mg IV q24h	
Amphotericin	0.5–1.0 mg/kg IV q24h	

IV = intravenously.
*These dosages are for patients with normal renal function.

common gram-positive and -negative organisms, is considered the first-line agent for treating SBP.

Most patients with SBP have sterile ascites fluid soon after beginning antibiotic therapy. Often, the ascites fluid becomes sterile after the initial dose of an antibiotic agent (10). In an evaluation of 90 patients with SBP and CNNA, who were randomized to receiving either 5 or 10 days of intravenous cefotaxime, no difference between the two groups was found in mortality, bacteriologic cure, or recurrence of infection (11). Although antibiotic therapy is often continued for 10 to14 days, a shorter course of therapy has been shown to be as effective, and certainly more cost-effective. Currently, 5 to 7 days of therapy is considered standard, so long as repeat paracentesis at 48 hours demonstrates resolution of infection and improved cell counts. If ascites-fluid neutrophil counts remain high or if resistant organisms are found on culture, then a longer course of therapy may be necessary.

Prophylaxis of Spontaneous Bacterial Peritonitis

Given that the recurrence of SBP is common and that the mortality associated with recurrence is high, preventing infection in the first place is the optimal goal. Both primary and secondary prevention strategies have been used with nonabsorbable antibiotics to selectively decontaminate the gut. Norfloxacin at 400 mg/d has been used for prophylaxis; however, although this has been shown to be effective in reducing the occurrence of SBP, it has the disadvantage of selecting for gram-positive organisms. Studies of both primary and secondary prophylaxis have shown a substantial decrease in the incidence of SBP, but no decrease in mortality or in the number of hospital admissions for the disease (2,6). Because patients with acute liver failure or gastrointestinal hemorrhage are likely to suffer the greatest morbidity from SBP, prophylaxis should be considered for these individuals.

Secondary Peritonitis

Pathogenesis

Secondary peritonitis is a distinct clinical entity that results from the rupture or spillage of an abdominal viscus into the normally sterile abdominal cavity. Predisposing factors include abdominal trauma, perforation, or intraperitoneal spread from an infected abdominal organ or abscess. Perforation of a gastric or duodenal ulcer, cholecystitis, rupture of diverticuli, rupture of the appendix, and penetrating abdominal wounds are all common causes. Subsequent infection may either be localized, as with an abscess, or consist of generalized peritonitis. Infection is common after rupture of a hollow viscus. Chemical peritonitis also may occur, especially after rupture of the stomach.

Clinical Manifestations

The signs and symptoms of secondary peritonitis are generally more pronounced than those of SBP. Most patients present with pain, either over a localized area (as can be seen with appendicitis) or as generally within the abdomen. Usually, the area of pain tends to extend as the inflammation progresses. Examination reveals tenderness over the involved area. Vomiting may be present at an early stage or may develop later if ileus or bowel obstruction develops. Fever and diarrhea also may be present, and abdominal rigidity, guarding, or rebound tenderness may be found on examination. Immunocompromised or elderly patients may have more subtle symptoms. SBP may be more difficult to diagnose in patients who are paralyzed and in those undergoing mechanical ventilation.

Diagnosis

Patients who present with abdominal pain should have the usual laboratory tests (as described previously in the section on Primary Peritonitis) to aid in establishing a diagnosis, including a complete blood count, electrolyte measurements, and plain radiography of the abdomen (*see* Tables 10.4 and 10.6). Although laboratory tests can be helpful in raising the index of suspicion for peritonitis, the definitive diagnosis can be made only surgically. Therefore, any patient suspected of having secondary peritonitis should undergo evaluation by a surgeon.

Microbiology

The number and types of bacteria increase progressively from the top to the bottom of the gastrointestinal tract. Therefore, the bacteria involved in secondary peritonitis depend on the level at which the rupture takes place. Proximally, there are sparse aerobes and oral anaerobes, whereas the colon contains the largest concentration of bacteria. The stomach in the fasting state contains relatively few microorganisms; however, multiple organisms are found after colonic perforation. If an organ ruptures below the ligament of Treitz, anaerobes constitute 99% of the organisms isolated. *Bacteroides fragilis* is the predominant anaerobe isolated from culture, and *E. coli* is the predominant facultative aerobe in gastrointestinal perforation (1). *B. fragilis* is present in approximately 75% of postoperative infections but accounts for less than 5% of fecal flora (12). Remember that the normal flora of the gut can be altered by prior antibiotic therapy or by antacids.

Meleney and coworkers (13) recognized early on that microbial synergy plays an important role in establishing infection within the peritoneum. It was noted that the clinical course of illness was much more severe if two or more organisms, as opposed to a single species, were found. Because synergy plays an important role in infection, it is usually not necessary to treat all the organisms that are isolated from a culture.

Treatment

Secondary peritonitis is usually a surgical disease. The most important aspect of its treatment is the evacuation of pus and fecal contamination from the abdominal cavity. The principles of therapy involve supportive measures, followed by operative intervention. The surgical approach involves controlling the source of infection, evacuating contaminated material, decompressing the abdomen, and preventing or treating persistent infection. Antimicrobial therapy should be aimed at potential organisms (e.g., gram-negative bacilli, anaerobes) (*see* Table 10.7). However, antimicrobial therapy is a temporizing measure only, and surgical intervention is the most important treatment modality in controlling infection. A wide variety of antibiotics can be used. Piperacillin-tazobactam, ticarcillin-clavulanate, or ciprofloxacin plus metronidazole are all good empirical choices that provide coverage for Enterobacteriaceae and anaerobes.

Because of the presence of mixed flora in peritonitis, it is difficult to establish a clinical correlation with intraoperative isolates. Patients with prolonged hospital stays or previous antibiotic therapy, both of which are likely to have altered the normal flora of the gastrointestinal tract, should have antibiotic regimens that include imipenem or meropenem, cefepime, fluoroquinolones, or an aminoglycoside (1). These drugs provide coverage of resistant nosocomially acquired pathogens.

The role of enterococci and *Candida* in uncomplicated peritonitis is controversial. Antimicrobial therapy aimed at *B. fragilis* and *E. coli* is generally sufficient when polymicrobial infection is present, because other microorganisms disappear as these bacteria are eradicated. Despite this, enterococci and *Candida* species have become important nosocomial pathogens. When either organism is isolated—whether in a single instance or persistently—antibiotic therapy should be adjusted to cover these species.

Tertiary Peritonitis

Definition

Tertiary peritonitis is a syndrome that occurs in patients who have inadequate host defenses and who often have multiple-organ failure. The term *tertiary peritonitis* was originally used in the 1980s to describe patients who died of sepsis and multiple-organ failure caused by a delay in management or by iatrogenic factors (14). These patients were sometimes found to have peritoneal fluid that was free of microorganisms or that contained low-grade pathogens at the time of surgery. The term *tertiary peritonitis* has been used largely to describe a situation that presents as sepsis late in the postoperative phase, but also can describe patients with complicated peritonitis associated with continuous ambulatory peritoneal dialysis (CAPD). Persistent peritonitis with systemic inflammation ensues after what usually would be an adequate course of antimicrobial therapy.

Pathogenesis

Microorganisms may gain access to the abdominal cavity by translocation of intestinal flora, which may result from 1) malnutrition, 2) alteration of the intestinal wall from CAPD, 3) intestinal ischemia, or 4) growth of resistant bowel flora through antibiotic selection pressure. Additionally, selection among the initial polymicrobial peritoneal inoculum may occur through antibiotic therapy, direct contamination during surgery, or direct access along peritoneal catheter devices. Patients develop a sepsis syndrome with hypotension, fever, low systemic vascular resistance, a high cardiac output, and multiple-organ failure. The mortality rate for patients with nonlocalized postoperative intra-abdominal sepsis approaches 100% when medical therapy alone is given (15). This mortality rate may be reduced somewhat by repeated laparotomy.

Microbiology

The microorganisms involved in tertiary peritonitis are often highly resistant nosocomial pathogens. Pathogens that can be involved include the following:

- Extended-spectrum, beta-lactamase–producing *K. pneumoniae* or *E. coli*
- *Pseudomonas aeruginosa*
- *Enterobacter* species
- Vancomycin-resistant enterococci
- *Candida* species
- *Staphylococcus epidermidis*
- *Stenotrophomonas maltophilia*
- *Acinetobacter* species

As previously discussed, peritoneal fluid culture also may be negative.

Treatment

Because tertiary peritonitis occurs postoperatively, after prolonged hospital stays, and usually after prior antibiotic therapy, the organisms involved are usually highly resistant. Empiric therapy (*see* Table 10.7) should include vancomycin, imipenem, meropenem, cefepime, a fluoroquinolone, or an aminoglycoside. Metronidazole is also often given empirically to provide coverage of resistant *Bacteroides* species. Antimicrobial therapy should be tailored to available cultures.

Peritonitis in Patients Undergoing Continuous Ambulatory Peritoneal Dialysis

Pathogenesis

Peritonitis in patients who are undergoing CAPD is a distinct clinical entity and is the main complication of CAPD. Its incidence is estimated to be approximately 1.0 to 1.3 episodes per patient per year (16-18). This incidence is lower in centers with more experience and higher in those with less. The mean period of peritonitis development after CAPD initiation is 8 to 9 months. Unlike with SBP, the recurrence of which is common, CAPD is estimated to recur in only approximately 25% of cases (18).

The main factor in the development of CAPD peritonitis is usually a violation of sterile technique during the four or five daily fluid exchanges that occur in CAPD. The pathogenesis of this infection is similar to that of infections that result from intravascular devices, when organisms migrate along the catheter groove and the catheter serves as an entry point for microorganisms into the normally sterile peritoneal cavity. Other host factors also may play a role; however, the incidence of CAPD peritonitis in diabetic and nondiabetic individuals is reported to be similar. Recurrent CAPD peritonitis is thought to be associated with some type of impairment in host bactericidal activity (19).

Clinical Manifestations

Although signs and symptoms of CAPD peritonitis are variable, the onset of the disease is usually noted by the presence of cloudy dialysate fluid. Additionally, most patients have abdominal pain and tenderness on examination. Other signs and symptoms of CAPD peritonitis are much less frequent. Only approximately 35% of patients have fever, and only approximately one quarter of patients have nausea and vomiting (18). CAPD patients are taught that they should be able to read newsprint through the dialysate fluid as a means of ensuring the absence of infection. If turbidity is present, it should always be taken seriously; the presence of infection should be assumed until proven otherwise.

Diagnosis

The diagnosis of CAPD peritonitis is established by evaluating the dialysate fluid, as discussed in the section on Laboratory Findings below. Laboratory evaluation of the dialysate fluid should be undertaken in any patient who notes a change in the appearance of this fluid.

Laboratory Findings
The initial evaluation of turbid dialysate fluid includes a white blood cell count with differential. Generally, a white blood cell count of 100 cells/cm^3 or more, with more than 50% polymorphonuclear leukocytes, is considered indicative of infection. It is important to obtain a differential count along with the white blood cell count because conditions such as eosinophilic peritonitis, which occurs as an allergic reaction to the dialysis catheter, also can cause cloudiness of the dialysate fluid.

A Gram stain is useful in evaluating peritonitis and is positive in 20% to 30% of cases. It is recommended that 10 to 20 mL of effluent be centrifuged for the Gram stain. Although the Gram stain is positive in less than 30% of cases, the procedure is simple and may give an early clue to the presence of fungal peritonitis.

Culture of infected peritoneal dialysate fluid is positive in more than 90% of cases (16). A variety of approaches have been tried for culture. As with SBP, 10 to 15 mL of fluid can be injected directly into blood culture bottles. Alternately, many dialysis centers send the entire bag of effluent to the microbiology laboratory, where the number of organisms can be concentrated either by filtration or by centrifugation. In contrast to other types of peritonitis, blood cultures in CAPD peritonitis are often negative and are not routinely helpful in making a diagnosis. In patients who are hospitalized with fever, blood cultures are indicated to rule out other sources of infection.

Microbiology

Given that they are consequences of a laxity in sterile technique, most infections are caused by skin flora. The most common isolates are *S. aureus* and coagulase-negative staphylococci, which are responsible for almost 60% of CAPD peritonitis (Table 10.8). Streptococci and diphtheroids account for an additional 15% of such infections. The remainder of cases are caused by gram-negative organisms, including *P. aeruginosa* in 5% to 10% of cases (17,18). Few cases are caused by fungi, but these are often very difficult to treat (*see* Table 10.6).

Table 10.8   Microorganisms Associated with Continuous Ambulatory Peritoneal Dialysis

Common Organisms	Rare Organisms
Coagulase-negative staphylococci	*Candida* species
Staphylococcus aureus	*Pasteurella multocida*
Streptococcus species	*Vibrio* species
Diphtheroids	*Aspergillus* species
Escherichia coli	*Rhodotorula* species
Pseudomonas aeruginosa	*Exophiala* species
Proteus species	*Penicillium* species
Acinetobacter species	*Fusarium* species
	Mycobacteria

Treatment

Empirical treatment of CAPD caused by coagulase-negative staphylococci and other gram-positive organisms involves the intraperitoneal administration of vancomycin in dialysate fluid. Empirical therapy also includes an aminoglycoside or third-generation cephalosporin to provide coverage of gram-negative organisms. Because nephrotoxicity is not an issue, aminoglycosides can be used (Table 10.9).

Vancomycin is usually administered at a dose of 2 g and allowed to dwell in the peritoneal cavity for at least 6 hours. This produces reasonable intraperitoneal levels of the drug for approximately 7 days; on day 7, a second dose is given. A loading dose of gentamicin (70-140 mg) is followed by maintenance therapy of a single daily exchange rate of 20 mg/L or by multiple daily exchanges at 4-8 mg/L. The clinical response of CAPD peritonitis to such therapy is generally rapid, and patients improve within 48 hours after treatment is begun. If the culture of the dialysate fluid is negative but the patient is responding to empirical therapy, the empirical therapy can be continued for the duration of therapy. Most cases of CAPD peritonitis can be treated with 7 to 10 days of intraperitoneal antimicrobial therapy; however, *S. aureus* and gram-negative organisms should be treated for 10 to 14 days. Uncomplicated CAPD peritonitis can be treated on an outpatient basis. Hospitalization is indicated when patients exhibit signs of sepsis, when there is suspicion of abscess formation or perforation, or when there is concern about resistant organisms.

Tunnel- or exit-site infections usually require the removal of the dialysis catheter and temporary hemodialysis. Certain microorganisms, including *P. aeruginosa* and fungi, are often associated with tunnel-site infections. Infection with these organisms tends to have a higher morbidity and usually does not resolve without the removal of the dialysis catheter. *Pseudomonas* peritonitis requires more aggressive therapy, and it is recommended that two antibiotics (e.g., aminoglycoside and ceftazidime) be given intraperitoneally. There have been anecdotal reports of successful treatment of fungal peritonitis with maintenance of the CAPD catheter; however, fungal peritonitis is associated with a high morbidity, and it is recommended that the catheter be removed. Fungal peritonitis also carries a high risk of adhesion formation, which may preclude

Table 10.9   Antibiotics in Continuous Ambulatory Peritoneal Dialysis

Vancomycin 2 g IP every 7 days (twice)
Gentamicin 20 mg/L IP for one exchange per day, then 4–8 mg/L on each subsequent day
Tobramycin (same as for gentamicin)
Ceftazidime 500 mg/L IP on day 1, then 125 mg/L with each exchange

IP = intraperitoneally.

future peritoneal dialysis. In addition to being relatively inefficacious in peritoneal dialysate fluid, amphotericin B is poorly tolerated intraperitoneally and causes severe inflammation in the patient. After catheter removal, patients with fungal peritonitis require a period of systemic antimicrobial therapy.

Tuberculous Peritonitis

The differential diagnosis of peritonitis should include consideration of TBP. This entity is not commonly seen in the United States, but is characterized by an insidious onset, often over a period of more than 1 month. Progressive ascites, fever, and abdominal pain are present. Night sweats, vomiting, chills, and weight loss also can occur. Active pulmonary tuberculosis is associated with TBP in approximately 20% of cases (20). A "doughy" abdomen caused by tuberculous adhesion can sometimes be found on physical examination, and an abdominal mass may be palpable in up to 50% of cases. TBP can present either as a chronic condition (plastic TBP)—in which there tends to be more abdominal pain, little ascites, and adhesions—or as a more acute condition (serous TBP) with ascites of rapid onset and fever.

Tuberculous peritonitis usually results from the rupture of a caseous necrotic abdominal lymph node whose contents spill into peritoneal fluid. Occasionally, a characteristic calcified abdominal node can be seen on plain radiographs of the abdomen. This entity should be suspected when a predominantly lymphocytic exudate is found on evaluation of ascitic fluid and in conjunction with an increased total protein concentration. The organism is rarely seen on a Ziehl-Neelsen stain but can be cultured in up to 69% of cases. The yield of culture is improved if a large volume of fluid is concentrated for culture. Culture of peritoneal fluid may give positive results in more than 80% of cases if 1 L of fluid is cultured (20). A polymerase chain reaction test probably aids in the diagnosis of TBP but has not yet been evaluated as a diagnostic tool in the disease. Peritoneoscopy and peritoneal biopsy often are used to examine the abdomen for evidence of characteristic pathology. Caseating granulomas, tissue that contains acid-fast bacilli, or granulomas (including epithelioid giant cells) must be found to make a definitive diagnosis histologically. When tubercles are seen studding the peritoneum, the yield on biopsy is approximately 75%. (Other chronic granulomatous diseases can produce an identical studding.) Because fluid cultures are often positive, it is recommended that they be performed even when no characteristic features are seen on peritoneoscopy.

Mortality from TBP has declined substantially since the advent of antituberculosis drugs. The treatment for this disease consists of standard antimycobacterial drugs in regimens that resemble those used for treating pulmonary tuberculosis.

REFERENCES

1. **Johnson CC, Baldessarre J, Levison ME.** Peritonitis: update on pathophysiology, clinical manifestations, and management. *Clin Infect Dis.* 1997;24:1035–47.

2. **Gilbert GA, Kamath PS.** Spontaneous bacterial peritonitis: an update. *Mayo Clin Proc.* 1995;70:365–70.

3. **Tito L, Rimola A, Gines P, et al.** Recurrence of spontaneous bacterial peritonitis in cirrhosis: frequency and predictive factors. *Hepatology.* 1988;8:27–31.

4. **Conn HO, Fessel JM.** Spontaneous bacterial peritonitis in cirrhosis: variations on a theme. *Medicine.* 1971;50: 161–9.

5. **Andreu M, Sola R, Sitges-Serra A, et al.** Risk factors for spontaneous bacterial peritonitis in cirrhotic patients with ascites. *Gastroenterology.* 1993;104:1133–8.

6. **Bhuva M, Ganger D, Jensen D.** Spontaneous bacterial peritonitis: an update on evaluation, management and prevention. *Am J Med.* 1994;97:169–75.

7. **Runyon BA, Hoefs JC.** Culture-negative neutrocytic ascites: a variant of spontaneous bacterial peritonitis. *Hepatology.* 1984;4:1209–11.

7a. **Such J, Runyon BA.** Spontaneous bacterial peritonitis. *Clin Infect Dis.* 1998;27:669–76.

8. **Runyon BA.** Care of the patient with ascites. *N Engl J Med.* 1994;330:337–42.

9. **Runyon BA, Umland ET, Merlin T.** Inoculation of blood culture bottles with ascitic fluid. *Arch Intern Med.* 1987;147:73–5.

10. **Akriviadis E, Runyon BA.** Utility of an algorithm in differentiating spontaneous from secondary bacterial peritonitis. *Gastroenterology.* 1990;98:127–33.

11. **Runyon BA, McHutchison JG, Antillon MR, et al.** Short-course versus long-course antibiotic treatment of spontaneous bacterial peritonitis. *Gastroenterology.* 1991;100: 1737–42.

12. **Wilson SE, Hopkins JA.** Clinical correlates of anaerobic bacteriology in peritonitis. *Clin Infect Dis.* 1995;20(Suppl 2):S251–6.

13. **Meleney FL, Harvey HD, Zaytseff-Jern H.** Peritonitis: the correlation of the bacteriology of the peritoneal exudates and the clinical course of the disease in one hundred six cases of peritonitis. *Arch Surg.* 1931;22:1–23.

14. **Wittman DH, Schein M, Condon RE.** Management of secondary peritonitis. *Ann Surg.* 1996;224:10–18.

15. **Munson JL.** Management of intra-abdominal sepsis. *Surg Clin North Am.* 1991;71: 1175–85.

16. **Bint AJ, Finch RG, Gokal R, et al.** Diagnosis and management of peritonitis in continuous ambulatory peritoneal dialysis. *Lancet.* 1987;1:845–8.

17. **Bernardini J, Piraino B, Sorkin M.** Analysis of continuous ambulatory peritoneal dialysis-related *Pseudomonas aeruginosa* infections. *Am J Med.* 1987;83:829–32.

18. **Saklayen MG.** CAPD peritonitis. *Med Clin North Am.* 1990;74;997–1010.

19. **Holmes CJ.** Peritoneal host defense mechanisms in peritoneal dialysis. *Kidney Int.* 1994;46(Suppl 48):S58–S70.

20. **Moreyra E, Rollhauser CA, Tenner SM.** Tuberculous peritonitis: clinical manifestations, diagnosis, and treatment. *Res Staff Phys.* 1994;40:29–32.

11

Intra-abdominal Abscesses

Farid F. Muakkassa, MD
Daniel P. Guyton, MD
William C. Papouras, MD

Intra-abdominal abscesses are walled-off collections of pus surrounded by inflammatory adhesions that occur either within or outside the abdominal viscera. In abscesses that occur outside the abdominal viscera, the abscess wall can be surrounded by adhesions, loops of small or large bowel and their mesenteries, or the omentum; sometimes they are retroperitoneal. The formation of a well-defined intra-abdominal abscess may take several days to a week, depending on the cause of the responsible insult. Formation of abscesses in the peritoneal cavity usually follows 1) the resolution of a diffuse peritonitis (of which a remaining small, infected focus becomes walled off by the host-defense system), 2) a perforation in a viscus, or 3) a postsurgical anastomotic leak. More than 80% of intra-abdominal abscesses occur after an abdominal operation. Postoperative intra-abdominal abscesses in the upper gastrointestinal tract are due largely to anastomotic leaks, whereas those in the lower tract are caused by the bacterial load in the colon. In contrast, most visceral abscesses result from hematogenous or lymphatic spread of organisms. Retroperitoneal abscesses can result from perforations of retroperitoneal organs, from the retroperitoneal portion of an organ, or from lymphatic or hematogenous seeding by infectious organisms.

The approach to the diagnosis and treatment of intra-abdominal abscesses may vary with the cause of the etiologic disease process and with the involved organs. Although this chapter takes an organ-focused approach to the diagnosis and management of intra-abdominal abscesses, a broader initial perspective sometimes is needed before focusing on a specific organ.

Liver Abscesses

Liver abscesses can be divided into two major categories—pyogenic and amebic abscesses—and share many clinical manifestations. Although liver abscesses are uncommon, their early diagnosis and management are crucial because of their high rate of mortality. Fortunately, the management of liver abscesses has improved over the years through advances in percutaneous drainage and laparoscopic techniques that have helped decrease the mortality rate from these lesions. The incidence of hepatic abscess is estimated to be eight to 15 cases per 100,000 population (1) or 13 to 20 per 100,000 hospital admissions (2). In the United States, approximately 80% of liver abscesses are pyogenic, 10% are amebic, 10% are due to superinfections, and less than 10% are due to fungal and other organisms (3). Liver abscesses are solitary in 50% to 60% of cases and multiple in the remainder. Multiple abscesses may coalesce into a larger abscess with or without the formation of septa. Pyogenic abscesses tend to be multifocal, especially when they originate from sepsis or pyelophlebitis, whereas amebic abscesses are usually solitary. Abscesses are more common in the right lobe of the liver (60%) than in the left lobe (10%–15%) and are bilobar in 20% of cases. Their high prevalence in the right lobe may be due to the laminar drainage of the superior mesenteric vein into this lobe of the liver. Pyogenic liver abscesses affect both sexes and all age groups; however, in a Los Angeles study, these abscesses were found to have a male-to-female predominance of 2:1 in young patients with AIDS. Amebic abscesses of the liver occur in 10% of cases of amebic colitis and in a male-to-female ratio that ranges from 9–10:1.

Etiology

The etiology of liver abscesses varies worldwide and is changing in some countries as a result of better health care and increased recognition through more advanced diagnostic techniques. Although pyogenic liver abscesses are the type preponderantly seen in most of the United States, amebic liver abscesses are endemic in many areas of the world. Other, less common abscesses involve cytomegalovirus, fungi, infected echinococcal cysts, and other organisms. Bacteria may spread to the liver through the following routes (2,4):

Biliary tree: from cholecystitis, choledocholithiasis, or cholangitis or from obstructing biliary or pancreatic malignancies
Portal vein: from appendicitis, diverticulitis, inflammatory bowel diseases, or pelvic inflammatory diseases
Hepatic artery: from hematogenous spread from other foci in the body
Adjacent organs: from direct extension from organs such as the gallbladder or from subhepatic or subdiaphragmatic infections

Direct trauma
Necrosis of hepatic neoplasms
Cryptogenic infection: infection without an identifiable source

The incidence of hepatic abscesses is rising, possibly as a result of increased instrumentation of the biliary tree, transplantation and immunosuppression, and improved diagnosis (5–7). In the beginning of the 20th century, the most common causes of pyogenic liver abscesses were appendicitis and diverticulitis (8). Lately, the leading cause of hepatic abscess has been biliary in origin.

The bacteriology of liver abscesses shows that most cases (79%) are polymicrobial, with enteric gram-negative bacilli (usually *Escherichia coli*) being the most common pathogen. Other facultative isolates are streptococci, enterococci, *Klebsiella pneumoniae*, and *Staphylococcus aureus* (9). With recent progress in anaerobic culture techniques, the frequency of anaerobe involvement in hepatic abscess has been found to be approximately 50% (10). The involved anaerobes include species of *Bacteroides*, *Fusobacterium*, *Actinomyces*, *Peptostreptococcus*, *Clostridium*, and *Prevotella* (9). Fungal liver abscesses, especially those caused by *Candida albicans* are usually multiple, stem from systemic fungemia, and are prevalent in patients with cancer and immune-deficiency syndromes (11). Rare causes of hepatic abscess are *Yersinia enterocolitica* and tuberculosis (12,13).

Clinical Manifestations

Symptoms of pyogenic liver abscesses are variable and, in some cases, entirely absent. Clinical findings include fever, chills, malaise, abdominal pain, nausea, anorexia, and weight loss usually of less than 2-weeks' duration but in some cases lasting several months. Because of the nonspecific symptoms of pyogenic liver abscesses, a significant number of patients with prolonged illness caused by such abscesses may have had a previous diagnosis of fever of unknown origin. Physical findings include right-upper-quadrant tenderness with hepatomegaly in 50% to 70% of patients, pleural dullness on percussion, and jaundice (2,14). Abscesses located high in the right upper lobe may cause respiratory symptoms, including cough, pleuritic pain that may radiate to the right shoulder, and a pleuritic rub. Chest radiography usually reveals an elevated right hemidiaphragm with basilar atelectasis and effusion.

Patients with amebic abscesses have a presentation similar to that of those with pyogenic abscesses but who additionally may have a history of diarrhea and radiographic chest findings and, in some series, have lacked the spiking temperature of the latter group. Rarely, patients with amebic abscesses may present with left-upper-quadrant pain if the abscess involves the left lobe of the liver and extends into the pericardium. Serologic tests for amebic infection help in differentiating amebic and pyogenic abscesses.

Most patients with liver abscesses have leukocytosis and increased liver enzyme activity, with alkaline phosphatase the enzyme most severely affected.

Half of patients with pyogenic abscesses have positive blood cultures. The presence of *Streptococcus viridans* and increased liver enzyme activities in the absence of endocarditis is an important clue to the diagnosis of pyogenic liver abscesses.

Diagnosis

Radiologic evaluation is the key to diagnosing liver abscesses in more than 95% of cases. Chest and abdominal radiography reveal nonspecific abnormalities in approximately 50% of cases, including right-lower-lobe atelectasis and infiltrates, right pleural effusion, and an elevated right hemidiaphragm; on most abdominal radiographs and some chest radiographs, extraluminal air can be seen in the right upper quadrant.

Ultrasonography is the most helpful screening test for liver abscess because of its high sensitivity (85%–95%), better biliary tree imaging than with computed tomography (CT), and therapeutic applicability to the biopsy or drainage of abscesses. Ultrasonography has its limitations in heterogeneous livers, lesions high in the chest cavity, and obese patients. CT is the most sensitive of all imaging modalities for liver abscess (95%–100%) and can be used for therapeutic intervention. It also can provide information about other abdominal lesions that may have caused a liver abscess. In some cases, CT reveals an enhancing rim around an abscess. Technetium-99m sulfur colloid scanning has been used widely to diagnose liver abscesses. Because the Kupffer's cells within the abscess and the Kupffer's cells that surround the abscess differ in their ability to engulf the Technetium-99m–labeled colloid, this technique can locate an abscess quite effectively. However, limitations of the technique include the inabilities to detect lesions smaller than 2 cm, to differentiate solid from cystic lesions, and to allow planning for therapeutic interventions. Although hepatic arteriography also has been used to image hepatic abscesses, it is invasive and does not offer any benefits over CT. Magnetic resonance imaging (MRI), although accurate in detecting liver abscesses, offers no advantage over CT scanning and does not allow percutaneous aspiration for diagnosis or treatment (1).

Amebiasis and amebic abscesses of the liver may be difficult to diagnose, because pathogens may not be recovered from pus. CT and ultrasonography can be used to aspirate these lesions for rapid diagnosis. Both aerobic and anaerobic cultures should be obtained. A sterile, brownish aspirate without a foul smell is characteristic of an amebic abscess. However, fluid in amebic abscesses can be yellow or green and secondarily infected with other organisms. Finding *Entamoeba histolytica* trophozoites on direct microscopy or culture is diagnostic of an amebic abscess. The diagnosis of amebic abscess can be confirmed by the finding of increased serum antiamebic antibody titers with an indirect hemagglutination test, for which results are readily available within 24 hours in most major medical centers. The serologic test for amebiasis indicates either past or current exposure to ameba and is positive in 90% of cases of amebic liver abscess; however, it could be misleading in areas of the world where such disease is endemic. If the diagnosis is in doubt, a trial of amebicidal therapy is helpful in reaching a conclusion.

Treatment

Pyogenic Liver Abscess

The keystones of treatment for pyogenic liver abscesses are drainage and antibiotic therapy in addition to eliminating the underlying source of the condition if it is known (15). Untreated pyogenic hepatic abscesses carry a 95% to 100% mortality rate. When a pyogenic hepatic abscess is suspected, the patient should be given broad-spectrum antibiotic therapy directed against gram-negative rods, *Streptococcus* species, and anaerobes. Appropriate initial antibiotics may include an aminoglycoside, clindamycin, or metronidazole for anaerobes and a penicillin. Antibiotic coverage is then adjusted according to the results of culture of the aspirated or drained abscess. The duration of antibiotic coverage can range from 2 weeks to 4 months, depending on the response of the patient. The mean duration of intravenous antibiotic therapy in one study was 19 days, with oral antibiotics given for long periods after hospital discharge because of their possible poor penetration into the abscess cavity (16). Once empirical antibiotic therapy is begun, CT or ultrasonography should be performed for diagnostic aspiration. If there is no intra-abdominal source of infection but there is at least one large abscess, then percutaneous drainage and antibiotic therapy may suffice.

In patients with multiple, small abscesses without intra-abdominal pathology, antibiotic therapy alone is a reasonable treatment choice, with surgical drainage reserved for cases of antibiotic failure if the clinical setting dictates the need. If on the initial CT scan an intra-abdominal source is found, then surgical drainage and surgical treatment of the source is recommended. Simple aspiration is useful as a diagnostic adjunct to antibiotic therapy in healthy young individuals and for draining multiple small abscesses. Most liver abscesses require continuous catheter drainage, with assessment by CT or ultrasonography once per week (sooner if there is no response to therapy). In the past, surgical drainage was the only available treatment option for hepatic abscesses. Currently, the indications for surgery include cases of liver abscess with an identifiable abdominal pathology and cases in which percutaneous drainage fails or cannot be performed. The availability of intraoperative sonography has been found to aid the detection and drainage of deep intrahepatic lesions; the mean time to defervesce was of 6 days, with more rapid defervescence in the group treated with antibiotics and catheter drainage than in the group treated with surgical drainage alone (16).

Recently, alternative approaches have been introduced for the treatment of pyogenic liver abscesses. Laparoscopic techniques have been used to drain hepatic abscesses and to identify and treat underlying abdominal pathology. This approach, in addition to antibiotic therapy, has been used for patients in whom percutaneous drainage has failed, thereby avoiding a laparotomy (17). Radiologic advances have allowed the drainage of pyogenic liver abscesses and the intracavitary instillation of antibiotics without the need for indwelling, percutaneously placed catheters (18). Endoscopic sphincterotomy with local antibiotic lavage via endoscopically placed nasobiliary catheters has been shown to be a safe and effective technique for completely resolving pyogenic abscesses of biliary origin, with only one of 19 patients requiring salvage surgical drainage (19).

Amebic Liver Abscess

The treatment of choice for amebic liver abscesses is an amebicidal agent. Metronidazole 750 mg orally for 7 to 14 days can be used effectively to treat both the hepatic and intestinal phases of most cases of amebiasis. In some cases, however, metronidazole may have to be continued for 4 to 6 weeks. In patients unable to take metronidazole orally, it can be given intravenously with similar results. Other agents used include emetine, dehydroemetine, and chloroquine; however, the toxicity of these drugs seldom makes them the primary agents of choice. Aspiration is rarely needed unless the diagnosis is suspect or a secondary bacterial infection is present. Surgical drainage has a role in suspected abscess rupture, adjacent structure perforation, and cases of erosion or poor response to medical therapy. Patients who fail to respond to antiamebic therapy may have a bacterial infection, and their treatment should be adjusted accordingly. In patients with perforated amebic abscesses, needle aspiration in combination with drug therapy is superior to drug therapy alone (20).

The prognosis of hepatic amebic abscess is good: Mortality from uncomplicated amebic abscesses is less than 5%. In cases in which there is erosion into the pericardium or free intraperitoneal rupture, the mortality rises to 30% to 50%.

Splenic Abscesses

Isolated splenic abscesses are rare and potentially lethal, and their diagnosis is often delayed. Fewer than 400 cases had been reported before 1986, but more case reports and smaller series have been reported recently, with a wider range of clinical conditions (21). The incidence of splenic abscesses in autopsy series ranges from 0.14% to 0.70% (22). Immunosuppression by AIDS and for organ transplantation, more aggressive chemotherapy for a wider variety of cancers, and efforts to conserve the spleen after trauma have contributed to the recent increase in splenic abscesses and to the change in pattern and bacteriology of these lesions (23). Splenic abscesses can appear *de novo* in patients in intensive care units (ICUs) and carry a high mortality rate (40%–100%), especially after surgery or trauma (24).

Etiology

The etiology of splenic abscesses can be divided into the following five major categories (21):

1. **Hematogenous spread from septic foci:** probably the most common; distant sources of infection that affect the spleen include endocarditis (25,26), pyelonephritis, disseminated tuberculosis (27), *Salmonella* bacteremia in AIDS patients (28), immunosuppression in cancer patients, intravenous drug abuse, intra-abdominal sepsis, chest infections, osteomyelitis, infected vascular access sites, infected ventriculoperitoneal shunts, and tooth extractions.
2. **Contiguous infection through direct spread from adjacent viscera:** such as in the case of colonic or gastric perforations and pancreatic and subphrenic abscesses
3. **Secondary infection of a splenic infarct:** such as those caused by emboli from the heart, lipid embolization in Weber–Christian disease, splenic artery embolization, and infarction due to splenic vein thrombosis from sickle cell disease or hemoglobinopathies (e.g., thalassemia).
4. **Splenic trauma:** including procedural or iatrogenic injury (29)
5. **Immunodeficiency:** especially when fungi or unusual organisms are involved.

Clinical Manifestations

The clinical presentation of splenic abscesses is nonspecific but includes abdominal pain in the left upper quadrant, fever, and leukocytosis (23,30). Most patients present with fever (69%–90%) and abdominal pain (56%–70%) (29). Other findings that may suggest splenic abscesses are pain referred to the left shoulder (from diaphragmatic irritation), elevation of the left hemidiaphragm, and left pleural effusion. Splenomegaly is present in 31% to 40% of patients (29).

Diagnosis

A high degree of clinical suspicion is essential for the early diagnosis of splenic abscesses. Diagnosis usually is delayed, with the duration of symptoms averaging 16 to 22 days (31). Plain radiography of the chest may reveal atelectasis of the left lower lobe, infiltrates, effusion, an elevation of the left hemidiaphragm, extraintestinal air-fluid levels, or diffuse air pockets in the left upper quadrant. Ultrasonography, CT, and MRI have been used successfully for diagnosing splenic abscesses. Ultrasonography is a good screening technique, especially when a 5-MHz linear-array transducer is used rather than a 3.5-MHz sector transducer (32). CT is superior to ultrasonography because it 1) can define the exact location of an abscess, 2) can demonstrate subcapsular or perisplenic pathology, 3) is unhindered by air in the left upper quadrant, and 4) has both a reported sensitivity and specificity of 96% (21,33). Leukocytosis has been reported in 60% to 100% of patients with splenic abscesses, depending on the series (21,29). Positive blood cultures have been found in 48% of patients, with only 24% having organisms similar to those obtained from their abscess pus (21). In their review, Ooi and Leong (21) found thrombocytosis (mainly due to splenic infarction) in 17% of cases; however, it was present in eight of nine patients in an ICU setting. It is worth mentioning that unexplained thrombocytosis in a septic ICU patient with persistent left pleural effusion is suggestive of splenic abscess (24).

Treatment

Once the diagnosis of a splenic abscess is made, treatment with broad-spectrum antibiotics should be instituted, because 25% of splenic abscesses are polymicrobial with anaerobes (23). Antibiotic therapy should be targeted against streptococci and staphylococci, which are the most common organisms seen in splenic abscesses and reflect the most common causes of abscesses that result from endocarditis or intravenous drug abuse. Gram-negative rods such as *Salmonella* and *Escherichia coli* account for 30% of cases of splenic abscess, whereas anaerobes account for 12%; both types of organism should be covered initially (21). Antibiotic therapy can then be tailored to the results of blood cultures, and surgical drainage can be performed (Table 11.1). Fungal splenic abscesses (especially those caused by *Candida*) have been on the rise, principally among patients who receive corticosteroids and those who undergo chemotherapy for cancer; antifungal coverage alone may be adequate for treating abscesses, particularly because most of those are caused by fungi and are small and multifocal. Antibiotic therapy alone, without drainage of a splenic abscess, carries a high mortality (*see* Table 11.1). Up to 90% of patients with unilocular, well-contained bacterial abscesses may be managed

Table 11.1   Common Causes and Recommended Antimicrobial Therapies for Various Intra-abdominal Abscesses

Condition	Common Etiologic Microorganisms	Antimicrobial Therapies*
Liver abscess		
Pyogenic	*Actinomyces* spp.	Single agents:
	Bacteroides spp.	Imipenem 500 mg IV q6h
	Clostridium spp.	*or*
	Enterococcus spp.	Beta-lactam or beta-lactamase-inhibitor combinations†
	Escherichia coli	Combination therapy:
	Fusobacterium spp.	Ampicillin 1–2 g IV q6h + gentamicin‡ 1 mg/kg IV q8h + either
	Klebsiella pneumoniae	metronidazole§ 500 mg IV q6h or clindamycin 600–900 mg IV q8h
	Peptostreptococcus spp.	*or*
	Pseudomonas spp.	Cefotetan 2 g q12h or cefoxitin 2 g q6h + gentamicin (as above)
	Staphylococcus aureus	For penicillin-allergic patients:
	Viridans-group	Clindamycin 600–900 mg IV q8h + ciprofloxacin 400 mg IV q12h
	Streptococcus	
Amebic	*Entamoeba histolytica*	Metronidazole 750 mg PO tid for 7–14 days¶
Splenic abscess	*Escherichia coli*	Single agents:
	Salmonella spp.	As with pyogenic liver abscesses
	Staphylococcus spp.	Combination therapy
	Streptococcus spp.	As with pyogenic liver abscesses
		For penicillin-allergic patients:
		As with pyogenic liver abscesses
		or
		Metronidazole 500 mg IV qh6 + aztreonam 2 g IV q8h**
Pancreatic abscess	*Bacteroides fragilis*	Single agents:
	Enterobacteriaceae	As with pyogenic liver abscesses
	Enterococcus spp.	Combination therapy:
	Escherichia coli	Ampicillin 1–2 g IV q6h + gentamicin‡ 1 mg/kg IV q8h + either
	Klebsiella pneumoniae	metronidazole 500 mg IV q6h§ or clindamycin 600–900 mg IV q8h
	Pseudomonas aeruginosa	For penicillin-allergic patients:
	Staphylococcus aureus	As with pyogenic liver abscesses
Appendiceal abscess	*Bacteroides fragilis*	Single agents:
	Escherichia coli	As with pyogenic liver abscesses
	Peptostreptococcus spp.	Combination therapy
	Pseudomonas aeruginosa	As with pyogenic liver abscesses
		For penicillin-allergic patients:
		As with pyogenic liver abscesses
Diverticular abscess	*Bacteroides fragilis*	Single agents:
	Escherichia coli	As with pyogenic liver abscesses
		or
		Cefotetan 2 g q12h or cefoxitin 2 g q6h IV
		Combination therapy:
		Ampicillin 1–2 g IV q6h + gentamicin‡ 1 mg/kg IV q8h + either
		metronidazole 500 mg IV q6h§ or clindamycin 600–900 mg IV q8h
		For penicillin-allergic patients:
		As with pyogenic liver abscesses

IV = intravenously; PO = orally.

* Antibiotic therapy should be directed toward the final culture results. Unless otherwise specified, treatment should last for 10–14 days until the patient is afebrile and has a normal leukocyte count. The antibiotic dosages should be adjusted according to the patient's renal and hepatic functions, with levels measured as necessary.

† These combinations include piperacillin–tazobactam 3.375 g IV q6h, ticarcillin–clavulanate 3.1 g q6h (has weak antienterococcal activity), and ampicillin–sulbactam (has no antipseudomonal activity).

‡ In patients with normal renal function, gentamicin dosage can be 5–7 mg/kg/d.

§ Has poor antistaphylococcal activity.

¶ In some cases, a duration of up to 4–6 weeks may be necessary.

** This combination does not have good activity against gram-positive cocci such as *Staphylococcus* and *Streptococcus* species.

with CT-guided percutaneous indwelling catheter drainage in addition to antibiotics (33). Splenectomy remains the treatment of choice for splenic abscesses and the gold standard for treating most of these lesions (34). Splenotomy with drainage is reserved for the most acutely ill patients, in whom extensive adhesions preclude the performance of a safe splenectomy. When untreated, splenic abscesses carry a mortality of close to 100% (35).

Pancreatic Abscesses

Infection of the pancreas is most often a consequence of secondary infection. The infection is usually bacterial and occurs in previously damaged pancreatic tissue. Most pancreatic cysts result from trauma and inflammatory diseases. The types of pancreatic cyst can be classified as infected pseudocyst, pancreatic abscess, and infected pancreatic necrosis (36). Each has different connotations for survival. An infected pseudocyst may be amenable to percutaneous drainage with minimal risk of mortality. Pancreatic abscess and infected pancreatic necrosis increase the risk of mortality two- and four-fold, respectively (36). Pancreatic abscess can be defined as a contained, intra-abdominal infection with purulent material close to the pancreas without any pancreatic necrosis. Infected pancreatic necrosis is defined as a diffuse or focal area of nonviable parenchyma with associated bacterial infection (37). The more severe the initial pancreatitis, the more likely it is that the patient will develop a secondary infection of the pancreas.

Etiology

As mentioned previously, most pancreatic abscesses occur as complications of pancreatitis (whatever the cause) and trauma. Additionally, endoscopic retrograde cholangiopancreatography is becoming a source of pancreatic abscesses. Acute pancreatitis has many causes (Table 11.2). Most cases are related to the biliary tract or to alcohol consumption. Gallstones obstruct the ampulla of Vater, which diverts bile flow into the pancreatic duct, causing injury and subsequent pancreatitis. The exact mechanism of alcohol-induced pancreatitis is unknown. The presence of acute necrotizing pancreatitis increases the likelihood of pancreatic infection and/or abscess. Infection develops in 40% of cases of pancreatic necrosis, usually in the second or third week of the disease (38).

Secondary pancreatic infections occur in 2% to 5% of cases of acute pancreatitis and represent serious complications (37). As a result, the pancreas becomes infected, either from the hematogenous spread of pathogens or from their transmural translocation from adjacent inflamed bowel.

Table 11.2   Etiologies of Acute Pancreatitis

Biliary tract disease	Ischemia
Alcohol	Pancreatic duct obstruction
Hyperlipidemia	Viral infection
Hypercalcemia	Scorpion venom
Familial	Idiopathic
Trauma	Drugs

Organisms cultured from pancreatic abscesses are predominantly gram negative and polymicrobial. They include *E. coli*, other Enterobacteriaceae organisms, and other aerobic fecal flora (39).

Clinical Manifestations

The clinical presentation of acute pancreatitis varies. The patient can present with a mild form of the disease or with hypovolemic shock, sepsis, or metabolic abnormalities (37). The pain typically begins in the mid-epigastrium and is constant. The pain itself is of varying intensity, and the patient may present with generalized peritonitis. The patient may complain of pain "boring into the back." Nausea and vomiting may accompany the abdominal pain. Abdominal distention resulting from paralytic ileus may be present. If hemorrhagic pancreatitis is present, Grey Turner's sign or Cullen's sign (i.e., a bluish discoloration of the flank or umbilicus, respectively) may be present, indicating severe pancreatitis. Jaundice may be present in patients with gallstone-induced pancreatitis.

A pancreatic phlegmon is palpable in a minority of patients. The patient with secondary infection may recover initially from a bout of acute pancreatitis only to deteriorate suddenly, or he or she may simply fail to respond to the initial therapy.

Diagnosis

The diagnosis of acute pancreatitis is based on the clinical presentation of the patient, laboratory values, and radiologic studies. An increased serum amylase is the laboratory parameter accepted most widely for assisting the diagnosis (40). A persistently increased amylase level beyond the first week usually reflects ongoing inflammation or may signal the development of complications such as a pseudocyst, phlegmon, or abscess (37). Persistent abdominal pain, fever, and leukocytosis also should alert the physician to the possibility of secondary infection.

Identifying a pancreatic pseudocyst, phlegmon, or abscess can be made in 80% to 90% of cases through imaging studies with ultrasonography, CT, or radionuclide scanning; however, CT is diagnostically superior to ultrasonography. Plain radiography may reveal a left pleural effusion, elevated hemidiaphragm, or retrogastric or retroperitoneal air. Contrast studies might show displacement of the stomach or duodenum. It can be difficult to distinguish sterile pancreatic necrosis from secondarily infected pancreatic abscesses. A CT scan alone may be beneficial in this regard, but CT-guided aspiration, Gram staining, and culture may be necessary to make the distinction (40). Ultrasonography also can be used for guided placement of drains or aspiration. Dynamic CT scanning can provide information about the viability of the pancreas through the uptake of intravenous contrast medium. MRI and radionuclide studies have not been beneficial in aiding in the diagnosis of pancreatic cysts (41).

Treatment

Appropriate empirical intravenous antibiotic coverage of pancreatic cysts should be started promptly (Table 11.1). Percutaneous drainage alone seems inadequate in most cases but can be considered as the initial treatment for culture-positive cysts (42,43). The indications for surgical drainage include demonstration of an infected pancreatic necrosis by bacterial cytology or dynamic CT scan or by a failure of a trial of percutaneous drainage. Some authors continue to recommend surgical drainage as the procedure of choice (40).

Several surgical options are available for the management of pancreatic cysts. Each has its proponents, and the surgeon should be familiar with all possible treatments. Reexploration is frequently needed in this group of patients. A midline abdominal or bilateral subcostal incision is used to gain access to the retroperitoneum, which is entered through the gastrocolic ligament.

All necrotic material must be debrided, which is performed with a blunt finger-fracture method to avoid injury to neighboring blood vessels. The pancreatic bed must be irrigated copiously. The pancreatic bed can be packed, and plans can be made for reoperation 48 hours later, with the absence or presence of healthy granulation used to determine a plan for subsequent laparotomies. After suction drains have been placed, the fascia are then closed.

Another operative plan is to leave several large-bore drains in place after adequate tissue debridement has been performed. Subsequently, these drains can be used for continuous postoperative lavage in the ICU. Large quantities of saline are instilled through one set of catheters, and the other set of catheters allows the saline to be collected.

Surgical debridement with closed-suction drainage is another option. With this method it is occasionally difficult to determine clinically when a repeat exploration is necessary. With the other methods described, reexploration is performed at 48-hour intervals to assess the viability of the tissue.

Recently, laparoscopic debridement of pancreatic abscesses has been performed successfully by placing trocars in the abscess cavity (44). Before the laparoscopic procedure is undertaken, percutaneous drainage is obtained with a size-16F catheter. Following the tract of the percutaneously placed catheter, a 5-mm trocar is positioned in the cavity and is subsequently replaced by an 11-mm trocar. The debridement is then performed, either under direct vision or by tactile sensation. The patient may have to make many trips to the operating room. With the future of surgery moving increasingly toward minimally invasive surgery, this laparoscopic debridement technique merits further investigation.

Appendiceal Abscess

The natural history of appendicitis includes perforation in 16% of cases (45). When an appendix perforates, a periappendiceal abscess, a phlegmon, or diffuse peritonitis develops. A periappendiceal abscess is a pus-containing periappendiceal mass, which usually lies in the right lower quadrant. A periappendiceal phlegmon is an inflammatory mass that comprises the appendix, adjacent viscera, and the omentum but does not contain purulent material (46). Diffuse peritonitis signifies a surgical emergency. These patients need to go to the operating room emergently. It is best to diagnose and treat appendicitis before perforation occurs to prevent the morbidity associated with the latter.

Etiology

Appendiceal abscesses result from the rupture of an acutely inflamed appendix. From 2% to 6% of cases of acute appendicitis are complicated by periappendiceal masses and/or abscesses (46). Obstruction of the lumen by a fecalith is the most common cause of appendicitis. The obstruction causes distention of the appendiceal lumen, which in turn increases the intraluminal pressure (45). Mucosal secretion and multiplication of bacteria continue, adding to the increased pressure. The intraluminal pressure eventually exceeds venous pressure, whereas arterial inflow continues, resulting in vascular congestion (45). As the distention progresses, the arterial inflow is compromised, causing areas of infarction and necrosis. Ultimately this leads to perforation, usually on the antimesenteric side of the appendix.

The bacteriology of appendiceal abscesses, as with most intra-abdominal abscesses, is polymicrobial. Anaerobes, aerobes, and facultative bacteria have been cultured from appendiceal abscesses (47). *Bacteroides fragilis* and *E. coli* are the most common organisms identified (47).

Clinical Manifestations

Abdominal pain is the most common complaint in appendicitis. The classic pain of appendicitis begins in the periumbilical region and, after a period of several hours, localizes to the right lower quadrant (45). This classic symptomatology is not always present: some people may have right lower-quadrant pain beginning with the onset of symptoms. The position of the appendix determines the clinical symptoms in cases of appendicitis. A long appendix in the pelvis may cause suprapubic pain, whereas a retrocecal appendix may cause back and right-flank pain. Malrotation causes pain on the left side of the abdomen that, in the elderly, may be confused with diverticulitis. Anorexia almost always accompanies appendicitis, and vomiting occurs in most patients. If vomiting occurs before the onset of pain, the diagnosis of appendicitis should be questioned (45).

The patient usually lies still, occasionally with the hips flexed to help relieve the peritoneal irritation. If the appendix lies anteriorly, then right-lower-quadrant pain is present in its characteristic fashion. Rebound and guarding are usually present, with maximal pain in the right lower quadrant. Leukocytosis is present and mild. A low-grade fever is present, with the temperature rarely exceeding 38.5°C (45).

Appendiceal rupture should be suspected in patients with a temperature above 39°C and with leukocytosis exceeding 18,000/mm^3 (45). Most appendiceal ruptures are contained, and generalized peritonitis is not present. If the rupture cannot be contained, generalized peritonitis occurs. In cases of appendiceal rupture, a mass may be palpable in the right lower quadrant. However, because of abdominal-wall guarding or obesity, the mass may not be palpable until the patient is anesthetized. Patients with an appendiceal mass and/or abscess tend to have longer periods of symptoms (usually lasting 5–7 days) before they present for treatment (46).

Diagnosis

Plain radiography of the abdomen in appendicitis patients reveals a nonspecific bowel gas pattern and only rarely reveals a fecalith. Ultrasonography has been used to diagnose acute appendicitis and appendiceal masses and abscesses. The diameter of the appendix is measured together with graded compression. The diagnosis of appendicitis can be made if the appendix is noncompressible and 6 mm in diameter (48).

The appendiceal mass can be seen more clearly on CT, which also allows one to assess the feasibility of percutaneous drainage. Contrast-enhanced CT is helpful in differentiating a phlegmon from an abscess.

Treatment

Broad-spectrum antibiotics that are targeted at the polymicrobial nature of appendiceal abscesses should be instituted in patients with these lesions. An antibiotic regimen consisting of an aminoglycoside with either clindamycin or metronidazole is effective (46) (Table 11.1).

Appendiceal abscesses can be treated in two ways: 1) immediate appendectomy with abscess drainage, or 2) initial nonoperative management with no oral intake, intravenous fluids, and intravenous antibiotics with or without percutaneous drainage. Proponents of immediate appendectomy state that it reduces hospital length of stay and spares the patient the risk of recurrent appendicitis. Those who propose initial nonoperative management state that the appendectomy-and-drainage procedure is technically difficult because of increased inflammation.

Most appendiceal masses resolve promptly with initial nonoperative treatment. If the mass and/or signs of infection persist, the causative abscess or phlegmon should be drained, preferably percutaneously. An interval appendectomy should be performed 6 to 8 weeks later. An interval appendectomy is performed to prevent recurrent episodes of appendicitis (46). In a recent report from the Harbor–University of California at Los Angeles Medical Center, nonoperative management failed in 5% of a simultaneously admitted series of patients with appendicitis (49). Failure consisted of progression of disease to peritonitis or simply failure to improve. Most of those patients who had recurrent appendicitis had it within the first 9 weeks after discharge (49).

Laparoscopic appendectomy is gaining favor among many surgeons as the treatment of choice for appendicitis (48). It permits a more complete examination of the abdomen and is especially useful for ruling out gynecologic diseases (48). Laparoscopically performed interval appendectomy has been proved to be safe to perform (50).

Patients 40 to 50 years of age or older who develop perforated appendicitis with a phlegmon or abscess and who initially were treated nonsurgically should have either a double-contrast enema or should undergo colonoscopy to rule out a malignant cecal tumor.

Diverticular Abscesses

The terminology for diverticular disease and associated inflammation or abscesses may be confusing. *Acute diverticulitis* implies an acute inflammatory process that results from an inflamed diverticulum. The inflammation is limited to the involved bowel wall and surrounding structures (most commonly the attached mesentery), and there is no confined collection of pus. In contrast, a *diverticular abscess* is a collection of pus usually associated with a perforated diverticulum. This abscess may be relatively contained by either the bowel wall mesentery or other structures in close proximity (e.g., lateral or anterior abdominal wall, urinary bladder, loops of small intestine). The perforation may spread freely within the peritoneal cavity, leading to generalized peritonitis, which is a surgical emergency.

Etiology

Diverticular abscesses arise from a diverticular perforation that may occur anywhere along the gastrointestinal tract. Diverticula are either congenital or acquired. Small bowel and cecum diverticula are congenital and may perforate, leading to multiple abscesses within a particular loop. The sigmoid colon is by far the most frequent point of origin of acquired diverticula, arising from a point of vascular egress within the hypertrophied muscular wall of the sigmoid colon. The following discussion focuses on abscesses associated with sigmoid diverticula (51).

Clinical Manifestations and Diagnosis

Patients who present with a diverticular abscess usually have concomitant fever, leukocytosis, and abdominal pain. The temperature may reach 39°C or higher, and a marked left shift is usually noted in the complete blood count. Findings on physical examination are highly variable and range from a dull but persistent abdominal pain to signs of frank peritonitis. The pain may be localized to the suprapubic region in the midline if the abscess is confined to the mesentery. In this situation, the sigmoid colon is pushed medially and anteriorly. The pain may be restricted to the left lateral abdominal wall if the abscess or inflammation is located between the colon and the lateral abdominal wall. Bowel movements may reflect either constipation or diarrhea, but the passage of formed, regular stool is the exception.

In some patients who present with acute diverticulitis, intensive antibiotic therapy may fail to resolve the inflammation and an abscess may develop. The clinical course of such patients is often characterized by unremitting fever, rising leukocytosis, and worsening abdominal pain.

Scanning with CT has proved an invaluable radiographic method both for the diagnosis of diverticular abscess and as a guide to its treatment. Pus or abscess formation may be readily distinguished from the more common mesenteric inflammation. Importantly, CT permits other diseases (e.g., perforated cancer of the colon, appendicitis [which often mimics the clinical presentation of diverticulitis with associated abscess]) to be evaluated. In patients with diverticular abscesses, it is important to remember that, as with all intra-abdominal abscesses, occult hypoxemia may be present. Thus, routine monitoring of oxygenation becomes important. Additionally, the overall nutritional status of the patient should be assessed at the time of hospital admission.

Treatment

Once diagnosed, a diverticular abscess is an indication for drainage. Diverticular abscesses do not resolve with antibiotic therapy alone. CT and CT-guided percutaneous drainage represent a huge step forward in the management of difficult, often elderly and frail, patients in whom many diverticular abscesses occur. A loculated abscess may be approached percutaneously, and effective drainage may be achieved. Usually, once defervescence and signs of systemic toxicity resolve, repeat CT is performed at 5 to 7 days, along with a sinogram to ensure closure of the diverticulum and the absence of any persisting fistulous tract. A repeat CT scan is also performed if the patient has not improved by 24 to 48 hours after drainage. This is used to assess any residual or ongoing abscesses. If at this point CT-guided drainage has been unsuccessful, surgical drainage via laparotomy should be instituted promptly. Broad-spectrum antibiotic coverage is begun, with the regimen usually consisting of an aminoglycoside and an agent effective against anaerobes (e.g., clindamycin, metronidazole). Aminoglycosides should be administered with caution in the elderly, particularly those with underlying renal dysfunction. Alternatively, initial therapy may begin as monotherapy with a broad-spectrum cephalosporin (*see* Table 11.1).

Once control of the abscess is achieved by nonoperative means, consideration should be given to elective colon resection with a primary anastomosis and a one-stage operation (52).

REFERENCES

1. **Branum GD, Meyers WC.** Pyogenic and amebic liver abscess. In Sabiston DC, Lyerly HK (eds). *Sabiston's Textbook of Surgery*, 15th ed. Philadelphia: WB Saunders; 1997:1061–8.

2. **Huang CJ, Pitt HA, Lipsett PA, et al.** Pyogenic hepatic abscess: changing trends over 42 years. *Ann Surg.* 1996;223:600–9.

3. **Barnes PF, Delock KM, Reynolds TN, et al.** A comparison of amebic and pyogenic abscess of the liver. *Medicine.* 1987;66:472–83.

4. **Branum CD, Tyson GS, Branum MA, et al.** Hepatic abscess: changes in etiology, diagnosis, and management. *Ann Surg.* 1990;212:655–62.

5. **Madariaga JR, Fung J, Gutierrez J, et al.** Liver resection combined with excision of vena cava. *J Am Coll Surg.* 2000;191:244–50.

6. **Kubo S, Kinoshita H, Hirohashi K, et al.** Risk factors for clinical findings of liver abscess after biliary-intestinal anastomosis. *Hepatogastroenterology.* 1999;46:116–20.

7. **Yu A, Mindelzum RE, Jeffrey RB Jr.** Hepatic abscess following transhepatic drainage of subphrenic abscess. *Abdom Imaging.* 1999;24:163–4.

8. **Ochsner A, DeBakey M, Murray S.** Pyogenic abscess of the liver. Part II: An analysis of forty-seven cases with review of the literature. *Am J Surg.* 1938;40:292.

9. **Brook I, Frazier EH.** Microbiology of liver and spleen abscesses. *J Med Microbiol.* 1998;47:1075–80.

10. **Perera MR, Kirk A, Noone P.** Presentation, diagnosis, and management of pyogenic liver abscess. *Lancet.* 1980;2:629–32.

11. **Thaler M, Pastakia B, Shawker T, et al.** Hepatic candidiasis in cancer patients: the evolving picture of the syndrome. *Ann Intern Med.* 1988;108:88–100.

12. **Rabson AR, Koornhof HJ, Notman J, et al.** Hepatosplenic abscess due to *Yersinia enterocolitica.* *BMJ.* 1972;4:341.

13. **Spiegel CT, Tuazon CU.** Tuberculous liver abscess. *Tubercule.* 1984;65:127–31.

14. **Barbour GL, Juniper K Jr.** A clinical comparison of amebic and pyogenic abscess of the liver in sixty-six patients. *Am J Med.* 1972;53:323–34.

15. **Gerzof SG, Johnson WC, Robbins AH, et al.** Intrahepatic pyogenic abscesses: treatment by percutaneous drainage. *Am J Surg.* 1985;149:487–94.

16. **Seeto RK, Rocky DC.** Pyogenic liver abscess: changes in etiology, management, and outcome. *Medicine* 1966;75:99–113.

17. **Tay KH, Ravintharan T, Hoe MN, et al.** Laparoscopic drainage of liver abscesses. *Br J Surg.* 1998;85:330–2.

18. **Miller FJ, Ahola DT, Bretzman PA, et al.** Percutaneous management of hepatic abscess: a perspective by interventional radiologists. *J Vasc Interv Radiol.* 1997;8:241–7.

19. **Dull JS, Topa L, Balgha V, et al.** Nonsurgical treatment of biliary liver abscesses: efficacy of endoscopic drainage and local antibiotic lavage with nasobiliary catheter. *Gastrointest Endosc.* 2000;51:55–9.

20. **Meng XY, Wu JX.** Perforated amebic abscess: clinical analysis of 110 cases. *South Med J.* 1994;87:988–90.

21. **Ooi LPJ, Leong SS.** Splenic abscesses from 1987 to 1995. *Am J Surg.* 1997;174:87–93.

22. **Chun CH, Raff MJ, Contreras L, et al.** Splenic abscess. *Medicine.* 1990;59:50–65.

23. **Nelken N, Isnatius J, Skinner M, et al.** Changing clinical spectrum of splenic abscess: a multicenter study and review of the literature. *Am J Surg.* 1987;154:27–34.

24. **Ho HS, Wisner DH.** Splenic abscesses in the intensive care unit. *Arch Surg.* 1993;128:842–8.

25. **Robinson SL, Saxe JM, Lucas CE, et al.** Splenic diseases associated with endocarditis. *Surgery.* 1992;14:781–6.

26. **Ting W, Silverman NA.** Splenic septic emboli in endocarditis. *Circulation.* 1990;82(Suppl IV):105–9.

27. **Khalil T, Uzoara I, Nadimpalli V, et al.** Splenic tuberculosis abscess in patients positive for HIV: report of two cases and review. *Clin Infect Dis.* 1992;14:1265–6.

28. **Tores JR, Rodriquez-Casas J, Balda E, et al.** Multifocal *Salmonella* splenic abscess in

an HIV-infected patient. *Trop Geogr Med.* 1992;44:66–8.

29. **Toevs CC, Beilman GJ.** Splenic abscess 10 years after splenic trauma: a case report. *Am Surg.* 2000;66:204–5.

30. **Gadacz T, Way LW, Dunphy JE.** Changing clinical spectrum of splenic abscess. *Am J Surg.* 1974;128:182–7.

31. **Phillips G, Radosevich M, Lipsett P.** Splenic abscess: another look at an old disease. *Arch Surg.* 1997;132:1331–6.

32. **Murray JG, Patel MD, Lee S, et al.** Microabscesses of the liver and spleen in AIDS: detection with 5 MHz sonography. *Radiology.* 1995;197:723–7.

33. **Gleich S, Wolin D, Herbsman H.** A review of percutaneous drainage in splenic abscess. *Surg Gynecol Obstet.* 1988;167:211–6.

34. **Starr MG, Zuidema GD.** Splenic abscess: presentation, diagnosis, and treatment. *Surgery.* 1982;92:480–5.

35. **Linos DA, Nagorney DM, McIlrath DC.** Splenic abscess: the importance of early diagnosis. *Mayo Clin Proc.* 1983;58:261–4.

36. **Bradley E.** Pancreatic Abscess. In Cameron J (ed). *Current Surgical Therapy,* 6th ed. St. Louis: Mosby; 1995:502–6.

37. **Yeo CJ, Cameron J.** Acute pancreatitis. In Zuidema G (ed). *Shackelford's Surgery of the Alimentary Tract,* 4th ed. Philadelphia: WB Saunders; 1996;18–37.

38. **Stiles GM, Byrne TV, Thommen VD, et al.** Fine-needle aspiration of pancreatic fluid collections. *Am Surg.* 1990;56:764–8.

39. **Shi ECP, Yeo BW, Ham JM.** Pancreatic abscesses. *Br J Surg.* 1984;71:689–91.

40. **Reber H.** Pancreas. In Schwartz S (ed). *Principles of Surgery,* 7th ed. New York: McGraw-Hill; 1999:1467–99.

41. **Paushter DM, Modic MT, Borkowski GP, et al.** Magnetic resonance: principles and applications. *Med Clin North Am.* 1984;68:1393–421.

42. **Rotman N, Mathien D, Anglade MC, et al.** Failure of percutaneous drainage of pancreatic abscesses complicating severe acute pancreatitis. *Surg Gynecol Obstetr.* 1992;174:141–4.

43. **Baril N, Ralls P, Wren S, et al.** Does an infected peripancreatic fluid collection or abscess mandate operation? *Ann Surg.* 2000;231:361–7.

44. **Alveroy J, Vargish T, Desai T, et al.** Laparoscopic intracavitary debridement of peripancreatic necrosis: preliminary report and description of the technique. *Surgery.* 2000;127:112–4.

45. **Kozar R, Roslyn J.** The appendix. In Schwartz S (ed). *Principles of Surgery,* 7th ed. New York: McGraw-Hill; 1999:1383–94.

46. **Nitecki S, Assalia A, Schein M.** Contemporary management of the appendiceal mass. *Br J Surg.* 1993;80:18–20.

47. **Thadepalli H, Mandal AK, Chuah SK, Lou MA.** Bacteriology of the appendix and the ileum in health and appendicitis. *Am Surg.* 1991;57:317–22.

48. **Pegoli W.** Acute appendicitis. In Cameron J. *Current Surgical Therapy,* 6th ed. St. Louis: Mosby; 1995:263–6.

49. **Oliak D, Yamani D, Udani V, et al.** Nonoperative management of perforated appendicitis without periappendiceal mass. *Am J Surg.* 2000;179:177–81.

50. **Vargas HI, Averbrook A, Stamos MJ.** Appendiceal mass: conservative therapy followed by interval laparoscopic appendectomy. *Am Surg.* 1994;60:753–8.

51. **Saini S, Kellum JM, O'Leary MO, et al.** Improved localization and survival in patients with intraabdominal abscesses. *Am J Surg.* 1983;145:136.

52. **Pruett TL, Rotstein OD, Crass J, et al.** Percutaneous aspiration and drainage for suspected abdominal infection. *Surgery.* 1984;96:731.

12

Urinary Tract Infections in Adults

Allan R. Ronald, OC, MD

A urinary tract infection (UTI) is the presence of microbes anywhere in the urinary tract, including the proximal urethra, bladder, prostate gland, ureters, and kidneys. UTIs are common in all populations, and their global annual incidence probably exceeds 250 million. The infection may be limited to asymptomatic superficial colonization of the epithelial lining of the urinary tract, or it may progress to invasive inflammatory injury to the renal parenchyma or suppuration of renal tissue, occasionally spreading through the renal capsule and creating a perinephric abscess. UTIs are categorized as uncomplicated if there is no known functional or anatomic abnormality of the urinary tract and no underlying host abnormalities. Approximately 80% of UTIs are "uncomplicated." UTIs are termed *complicated* whenever any of the entities listed in Table 12.1 is present (1). Although many infections that are categorized as complicated can be readily cured, a proportion of complicated UTIs will be persistent, difficult-to-treat infections with frequent recurrences. As a result, the categorization of a UTI as complicated is important for patient management.

Etiology

The vast majority of UTIs are due to rapidly growing pathogens, with a predominance of *Escherichia coli*. Table 12.2 compares the prevalence of organisms in community-acquired infections, most of which are uncomplicated, and in hospital-acquired infections, many of which are complicated. The *E. coli*

Table 12.1　Classification of Causes of Complicated Urinary Tract Infections

---

Structural Abnormalities
  Obstruction
  Vesicouretal reflux
  Neurogenic bladder
  Calculi
  Renal abscess(es)
  Fistula to intestine or other sites
  Urinary diversion procedures
  Infected cysts
  Urinary catheters
Metabolic or Hormonal Abnormalities
  Diabetes mellitus
  Pregnancy
  Renal impairment
Impaired Host Response
  Post-transplantation
  Neutropenia
  HIV/AIDS
Unusual Pathogens
  Pseudomonas aeruginosa and other multiresistant organisms
  Calculi-associated bacteria
  Yeasts, fungi, mycobacteria

AIDS = acquired immune deficiency syndrome; HIV = human immunodeficiency virus.

strains that cause most community-acquired infections originate from colonic flora. Women with increased susceptibility to infections are more often colonized in the perineal areas and the vagina with *E. coli*, and this facilitates UTIs caused by *E. coli*. P-fimbriated *E. coli* of the pap+ genotype are more frequently associated with acute pyelonephritis. These organisms adhere to colonic, vulvovaginal, and uroepithelial cells, and thereby colonize and infect susceptible patients (2). Bacterial multiplication in the urinary tract results in cytokine generation, with the production of interleukins (ILs) IL-6 and IL-8 by mucosal cells (3). IL-6 activates acute-phase reactants and produces fever and other systemic symptoms. IL-8 is a chemoattractant for neutrophils.

Among sexually active women, *Staphylococcus saprophyticus* is in most settings the second most common urinary pathogen. Its epidemiology is not well understood. Group B streptococci, *Klebsiella* spp., *Proteus* spp., and other gram-negative organisms occur, also in UTIs, but are less frequent among patients with community-acquired infections. Patients receiving antimicrobial therapy often acquire more resistant infections, usually from altered flora within their gastrointestinal (GI) tract that develop as a result of antimicrobial pressure (4).

Table 12.2   Microbiology of Urinary Infection

	Uncomplicated	Complicated*
Escherichia coli	80–85%	40–60%
Klebsiella spp.	1–3%	5–10%
Enterobacter spp.	1–3%	5–10%
Proteus spp.	1–3%	5–10%
Pseudomonas spp.	<1%	5–10%
Staphylococcus saprophyticus	5–10%	1–2%
Staphylococcus epidermidis	1–3%	5–10%
Enterococci	1–3%	5–10%
Group B streptococci	1–3%	1–3%
Staphylococcus aureus	<1%	1–3%
Candida spp.	<1%	5–10%

*Many isolates of gram-negative rods in complicated urinary tract infections are multiresistant to urinary tract antimicrobial agents, and most have been acquired in an institutional setting (i.e., nosocomial).

Among patients with complicated infections, a variety of more resistant organisms occur. In the hospital setting, nosocomial infections are more common, and are often caused by difficult-to-treat pathogens such as *Pseudomonas aeruginosa*, other resistant gram-negative rods, and *S. epidermidis*. Among older men, *Enterococcus faecalis* is the second most common pathogen after *E. coli*. Institutionally acquired pathogens are often transmitted from other patients with nosocomial urinary infection. *Candida albicans* is commonly acquired within institutions, usually by patients with indwelling catheters and receiving antibacterial treatment regimens.

Fastidious organisms including anaerobes, *Ureaplasma urealyticum*, and invasive fungal infection caused by organisms other than *Candida* are all occasional pathogens. Viruses are sometimes present in urine (viruria), and occasionally propagate in renal tissue, producing local or systemic symptoms. However, viral UTIs are rarely diagnosed. Outbreaks of hemorrhagic cystitis due to adenovirus have been described (5). *Brucella* spp. and *M. tuberculosis* would not be considered among mixed *Mycobacterium* species (per Bergey's manual) should be considered in patients with persistent signs of infection and negative conventional urine cultures. However, these pathogens are unusual and, even in developing countries, are responsible for less than 1% of urinary infections.

Epidemiology

Approximately 150,000 individuals, or 1 per 1000 adults/year, are admitted to hospitals with acute pyelonephritis (6). UTIs are the most common nonsocomial-acquired infection, and their acquisition increases health care costs substantially. Renal infection was identified as the cause of death in 896 individuals in the United States in 1996 (7). Septicemia, which arises from the urinary tract in about one-third of instances, was responsible for 21,420 deaths (7).

The epidemiology of urinary infection varies with age, gender, and underlying risk factors (8). During the first year of life, the cumulative prevalence of UTI in males is about 0.2%. These infections are frequently symptomatic, and require urologic investigation because of the possibility of underlying congenital anomalies. Urinary infections are subsequently rare in male children, with a cumulative incidence by the age of 10 years of less than 1%. The presence of a foreskin increases by at least five-fold the probability of urinary infection during childhood and adolescence (9). Among girls, the cumulative incidence of UTI during the first 10 years of age is 3%. UTIs in infancy and early childhood can be associated with symptomatic pyelonephritis, persisting renal infection with failure of renal growth, and extensive renal scarring. As a result, urinary infections in early childhood are investigated and managed more aggressively. Treatment is usually prescribed, and follow-up cultures should be done to ensure cure. However, asymptomatic bacteriuria in a normal urinary tract in older girls is often benign, and management is controversial.

Acute cystitis is by far the most common clinical presentation of urinary infection in adults. Urinary infections are extremely common in sexually active women, with at least one-third of women having had an episode of symptomatic UTI within 10 years of the onset of sexual activity. In a prospective study of sexually active women, the annual incidence of cystitis was 50 for every 100 women in a health management organization, and 70 for every 100 women attending a university (10). Extrapolating from these data would suggest that at least 25 million episodes of cystitis occur each year in the United States. Most of these infections are treated by physicians.

Studies have shown that sexual intercourse and the use of spermicides, with or without a diaphragm, are predisposing factors for UTIs among sexually active women (10,11). Condoms coated with nonoxyl-9 also increase the risk of cystitis. Numerous other factors have been studied prospectively and appear not to be significant in predisposing to UTI. These include voiding habits, bathing, intake of fluid, voiding following intercourse, the direction of wiping after defecation, douching habits, types of menstrual protection or perineal hygiene (10). However, recent antecedent antimicrobial use, and in particular the use of beta-lactam antibiotics, alters vaginal flora and predisposes women to cystitis (4).

Factors that predispose women to an initial episode of acute cystitis also predispose to recurring bouts. About 5% of women are UTI-prone and experience multiple, closely spaced episodes of infection (10). Most of these women have uroepithelial cells to which invasive strains of *E. coli* are more readily adherent. No other functional abnormalities or defects in host response have been identified in these infection-prone women, and urologic investigation or treatment has no proven role in their management.

A proportion of patients who present with acute cystitis have renal involvement. Table 12.3 identifies factors that have been shown to increase the probability of upper tract infection in patients with symptoms confined to the bladder.

Both acute and recurrent cystitis are common in postmenopausal women. The risk factors for such cystitis are not well understood, but at least one study has suggested it may occasionally be due to estrogen deficiency (12). Additionally, older women with recurring UTIs may often have increased residual urine or other functional abnormalities of the urinary tract.

Acute pyelonephritis usually occurs among patients who are susceptible to acute cystitis. Pregnancy, diabetes, immunosuppression, and obstruction predispose both men and women to acute pyelonephritis. Among patients with diabetes, the incidence of acute hospitalization for pyelonephritis is 10 times that for controls without diabetes for both men and women (6).

The epidemiology of complicated UTIs has not been well studied. In a survey of nosocomial UTI, the incidence was 4.3/1000 patient days, and 88% of these infections were catheter related (13). However, UTIs are common in a wide range of patients with abnormalities of the urinary tract. In men under the age of 60, prostatic symptoms account for 25% of visits to urologists (14). Although less than 10% of these men are proven to have bacterial prostatitis, the diagnosis in such cases must be made with care, because treatment is expensive and prolonged (14). All patients with chronic indwelling catheters have bacteriuria, but most remain asymptomatic unless obstruction occurs. However, over decades of urinary drainage with a catheter, patients with cord injuries often experience complications caused by urinary stones or abscess formation, and a few progress to having end-stage renal disease. Complications are at least three times more common in chronically catheterized men than in chronically catheterized women.

Table 12.3   Factors that Predict Renal Involvement in Patients Presenting with Cystitis or Asymptomatic Bacteriuria

Vesicouretal reflux
Pregnancy
Upper tract pathology (known or unknown)
Diabetes
Relapse (rapid recurrence with identical pathogen)
Unusual or resistant pathogen
Older age
Nosocomially acquired infection

UTIs in pregnancy cause preterm labor and low birth weight (15). Also, almost one-half of patients with asymptomatic infections, if not treated, will develop pyelonephritis during pregnancy. Presumably, this is due to physiologic and anatomic changes in the urinary tract during pregnancy. Screening for and treating asymptomatic bacteriuria in all pregnant patients during the first trimester will prevent about 80% of episodes of acute pyelonephritis during pregnancy, and this intervention has been shown in prospective studies to decrease the incidence of prematurity by 10% to 20% (15).

Asymptomatic UTIs are common, and their prevalence is increased among patients who are prone to symptomatic infections. The prevalence of asymptomatic bacteriuria has been studied in many populations, and relevant data are summarized in Table 12.4. Asymptomatic bacteriuria has been a controversial diagnosis. Is it a benign happening or is it a *disease burden* with links to other illness or consequences? Studies done during the past decade have determined that, with the exception of its occurrence during pregnancy, asymptomatic UTI in the healthy adult urinary tract has limited significance for the patient's ongoing health, and rarely alters renal function or overall morbidity (16). As a result, asymptomatic UTI should not be routinely sought and treated. In particular, asymptomatic bacteriuria is extremely common among the elderly, and its treatment is usually futile and unnecessary (17). The known factors predisposing to asymptomatic infection are similar to those for symptomatic urinary infection, and include diabetes, residual urine, and urinary instrumentation, as well as sexual intercourse (8).

Clinical Manifestations and Differential Diagnosis

UTIs present clinically as cystitis with urgency, burning, frequency, and lower abdominal pain, or as pyelonephritis with fever, chills, flank pain, and symptoms of a systemic inflammatory response.

Acute cystitis, particularly when the urethral symptoms are prominent, must be differentiated from sexually transmitted infections such as those

Table 12.4   Prevalence of Asymptomatic Bacteriuria

Population Screened	
Males 1–12 years old	0.1%
Females 1–12 years old	1%
Females 20–40 years old (including pregnant women)	3–6%
Males 20–40 years old	0.1%
Elderly ambulatory patients (men and women)	5–15%
Elderly bedridden patients (men and women)	10–50%
Chronically catheterized patients (men and women)	100%

caused by *Chlamydia trachomatis, Neisseria gonorrhoeae*, and herpes simplex, which can also present with urethral symptoms. Some women may have difficulty differentiating symptoms originating from the genital tract from those due to urinary infection. In particular, the symptoms of urinary infection can be confused by patients with vulvovaginal moniliasis and other illnesses that manifest with predominantly vaginal symptoms. All women with a first diagnosis of urinary infection should have some laboratory investigation, usually including urinalysis and urine culture, and a sexual risk assessment. If the last of these is positive, further studies for sexually transmitted diseases (STDs) and vaginal pathogens are indicated.

Interstitial cystitis (IC) is a diagnosis that is poorly understood, difficult to confirm, and confused with recurring bacterial cystitis (18). This diagnosis is optimally made through a combination of features that include negative urine cultures (see section on Laboratory Testing), a lack of pyuria during symptomatic episodes, absence of a response to antibacterial treatment, and frequent recurrences. IC is at least 10 times as common in women as in men. On occasion, cystoscopy with dilatation of the bladder leads to the observation of petechiae on the bladder mucosa. However, the sensitivity and specificity of this cystoscopic diagnosis is still undetermined. At present, IC is a diagnosis of exclusion, and should be made only with serial observations over a patient's course. It is also uncommon in men. Additional investigation is required to establish diagnostic parameters and develop approaches for the care of these patients. Too often they are shunted from primary care physician to urologist and back with no adequate direction for long-term care.

Acute pyelonephritis must be an exact diagnosis, since it is frequently misdiagnosed. About one-fifth of patients initially diagnosed with pyelonephritis are proven to have alternate diagnoses including surgical conditions, acute pelvic inflammatory disease, ectopic pregnancy, diverticulitis, renal calculi, and other conditions that require a specific diagnosis. As a result, patients with clinically presumed acute pyelonephritis should be followed carefully until the diagnosis is confirmed by laboratory results. In addition, further investigation may be indicated to exclude obstruction and suppurative processes.

The complications of acute pyelonephritis are outlined in Table 12.5. Most of these occur because of infection in a host with an anatomic or functional abnormality of the urinary tract, although acute uncomplicated pyelonephritis occasionally leads to septic shock and multiple organ failure. As a result, pyelonephritis must be regarded as a relative medical emergency and treated promptly, and the patient observed until initial improvement.

Men may present with urethritis and/or cystitis due to urinary infection as well as with prostatic symptoms. The clinical features of acute prostatitis include fever, an acutely tender, warm prostate, and rectal or perineal pain. With this diagnosis, prostatic massage should not be done and prostatic ex-

Table 12.5   Complications of Acute Pyelonephritis

Hypotension, septic shock, multiple organ failure, death
Renal or perinephric abscesses
Metastatic infections at other sites
Papillary necrosis
Acute renal failure
Emphysematous pyelonephritis
Renal gangrene
Localized or generalized atrophy/permanent loss of function

amination should be performed with care. Recurring prostatic symptoms are a frustrating and common presentation to both family physicians and urologists (14). Men with presumed prostatic symptoms may have perineal discomfort, irritative symptoms on voiding, or rectal pain. Sometimes, impotence or other problems relating to coitus may predominate. Careful investigation before antibacterial treatment is essential in order to make a correct diagnosis and to avoid empiricism. Nonbacterial prostatitis, (i.e., inflammation without pathogens) is more common than bacterial prostatitis, and does not respond to anti-infectious agents (14). However, the pelviperineal pain syndrome or prostatodynia is the most common diagnosis made in men with pain localized to the prostate, groin, or perineum, and these patients do not have inflammation or infection in the prostate. Studies to sort out the etiology and influence the course of these common *symptom complexes* are currently underway.

Laboratory Testing

Laboratory diagnosis of UTI is usually straightforward. Pyuria is present in over 90% of patients with a UTI, and in its absence, the diagnosis should be reconsidered. Pyuria is ideally assessed with a leukocyte count made with a hemocytometer. The widely used leukocyte esterase test has a sensitivity of about 85% and a specificity of 90% for 10 or more leukocytes per high-power field. Microscopic hematuria is present in 20% to 40% of patients with acute cystitis. The observation is unusual in vaginitis. A urine gram stain or direct bacterial visualization has a low sensitivity (60%–70%) in identifying cystitis in women due to low bacterial numbers in one-third of patients. Of particular importance is that from 10% to 30% of patients with acute symptoms will have bacterial counts of $<10^8$ cfu/L (10^5 cfu/mL) (19). *Low count* bacteriuria occurs in both men and women with both acute cystitis and acute pyelonephritis. As a result, quantitatative counts cannot be used to exclude the diagnosis of UTI, particularly in patients with symptoms and pyuria.

Conversely, asymptomatic bacteriuria is a diagnosis made by the laboratory, and requires at least two urine cultures with $>10^8$ cfu/L (10^5 cfu/mL) unless the specimen is obtained through a catheter.

A positive microscopic examination of a properly collected, stained, and interpreted urine specimen is specific and may influence empiric treatment choices in patients with acute pyelonephritis (20). Urine culture requires proper collection and transport of the specimen in order to provide a definitive diagnosis. The specimen is usually cultured quantitatively on both blood agar and a selective medium. Although a number of so-called improved technologies have been evaluated for urine culture, few if any have proven to be less expensive or more definitive than the conventional urine culture technology.

Prostatitis is a particularly difficult diagnosis to confirm microbiologically. Because less than 10% of men who present to a physician with prostatic symptoms will be proven to have bacterial prostatitis, accurate diagnosis is a priority (14). Men with presumed acute prostatitis should have the condition diagnosed on the basis of clinical features together with a positive urine culture and occasionally a positive blood culture. Prostatic massage is contraindicated whenever acute prostatitis is the probable diagnosis. However, men with chronic prostatitis require a localization procedure initially described by Meares and Stamey (Table 12.6) (21). Quantititative counts need to be made on all specimens. Frequently, prostatic secretions are not obtained, and the VB3 voided bladder urine (*see* Table 12.6) specimen becomes critical for determining whether prostatic infection is present. Concomitant bacteriuria with counts over 10^5/mL prevents bacterial localization to the prostate. A 5-day course of nitrofurantoin before a localization procedure may assist by eradicating bacteriuria transiently but allowing persistence of bacteria in the prostate. The VB3 specimen or expressed prostatic secretion (EPS) will usually be culture positive within 24 hours after stopping nitrofurantoin if infection is present in the prostate. No pathogens have been consistently identified from men with *nonbacterial prostatitis*, and investigation for either *Chlamydia* spp. or *Mycoplasma* spp. is of no proven value (for a more detailed discussion, see *Chapter 17*, "Prostatitis and Epididymitis".)

Table 12.6   Localization Steps to Diagnose Prostatic Infection

Step 1:	Retract the foreskin, clean the glans penis, and obtain 5 ml of urine (VB1)
Step 2:	Obtain 20 ml of midstream urine *without* completion of voiding (VB2)
Step 3:	Massage prostate and collect expressed prostatic secretions
Step 4:	Collect 5 ml of urine (VB3)

All specimens should be cultured quantitatively and gram stains performed.
Wright's stain should be prepared from EPS and VB3 to examine cells.
EPS and/or VB3 must have bacterial counts at least one log greater than that of VB2 to diagnose prostatic infection.

Men presenting with urethritis, epididymitis, or infection within the scrotal sac should have a urine culture, *N. gonorrhoeae* and *C. trachomatis* studies, and if possible, prostatic fluid cultures. Bacterial epididymo-orchitis is common in elderly men, particularly in the presence of an indwelling catheter. Occasionally, a needle aspirate of a suppurative process in the scrotal sac may lead directly to microbiologic diagnosis.

In both men and women with symptoms confined to the bladder, localization of infection to one or both kidneys has been an unrealized goal. Efforts to localize infection urologically with ureteral catheterization are difficult, and expensive, and carry significant risk. The bladder washout technique of Fairley is unpleasant and often gives uncertain results. The antibody-coated bacteria test has failed to be a definitive test for the individual patient. As a result, no procedure is currently recommended for the vast majority of patients who present either without symptoms or with lower tract symptoms. However, relapse with the identical infecting pathogen within 2 weeks after following a short (3 day) course of treatment in women, and probably also in men, usually means more established persistent infection either at a renal or a prostatic site (22). Unfortunately, no prospective study has recently addressed the usefulness of this therapeutic maneuver to diagnose upper tract infection.

The microbiology of complicated urinary infections is less well characterized than that of uncomplicated infections. Multiple pathogens are often present, and one particular pathogen may initially predominate in culture. Often, suppression of one pathogen with a treatment regimen permits others to appear. Both microbial numbers in complicated UTI and correlates with abnormalities of the urinary sediment, including pyuria, are largely unstudied.

Blood cultures should be obtained for patients with presumed acute prostatic or renal infection, and are positive in 15% to 30% of cases. A positive blood culture has not been shown prospectively to alter the outcome of therapy for complicated infections.

Antimicrobial susceptibility testing should be done routinely of urine isolates from patients with pyelonephritis and those with complicated infections. However, this additional expense is not warranted for patients with cystitis, unless the patient has a history of previous treatment failure.

Follow-up urine cultures need be obtained only if patients have symptoms or have complicated UTIs. Historically, too much emphasis has been given to follow-up of adults with normal urinary tracts. In the absence of symptoms, follow-up has not been shown to be useful.

Imaging Studies

Imaging of the urinary tract has changed dramatically over the past decade. Intravenous pyelography is less useful than computed tomography (CT) scanning (23). Sonography is particularly useful for rapid evaluation for obstruction or abscesses, but is less sensitive than CT for recognizing calculi or renal abnormalities in acute pyelonephritis. Helical CT, if available, has become the procedure of choice for excluding obstruction, identifying suppurative processes, excluding other intraabdominal conditions that may mimic acute pyelonephritis, and diagnosing acute changes in patients with pyelonephritis (23). Helical CT has an accuracy of 97% in depicting ureteral calculi (23). It can also contribute to the diagnosis of renal tuberculosis and xanthogranulomatous pyelonephritis or other upper tract abnormalities that may present with symptoms that mimic recurrent urinary infection. Although helical CT requires a substantial initial investment of capital, the net marginal cost is less than excretory urography (intravenous pyelography [IVP]) and should, in most instances, replace this technology (23).

Nuclear imaging studies are of less use (23). The radiotracer Dimercaptosuccinic acid will be abnormal in patients with acute pyelonephritis, but appears to add nothing to a CT scan. A gallium- or indium-labeled white blood cell (WBC) scan will usually be positive in patients with acute pyelonephritis, but these technologies are rarely necessary. Occasionally, in the search for fever of unknown origin, indium or gallium studies will localize infection to the kidney.

Treatment

Drug choices and doses are summarized in Table 12.7.

Acute Cystitis

The treatment of acute cystitis has been extensively studied in numerous randomized controlled trials. Other urinary infection syndromes are less well investigated, with small numbers of patients and frequently inappropriate comparator arms. On the basis of more than 20 studies of women with acute bacterial cystitis, trimethoprim/sulfamethoxazole (TMP/SMX) is the drug of choice for acute cystitis (24,25). Single-dose treatment with TMP/SMX eradicates bacteriuria in about 85% of women with acute cystitis; a 3-day regimen eradicates bacteriuria in significantly more women (over 90%), and is equivalent to longer, 7- to 10-day courses of therapy. Longer courses of therapy are associated with greater adverse effects and increase the propensity to TMP/SMX-resistant recurrences (24,25). Trimethoprim alone is equivalent to the combination, and avoids the adverse effects associated with the use of sulfonamides. Beta-lactam drugs have also been well studied in randomized controlled trials of acute cystitis. Overall, they have a significantly lower eradication

Table 12.7   Drug Choice and Dose for Urinary Tract Infection

Acute Bacterial Cystitis and Asymptomatic Bacteriuria

Women

Trimethoprim/sulfamethoxazole	100 mg/800 mg	b.i.d.	3 days
Ciprofloxacin*	500 mg	b.i.d.	3 days
Ofloxacin*	400 mg	b.i.d.	3 days
Levofloxacin*	500 mg	Daily	3 days
Nitrofurantoin	100 mg	q.i.d.	7 days
Cephalexin	500 mg	q.i.d.	7 days

Men

Trimethoprim/sulfamethoxazole	160mg/800 mg	b.i.d.	7 days
Ciprofloxacin*	500 mg	b.i.d.	7 days
Ofloxacin*	400 mg	b.i.d.	7 days
Levofloxacin	500 mg	Daily	7 days
Cephalexin	500 mg	q.i.d.	7 days

Acute Pyelonephritis (Men and Women)

Oral trimethoprim/sulfamethoxazole	160 mg/800 mg	b.i.d.	14 days
Ciprofloxacin*	500 mg	b.i.d.	7 days[†]
Ofloxacin*	400 mg	b.i.d.	7 days[†]
Levofloxacin	500 mg	Daily	7 days[†]
Cephalexin	500 mg	q.i.d.	14 days

Intravenous Therapy/Hospitalization* (Usually for 2–4 Days Followed by an Oral Regimen for 14 Days

Gentamicin	5 mg/kg	Daily	2–4 days
with ampicillin	2 g	q6h	2–4 days
Ceftriaxone	1 g	Daily	2–4 days
Imipenem	500 mg	q6h	2–4 days
Piperacillin/tazobactam	3.375 g	q8h	2–4 days
Ciprofloxacin*	400 mg	q12h	2–4 days
Ofloxacin*	500 mg	q12h	2–4 days
Levofloxacin*	500 mg	Daily	2–4 days

* Identified fluoroquinolone antimicrobial agents. Other members of this class may be equally effective.
[†] A 7-day regimen of ciprofloxacin has been effective in curing most women with acute uncomplicated pyelonephritis. Similar studies in men or with other fluoroquinolones are not available.

rate than TMP/SMZ, particularly if prescribed for 3 days, and are associated with more adverse effects and recurrences with resistant pathogens (25).

Fluoroquinolones have been compared in 3-day and 7- to 10-day regimens (25,26). All fluoroquinolone regimens eradicate infection in at least 90% of premenopausal women with acute bacterial cystitis. A 3-day course is probably the optimal duration of therapy for achieving the greatest efficacy with the fewest side effects. However, fluoroquinolones that have more prolonged urinary excretion may be as effective as single-dose agents.

Nitrofurantoin has been used for four decades in treating acute cystitis, and almost all *E. coli* strains remain susceptible to this agent. Unfortunately, nitrofurantoin has not been well studied in controlled trials. A 7-day course of treatment is probably required in order to achieve a 90% success rate in acute cystitis (25,27).

Fosfomycin is a new agent recently marketed for single-dose treatment of acute cystitis. It is a unique antimicrobial and has been used successfully for over a decade in Europe. However, it has a success rate of only 85% to 90% in acute bacterial cystitis, and is relatively expensive (25).

TMP and sulfonamide resistance is emerging in many areas of the world, including the United States (28). Once community resistance to TMP/SMX among *E. coli* exceeds 10%, alternative agents, and specifically the fluoroquinolones, should be selected. Although each of the fluoroquinolones is efficacious, ciprofloxacin is the most effective agent for gram-negative rods and probably should be the fluoroquinolone of initial choice on the basis of existing evidence. Unfortunately, fluoroquinolones cannot be routinely prescribed for acute bacterial cystitis in children or pregnant or breast-feeding women. As a result, TMP/SMX, the nitrofurantoins, and some of the beta-lactams are the drugs of choice, in descending order, for these patients.

Large adequately designed therapeutic trials involving older postmenopausal women with acute cystitis, or for etiologic organisms other than *E. coli*, have not been well conducted.

Acute Pyelonephritis

Patients with acute pyelonephritis are now being stratified according to their comorbidities and the severity of the presenting illness. Complications of acute pyelonephritis occur in 5% to 10% of patients, and are listed in Table 12.5. These complications are about three times as common in patients with diabetes.

Numerous studies have shown that patients with acute, presumably uncomplicated pyelonephritis, and even patients who are pregnant without severe symptoms, can be managed as outpatients with a 2-week course of oral antimicrobial therapy. The indications for hospitalization are listed in Table 12.8. TMP/SMX has been the empiric initial treatment of choice, with TMP alone presumably equivalent. However, if resistance exceeds 10% in the community, alternative agents should be selected (28). In a recent study, Talan et al. showed that the failure rate for TMP/SMX in acute pyelonephritis is about 50% if the infecting organism is resistant (29). In nonpregnant patients, the fluoroquinolones are an appropriate alternative choice. In the study al-

Table 12.8   Indications for Hospitalization in Patients with Pyelonephritis

Sepsis syndrome
Uncertain diagnosis
Structural abnormalities in urinary tract
Diabetes
Immunocompromised host
Pregnancy*
Multiresistant pathogens
Failure of oral regimen
Lack of home supports
Concerns about compliance

* Several studies have shown that 60% to 80% of pregnant patients can be treated safely for acute pyelonephritis as outpatients with oral antibiotics.

ready noted, Talan and coworkers found that ciprofloxacin prescribed for 1 week achieved a cure rate in excess of 90% in women with uncomplicated acute pyelonephritis (29).

Although the beta-lactams are used both parenterally and orally for treatment of acute pyelonephritis, they have a lower eradication rate and should be reserved for populations in whom TMP/SMZ or the fluoroquinolones are not optimal choices. Also, if the urine gram stain shows gram-positive cocci, amoxicillin or piperacillin with a beta-lactamase inhibitor should be included until the culture results are available.

Patients who are very ill, who have nosocomially acquired or complicated urinary infections (Table 12.1), or who fail to respond to oral treatment require hospital admission for parenteral therapy (Tables 12.8 and 12.9). An aminoglycoside with ampicillin, a third-generation cephalosporin, a fluoroquinolone, a beta-lactam/beta-lactamase inhibitor combination, or a carbapenem are all recommended empiric regimens. Randomized controlled trials have generally been of inadequate size to have the power to show superiority of one regimen over another, but there is considerable clinical experience with most of these regimens. For patients in whom *Pseudomonas* is a possible pathogen, imipenem, ceftazidime, ciprofloxacin, or piperacillin are preferred initial treatment choices.

Most patients initially given parenteral therapy can have it changed to oral therapy within 1 to 4 days. Two weeks is an optimal treatment regimen for more severe or complicated pyelonephritis in women, and longer courses have not been shown to be more effective. Men are often treated for 4 to 6 weeks with an oral regimen because of the possibility of concomitant prostatic infection.

Table 12.9   Reasons for Failure to Respond in Patients with Acute Pyelonephritis

Misdiagnosis (common)
Pathogen resistant to prescribed antimicrobial (multiple pathogens may be present)
Resistant pathogen emergent during therapy (unusual)
Intercurrent infection or superinfection (particularly in a catheterized patient)
Infection proximal to obstructed urinary tract
Renal or perinephric abscess(es)
Infected cyst
Drug fever
Metastatic infection elsewhere

Patients with acute pyelonephritis usually respond to antibacterial therapy within 24 to 48 hours with resolution of fever and symptom improvement. If there is no response by 72 hours, further investigation is required to ensure that the initial diagnosis was correct, the organism is susceptible, and no obstructing or suppurative lesions are present. The common reasons for treatment failure in patients with acute pyelonephritis are outlined in Table 12.9.

Asymptomatic Bacteriuria

Except for those done with pregnant women, few studies have identified optimal treatment regimens for asymptomatic patients with bacteriuria. Treatment should be initiated only after a repeat culture confirms the presence of bacteriuria, and usually after a urinalysis to confirm the presence of pyuria. An indication for treatment should also be present (Table 12.10).

A 3-day regimen of TMP/SMX or, in nonpregnant patients, of a fluoroquinolone followed by a urine culture 2 weeks later will determine whether treatment has eradicated the infection (Table 12.7). About 70% of women are cured with a 3-day regimen. Patients in whom therapy fails should be further evaluated for a longer 2-week course of therapy, and a decision should be made about investigation for underlying complications.

Bacterial Prostatitis and Epididymitis

Acute bacterial prostatitis should be treated initially with a parenteral regimen similar to that for acute pyelonephritis, and once improvement has occurred, with a 6-week course of an oral regimen usually of either TMP/SMX or ciprofloxacin prescribed on the basis of susceptibility tests. Cure rates are usually in excess of 80%. Oral therapy can be prescribed if patients can be treated out of the hospital.

Table 12.10   Indications for Treating Asymptomatic Bacteriuria*

Pregnancy
Infancy and childhood
Diabetes[†]
Infection with stone-forming pathogens, particularly *Proteus mirabilis*
Prior to surgery at any site and in patients undergoing urethral manipulation
Immunocompromise or neutropenia
Following renal transplantation
Following catheter removal with recently acquired infection

*The diagnosis should be substantiated with significant quantitative cultures.
[†] Further studies required.

Men with a proven diagnosis of chronic bacterial prostatitis require a prolonged course of therapy. TMP/SMX or ciprofloxacin are drugs with proven efficacy. A 12-week regimen will cure about 80% of men without recurrence of symptomatic infection and with sterile EPS. However, it is important that follow-up studies be performed at least 2 weeks after completion of therapy in order to identify bacterial relapse within the prostatic milieu. Nitrofurantoin, aminoglycosides, and beta-lactams are less efficacious for eradication of prostatic infection because of their limited ability to diffuse into the prostate as a result of the unique pK of this organ.

Acute epididymitis caused by pathogens responsible for UTI should be treated initially with the empiric oral or parenteral regimens used for acute pyelonephritis. Ofloxacin is also effective for UTI pathogens, and will eradicate the sexually transmitted pathogens *C. trachomatis* and *N. gonorrhoeae*. Men with epididymitis caused by UTI pathogens should have a prostatic localization test done after treatment, since the prostate may be a continuing focus of residual infection.

Complicated Urinary Infections

The treatment regimens shown in Table 12.7 are largely empiric and untested in well-designed trials. Many patients who have complicated UTIs can be treated with ordinary courses of oral antibacterials with expectations of high cure rates, although a proportion of these patients will have difficult-to-treat UTIs (1). Also, many patients with complicated UTIs have two or more underlying factors that predispose them to UTIs, and these may be additive or synergistic.

Complications can 1) increase the potential of an infection to be symptomatic or lead to serious outcomes, 2) increase the risk and incidence of a new infection occurring, and 3) increase the probability of treatment failure with an existing infection. These outcomes vary with the underlying reasons for complicated UTI, and probably should be assessed independently as well as within the overall context of treatment indications and expected outcome.

Urologic review is usually indicated in patients with complicated UTI. However, most surgical procedures for complicated UTI have not been validated by well-performed trials. The literature on complicated UTI is littered with unsatisfactory interventions that have often created their own estrogenic problems. In almost all instances, obstruction should be relieved, calculi removed, and pus drained. However, in selected patients, these desired interventions may not be possible, and antimicrobial treatment can occasionally achieve adequate outcomes despite difficult scenarios.

Infections in the lower male genital tract and infections in pregnant women have been previously discussed. In the present section, seven categories of complicated UTI are further discussed.

Suppurative Renal Infections

Suppurative infections are categorized as renal cortical abscesses, corticomedullary abscesses, and perinephric abscesses (30).

Renal cortical abscesses are caused by hematogenous infection, usually with *S. aureus* from a remote site. Corticomedullary abscesses are caused by classical urinary tract pathogens, and often occur in patients with complicated urinary infections in the presence of obstruction. The sequence appears to begin with a focal or sometimes multifocal acute bacterial pyelonephritis that proceeds to tissue liquefaction, often because of delayed or inappropriate treatment, obstruction, or concomitant xanthogranulomatous pyelonephritis. Perinephric abscesses often originate from a hematogenous site, and these are most commonly due either to *S. aureus* or *C. albicans*. They also can develop from an ordinary episode of acute pyelonephritis or from extension of an intestinal perforation. The latter complication will usually create an abscess with multiple pathogens, including anaerobes.

Suppurative renal diseases are too often diagnosed very late or at postmortem. CT evaluation is the procedure of choice for early diagnosis, and should be considered in all patients with persisting fever and possible renal abscesses (23).

Treatment requires specific parenteral antimicrobial regimens directed at the presumed or proven pathogens, together with drainage procedures as indicated and vigorous management of often accompanying comorbidities either within the urinary tract or at other sites. Empiric treatment with anti-staphylococcal, enterococcal, and antigram-negative regimens should usually be initiated for all patients with abscesses until the etiology is established. Often percutaneous drainage is adequate, but surgical drainage may be required if fever persists and the patient does not begin to rapidly recover.

The fluoroquinolones and TMP/SMX are ordinarily excellent treatment choices for urinary tract pathogens, but need to be complemented with more specific anti-staphylococcal and anti-anaerobic agents if these are deemed to be necessary.

Infected Renal Cysts

Both polycystic kidneys and solitary renal cysts can become infected, usually with aerobic gram-negative pathogens. These can be difficult to eradicate, and in multicystic kidneys, surgical drainage is often impossible and can be disastrous if attempted. Fortunately, long-term suppression and even cure can be achieved with the fluoroquinolones, which diffuse widely and are not inhibited by pus or a low pH within the cyst milieu. As a result, the fluoroquinolones, or occasionally TMP/SMX, can be prescribed for 6 to 12 weeks and, if necessary, for even longer periods to suppress and perhaps cure infection localized to one or more infected cysts (See Table 12.7 for dosages).

Renal Impairment

UTIs are common complications of renal impairment, even though they are only rarely the sole cause of renal failure. Despite the observation that half of patients with renal failure at some time have a urinary infection, the optimal management of infections in these patients remains largely obscure.

In patients with bilaterally disparate renal function or with significant areas of impaired function within a single kidney, blood flow is preferentially increased to functioning renal tissue, and levels of an antimicrobial agent within the poorly perfused tissue may be inadequate to inhibit bacterial growth. However, urinary levels of an antimicrobial agent in these patients will often be very substantial, and urine cultures will be sterile despite persisting active infection in the area of renal injury.

In general, antibacterial agents that could further impair renal function, including the aminoglycosides, should be avoided in these patients. Also, therapeutic agents such as the tetracyclines and nitrofurantoin are contraindicated, since too little of these agents is filtered in areas of impaired renal function to effectively suppress bacterial multiplication. However, the quinolones, trimethoprim alone, and most beta-lactam agents are effective in the presence of renal impairment, and are the therapeutic agents of choice for patients with impaired renal function. However, drug dosages should be modified according to the level of renal impairment.

Patients with impaired renal function and asymptomatic infection constitute a particularly problematic group. No good studies of this population have been done, and in most patients the infection is probably not contributing to renal failure. However, many physicians choose to treat asymptomatic infection in patients with renal impairment in case infection is contributing to reduced renal function.

Diabetes Mellitus

UTIs are five to 10 times more common among patients with diabetes mellitus than among controls (31). About 20% of patients with diabetes have histologic evidence of pyelonephritis at postmortem. Most prospective studies suggest multiple reasons for the increased frequency, morbidity, and mortality of urinary infections among patients with diabetes. The complications of UTI in patients with diabetes include bacteremia, papillary necrosis, emphysematous cystitis and pyelonephritis, renal and perinephric abscesses, and ketoacidosis.

No substantive studies have shown that treatment of asymptomatic infection in patients with diabetes will prevent these complications. As a result, the management of both asymptomatic bacteriuria and symptomatic infections in patients with diabetes is identical to that in other populations. However, studies are underway to determine whether diabetes creates a milieu in which infections should be treated differently.

Catheterization

All patients with long-term (>30 days) indwelling catheterization have infections, often with multiple pathogens that grow both in the urinary tract and on the catheter surface. Usually, one pathogen is predominant, but if it is suppressed with treatment, others may emerge. The complexity of infection in catheterized patients is not well understood, but more than 200,000 patients in the United States are chronically catheterized, and infections originating from their urinary tracts have substantial morbidity. Although most episodes of bacteriuria are asymptomatic, systemic symptoms, including fever, occur in 15% to 25% of patients per year of catheterization, and UTIs due to catheterization account for about 15% of nosocomial bloodstream infections (32). It is estimated that about half of febrile episodes in chronically catheterized patients are due to UTI. At postmortem, about one-third of chronically catheterized patients have evidence of acute pyelonephritis. Other complications of chronic catheterization include renal stones, penile and scrotal abscesses, prostatic abscesses, and bladder cancer.

Asymptomatic infection in chronically catheterized patients should not be treated (16,17,32,33). Treatment has no effect on the incidence of complications, and leads to an increase in drug-resistant organisms (8,16,17,33,34). Some physicians consider *Proteus mirabilis* a particularly dangerous catheter colonist, since it leads to encrustation of the catheter and bladder and to renal calculi. Unfortunately, eradication of *P. mirabilis* is usually impossible in patients with indwelling catheters.

Patients with symptoms caused by urinary invasion in the presence of a catheter do require treatment. In most instances a broad-spectrum agent should be chosen and treatment should be limited, probably to 7 days, with the intention of suppressing the infection without attempting to eradicate it (Table 12.7). Longer courses of therapy lead only to the selection of multiply resistant organisms that will be increasingly difficult to treat and likely to spread to other catheterized patients.

Candida spp. are common pathogens that result from chronic catheterization and antibacterial use. In the absence of symptoms, *Candida* spp. should not be treated (35). In patients with symptoms, a short course of fluconazole constitutes optimal treatment and is superior to irrigation with amphotericin B. However, in most instances candiduria should be allowed to persist, and usually disappears once antibacterial regimens are stopped and the catheter is removed.

Renal Transplants

UTI follows renal transplantation in about 50% of patients, and is multifactorial, stemming in part from the initial use of a urinary catheter, surgical trauma, and immunosuppression (36). Urinary infection in the renal transplant patient can lead to pyelonephritis in the transplanted kidney or in native kidneys, and to reactivation of latent CMV infection in the allograft. As a result, early recognition and treatment of urinary infection, including yeast infection, is essential. TMP/SMX and fluoroquinolones are the treatments of choice for bacterial infection, and should be prescribed for 2 weeks.

Ileal Conduit

A ureteroileal conduit diversion is required whenever malignancy, congenital anomalies, or other processes require removal of the bladder. These diversions are always infected with a variety of pathogens, and three or more species are often present. No prophylactic regimens have been shown to be effective in such cases. Treatment leads only to increasingly resistant pathogens, and the patient ultimately becomes infected with pathogens that are very difficult to treat. Obstruction, calculi, and other problems require frequent imaging and urologic investigations, and most patients have intermittent episodes of symptomatic invasive infection. These should be treated with a broad-spectrum empiric regimen for 7 to 10 days, with no attempt being made to eradicate the pathogen with prolonged treatment (Table 12.7). Unfortunately, management is problematic, and prospective controlled studies are required to determine what, if any, strategies will reduce the burden of disease caused by infection.

Prevention

Many urinary infections can be prevented. Unfortunately, no vaccine has been shown to be useful for preventing UTI. However, several strategies have been shown in prospective studies to reduce the incidence and the disease burden of urinary infections.

Among premenopausal women with recurring cystitis, antimicrobial prophylaxis, either used regularly or with intercourse, is effective. TMP/SMX in a dose of 80 mg/400 mg three times a week, or a fluoroquinolone (i.e., ciprofloxicin) at 500 mg three times weekly, reduces the number of recurrences by tenfold (27). Nitrofurantoin taken daily is also effective (27). Because many infections follow intercourse, postcoital antibacterial treatment is a possible option. Usually, prophylaxis is prescribed for 1 year, and patients are thereafter followed without prophylaxis to determine whether susceptibility to UTIs persists.

Antimicrobial prophylaxis can be prescribed with similar efficacy for postmenopausal women. However, at least one controlled study has shown that many postmenopausal women are estrogen-deficient, and that topical intravaginal estradiol markedly decreases the rate of infection, by about 10-fold (12). Additional studies are required to determine whether restoration of vaginal lactobacilli in populations of patients whose vaginal microbial ecosystem is disturbed because of estrogen deficiency, antimicrobial use, or bacterial vaginosis can prevent recurrences of urinary infection. All women who experience recurrent infections should be cautioned with regard to the use of spermicides, including nonoxynol-9-impregnated condoms. Other interventions, including daily ingestion of 300 ml of cranberry juice, may be of value, but have not been adequately studied.

Prevention of infection in catheterized patients is an effective initiative measure, and should be a priority for all patients catheterized for 30 days or less. If proper measures are taken to maintain a closed drainage system, the risk of infection ranges from 3% to 10%/day. Most patients with short-term catheter placement (less than 2 weeks) should be free of bacteriuria when the catheter is removed. Although some studies have suggested that systemic antibiotic therapy prevents infection in patients with short-term catheterization, its use will predictably lead to resistant infection, and most experts do not advise antibiotics for preventing bacteriuria during catheterization. If, however, bacteriuria is present after the catheter is removed, a short course of therapy is indicated even in the absence of symptoms, in order to prevent subsequent symptomatic infection from occurring (38). Condom catheter drainage can reduce some of the infectious complications of catheterization in men, but the incidence of infection remains increased with these appliances, and penile maceration is common.

All patients undergoing urologic manipulation or surgery should have urine cultures done before the procedure, and any infection should be treated. Short-term or single-dose therapy with agents effective against gram-negative pathogens and enterococci should also be prescribed at the time of urologic surgical procedures.

Summary

Urinary infections are common everyday events in medical practice. Many can be prevented. Most can be well treated outside the hospital with relatively inexpensive management programs. However, UTIs can on occasion be very serious and life-threatening infections. Appropriate investigation, specific therapy, and patient education usually can lead to a satisfactory outcome for what can otherwise be a frustrating, recurrent, and problematic illness.

REFERENCES

1. **Ronald AR, Harding GKM.** Complicated urinary tract infections. *Infect Dis Clin North Am.* 1997;11:583–592.

2. **Svanborg C, Godaly G.** Bacterial virulence in urinary tract infection. *Infect Dis Clin North Am.* 1997;11:513–529.

3. **Hedges S, Agace W, Svensson M.** Uroepithelial cells are a part of a mucosal cytokine network. Infect Immun. 1991;62;2315–2321.

4. **Smith HS, Hughes JP, Hooten TM, et al.** Antecedent antimicrobial use increases the risk of uncomplicated cystitis in young women. *Clin Infect Dis.* 1997;25:63–68.

5. **Numazaki Y, Kumasaka T, Yano N.** Further study on acute hemorrhagic cystitis due to adenovirus type 11. *N Engl J Med.* 1975;289:344–347.

6. **Nicolle LE, Friesen D, Harding GKM, Roos LL.** Hospitalization for acute pyelonephritis in Manitoba, Canada, during the period from 1989 to 1992: impact of diabetes, pregnancy, an aboriginal origin. *Clin Infect Dis.* 1996:22:1051–1056.

7. **Peters KD, Kochanek K, Murphy SH.** Deaths: final data for 1996. *Natl Vital Stat Rep.* 1998;47:51–52.

8. **Nicolle LE, Henderson EE, Bjornson J.** The association of bacteriuria with resident characteristics and survival in elderly institutionalized men. *Ann Intern Med.* 1987;106:682–686.

9. **Wiswell TE, Hockey WE.** Urinary tract infections and the uncircumcised state: an update. *Clin Pediatr.* 1993;32:130–134.

10. **Hooten, TM, Scholes D, Hughes JP, et al.** A prospective study of risk factors for symptomatic urinary tract infection in young women. *N Engl J Med.* 1996;335:468–476.

11. **Hooten TM, Roberts PL, Stamm WE.** Effects of recent sexual activity and use of diaphragm on the vaginal microflora. *Clin Infect Dis.* 1994;19:274–278.

12. **Raz R, Stamm WE.** A controlled trial of intravaginal estrogen in postmenopausal women with recurrent urinary tract. *N Engl J Med.* 1993;329:753–756.

13. **Bronsema DA, Adams JR, Pallares R, et al.** Secular trends in rates and etiology of nosocomial urinary tract infections at a university hospital. *J Urol.* 1993;150:414–146.

14. **Pewitt EB, Schaeffer AJ.** Urinary tract infection in urology, including acute and chronic prostatitis. *Infect Dis Clin North Am.* 1997;11:623–646.

15. **Patterson TF, Andriole VT.** Detection, significance, and therapy of bacteriuria in pregnancy: update in the managed health care era. *Infect Dis Clin North Am.* 1997;11: 593–608.

16. **Abrutyn E, Mossey J, Berlin JA, et al.** Does asymptomatic bacteriuria predict mortality and does antimicrobial treatment reduce mortality in elderly ambulatory women. *Ann Intern Med.* 1994;120:827–33.

17. **Nicolle LE.** Consequences of asymptomatic bacteriuria in the elderly. *Int J Antimicrob Agents.* 1994;4:107–111.

18. **Jones CA, Nyberg L.** Epidemiology of interstitial cystitis. *Urology* 1997;49:2–9.

19. **Stamm WE, Counts GW, Running KR, et al.** Diagnosis of coliform infection in acutely dysuric women. *N Engl J Med.* 1982;307:463–9.

20. **Jenkins RD, Fenn JP, Matsen JM.** Review of urine microscopy for bacteriuria. *JAMA.* 1986;225:3397–3403.

21. **Meares EM Jr, Stamey TA.** Bacterial localization patterns in bacterial prostatitis and urethritis. *Invest Urol.* 1968;5:492.

22. **Ronald AR, Boutros P, Mourtada H.** Bacteriuria localization and response to single-dose therapy in women. *JAMA.* 1976;235:1854.

23. **Kaplan DM, Rosenfield AT, Smith RC.** Advances in the imaging of renal infection. *Infect Dis Clin North Am.* 1997;11:681–705.

24. **Hooten TM, Winter C, Tiu F, et al.** Randomized comparative trial and cost analysis of 3-day antimicrobial regimens for treatment of acute cystitis in women. *JAMA.* 1995;273:41.

25. **Warren JW, Abrutyn E, Hebel JR, et al.** Guidelines for antimicrobial treatment of uncomplicated acute bacterial cystitis and acute pyelonephritis in women. *Clin Infect Dis.* 1999;29:745–758.

26. **Hooten TM, Johnson C, Winter C, et al.** Single-dose and three-day regimens of ofloxacin versus trimethorpin-sulfamethoxazole for acute cystitis in women. *Antimicrobial Agents Chemother.* 1991;35:1479–83.

27. **Brumfitt W, Hamiliton-Miller JMT.** Efficacy and safety profile of long-term nitrofurantoin in urinary infections: 18 years experience. *J Antimicrob Chemother.* 1998;42: 363–371.

28. **Gupta K, Scholes D, Stamm WE.** Increasing prevalence of antimicrobial resistance among uropathogens causing acute uncomplicated cystitis in women. *JAMA.* 1999;281:736–738.

29. **Talan DA, Stamm WE, Hooten TM, et al.** Comparison of ciprofloxacin (7 days) and trimethoprin/sulfamethoxazole (14 days) for acute uncomplicated pyelonephritis in women: a randomized trial. *JAMA.* 2000;283:1583–1590.

30. **Dembry LM, Andriole VT.** Renal and perirenal abscesses. *Infect Dis Clin North Am.* 1997;11:663–680.

31. **Zhanel GG, Nicolle LE, Harding GKM, and the Manitoba Diabetic Urinary Infection Study Group.** Prevalence of asymptomatic bacteriuria and associated host factors in women with diabetes mellitus. *Clin Infect Dis.* 1995;21:316–322.

32. **Warren JW.** Catheter-associated urinary tract infections. *Infect Dis Clin North Am.* 1997;11:609–627.

33. **Weiner J, Quinn JP, Bradford PA, et al.** Multiple antibiotic resistant Klebsiella Escherichia coli in nursing homes. *JAMA.* 1999;281:517–523.

34. **Swartz MN.** Use of antimicrobial agents and drug resistance. *N Engl J Med.* 1997;337:491–492.

35. **Sobel JD, Kauffman CA, McKinsey D, et al.** Candiduria: A randomized double-blind study of treatment with fluconazole and placebo. *Clin Infect Dis.* 2000;30:19–24.

36. **Tolkoff-Rubin NE, Rubin RH.** Urinary tract infection in the immunocompromised host. *Infect Dis Clin North Am.* 1997;11:707–717.

37. **Stapleton A, Stamm WE.** Prevention of urinary tract infection. *Infect Dis Clin North Am.* 1997;11:719–733.

38. **Harding GKM, Nicolle LE, Ronald AR, et al.** How long should catheter-acquired urinary tract infection in women be treated? A randomized controlled study. *Ann Intern Med.* 1991;114:713–719.

13

Prostatitis and Epididymitis

Keith B. Armitage, MD
Catherine Markin Colecraft, MD

Prostatitis

Prostatitis is one of the most frequently encountered urogenital conditions in primary care (1,2). The term *prostatitis* is applied to a range of symptomatology referable to the male urogenital tract and perineum. Symptoms referable to prostatitis include low back pain, perigenital pain, irritative voiding, and voiding dysfunction (2–4). In the late 1970s, Stamey and coworkers advanced the understanding of prostatitis by dividing voided urine into three portions: a first void or urethral portion (VB1), a midstream void (VB2) or bladder portion, and postprostatic massage urine (VB3) or expressed prostatic secretion (3). This system allowed differentiation not only between urethral and prostatic infections in the presence of sterile midstream urine but also between bacterial and nonbacterial forms of prostatic infection (2–4). This process was named the *localization technique* and was described in the 1970s by Meares (4a). On the basis of this approach, prostatitis has been separated into four categories: 1) acute bacterial prostatitis (ABP), 2) chronic bacterial prostatitis (CBP); 3) chronic abacterial prostatitis (CAP); and 4) prostatodynia. Figure 13.1 illustrates the frequency of occurrence of the four types of prostatitis.

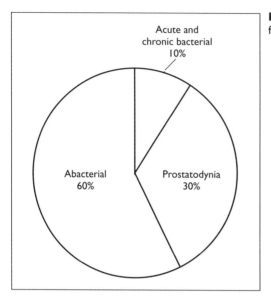

Figure 13.1   Frequency of differing forms of prostatitis.

Etiology and Pathogenesis

Despite progress made in the past 30 years in understanding the syndrome of prostatitis on the basis of localization technique and other methods, prostatitis is often difficult to diagnose accurately, and the etiologic agent is often difficult to identify. In 1980, Stamey (4b) stated that "little more is known about prostatitis than was reported by Hugh Young and associates in 1906." In clinical practice, prostatitis is often treated on the basis of clinical signs and symptoms without the use of the localization technique. Although efficient, this approach may lead to over- or undertreatment owing to the inaccuracy of clinical diagnosis. Differentiating between the four classifications of prostatitis solely on the basis of clinical presentation or impression (with the possible exception of the acute bacterial form) is problematic. In cases of symptoms of recurrent or complicated prostatitis, it is crucial to use the localization technique described above to make an accurate diagnosis.

The precise pathogenesis of prostatitis is not clear, and this contributes to the confusion about its optimal management. In bacterial prostatitis, it has been hypothesized that infection may result from an ascending urethral infection, either by extension subsequent to vaginal (or rectal) inoculation of the urethral meatus during intercourse or via hematogenous or lymphatic spread of coliform microorganisms (1,5). Some have suggested that the reflux of urine into the prostatic ducts causes prostatic calculus formation, with the calculi then forming a nidus for bacterial infection (1,3,6). Others have described bacterial prostatitis as being associated with a urinary tract infection (4,6). The primary pathogens that have been implicated are enteric, aerobic, gram-negative rods that colonize the gastrointestinal tract and commonly infect the urinary tract, with *Escherichia coli* being the most frequently isolated organism. Enterococci, *Pseudomonas* and other nonenteric gram-negative rods also are seen in acute and chronic prostatitis. Foreign bodies (e.g., indwelling Foley catheter, obstruction caused by benign prostatic hypertrophy) have been implicated as cofactors in the development of prostatitis (7). Genital pathogens such as *Neisseria gonorrhoeae* and *Chlamydia trachomatis* also have been implicated in prostatitis and are the most likely agents of this condition in men aged 35 years or younger (7,8).

The cause may differ according to the category of prostatitis and the age of the patient. In older men, CAP, prostatodynia, and bacterial epididymo-orchitis are among the most common presentations of prostatic disease; however, despite their frequency, the etiology and pathogenesis of these diseases are not well characterized. In the case of CAP, molecular probe data suggest an infectious cause (8).

Clinical Manifestations

As mentioned earlier, patients with syndromes of prostatitis usually present with a range of symptomatology referable to the male urogenital tract and the perineum. This primarily consists of symptoms of irritative and dysfunctional voiding, such as urgency, hesitancy, dysuria, frequency, incomplete emptying of the bladder, fever, perigenital pain, ejaculatory discomfort, low-back pain, or low-abdominal pain. Constitutional signs and symptoms may or may not be present, depending on the type of prostatitis.

Diagnosis

The diagnosis of prostatitis is often based on symptoms and prostatic tenderness on examination, but bacterial prostatitis can be differentiated from nonbacterial prostatitis only by urinary localization cultures or by the localization studies previously cited (1). The finding of bacterial pathogens in the urine after prostatic massage and in the presence of sterile urethral and midstream urine specimens is highly diagnostic of bacterial prostatitis (1). The prostatic localization technique demonstrates the contribution of urethral, prostatic, and bladder organisms to bacteriuria in specimens of voided urine and is the diagnostic "gold standard" for bacterial prostatitis.

Additional studies for the diagnosis of prostatitis are available but typically are used only in cases that do not respond to treatment or in which prostatitis is recurrent or complicated. Plain radiography, ultrasonography, and intravenous urography can be used to rule out other conditions (e.g., osteitis pubis and urolithiasis, both of which mimic prostatitis) and, in the case of ultrasonography, to diagnose prostatitis (3). Both specific and nonspecific echogenic qualities have been described in prostatitis; however, nonbacterial prostatitis cannot be diagnosed with certainty by transrectal ultrasonography, and a normal ultrasound examination does not exclude its diagnosis (3). In contrast, the sonographic features of acute bacterial prostatitis are well documented and consist of an enlarged rounded prostate (usually with a symmetrical capsule), a decrease in echogenicity, and an increase in sound transmission within the gland parenchyma (which is believed to indicate edema) (9).

Other studies that may aid in the diagnosis of prostatitis include uroflowmetry (in which abnormalities are reported in only 30% of cases) and urine cytology (which lacks clinical data to support its value in the screening of patients with prostatitis). The value of the outcome of cytologic screening of patients with prostatitis depends exclusively on the experience of the investigator (3). The level of prostate specific antigen is often increased in the setting of acute and chronic prostatitis, and screening for prostate cancer should not be performed when these conditions are suspected.

Management

It is often difficult to differentiate between the various forms of prostatitis, which makes therapeutic decisions problematic. No specific therapy exists for nonbacterial and chronic prostatitis, and antimicrobial therapy is often ineffective.

When using antimicrobial agents to treat prostatitis, it is important to consider the capacity of a particular drug to cross the prostate–blood barrier, and the performance of the drug in the relatively alkaline environment of the prostate. For an antimicrobial drug to enter the prostate, it must be lipid soluble and have a low protein-binding affinity, because drug-bound proteins do not pass freely into the prostatic fluid. The drug also should have a high dissociation constant at a high pH (i.e., $pK_a > 8.6$) and optimal activity against gram-negative rods at a pH > 6.6 (4,6). Many of the available antimicrobial agents lack these penetration characteristics, most notably the beta-lactam drugs. Trimethoprim with or without sulfamethoxazole is an attractive option, because trimethoprim achieves high levels in the prostate and has good activity against primary pathogens. Trimethoprim alone is an attractive alternative to trimethoprim–sulfamethoxazole, because it is not commonly associated with

Table 13.1   Pharmacokinetic Characteristics of Antibiotics Used in Treating Prostatitis

Drug	Lipid Solubility	Chemical Nature	pK_a	Percentage Bound to Plasma Proteins	Relative Penetration
Ampicillin	Negative	Acidic	2.5	20%	Poor
Cephalothin	Negative	Acidic	2.5	60%	Poor
Penicillin G	Negative	Acidic	2.7	60%	Poor
Nitrofurantoin	Slight	Acidic	7.2	95%	Good to Poor
Doxycycline*	Positive	Amphocytic	3.4, 7.7, 9.7	82%	Very Good
Erythromycin*	Positive	Basic	8.8	73%	Good
Minocycline*	Positive	Amphocytic	7.8, 9.3	75%	Very Good
TMP-SMX	Positive	Amphocytic	7.3, 6.1	10%/70%	Very Good
Ciprofloxacin	Negative	Basic	6.0, 8.8	20%–40 %	Very Good

TMP-SMX = trimethoprim–sulfamethoxazole.
* Degree of lipid solubility: minocycline 5× > doxycycline 5× > tetracycline.
Adapted from Cunha BA, Marx J, Gingrich D. Managing prostatitis in the elderly. *Geriatrics.* 1991;46:50–63.

hypersensitivity reactions and is inexpensive. Table 13.1 lists selected pharmacokinetic characteristics of various drugs used in treating prostatitis.

The failure of antibiotics in treating some forms of prostatitis has led to the use of other treatment modalities. Several supportive and symptomatic modalities have been tried (6,10,11). Hyperthermia (e.g., hot sitz baths, transurethral microwave thermotherapy) has been used with limited success (10). Prostatic massage to break down loculi of infected prostatic secretions and/or fluid improves drainage but may have limited value in CBP. Anticholinergic agents effectively reduce urinary frequency and urgency but probably are best reserved for benign prostatic hypertrophy and bladder-neck dyssynergia, because they may inhibit the flow of prostatic fluid (6). Nonsteroidal anti-inflammatory agents provide symptomatic relief for chronic prostatitis and prostatodynia, and the use of steroids has been tried during severe, acute symptomatic exacerbations of chronic prostatitis (6). All of these measures afford only temporary relief, and few objective data are available to indicate that any of them alter the natural course of the disease.

Primary care physicians can manage most cases of prostatitis, but urologic consultation should be considered for patients with recurrent or refractory symptoms. Surgical options have been proposed since the early 1970s for the management of chronic prostatitis that is unresponsive to medical management. In 1973, Warwick and coworkers (12) advocated open prostatectomy and posterior capsulectomy. Transurethral prostatectomy has been reported to alleviate symptoms of chronic prostatitis, even in the absence of outflow obstruction (13). However, this approach has lost favor because it does not provide lasting symptomatic relief, and it is now seldom recommended, particularly in view of the risk of impotence and incontinence associated with the procedure. Bladder-neck incision has been proposed for younger patients with refractory prostate pain. This approach has been reported to have less morbidity than transurethral prostatectomy (6). It is said to be curative in approximately one third of patients with proven chronic bacterial prostatitis. Retrograde transurethral balloon dilation has been introduced as an alternative treatment for patients with benign prostatic hypertrophy, CAP, or prostatodynia (6).

Acute Bacterial Prostatitis

In contrast to the other forms of prostatitis, ABP is an easily recognized clinical entity that is dramatic in its presentation. The patient may present in the throes of an acute septic process, with irritative and obstructive voiding symptoms, including low-back and perineal pain. Fever of sudden onset, chills, rigors, myalgias (associated with dysuria, frequency, urgency, hesitancy), a sensation of rectal fullness, and suprapubic discomfort often accompany the presentation. The signs and symptoms of ABP are both highly reliable and diagnostic.

A complete genitourinary examination, including digital rectal examination, should be performed judiciously on patients with suspected ABP to detect urethral discharge and evaluate scrotal content (to rule out concurrent urethritis and epididymitis). The digital rectal examination may provoke intense pain; conversely, a nontender prostate rules out ABP. It is important to note that prostatic massage is strongly contraindicated in ABP because of the very high risk of inducing a heavy bacterial load into the bloodstream and thus precipitating septicemia. Blood and urine cultures should always be a part of the routine workup in ABP.

The severity of illness in ABP often leads to hospitalization and the initiation of parenteral antimicrobial therapy to cover major potential pathogens such as aerobic gram-negative rods. It is appropriate to complete the course of therapy with oral antibiotics once the patient has stabilized.

Numerous antimicrobial regimens are available for empirical therapy pending identification and recognition of the sensitivity patterns of the organism(s) obtained from culture specimens (Table 13.2). These options include the combination of a beta-lactam and an aminoglycoside, a fluoroquinolone, or trimethoprim–sulfamethoxazole. Antibiotic therapy should be given for at least 2 weeks and even longer, depending on the severity of the presentation and the response to therapy (1,2,14). ABP usually responds well to antibiotic

Table 13.2   Prostatitis Syndromes

	Clinical Manifestations	Diagnosis	Common Bacterial Etiology	Management and Treatment
Acute bacterial prostatitis	Dramatic and sudden onset; irritative and dysfunctional; voiding symptoms; urinary obstruction (for 2–3 weeks); systemic symptoms (e.g., fever, chills, rigors)	Hard, exquisitely tender, and warm prostate on digital exam (Note: prostatic massage is contra-indicated); inflammatory cells in EPS/urine; positive culture and microbiologic data from EPS/urine	Enterobacteriaceae (Escherichia coli most common)	Pharmacologic: initial parenteral antimicrobial (e.g., ciprofloxacin, ofloxacin, TMP-SMX, tetracycline, penicillin + aminoglycoside) followed by oral antimicrobial for a total of 3–6 weeks Supportive: analgesia, bedrest, antipyretic, stool softener, suprapubic catheterization (if obstruction present)
Chronic bacterial prostatitis	Hallmark: relapsing or recurrent UTIs and intervening asymptomatic periods Very variable; irritative; voiding signs + symptoms; afebrile or low grade fever	Usually normal prostate examination; inflammatory cells in EPS/urine; positive culture and microbiologic data from EPS/urine	Enterobacteriaceae (including Klebsiella, Serratia, Pseudomonas, and Proteus species) Enterococcus species	Oral fluoroquinolone for 4–6 weeks, oral TMP-SMX for 1–3 months, oral TMP for 1–3 months, chronic suppressive therapy
Chronic abacterial prostatitis	Chronic irritative voiding symptoms; afebrile	Normal prostate examination; inflammatory cells in EPS/urine; negative culture and microbiologic data from EPS/urine	Unknown; Chlamydia and Ureaplasma are suspected	Counseling ± antibiotics: ?Doxycycline for 2 weeks or erythromycin for 2 weeks
Prostatodynia	Chronic low-back, perineal, and suprapubic pain; psychological disturbances	Normal prostate examination; usually no inflammatory cells in EPS/urine; negative culture and microbiologic data from EPS/urine	Unknown; noninfectious	Counseling; alpha-adrenergic–blocking agent

EPS = expressed prostatic secretion; TMP-SMX = trimethoprim–sulfamethoxazole; UTIs = urinary tract infections.

therapy despite the lack of optimal penetration characteristics for most of the antimicrobial agents used to treat it, as discussed previously, and their usually consequent failure to achieve therapeutic concentrations in prostatic fluid. Antimicrobial agents that are not normally effective in the prostate are effective in acute prostatitis because the acute inflammation in the disease renders the blood–prostate barrier more permeable, which is analogous to the situation of the blood–brain barrier during acute meningitis (4,14).

Management of patients with ABP also should include supportive care with intravenous fluid resuscitation, bed rest, analgesia, and stool softeners.

When urinary retention is a complicating factor, placing a suprapubic catheter is preferred to using a transurethral catheter so as to avoid blocking the drainage of infected prostatic secretions into the urethra (5).

Aggressive treatment of ABP can prevent complications such as prostatic abscess, CBP, persistent asymptomatic bacteriuria, granulomatous prostatitis (i.e., the histologic stage of resolving ABP, which manifests on examination as an area of induration that is suspicious for malignancy), and prostatic infarction (1,2,6,14).

Chronic Bacterial Prostatitis

Chronic bacterial prostatitis is a more subtle disease than ABP and is characterized by relatively asymptomatic periods that are punctuated by episodes of recurrent symptomatic bacteriuria. Patients often present with a long-standing history of irritative voiding symptoms with a persistence of urinary pathogens and the presence of inflammatory cells in the expressed prostatic secretion. In CBP, the diagnosis is more difficult, the response to therapy is less certain, and relapse is more common than with ABP.

In contrast with ABP, lower urinary tract localization studies should be preformed before antimicrobial therapy is begun for CBP. Trimethoprim–sulfamethoxazole or trimethoprim alone are cost-effective antibiotics for treating CBP; the cure rate with these drugs is approximately 30% to 40% (1). The quinolones are also efficacious but are more expensive. Clinical trials with the fluoroquinolones norfloxacin and ciprofloxacin have achieved cure rates of 60% to 92% (1). These trials were criticized for having only short-term follow-up, which may have underestimated the number of relapses. In an attempt to assess the long-term efficacy of these drugs, Weidner and coworkers (14a) reported cure rates with ciprofloxacin and norfloxacin of 53% and 64%, respectively, after 6 to 12 months of follow-up (1).

Chronic, low-dose, suppressive therapy may be tried in an attempt to control the symptoms of patients with multiple relapses of ABP. Antimicrobial recommendations for chronic suppressive therapy include trimethoprim, nitrofurantoin, minocycline, and the fluoroquinolones, all of which have to some degree the characteristics favorable for penetration into and entrapment within the prostate. All of the fluoroquinolones have low protein-binding affinities, small molecular sizes, high lipid solubility, and basic properties (1).

Chronic Abacterial Prostatitis

Chronic abacterial prostatitis is a common form of prostatitis; however, despite its frequency, it is attended by a lack of scientific data (3,6). Patients with CAP are usually between the ages of 20 and 35 years. CAP may represent a noninfectious disease entity that results from the urethral reflux of urine into the prostatic ducts, causing a chemical prostatitis. Alternatively, an unidentified infectious agent may cause CAP, and there are molecular probe data to suggest this (8). The role of *C. trachomatis* (and other bacteria implicated in nongonococcal urethritis) in the pathogenesis of CAP has been a topic of debate since the early 1970s (2).

Chronic abacterial prostatitis has no pathognomonic or characteristic histopathologic features; the only marker of the disease is a modest increase in chronic inflammatory cells. The symptoms resemble those of other prostatitis syndromes except for fluctuation with remission followed by recrudescence in 3- to 6-week cycles (6). Because of the cyclic nature of the condition, the efficacy of antimicrobial therapy is difficult to assess.

In the literature, the approach to the role of antimicrobial drugs in CAP has changed over the years. In 1978, Meares (4a) and Stamey (4b) opposed the use of antimicrobial therapy because no infectious agent could consistently be isolated, and empiric use of various antibiotics had proven to be ineffective. In 1985, Simmons and Thin (14b) advocated the use of minocycline, which not only has the desirable penetration characteristics for permeability into prostatic tissue but also seemed to be clinically efficacious in treating CAP. In the 1980s and early 1990s, there was a revival of enthusiasm for antimicrobial therapy in CAP, perhaps reflecting the belief in the potential role of pathogens such as *C. trachomatis* and *Ureaplasma urealyticum* in causing the disease (6). A 1991 review of the available data indicated that some patients with CAP did improve with antimicrobial therapy, and the authors highlighted trimethoprim–sulfamethoxazole as the antibiotic of choice for prolonged therapy (6). Doxycycline and erythromycin also have been recommended for treating CAP (*see* Table 13.2) (6).

Psychological factors can be an important aspect of the management of CAP and other forms of chronic prostatitis. Many patients benefit from a candid discussion of the enigmatic nature of the disease. Reassurance that in most cases it is not a sexually transmitted disease (STD), that it is not hereditary, and that it does not cause infertility may help prepare the patient to cope with what can be a chronic illness. Honesty about the current therapeutic limitations for CAP should be emphasized to the patient (6).

Prostatodynia

The term *prostatodynia* literally means "pain in the prostate." Clinically, the term is used to refer to a prostate pain syndrome for which no cause can be established and for which there is no objective evidence of it being due to infection or inflammation. Patients with prostatodynia constitute approximately one third of patients who present with chronic prostatitis syndromes.

Despite the lack of evidence of inflammation, patients present with many of the symptoms associated with prostatitis, including perineal, low-back, and suprapubic pain. Generally, irritative voiding symptoms such as dysuria and urinary frequency are absent. The prostate is normal and without tenderness on physical examination. A normal examination and the lack of inflammatory cells distinguishes prostatodynia from CAP, in which white blood cells and lipid-laden macrophages are characteristically found. Localization cultures are also negative in prostatodynia. Possible mechanisms of prostatodynia include neuromuscular abnormalities such as detrusor sphincter dyssynergia or overactivity of the pelvic sympathetic nerves at the level of the external urethral sphincter (1,2,6). These suggested mechanisms are based on observations of attenuated urinary flow rates with incomplete relaxation of the bladder neck and narrowing of the urethra proximal to the external urethral sphincter (2). Therapeutic agents of potential benefit include alpha-blockers such as phenoxybenzamine and prazosin, which reduce spasm and intraurethral pressure. This effect should prevent intraprostatic urinary reflux that could result in chemical prostatitis. Psychological issues also should be addressed in these patients.

Table 13.2 provides a summary of the salient features of the four prostatitis syndromes.

Epididymitis

Epididymitis is a common clinical syndrome in primary care, accounting for 600,000 visits to physicians per year (5). From 1990 to 1991, epididymitis was estimated to be responsible for approximately 20% of urologic inpatient admissions (15,16). In developing nations, it has been cited as a common cause of infertility because concurrent orchitis is frequent in this setting (presumably as a consequence of lack of treatment, inadequate treatment, or delay in treatment, resulting in testicular involvement) (17). Infertility is an uncommon complication of unilateral orchitis but occurs in up to 50% of cases of bilateral orchitis. When treatment is lacking or delayed, other major sequelae of acute epididymitis and epididymo-orchitis include testicular atrophy (~67% of patients), testicular abscess, and infarction or necrosis (~5%) (14–17).

Etiology

Inflammation of the epididymis can result from trauma or other noninfectious insults but is most often caused by infection. Urine has been postulated as the precipitating irritant in some cases of epididymitis, and drugs have been implicated on rare occasions. Epididymitis caused by amiodarone has been well described, and clinicians who care for patients that received this drug need to be aware of this adverse reaction to prevent subjecting the patient to unneeded work-up and antimicrobial therapy. Epididymitis caused by amiodarone is a benign and self-limited sterile epididymitis that requires no treatment other than cessation of the amiodarone (15,18).

When an infectious cause is identified in acute epididymitis, the etiologic organisms usually fall into one of two categories: genital or sexually acquired pathogens (e.g., gonococcus, *Chlamydia*, *Ureaplasma*) or urinary tract pathogens (aerobic gram-negative rods, enteric coliforms such as *E. coli*, *Klebsiella*, *Proteus*, *Pseudomonas*). The likelihood of isolating one type over another from a particular patient is related to age, sexual activity, and the presence of anatomical or functional genitourinary pathology (19).

Sexually transmitted causes of epididymitis are rare in the prepubertal child, and the isolation of an STD organism should alert the clinician to the probability of sexual abuse. The most likely causes of urinary tract infection in this age group are coliform organisms or *Pseudomonas*. STDs are the most common cause of epididymitis in heterosexual men under 35 years of age (20), possibly via an ascending infection from the urethra. However, epididymitis as a complication of urethritis occurs only rarely (estimated frequency 1%–2%) (21). Urinary pathogens are an infrequent cause of epididymitis in anatomically intact, heterosexual, young adult men. Conversely, in sexually active homosexual men of similar age, the most common etiologic agents are enteric pathogens acquired during anogenital intercourse and then introduced into the urogenital tract. In older men and in men with structural or functional defects (e.g., benign prostatic hypertrophy, bladder-neck obstruction), urinary tract pathogens are the likely culprits.

Clinical Manifestations

Epididymitis typically presents with unilateral testicular pain, swelling, erythema, and tenderness of an acute or subacute onset. Inflammation of the epididymis in severe cases often extends to the testicle itself or the scrotum. Patients present with an "acute scrotum," the differential diagnosis of which is listed in Table 13.3. These scrotal signs and symptoms may present in the absence of urogenital symptomatology, such as urethral discharge and/or dysuria. Constitutional symptoms such as fever or chills may or may not be associated with the scrotal signs and symptoms, depending on the severity of illness. Less frequently, the patient may present only with vague lower abdominal and inguinal complaints of sudden onset (*see* Table 13.3). Testicular torsion, epididymitis, and epididymo-orchitis have a similar presentation, and differentiation between the conditions on clinical grounds alone is often difficult.

Table 13.3   Differential Diagnosis of the Acute Scrotum

Testicular torsion	Inguinal hernia
Epididymo-orchitis	Traumatic hematoma
Torsion of appendix testis	Henoch–Schönlein purpura
Hydrocele	Idiopathic scrotal edema

Modified from Petrack EM, Hafeez W. Testicular torsion versus epididymitis: a diagnostic challenge. *Pediatr Emerg Care.* 1992;8:347–50.

Table 13.4   Diagnostic Criteria for Urethritis

≥4 PMNLs per oil-immersion field (of urethral specimen per sediment of 10–15 mL of first-catch urine specimen) (14)
Or
>5 PMNLs per high-power field (×1000) on microscopic evaluation of urethral smear (25)
Or
≥15 PMNLs per field (×400) on microscopic evaluation of resuspended sediment of a centrifuged 10–15 mL first-catch urine specimen (23)
Or
Mucopurulent or purulent urethral discharge (26)

Diagnosis

Clinically, the diagnosis of epididymitis can be made easily, with an extremely tender epididymis usually being confirmatory. As mentioned previously, diagnostic confusion can arise when epididymitis is accompanied by significant orchitis, in which case other acute testicular conditions need to be considered. In epididymitis without orchitis, the need for radiographic studies is unusual and probably should be limited to situations in which the etiologic diagnosis cannot be ascertained. Radiodiagnostic tools (e.g., ultrasonography, intravenous pyelography) often yield indecisive results with regard to epididymitis, making them unreliable. Their role should be to rule out other noninfectious or noninflammatory causes of a tender, swollen scrotum. In situations in which structural abnormalities of the lower urinary tract are a concern (e.g., in infants, in elderly patients), studies such as intravenous pyelography may help in providing objective data.

When orchitis is present and cannot be differentiated from torsion by clinical examination, radiographic diagnostic tools that are potentially useful include radionuclide scanning (99m-technetium) and Doppler ultrasonography.

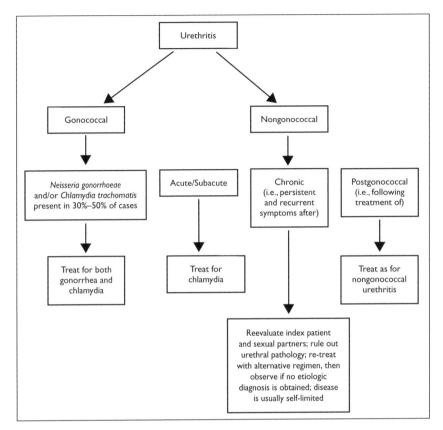

Figure 13.2 Algorithm for the management of urethritis.

Both of these tests are sensitive in revealing decreased blood flow through the spermatic cord (an observation indicative of testicular torsion) (22). In epididymitis, radionuclide scanning demonstrates increased perfusion around the testicle. Doppler ultrasonography demonstrates brisk blood flow. Ultrasonography easily reveals structural testicular abnormalities and intra- or extra-testicular lesions; however, differentiating between an infection and a tumor is more difficult with this technique (22–24).

Torsion is a surgical emergency and, if strongly suspected clinically, should prompt an immediate consult with a urologist. Optimal recovery of gonadal viability is achieved with operative intervention within 6 hours of torsion onset. Within this time frame, the salvage rate is 80%. After a period of 10 to 12 hours, the salvage rate drops precipitously to less than 20% (24).

Table 13.5   Distinguishing Features of Urethritis Syndromes

	Pathogens	Incubation Period	Epidemiology and Distinguishing Aspects	Principles of Management (Treatment and Prevention)	Suggested Antibiotic Regimens
Gonococcal	*Neisseria gonorrhoeae* ± *Chlamydia trachomatis* (15%–25% of heterosexual men, 5% of homosexual men)	<1 week	Florid, purulent urethral discharge (usually)	Treat for both gonorrhea and chlamydia; evaluate and treat sexual partners for both; counsel patients about total compliance (including sexual abstinence until treatment is completed)	For *N. gonorrhoeae* (all as a single dose): Ceftriaxone 125 mg IM *or* Cefixime 400 mg PO *or* Cefotaxime 500 mg IM *or* Ciprofloxacin 500 mg PO *or* Ofloxacin 400 mg PO *Plus* For *C. trachomatis*: Doxycycline 100 mg PO bid for 7 days *or* Azithromycin 1 g PO as a single dose
Nongonococcal	*C. trachomatis** *Ureaplasma urealyticum* ?*Mycoplasma hominis* ?*M. genitalium* Trichomonas Herpes simplex virus Yeast (*Candida albicans*)	Peaks at 2–3 weeks	2–3 times more prevalent; scant, mucoid, whitish discharge	Thorough reevaluation, including urethroscopy to rule out urethral pathology; alternate regimen; tincture of time; no further antibiotic therapy	Doxycycline 100 mg PO bid for 7 days *or* Azithromycin 1 g PO single dose *or* Erythromycin 500 mg PO qid for 7 days *or* Ofloxacin 300 mg PO q12h for 7 days *or* Trovafloxacin 200 mg PO qd for 5 days

* Most commonly isolated.

In cases of recurrent disease or in other settings in which establishing an exact etiologic diagnosis may be important, evaluation should be directed at both genital and urinary sources of infection. A common clinical practice when evaluating genitourinary diseases is to obtain a midstream urine specimen from a patient before examination. In the setting of the epididymitis, this practice results in the loss of potentially diagnostic urethral data. A urethral swab before voiding or at least a first-void urine specimen (i.e., the first 7–8 mL of urine) reveals evidence of urethritis in most instances if it is present (Table 13.4). In addition to performing a complete genitourinary examination, both urethral and urinary specimens should be examined microscopically.

Table 13.6 Suggested Regimens for Epididymo-orchitis

Types of Epididymitis	Associated Features	Pathogens	Recommended Regimens
Sexually transmitted	Age <35 years	Gonococci, *Chlamydia* (heterosexual)	Ceftriaxone 250mg IM in a single dose + doxy-cycline 100 mg PO bid for 10 days
Non–sexually transmitted	Age >35 years	Enteric organisms (homosexual)	Ofloxacin 300mg PO bid for 10–14 days (200 mg IV bid for 10–14 days)
		Enteric organisms, urinary pathogens	Ofloxacin 300 mg PO bid for 10–14 days (200 mg IV bid for 10–14 days) *or* Ciprofloxacin 500 mg PO bid for 10–14 days (400 mg IV bid for 10–14 days)

Adapted from Centers for Disease Control and Prevention. 1998 guidelines for treatment of sexually transmitted diseases. *MMWR Morb Mortal Wkly Rep.* 1998;47(RR-1):49–55,86–87; and Gilbert DN, Moellering RC Jr, Sande MA. *The Sanford Guide to Antimicrobial Therapy*, 31st ed. 2001:5,26.

Treatment

When a diagnosis of epididymitis is considered, prompt initiation of antimicrobial therapy is indicated. Delaying the initiation of treatment risks progression to epididymo-orchitis with potential loss of gonadal function. When orchitis does occur, it must be treated promptly and aggressively to prevent or minimize the risk of this and other complications discussed previously. Severe disease usually merits the use of parenteral therapy; otherwise, an oral agent such as trimethoprim–sulfamethoxazole or a fluoroquinolone is often adequate.

Epididymitis usually responds readily to therapy with antimicrobial agents, with the choice of drug based on the age of the patient. Antimicrobial agents with activity against enteric pathogens are prescribed for older men, and treatment directed against pathogens associated with STD is used in sexually active younger men. If there is any indication of a concomitant urethritis (either microscopically or clinically), then treatment should be directed against the STD genital pathogens *N. gonorrhoeae* and *C. trachomatis* (Fig. 13.2 and Table 13.5) (15). If a urethral discharge is absent or if microscopy reveals lack of polymorphonuclear leukocytes and the urine specimen reveals inflammation and bacteria, treatment should be as that given for a complicated urinary tract

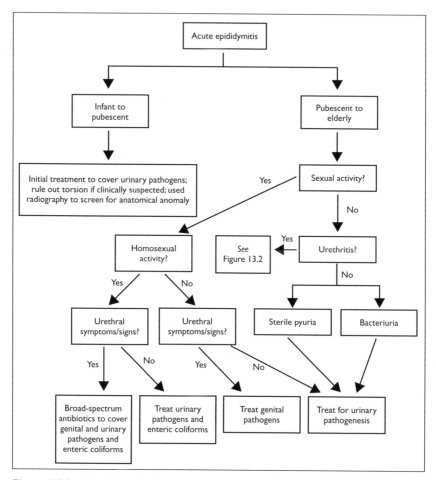

Figure 13.3   Algorithm for the management of epididymitis.

infection. Table 13.6 lists some suggested regimens, and Figure 13.3 is an al-gorithm for the treatment of epididymitis.

Symptomatic treatment of the patient with epididymitis is often indicated and remains an integral part of management of the disease in severe cases. Management may include bed rest, analgesics, scrotal elevation to allow max-imal lymphatic drainage, avoidance of constricting clothing, and local applica-tion of ice packs (14,15).

In the preantibiotic era, surgery was often used to treat epididymitis, which produced immediate analgesia, prompt resolution of fever, reduced incidence of sterility, increased testicular salvage rate, decreased recurrence rate, and a shorter recovery time. With the advent of antibiotics, the degree of morbidity

Table 13.7   Indications for Surgical Intervention for Epididymitis

Absolute Indications	Relative Indications
Abscess formation	Failure to respond clinically to medical therapy within 48 hours
Testicular ischemia	
Testicular torsion	Situations in which rapid convalescence is of primary concern (e.g., in an elderly patient); prolonged bedrest is contraindicated
Solitary testicle	
Scrotal fixation (indicates severe inflammation and potential suppuration)	

associated with epididymitis decreased substantially, as did the status of surgery as the treatment of choice. Today there are both absolute and relative indications for surgery in treating epididymitis (17), which are listed in Table 13.7.

Summary

Prostatitis and epididymitis represent heterogeneous conditions that are commonly encountered in the primary care setting. With the exception of its acute form, prostatitis can be difficult to diagnose and treat; hence, it is important to evaluate patients with prostatitis for both infectious and noninfectious causes. In contrast, the clinical presentation of epididymitis is usually clear cut, and management options for this condition are well defined.

REFERENCES

1. **Schaeffer AJ.** Diagnosis and treatment of prostatic infections. *Urology.* 1990;36(Suppl): S13–S7.

2. **Aagard J, Madsen PO.** Diagnostic and therapeutic problems in prostatitis: therapeutic position of ofloxacin. *Drugs Aging.* 1992;2:196–207.

3. **De La Rosette JM, Debruyne FM.** Diagnostics and treatment of prostatitis: an actualized overview. *Rev Med Suisse Romande.* 1992;112:757–63.

4. **Cunha BA, Marx JD, Gingrich D.** Managing prostatitis in the elderly. *Geriatrics.* 1991;46:50–63.

4a. **Meares EM.** Prostatitis syndromes: new perspectives about old woes. *J Urol.* 1980; 123:141–7.

4b. **Stamey TA.** *Pathogenesis and Treatment of Urinary Tract Infections.* Baltimore: Williams & Wilkins; 1980:1–342.

5. **Krieger, JN.** In Mandell, Douglas, Bennett (eds). *Principles and Practice of Infectious Diseases,* 4th ed. 1995:1098–103.

6. **Evans DTP.** Treatment of chronic abacterial prostatitis: a review. *Int J Sex Trans Dis Acq Immun Defic Syndr.* 1994;5:157–64.

7. **Eisenstein BI.** In Mandell, Douglas, Bennett (eds). *Principles and Practice of Infectious Diseases*, 4th ed. 1995:1970–1.

8. **Gilbert DN, Moellering RC Jr, Sande MA.** *The Sanford Guide to Antimicrobial Therapy*, 31st ed. Hyde Park, VT: Antimicrobial Therapy, Inc.; 2001:18–19.

9. **Doble A, Carter SS.** Ultrasonographic findings in prostatitis. *Urol Clin North Am.* 1989;16:763–72.

10. **Servadio C, Leib Z, Lev A.** Diseases of the prostate treated by local microwave hyperthermia. *Urology.* 1987;30: 97–9.

11. **Choi NG, Soh SH, Yoon TH, Song MH.** Clinical experience with transurethral microwave thermotherapy for chronic nonbacterial prostatitis and prostatodynia. *J Endourol.* 1994;8:61–4.

12. **Warwick RT, Whiteside CG, Arnold, EP, et al.** A urodynamic view of prostatic obstruction and the results of prostatectomy. *Br J Urol.* 1973;45:44–59.

13. **Stamey TA.** *Pathogenesis and Treatment of Urinary Tract Infections.* New York: Williams & Wilkins; 1980:124–36.

14. **Bowie WR.** Approach to men with urethritis and urologic complications of sexually transmitted diseases. *Med Clin North Am.* 1990;74:1543–57.

14a. **Weidner W, Shiefer HG, Dalhoff A.** Treatment of chronic bacterial prostatitis with ciprofloxacin, results of a one-year follow-up study. *Am J Med.* 1987;82(Suppl rA):280–3.

14b. **Simmons PD, Thin RN.** Minocycline in chronic abacterial prostatitis: a double-blind prospective trial. *Br J Urol.* 1985;57:43–5.

15. **Berger RE.** Acute epididymitis: etiology and therapy. *Semin Urol.* 1991;9:28–31.

16. **Kaver I, Matzkin H, Braf ZF.** Epididymo-orchitis: a retrospective study of 121 patients. *J Fam Pract.* 1990;30:548–52.

17. **Vordermark JS, Deshon GE, Jones TA.** Role of surgery in management of acute bacterial epididymitis. *Urology.* 1990;35:283–7.

18. **Sadek I, Biron P, Kus T.** Amiodarone-induced epididymitis: report of a new case and literature review of 12 cases. *Can J Cardiol.* 1993;9:833–6.

19. **Oriel JD.** Male genital *Chlamydia trachomatis* infections. *J Infect Dis.* 1992;25(Suppl 1):35–7.

20. **Petrack EM, Hafeez W.** Testicular torsion vs. epididymitis: a diagnostic challenge. *Pediatr Emerg Care.* 1992;8:347–50.

21. **Lucas LM, Smith DL.** Nongonococcal urethritis: diagnosis and management. *J Gen Intern Med.* 1987;2:199–203.

22. **Petrack EM, Hafeez W.** Testicular torsion vs. epididymitis: a diagnostic challenge. *Pediatr Emerg Care.* 1992; 8:347–50.

23. **Hsu CF, Wang CC, Chu CC, et al.** Epididymo-orchitis in an infant resulting from *Escherichia coli* urinary tract infection. *Chung-Hua Min Kuo Hsiao Erh Ko i Hsueh Hui Tsa Chih.* 1996;37:48–51.

24. **Rosenson AS, Ali A, Fordham EW, Chaviano A.** A false-positive scan for testicular torsion and false-negative scan for epididymitis. *Clin Nuclear Med.* 1990;15:863–4.

25. **Cheong WK.** The management of chronic non-gonococcal urethritis. *Singapore Med J.* 1990;31:378–80.

26. **Centers for Disease Control and Prevention.** 1998 guidelines for treatment of sexually transmitted diseases. *MMWR Morbid Mortal Wkly Rep.* 1998;47(RR-1):49–55,86–7.

14

Common Sexually Transmitted Diseases

Barbara M. Gripshover, MD
Hernan Valdez, MD

S exually transmitted diseases (STDs) are among the oldest and most prevalent infectious diseases of humans. The Old Testament of the Bible and writings of ancient China contain references to gonorrhea. Today, one fourth of all adults in some parts of sub-Saharan Africa are infected with HIV. Genital ulcerative diseases (GUDs), cervicitis, and urethritis all facilitate the transmission of HIV infection, and the treatment of these STDs can decrease the rate of new HIV infection.

The major STD syndromes and their most common etiologies are listed in Table 14.1. Because many of these conditions are covered elsewhere in this text, this chapter discusses only the most common pathogens that cause urethritis in men (*Neisseria gonorrhoeae*) and cervicitis in women (*Chlamydia*) and the common causes of GUD in developed countries (1)

A few unifying principles apply to the treatment of any patient with an STD (Table 14.2). The first is that patients with one STD are at risk for other STDs and should be screened for gonorrhea, chlamydia, syphilis, and HIV. No commercially available screening test exists for herpes. Women should have a Pap smear to exclude lesions caused by cervical infection with human papillomavirus. All sexual partners of patients with a diagnosed STD must be treated, and the patient must be reminded to refrain from sexual intercourse until he or she and his or her partner(s) have completed a course of therapy to prevent reinfection.

271

Table 14.1   Common Sexually Transmitted Disease Syndromes

Syndrome	Symptoms	Pathogens
Urethritis	Urethral discharge, dysuria	*Neisseria gonorrhoeae* *Chlamydia trachomatis* *Uraplasma urealyticum* *Trichomonas vaginalis* (rare)
Cervicitis	Often asymptomatic, vaginal discharge, dysuria	*Neisseria gonorrhoeae* *Chlamydia trachomatis* Unknown (>80%)
Genital ulcer disease	Single or multiple ulcers in genital area	Herpes simplex *Treponema pallidum* *Hemophilus ducreyi*
Warts (condyloma)	Asymptomatic raised plaques	Human papilloma virus
Molluscum contagiosum	Asymptomatic papules with central umbilication	Pox virus
Hepatitis	Fever, malaise, anorexia, jaundice	Hepatitis A virus Hepatitis B virus
Primary human immuno-deficiency virus (HIV) infection	Fever, lymphadenopathy, pharyngitis, rash	HIV

Table 14.2   Evaluation of Patients with a Sexually Transmitted Disease

1. Screen for other sexually transmitted diseases including gonorrhea culture, *Chlamydia* detection, serologic test for syphilis, and antibody to human immunodeficiency virus.
2. All sexual partners of patient must be evaluated and treated.
3. Advise temporary abstinence from sexual intercourse until patient and all other affected persons have completed therapy.
4. Advise use of condoms to prevent further infection.
5. Consider hepatitis B vaccine for patient and all sexual contacts, and hepatitis A vaccine as well if patient is a homosexual male.

Gonorrhea in Adults

Gonorrhea is a common bacterial illness that is transmitted sexually and peri-natally. It primarily affects mucous membranes of the lower genital tract and, less frequently, those of the rectum, oropharynx, and the conjunctivae (2).

Etiology

Gonorrhea is caused by *N. gonorrhoeae*, a gram-negative diplococcus that has complex growth requirements, growing best at 35° to 37°C and with 5% carbon dioxide added. Many gonococci have a conjugative plasmid that enables them to acquire non–self-plasmids, which may be a mechanism for the acquisition of antimicrobial resistance.

Clinical Manifestations

Asymptomatic Infection
The prevalence of asymptomatic urethral *N. gonorrhoeae* infection in military recruits or otherwise unselected men ranges from 1% to 2%; if contacts of patients with gonorrhea are cultured, the prevalence can be as high as 50%. In women, the prevalence of asymptomatic *N. gonorrhoeae* infection ranges from 19% to more than 50% (3,4).

Genital Infection in Men
Urethritis is the most common clinical manifestation of gonorrhea in men. A purulent discharge and dysuria are frequent. As shown in Table 14.3, one cannot differentiate gonococcal from nongonococcal urethritis on the basis of clinical findings. Between 15% and 30% of male patients with gonorrhea have coexistent *Chlamydia trachomatis* urethritis. Less than 1% of cases are complicated by epididymitis (5,6).

Genital Infection in Women
Women with symptomatic gonorrhea may present with a vaginal discharge, dysuria, or intermenstrual bleeding (4). Close to 50% of patients with positive endocervical cultures for *N. gonorrhoeae* (the endocervix is the site most often affected in women) have positive urethral cultures (the urethra is the site most frequently involved by gonorrhea in hysterectomized patients). Coinfection with *C. trachomatis* is twice as common in women with gonorrhea as it is in men with gonorrhea. Less frequently, women may present with infection of Skene's or Bartholin's glands. Pelvic inflammatory disease, a potentially severe complication of gonococcal infection, is discussed in Chapter 14 (7,8).

Pharyngeal and Rectal Infections and Gonococcal Conjunctivitis
Pharyngeal infection with *N. gonorrhoeae* occurs most commonly in women and men who have sex with men and is symptomatic in less than 5% of patients (5). Microbiologic cure rates of pharyngeal gonorrhea are consistently lower than for gonococcal infections at other anatomic sites.

Table 14.3   Gonococcal and Nongonococcal Urethritis: Clinical Picture

Characteristic	Gonococcal	Nongonococcal
Mean incubation period, days	5	10
Symptoms		
Discharge and dysuria	48–71%	38%
Discharge or dysuria	29%	62%
Signs		
No discharge	0%	19%
Purulent discharge	91%	23%
Mucoid discharge	9%	58%

Although frequently asymptomatic, patients with rectal gonococcal infection may present with pain, tenesmus, a purulent discharge, or rectal bleeding. Infections with *C. trachomatis* and herpes simplex virus (HSV) should be considered in the differential diagnosis (5).

Adult gonococcal conjunctivitis results from manual or direct contamination of the conjunctiva with infected genital secretions. If inadequately treated, it may progress to sight-threatening ulcerative keratitis. Patients present with severe conjunctival inflammation and a copious purulent discharge, which is unilateral in 60% of cases. Although 60% of adult patients with gonococcal conjunctivitis have urogenital cultures positive for *N. gonorrhoeae*, most are unaware of eye contamination with genital secretions. The diagnosis of gonococcal conjunctivitis is easily made by Gram staining the conjunctival secretions. The visual outcome of the disease is related to the severity of disease at the time adequate therapy begins (11).

Disseminated Gonococcal Infection

Disseminated gonococcal infection (DGI) is an uncommon complication of infection with *N. gonorrhoeae* (<1% of infected patients) that results from a complex interaction between bacterial (e.g., resistance to complement-mediated killing, presence of Por IA, and AHU⁻ auxotype) and host (e.g., complement deficiency, perimenstrual period) factors (12–14).

Patients with DGI usually present after a few days of malaise, fever, and asymmetric polyarthralgia or monoarthralgia. The frequency of urogenital symptoms varies, and only a minority of patients present with cutaneous complaints. On examination, most patients are found to have polyarthritis (involving the knees, elbows, or distal joints), and only a quarter have monoarthritis (most commonly of the knee or ankle). Purulent joint effusions seldom result in permanent articular damage. Tenosynovitis and skin lesions that consist of papules or pustules on the torso or limbs are commonly present.

The diagnosis of DGI is usually made on the basis of clinical features and positive cultures from a mucosal site or normally sterile body fluid (e.g., blood, synovial fluid). The laboratory and microbiologic findings in DGI are shown in Table 14.4.

Other Infections
Perihepatitis (15,16) and endocarditis (17) are uncommon complications of infection with *N. gonorrhoeae*. The discussions of these two conditions are beyond the scope of this chapter.

Diagnosis

A Gram stain of urethral secretions and a direct-detection method for *N. gonorrhoeae* and *C. trachomatis* should be performed for all patients who present with urethritis (urethral discharge, dysuria, or both). If facilities for Gram staining are unavailable, direct detection methods for both *N. gonorrhoeae* and *C. trachomatis* should be used, and the patient should be treated for both infections (18).

Direct Visualization
The Gram-stained smear has the advantages of low cost and rapidity but requires technical skill and does not provide information about the antibiotic sensitivity of the stained organism. The Gram stain is a good, quick, and inexpensive method for making a positive diagnosis of gonorrhea in symptomatic men, but the absence of typical Gram-negative intracellular diplococci from the stained smear cannot be used to exclude the diagnosis.

Direct Detection of N. gonorrhoeae Cell Components
DNA PROBE
The DNA-probe technique rapidly detects gonococcal rRNA and may be useful when proper culture conditions are unavailable because it can detect nonviable organisms. However, this technique may be inhibited nonspecifically by genital secretions (19).

Table 14.4   Laboratory Findings in Disseminated Gonococcal Infection

Peripheral white blood cell (WBC) count	$10–12 \times 10^9$/L
Synovial fluid WBC count*	$20–50 \times 10^9$/L
Culture (% positive)	
Urogenital site	80–90%
Synovial fluid	40–50%
Blood	20–40%
Skin	<5%

*The rate of synovial culture positivity directly correlates with synovial WBC count.

LIGASE CHAIN REACTION

With the advent of the LCR technique, gonorrhea is confirmed either by a positive culture and/or by an LCR that yields positive results for two different amplification targets. The LCR assay of either urethral or cervical swab specimens (from men and women, respectively) seems to be more sensitive than does the culture of these sites. Furthermore, the LCR technique seems to be applicable to swabs taken from pharyngeal and rectal sites. Whether or not the additional number of cases of detected gonorrhea justifies the expense of this recent technique remains to be determined (20–23).

MULTIPLEX POLYMERASE CHAIN REACTION

The recent kit-based multiplex polymerase chain reaction (PCR) assay (AMPLICOR) developed for amplification of the DNA of both *C. trachomatis* and *N. gonorrhoeae* has not undergone extensive clinical testing. Potential drawbacks of this technique are the presence of inhibitors in genital secretions and, as with all other tests developed for detecting bacterial components, the failure of the technique to provide antibiotic sensitivity data for the organisms it identifies (24,25).

Culture

Culture has a sensitivity of 50% to 95% for *N. gonorrhoeae*, depending on the site tested and the criterion used as a standard (25a). The advantages of culture are a high specificity and the availability of information about antibiotic sensitivity. Because gonorrhea is a reportable disease and culture offers antibiotic sensitivity information about the strain of organism causing it, a culture for *N. gonorrhoeae* should be performed for every patient who presents with urethritis.

The disadvantages of culture are the inevitable delay before it provides results and its requirement for organisms to remain viable (e.g., carbon dioxide, moisture, nutrients). The incremental yield of culturing additional sites after having cultured the urethra in men and the endocervix in women is too low to justify routinely recommending such additional culture for all patients (18). A comparison of the different diagnostic methods for gonorrhea is shown in Table 14.5.

Treatment

Single-dose treatment should always be used for uncomplicated gonococcal infections (26–30). Additionally, treatment for *C. trachomatis* should always be given to patients being treated for any infection caused by *N. gonorrhoeae*. The reasons for this recommendation are the high coinfection rate of the two organisms, the consistently low return rate for treatment of patients not treated

Table 14.5 Sensitivity and Specificity of Different Diagnostic Methods for Genital Specimens for Gonorrhea Obtained from Symptomatic Individuals Relative to Culture

Test	Site	Sensitivity (%)	Specificity (%)
Gram stain	Male urethra	95–100	95–100
	Endocervix	40–60	95–100
Deoxyribonucleic acid probe	Male urethra	92	96
	Endocervix	86	96
Ligase chain reaction	Male urine	89–98 (72–95)*	99–100
	Female urine	50–95 (50–84)	99–100

*Values in parentheses indicate the percent of culture-positive samples obtained by urethral and endocervical swab.

during their initial visit, and the decreased complication rate and cost effectiveness of this measure (8,31). Ceftriaxone is the only commonly used antimicrobial agent for gonorrhea that is partly effective for treating incubating syphilis; however, because incubating syphilis is rare among patients being treated for gonorrhea, it should not be a major consideration in the choice of an antimicrobial agent for this population (32). Although many antimicrobial agents are effective as single-dose therapy for uncomplicated gonococcal infections, Table 14.6 shows the agents that offer the best balance of efficacy and safety.

N. gonorrhoeae is eliminated from the male urethra within 24 hours after treatment with either ceftriaxone, cefixime, or ciprofloxacin (33). Tests of cure are not recommended for asymptomatic patients because 1) the modern treatment of urogenital gonorrhea is highly efficacious, 2) most treatment failures are symptomatic, and 3) culture of the anatomic sites at which failure is most likely to occur (the pharynx and rectum) is relatively insensitive (30,34). Nevertheless, all sexual contacts of a patient with gonorrhea should be treated if their last sexual contact with the patient took place within the 60 days preceding the patient's treatment.

Mass Treatment
Mass treatment of high-risk groups has low to moderate effectiveness in decreasing the prevalence of gonorrhea, but the effect is short-lived (41). Whether repeated mass treatment followed by frequent screening of core groups is more effective remains unknown, but it seems clear that every effort to eradicate gonorrhea needs to be sustained over prolonged periods.

Table 14.6   Recommended Treatment of Gonococcal Infections in Adults

Uncomplicated urogenital infection	Ceftriaxone 125 mg intramuscularly; or
	Cefixime 400 mg orally; or
	Ciprofloxacin 500 mg orally*†; or
	Ofloxacin 400 mg orally*†; or
	Spectinomycin 2 g intramuscularly‡
Uncomplicated pharyngeal infection	Ceftriaxone 125 mg intramuscularly; or
	Ciprofloxacin 500 mg orally*†; or
	Ofloxacin 400 mg orally*†
Disseminated gonococcal infection	Ceftriaxone 1 g/day intravenously until defervesence, then complete 10 days with either
	Cefixime 400 mg orally twice daily; or
	Ciprofloxacin 500 mg orally twice daily†
Conjunctivitis	Ceftriaxone 1 g intramuscularly once and irrigation of affected eye(s) with saline once
To any of the above treatments add	Azithromycin 1 g orally; or
	Doxycycline 100 mg orally twice daily for 7 days†

*Increasing number of isolates with decreased quinolone susceptibility and a few therapeutic failures have been reported (35–37).
†Contraindicated in pregnancy.
‡Should be used only in pregnant patients allergic to penicillin.

Prevention

Condoms

Condoms are an effective means for decreasing the transmission of *N. gonorrhoeae* (35) and other STDs. Their use should always be recommended to patients who present with an STD.

Screening

As mentioned earlier, the prevalence of asymptomatic gonococcal infection in men is less than 3%. Testing of first-catch urine specimens for leukocyte esterase in male populations that are at high risk for such infection (e.g., adolescent male detainees, minorities attending an emergency department) has positive and negative predictive values of 13% to 30% and 99% to 100%, respectively (36,37). Unfortunately, only 20% to 60% of patients with positive screening cultures for *N. gonorrhoeae* return for treatment (36,38). As a measure for decreasing the transmission of gonorrhea, it is not yet clear if it is cost effective to treat every asymptomatic man who has a positive leukocyte esterase screen. All pregnant women and any woman who presents to an STD clinic should be screened for gonorrhea; young unmarried women also should be considered candidates for screening (39,40).

Vaccination

Although many formulations have been tried, there is no currently effective vaccine for gonorrhea (42).

Chlamydial Infections in Adults

Chlamydial infections are the most common bacterial STDs in the United States (43–45). They are caused by *C. trachomatis*, a species of bacteria that grows intracellularly. Infection with *C. trachomatis* manifests as nongonococcal urethritis in men and as mucopurulent cervicitis in women. Chlamydial infections and their complications are estimated to result in 2.7 billion dollars of health care costs in the United States each year (46).

Etiology

C. trachomatis is an obligate intracellular bacterium with a biphasic life cycle (43,44). The infectious elementary-body (EB) form of the organism is taken into squamocolumnar cells of the endocervix, urethra, rectum, and conjunctiva by endocytosis. Once inside the cell, the EB reorganizes to become the metabolically active reticulate body (RB), which replicates by binary fission within the intracellular inclusion (45). As the RB matures to the infectious EB form, the inclusion ruptures, killing the host cell and releasing EBs in a free state to infect other cells. Previous infection with *C. trachomatis* does not provide immunity (44).

Sexually active adolescents have the highest prevalence of chlamydial infection, with approximately 10% of screened asymptomatic adolescents testing positively in several series (47). Because chlamydial infections are often asymptomatic, the duration of untreated disease is longer than that of treated disease, facilitating its transmission into broader demographic groups than is the case with gonorrhea.

As many as 20% to 30% of men with gonococcal urethritis are coinfected with *C. trachomatis* (43), and the incidence of coinfection with the two organisms is even greater among women.

Clinical Manifestations

Asymptomatic Infection

Nearly 25% of chlamydial urethral infections in men are asymptomatic (43), whereas approximately 60% to 70% of chlamydial endocervical infections in women are asymptomatic.

Genital Infection in Men

Urethritis is the most common manifestation of *C. trachomatis* infection in men, and such disease represents from 30% to 50% of all cases of nongonococcal urethritis (43,48–50). The discharge is classically less copious and less purulent than that of gonococcal urethritis (51); it is often noted only in the morning and in association with mild dysuria. However, the spectrum of symptoms of chlamydial urethritis overlaps that of gonococcal urethritis (*see* Table 14.3). Only a Gram stain that reveals intracellular gram-negative diplococci can establish a clinical diagnosis of gonococcal urethritis reliably and, as mentioned earlier, does not exclude concurrent chlamydial infection.

 C. trachomatis is the most frequent cause of epididymitis in men under 35 years of age (44). Chlamydial urethritis is also the most common trigger of the reactive arthritis of Reiter's syndrome. Approximately 1% of men with nongonococcal urethritis develop acute aseptic arthritis. The arthritis associated with chlamydial infection improves with treatment of this infection.

Genital Infection in Women

Although most chlamydial infections in women are asymptomatic, manifestations of the infection in other cases include vaginal discharge (from endocervical infection), intermenstrual bleeding, and dysuria (44,52,53). Examination with a speculum may reveal a mucopurulent discharge in the cervical os; however, this is neither sensitive nor specific for infectious cervicitis. As many as 20% of women with genital chlamydial infections may have only a urethral infection.

 Ascending infection that leads to endometritis and salpingitis is much more common with chlamydial infection than with gonorrhea, and its effects range from acute severe abdominal pain to asymptomatic salpingitis. Evidence of chlamydial infection is found in approximately 20% of cases of acute pelvic inflammatory disease (44). Sequelae of chlamydial salpingitis include tubal infertility, pelvic pain, and ectopic pregnancy. Multiple studies have shown an association between serologic evidence of previous chlamydial disease and tubal infertility; however, most of the women affected were not aware of having had chlamydial infections (54).

Inclusion Conjunctivitis

In adults, chlamydial eye infection presents with hyperemia, mucoid discharge, and the sensation of a foreign body in the eye (44). If untreated, chlamydial inclusion conjunctivitis may persist for months but rarely causes conjunctival scarring. More than 50% of chlamydial eye infections in adults are associated with concurrent genital infections (44).

Diagnosis

The choice of tests for diagnosing genital chlamydial infections is not simple. In addition to considering the performance characteristics of a particular test, the treating physician needs to consider the type of population to whom the test is being applied (i.e., symptomatic vs. asymptomatic), the volume of samples to be assayed, and the cost of the assay (48,55–57). Table 14.7 summarizes some characteristics of the currently available assays for diagnosing genital chlamydial infections. Enzyme immunoassay of urethral or endocervical secretions to detect chlamydial antigens is probably the most cost-effective way of diagnosing symptomatic chlamydial infections in the office setting.

Detection of C. trachomatis Cell Components

DIRECT FLUORESCENT ANTIBODY TEST

The direct fluorescent antibody test uses specific fluorescinated monoclonal antibodies to *C. trachomatis* to detect extracellular EBs of the organism. It is a rapid and relatively specific test, and specimens can be evaluated for adequacy of cells in the sample. Its disadvantages are that it is tedious, is subject to the expertise of the observer, and requires a fluorescence microscope. It is best suited for populations with a high prevalence of disease in which a small volume of samples are to be processed.

ENZYME IMMUNOASSAY FOR CHLAMYDIAL ANTIGENS

The enzyme immunoassay for chlamydial antigens is simple and objective and may be used to process large amounts of batched samples. It is an acceptable method for diagnosing genital *C. trachomatis* infections in both male and female patients, but its use for identifying infections at other sites is not recommended because of the potential for nonspecific reactions. Urine is a suitably sensitive specimen for the enzyme immunoassay screening of male but not of female populations. The use of blocking antibodies to confirm positive reactions substantially increases the specificity of the test, making it better for screening low prevalence populations.

Table 14.7   Characteristics of Tests to Diagnose Chlamydia trachomatis Genital Infections in Adults

Test	Population	Sensitivity		Specificity		Suggested Use
		Male	Female	Male	Female	
Culture	Symptomatic	65–75%	55–81%	100%	100%	Confirmatory in cases with legal implications.
	Asymptomatic[†]	61–74%	30–65%	100%	100%	
Direct fluorescence antibody (DFA)*	Symptomatic	92% (90–100)	90% (88–99)	97% (72–99)	95% (89–99)	Diagnosis of symptomatic patients in settings with low sample volumes.
	Asymptomatic[†]	NA	77% (61–96)	NA	97% (94–99)	
Enzyme immunoassay (EIA)*	Symptomatic	79% (62–95)	89% (70–98)	97% (96–100)	80% (61–94)	Diagnosis in settings with high sample volumes.
	Asymptomatic[†]	49% (48–50)	85% (60–96)	95% (90–100)	70% (45–80)	Screening.
Ligase chain reaction (LCR)[¶]	Symptomatic	98.8%	81–100%	99.6%	99.5–100%	Screening.
	Asymptomatic	93.3%	84–90%	100%	99.5–100%	Diagnosis when costs decrease.

*Sensitivity and specificity using culture as gold standard.
[†]Asymptomatic patients or patients at low to intermediate risk of infection.
[¶]Performance using expanded definition (culture positive or LCR and either DFA or LCR using other positive primary test).

DNA-PROBE ASSAY

The DNA-probe assay for chlamydial infection uses a DNA probe that hybridizes with rRNA of *C. trachomatis*. This test is specific, and samples can be batch-processed.

AMPLIFICATION TESTS

The LCR for *C. trachomatis* amplifies the cryptic plasmid of the organism (58–65). This is the most sensitive test for the diagnosis of *C. trachomatis* infections, identifying 30% more cases than by culture. Approximately 5% of cases identified by culture are negative for *C. trachomatis* with the LCR test because of the presence of inhibitors. The specificity of the LCR test is close to that of culture. Another important advantage of the LCR test, especially when using this test as a screening tool, is that its sensitivity for infection in men when applied to urine is close to the sensitivity of the LCR method as applied to urethral swabs and is much higher than that of urethral swab culture. Although the urine LCR is probably not as sensitive a screening method for chlamydial infection in women as is the LCR of endocervical swab specimens, it is at least as sensitive as the combination of culture of urethral and endocervical swab specimens. The major drawbacks of the LCR test are its high cost and the stringent precautions required to avoid cross-contamination. The LCR test should not be used as a test for the cure of chlamydial infections because its results may remain positive even after 2 weeks of effective therapy.

Isolation Tests

C. trachomatis is most commonly grown in McCoy cells. The inoculum is centrifuged into the tissue culture monolayer, and the resulting culture preparation is incubated for 48 to 72 hours. Intracytoplasmic inclusions of *C. trachomatis* are detected by staining with Giemsa stain, iodine, or fluorescent antibodies. Several factors, including improper specimen collection and a low number of viable organisms, can decrease the sensitivity of culture for *C. trachomatis*. Nevertheless, this method is the most specific method for diagnosing chlamydial infections, and it can be used to test for infection at most anatomic sites.

Treatment

The mainstay of treatment for uncomplicated chlamydial urethritis and cervicitis has been doxycycline (or erythromycin in pregnancy) given for a week (Table 14.8) (1). A great advance in simplifying treatment for people at risk (e.g., adolescents who are so disproportionately affected by chlamydial infections) has been the recognition of the fact that a single 1-g dose of azithromycin eradicates chlamydial infection (52,66). Unfortunately, azithromycin is a signif-

Table 14.8   Treatment for Chlamydial Cervicitis and Urethritis

Doxycycline 100 mg orally twice a day for 7 days, or
Azithromycin 1000 mg orally once, or
Ofloxacin 300 mg orally twice a day for 7 days

For pregnant patients:
Erythromycin 500 mg four times a day for 7 days, or
Amoxicillin 500 mg orally three times a day for 7 days, or
Azithromycin 1 g orally taken once

icantly more expensive antibiotic than doxycycline or erythromycin; however, in one analysis, the decrease in late complications of chlamydial cervicitis in people treated with azithromycin versus doxycycline (with some instances of failure estimated to result from noncompliance) made azithromycin more cost effective to the medical system (67). Ofloxacin has activity against *C. trachomatis* but, like doxycycline or erythromycin, requires a week of therapy. However, one situation in which this costly drug might be helpful is in epididymitis, because of its coverage of both *C. trachomatis* and enteric pathogens.

Prevention

As with all STDs, the use of condoms and the treatment of sexual partners of infected people can decrease the rate of transmission of chlamydial infections. In a managed care population in Seattle, screening of women at high risk for chlamydial infection (i.e., unmarried, aged <24 years, and having had more than two sexual partners in the past 12 months) for chlamydial cervicitis decreased the incidence of pelvic inflammatory disease (68). Additionally, treating pregnant women may decrease premature labor, premature rupture of membranes, and birth rates of infants who are small for their gestational age (69).

Genital Herpes Infection

Etiology and Epidemiology

Genital herpes, a sexually transmitted viral infection, is the most common cause of GUD in the United States. In 80% to 90% of cases, genital herpes is caused by infection with HSV type 2 (HSV-2), with the remaining 10% to 20% of cases caused by HSV type 1 (HSV-1), which more commonly causes orolabial disease (70). Both types of HSV are DNA viruses, and, like all members of the herpes virus family, HSV establishes a lifelong, latent infection in its human host. Latent HSV resides in sensory nerve ganglia and, in genital herpes, resides particularly in the sacral nerve ganglion.

Seroepidemiologic studies in the United States have indicated that up to 21.7% of U.S. citizens between the ages of 13 and 74 years are infected with HSV-2—an increase of 32.3% in the prevalence of infection from the late 1970s to the late 1980s (71). Multiple studies have shown that most people infected with HSV-2 are unaware of being infected (72–77), which indicates that asymptomatic viral shedding is the major mode of transmission of such infection.

In prospective studies of couples discordant for anti–HSV-2 antibody (75,76), the transmission of infection was detected in 10% of couples per year. Transmission was higher when the male partner was the infected source partner and also when the previously uninfected partner was seronegative for HSV-1 and HSV-2. A study of patients at private obstetric offices in California found that 10% of pregnant women were at risk for contracting HSV-2 from their spouses despite a mean duration of exposure of 6.1 years (73). Unfortunately, type-specific serologic tests for HSV are not yet commercially available.

Clinical Manifestations

Asymptomatic Infection

As mentioned previously, most HSV-2 infections are asymptomatic. These may be first recognized by transmission to another person who develops symptomatic disease.

First-Episode Genital Herpes

Patients with a first episode of genital herpes and without serologic evidence of previous HSV infection have a more severe course of disease than do those with previous HSV-1 infection (70). The incubation period after sexual exposure is usually 3 to 7 days. Primary infection often begins with systemic symptoms, including headache, fever, and myalgia for the first few days of the illness. Pain and itching in the genital area are the first local symptoms noted, followed by the development of painful vesicles on the vulva and labia in women and on the penile shaft and glans in men. Usually the vesicles have ulcerated by the time the patient seeks medical care. Pain peaks approximately 1 week into the illness, then gradually resolves as lesions heal. New lesions develop in most patients well into the first week of clinical illness, and typically all lesions resolve by 3 weeks after the start of the illness. Bilateral, tender, nonfluctuating inguinal adenopathy develops in the second week and is one of the last symptoms to resolve. Cervicitis occurs in almost 90% of primary genital HSV infections in women; urethritis occurs in 80%. Complications of primary genital HSV include meningitis, which occurs in one third of women and in 13% of men approximately 1 week into the illness, and autonomic dysfunction (including urinary retention), which is rare.

Recurrent Infection

Constitutional symptoms infrequently accompany recurrent episodes of genital HSV, and the duration of lesions in such episodes is much shorter than in cases of primary disease, with healing typically occurring after 7 to 10 days. Almost half of episodes of recurrent HSV infection are preceded by a prodrome of tingling paresthesias, sometimes radiating to the buttocks or hips. Recurrences are 20% more common in men than in women and are more common in people who have a severe primary episode of genital infection (78). Treatment of the primary episode does not decrease the rate of recurrence (79). Recurrence of genital HSV-1 infection is less likely than that of genital HSV-2 infection (80).

Diagnosis

The diagnosis of genital HSV infection is often clinically apparent when patients present with classically clustered vesicles or ulcers; however, confirmatory tests are available and especially important for patients with atypical lesions. Because the diagnosis of genital herpes can cause significant psychological trauma, confirmatory tests in the office are helpful in eliminating any uncertainty. Culturing the base of a fresh vesicle gives the highest yield of virus.

Culture

Herpes simplex virus grows readily in cell culture, with a cytopathic effect noted within 24 to 48 hours (81). Titers of virus are highest in clinical specimens from early vesicles and wet ulcers; virus also can be cultured from the cervix (88% of primary infections) and rectum (the most common site of asymptomatic shedding of virus in women, and from which shedding is not correlated with anal intercourse). Culture is the "gold standard" test for HSV infection, but the yield decreases in older lesions.

Tzanck Smear

A more rapid but less sensitive test for HSV infection is the Tzanck smear (82), in which a scalpel blade is used to scrape cells from the base of a vesicle and to spread them on a slide that is then stained with Wright or Giemsa stain. In the presence of infection with HSV or varicella zoster virus, multinucleated giant cells are seen. Tzanck smears have a sensitivity of 50% to 60%

for HSV and are more likely to be positive when made from fresh lesions. However, they cannot distinguish infection caused by HSV from that caused by varicella zoster virus, but this is often clinically apparent.

Herpes Simplex Virus Antigen Detection
Monoclonal antibodies are available to detect HSV antigens, and they can distinguish HSV-1 and -2 from each other (81). Fluorescence-labeled antibodies can be used to detect HSV antigens in cells scraped from the base of an ulcer and dried on a slide. This method is less sensitive than culture but constitutes a rapid test specific for HSV.

Polymerase Chain Reaction for Herpes Simplex Virus DNA
The PCR for detecting HSV infection is based on DNA amplification of the virus from a vesicle or ulcer. Although this has been shown to be more sensitive than culture for detecting HSV (83), its role in routine clinical practice has yet to be established.

Treatment

First-Episode Genital Herpes
In the early 1980s, acyclovir therapy was first shown to decrease the duration of viral shedding, pain, development of new lesions, and time to complete healing of lesions in first-episode genital herpes (84,85). Although topical acyclovir can reduce the duration of viral shedding, it is clearly inferior to systemic therapy (85). Treatment does not prevent further recurrences.

The newer antiviral agents famciclovir and valacyclovir are also active against HSV (86,87). They have better bioavailability and a longer half-life than does acyclovir, thereby permitting less-frequent dosing. For initial episodes of genital HSV, valacyclovir 1000 mg given twice per day was just as efficacious as acyclovir 200 mg given five times per day (Table 14.9).

Episodic Recurrent Therapy
Studies with acyclovir, famciclovir, and valacyclovir have all shown that treatment initiated at the first symptom of recurrence of genital HSV infection can decrease the duration of pain, viral shedding, and lesions by approximately 1 day (85–87). Unless the recurrence is exceptionally painful, treating episodic recurrences is not usually indicated in otherwise normal hosts.

Suppressing Recurrent Genital Herpes Simplex Virus
Patients who have more than six recurrences in a year can benefit from continuous suppressive therapy for symptomatic recurrent genital HSV. Acyclovir has the longest track record for suppressive therapy, being safe and

Table 14.9   Treatment for Genital Herpes Simplex Virus Infection

First episode genital herpes	
Acyclovir	400 mg three times a day for 7–10 days
	200 mg five times a day for 7–10 days
Famciclovir	250 mg twice a day for 5 days
Valacyclovir	1000 mg twice a day for 7–10 days
Episodic recurrent therapy	
Acyclovir	400 mg three times a day for 5 days
	200 mg five times a day for 5 days
Famiciclovir	125 mg twice a day for 5 days
Valacyclovir	500 mg twice a day for 3 days
Continuous suppressive therapy	
Acyclovir	400 mg twice a day
Famiciclovir	250 mg twice a day
Valacyclovir	500 mg once a day (if <9 recurrences in a year)
	1000 mg once a day (if >9 recurrences in a year)

effective for patients who require treatment for as long as 6 years (88,89). Famciclovir and valacyclovir are also effective in suppressing recurrences of genital HSV but, at the time of this writing, have been studied for only 1 year each. Patients in whom suppressive therapy is started should have it stopped on a yearly basis to see whether continued therapy is needed, because the frequency of recurrence does decrease with time. Suppressive therapy also decreases asymptomatic shedding of HSV-2, but not completely (89).

Prevention

Patients with genital HSV infections should be advised to refrain from intercourse when they have lesions. To avoid transmission of infection by asymptomatic shedding of the virus, infected patients should use condoms at all times.

Syphilis

Syphilis is an STD caused by infection with the bacterial spirochete *Treponema pallidum* (90,91). Traditionally, syphilis has been divided into three stages. Primary syphilis (a GUD), secondary syphilis (caused by dissemination of *T. pallidum* from the primary site of infection and characterized by a generalized rash and lymphadenopathy), and tertiary syphilis (the result of long-standing untreated end-organ disease).

Etiology and Epidemiology

T. pallidum is a thin, unicellular, coiled bacterium that can be recognized under a darkfield microscope by its characteristic corkscrew motility with flexion about the center of the organism (90,91). Because *T. pallidum* cannot be cultured *in vitro*, the test for viable organisms requires injection of a specimen into rabbit testes. The rabbits are then monitored for the development of orchitis and serologic evidence of infection (92).

Although its incidence has been decreasing recently in the United States, syphilis remains the second most common GUD. Its incidence is higher among blacks than among other racial groups. Recent epidemics have been associated with crack cocaine use and the exchange of sex for drugs (93).

People with early syphilis are infectious to their sexual partners (90). All partners who have had sex within 3 months of diagnosis with a patient who has primary syphilis and anyone who has had sex within 6 months of diagnosis with a patient who has secondary syphilis should be considered at risk for contracting the disease and should be referred for treatment (1).

Clinical Manifestations

For a more exhaustive discussion of the clinical manifestations of syphilis, *see* references 90, 91, and 93.

Primary Syphilis
Approximately 3 weeks (range 10–90 days) after exposure to *T. pallidum*, an ulcer develops at the site of organism inoculation (90,91,93). This chancre is typically painless with indurated edges and may be found on the penis, vagina, lip, mouth, or anus. Firm, nontender, bilateral inguinal adenopathy is often present. The chancre heals spontaneously in 3 to 6 weeks.

Secondary Syphilis
Symptoms of secondary syphilis develop from 4 to 10 weeks after the appearance of the chancre of primary syphilis. The most common of these symptoms is a rash that is usually accompanied by constitutional symptoms, including malaise, low-grade fever, arthralgias, and generalized lymphadenopathy. The rash is typically nonpruritic and maculopapular, originating on the trunk and proximal extremities but then spreading to include the palms of the hands and

soles of the feet. However, the rash also can be pustular, nodular, or eczematous. Other skin manifestations of secondary syphilis include patchy alopecia (5%); condyloma lata (10%–20% of cases), which are heaped gray plaques in moist skin folds that teem with spirochetes; and pharyngeal mucous patches (6%–30%), which are gray erosions surrounded by an erythematous border. None of these lesions is painful. Involvement of the central nervous system in secondary syphilis can be manifested as aseptic meningitis (with headache, photophobia, and neck stiffness), cranial neuropathy (especially that which involves the VIII nerve), and eye involvement (especially in the form of anterior uveitis). Rare complications include hepatitis, glomerulonephritis, arthritis, and periostitis.

Latent Syphilis
As with the chancre of primary syphilis, the manifestations of untreated secondary syphilis resolve, and the patient enters a prolonged period of asymptomatic infection. For treatment purposes, latent syphilis is infection that is present for more than 1 year or nonprimary and nonsecondary disease that occurs with an infection of unknown duration. The diagnosis of latent syphilis is a serologic diagnosis, because the patient is by definition asymptomatic.

Tertiary Syphilis
Late complications of syphilis are rare in today's antibiotic era. One third of individuals with untreated syphilis develop late complications on an average of 10 to 20 years after infection. Gummata (chronic necrotizing inflammatory lesions found predominantly in skin, subcutaneous tissue, and bone) are the most common manifestation of tertiary syphilis, occurring in 15% of untreated patients. Syphilitic aortitis, which results from endarteritis obliterans in the vasa vasorum of the aorta, causes aneurismal dilatation of the ascending aorta and is clinically apparent in 10% of individuals with long-standing syphilis. The late neurological sequelae of untreated syphilis include tabes dorsalis (in which demyelination of the posterior columns and dorsal roots results in shooting pains and ataxia), generalized paresis, and loss of parenchymal nerve cells (which results in dementia, hyperactive reflexes, pupillary abnormalities [accommodation without reactivity], and slurred speech).

Neurosyphilis
The nervous system can be involved at all stages of infection by *T. pallidum* (94). In fact, the organism can be found in the cerebrospinal fluid (CSF) of 29% of patients with primary syphilis (95). As mentioned previously, meningitis is an early manifestation of neurosyphilis, occurring in the first year or two after infection, commonly with secondary syphilis. Meningovascular syphilis occurs from 4 to 7 years after infection and is caused by endarteritis

obliterans in the small vessels of the meninges, brain, and spinal cord; it presents with strokes and seizures. Tabes dorsalis and generalized paresis occur decades after infection.

Syphilis and HIV infection

Several reports have suggested that syphilis progresses more rapidly in people who are coinfected with HIV. A higher incidence of chancre is found in HIV-infected individuals with secondary syphilis (43% vs. 15% in HIV-negative people). HIV-infected individuals who are treated appropriately for early syphilis have still developed neurosyphilis (92). Meningovascular syphilis also occurs earlier in HIV-infected individuals (96,97). These findings have led to the recommendation for a CSF examination to exclude asymptomatic neurosyphilis in all HIV- infected individuals who have latent syphilis (1).

Diagnosis

Detection of Treponema pallidum in Clinical Specimens

Mucosal lesions of primary and secondary syphilis (e.g., chancres, mucous patches, condyloma lata) can be scraped and examined under a darkfield microscope to detect treponemes moving in their characteristic spiral manner (90). No studies address the sensitivity or specificity of this test; both depend in part on the skill of the microscopist. Furthermore, the sample must be examined immediately, because the organisms must remain viable for their motion to be detected. Fluorescent antibodies are available for detecting treponemal antigens (DFA) in slide preparations of scrapings from lesions and have the advantage of binding with antigens in dried specimens so that the latter can be sent to a central laboratory. The PCR technique for amplifying treponemal DNA in a lesion has a sensitivity similar to that of darkfield microscopy and DFA testing (98,99).

Serologic Tests

Two classes of serologic tests have been the mainstay of diagnosis for syphilitic infections and are used to monitor the response to treatment (90,93,100,101). Nontreponemal tests detect antibodies to the lipid antigens of *T. pallidum*, and treponemal tests detect antibodies directed at treponemal antigens (90,93,100,101). Nontreponemal serologic tests (e.g., rapid plasma reagin [RPR] test, Venereal Disease Reference Laboratory [VDRL] test) are technically easier to perform than are the treponemal tests (e.g., fluorescent treponemal antibody-absorption test, microhemagglutination assay for *T. pallidum*). Moreover, the antibody titer in the RPR and VDRL tests changes in response to therapy. However, all positive results of nontreponemal serologic tests must be confirmed as true positives by verifying them with a treponemal test. Table 14.10 shows the common causes of false-positive results to VDRL tests. The treponemal tests first become positive during primary syphilis and, once positive, usually remain so for the life of the patient despite appropriate therapy. By 1 week after occurrence of the chancre in primary syphilis, the results of the VDRL or RPR test should be positive, and 100% of results of these two tests are positive during secondary syphilis. The titers are highest in secondary syphilis and decrease in time even without therapy, so that approximately 25% of cases of latent syphilis culminate as seronegative with the VDRL and RPR tests. In response to therapy, the titers with the two tests should decline by fourfold at 6 months for primary and secondary disease; latent disease takes longer to respond, and titers should be fourfold lower by 12 months (100,102).

Unfortunately, tests for neurosyphilis are not sensitive. Both the VDRL test of CSF and the PCR test for treponemal DNA are specific for neurosyphilis but are negative in 30% to 70% of cases (93). The treponemal tests are more sensitive but are not routinely recommended for application to CSF because of the high occurrence of false-positive results (101). Abnormalities of the CSF (e.g., mononuclear pleocytosis, increased protein concentration) support the diagnosis of neurosyphilis in a seropositive patient.

Treatment

Penicillin remains the drug of choice for treating syphilis at all stages (Table 14.11) (1). Doxycycline is an alternative for penicillin-allergic patients; however, there is no alternative to penicillin therapy for pregnant women and people with neurosyphilis, and desensitization must be performed. As already noted, serologic testing should be repeated at 6 and 12 months of treatment to assess the adequacy of response; titers should decrease by fourfold within 12 months after treatment is begun.

Table 14.10   Common Causes of False-Positive Non-Treponemal Tests

Infectious	
Bacterial:	Endocarditis, pneumococcal pneumonia, tuberculosis, chancroid, scarlet fever, leptospirosis, mycoplasma, rickettsial disease
Viral:	Varicella, hepatitis, measles, infectious mononucleosis, human immunodeficiency virus infection, mumps
Noninfectious	
	Pregnancy
	Chronic liver disease
	Intravenous drug use
	Advancing age
	Connective tissue disease (especially systemic lupus erythematosis)
	Cancer
	Multiple blood transfusions

Table 14.11   Treatment of Syphilis*

Primary	Benzathine penicillin G 2.4 million units intramuscularly once
	For penicillin allergic patients: Doxycycline 100 mg orally twice a day for 2 weeks, or tetracycline 500 mg orally four times a day for 2 weeks
Secondary	Benzathine penicillin G 2.4 million units intramuscularly once
	For penicillin allergic patients: Doxycycline 100 mg orally twice a day for 2 weeks, or tetracycline 500 mg orally four times a day for 2 weeks
Latent	Benzathine penicillin G 2.4 million units intramuscularly each week for 3 weeks
(asymptomatic infection for more than 1 year)	For penicillin allergic patients: Doxycycline 100 mg orally twice a day for 4 weeks, or tetracycline 500 mg orally four times a day for 4 weeks.
Neurosyphilis	Aqueous penicillin G 18–24 million units a day, given as 3–4 million units IV every 4 hours for 10–14 days, or procaine penicillin 2.4 million units intramuscularly each day with probenecid 500 mg orally four times a day, both for 10–14 days

*Pregnant women and persons with neurosyphilis must be treated with a penicillin-containing regimen, and therefore need desensitization if they are penicillin-allergic.

People who should have a CSF examination before being treated for latent syphilis include those with 1) neurological or ophthalmic symptoms, 2) evidence of active tertiary syphilis (e.g., aortitis, gumma), 3) failure of previous treatment (with increasing VDRL test titers or a high titer [>1:32] that does not decrease), and 4) HIV infection (1).

Prevention

All sexual partners of syphilis patients and any contacts of these individuals, must be identified so that they can be treated with an effective antimicrobial regimen. Individual eradication of syphilis, whether symptomatic or asymptomatic, is important. Education should be given to patients and their contacts about abstinence and the use of condoms. Patients and others at risk for syphilis should be made aware that the presence of genital ulcers increases the risk of acquiring HIV infection.

Chancroid

Chancroid is a sexually transmitted GUD caused by *Haemophilus ducreyi*, a fastidious, pleomorphic gram-negative coccobacillus that requires carbon dioxide, hemin, and nicotinamide adenine dinucleotide for growth in culture. Chancroid is the most common GUD in underdeveloped countries but is infrequent in North America and occurs most commonly in outbreaks (103,104). Chancroid has been proven to increase the transmission of HIV.

Clinical Manifestations

The classic description of chancroid is a tender, purulent ulcer (or ulcers) that invades beneath or undermines the border of normal tissue (83,105–106). This lesion usually appears after a median incubation period of 5 to 7 days. Common locations of chancroid lesions, in order of frequency, are the preputial orifice, coronal sulcus, and the frenulum of the penis (in men) or the fourchette, vestibule, and labia minoris of the vagina (in women). It is now known that the classic presentation of chancroid is uncommon (107–109); however, lymphadenopathy is common in chancroid, is unilateral half of cases, and evolves into a fluctuant abscess or bubo in many cases.

The clinical diagnosis of GUD suffers from inaccuracy. There is broad overlap in clinical features among HSV, chancroid, and syphilis, and the likelihood that a certain constellation of signs reflects a given entity depends heavily on the relative prevalence of each of the GUD entities in the location in which the finding is made. Thus, single clinical features that are highly specific for a particular GUD are not sufficiently sensitive for its diagnosis (e.g., ulcer induration was found to be 95% specific for syphilis in one study but was only 47% sensitive). Furthermore, as many as 25% of patients have mixed infections (primary syphilis and chancroid are the most common ulcerative infections [109]); thus, diagnostic tests are needed to ascertain the cause of most cases of GUD.

Because the male-to-female ratio for chancroid ranges from 3:1 to 25:1, it has been suggested that women may be asymptomatic carriers of *H. ducreyi*. However, a study performed with molecular amplification techniques found that only 2% to 4% of female prostitutes in Africa carried *H. ducreyi* asymptomatically (110). Men with chancroid frequently give a history of a recent exposure to female prostitutes. Asymptomatic female partners may provide an alternative explanation for this finding.

Diagnosis

The minimal procedures needed to make an etiologic diagnosis in patients who present with GUD include a darkfield microscopic examination and serologic testing for syphilis and cultures for chancroid and HSV infection (108,109). Even when all of these tests are performed, a diagnosis cannot be made in 20% to 40% of patients. In a survey of facilities that treat patients with STDs, 88% performed a serologic test for syphilis and 25% performed either a darkfield microscopic examination or a DFA test for *T. pallidum*. Only

50% collected specimens for HSV culture and 8% for culture of *H. ducreyi* (111). When a patient presents with GUD, the minimal evaluations listed above should be performed. If these tests are unavailable and the patient's lesions are not typical for herpes, therapy for chancroid, syphilis, and herpes (if indicated) should be prescribed. The performance characteristics of diagnostic tests for chancroid are described below.

Direct Visualization and Culture

Gram staining of ulcer secretions to identify the *school-of-fish* appearance of *H. ducreyi*, which causes the disease, is insensitive for the diagnosis of chancroid (40%–60%). One reason for this is that there are other bacteria that may resemble *H. ducreyi*.

Two media are preferred for culturing *H. ducreyi* in making a diagnosis of chancroid: gonococcal-based agar with fetal calf serum and bovine hemoglobin (GC-HgS) and Mueller–Hinton agar with horse blood (MH-HB) (112). The sensitivity of culture in patients with clinically diagnosed chancroid ranges from 30% to 90%. Factors that may explain the lack of sensitivity of the technique are previous antibiotic use by the patient, improper sample handling, strain differences in nutritional requirements of the causative *H. ducreyi*, and rare cases of *H. ducreyi* sensitivity to vancomycin (which is present in culture media).

Detection of Microbial Components

A multiplex PCR has been developed for detecting *T. pallidum*, *H. ducreyi*, and HSV (113,114). It seems to be much more sensitive and only slightly less specific than culture-based methods for the diagnosis of GUD. Nevertheless, the method fails to detect GUD in 20% of patients, and its applicability to routine clinical practice remains to be determined.

Treatment

As mentioned previously, the clinical presentation of GUD often prevents an etiologic diagnosis in presenting patients, and many centers do not perform the minimal tests needed to establish such a diagnosis. Fortunately, syphilis is relatively uncommon in North America (115), and most cases of chancroid occur in specific geographic areas (84% of the 386 cases of chancroid reported in 1996 occurred in New York State, Louisiana, Texas, and Illinois [115]). Thus, if a patient presents with vesicular lesions or with a constellation of symptoms and signs highly suggestive of HSV infection (the most common cause of GUD in North America), then a diagnosis of such infection is likely. The patient should be treated for HSV infection if indicated, and a serologic test for syphilis should be performed. If the diagnosis is uncertain, then the

Table 14.12   Recommended Regimens for the Treatment of Chancroid

Azithromycin 1 g orally once, or
Ceftriaxone 250 mg intramuscularly once, or
Ciprofloxacin 500 mg orally twice a day for 3 days, or
Erythromycin 500 mg orally four times a day for 7 days

patient should be treated for syphilis (and for chancroid if the patient resides in a community in which *H. ducreyi* is a significant cause of GUD) and a serologic test for syphilis should be performed.

Many antibiotics are effective for treating chancroid (1,116). Recommended options for antibiotic treatment are shown in Table 14.12. Ulcers are usually culture negative after the third day of treatment, and patients have to be reevaluated after 5 to 7 days of therapy. Objective signs of improvement are decreased purulence at the ulcer base and epitheliazation of the ulcer (116). Most ulcers heal within 10 days, but some may take as long as 28 days. Healing may be slower in uncircumcised patients or in patients coinfected with HIV. If no signs of improvement are seen after 7 days of treatment, the clinician must consider either an incorrect diagnosis or coinfection with another STD as possible explanations for treatment failure.

The fluctuant adenopathy of chancroid may take longer than ulcers to resolve, and its failure to resolve by 7 days after the beginning of treatment should not be considered treatment failure. Drainage of chancroid lesions is often needed, and there is evidence that incision and drainage of these lesions may entail less re-treatment than does needle aspiration (117).

Prevention

As with other STDs, the prevention of chancroid involves identifying and treating the sexual contacts of patients. Condoms and careful partner selection may reduce the transmission of *H. ducreyi*. It is important to stress once again that genital ulcers increase the chances of acquiring HIV disease.

REFERENCES

1. **Centers for Disease Control and Prevention.** 1998 Guidelines for treatment of sexually transmitted diseases. *MMWR Morbid Mortal Wkly Rep.* 1998;47:1–119.

2. **Handsfield HH, Sparling PF.** *Neisseria gonorrhoeae.* In Mandell GL, Bennett JE, Dolin R (eds). *Principles and Practice of Infectious Diseases*, 4th ed. Philadelphia: Churchill Livington; 1995:1909–26.

3. **Handsfield HH, Lipman TO, Harnisch JP, et al.** Asymptomatic gonorrhea in men. *N Engl J Med.* 1974;290:117–23.

4. **McCormack WM, Johnson K, Stumacher RJ, Donner A.** Clinical spectrum of gonococcal infection in women. *Lancet.* 1977;1:1182–5.

5. **Sherrard J, Barlow D.** Gonorrhoea in men: clinical and diagnostic aspects. *Genitourin Med.* 1996;72:422–6.

6. **Jacobs NF, Kraus SJ.** Gonococcal and nongonococcal urethritis in men: clinical and laboratory differentiation. *Ann Intern Med.* 1975;82:7–12.

7. **Platt R, Rice PA, McCormack WM.** Risk of acquiring gonorrhea and prevalence of abnormal adnexal findings among women recently exposed to gonorrhea. *JAMA.* 1983;250:3205–9.

8. **Stamm WE, Guinan ME, Johnson C, et al.** Effect of treatment regimens for *Neisseria gonorrhoeae* on simultaneous infection with *Chlamydia trachomatis. N Engl J Med.* 1984;310:545–9.

9. **Collier AC, Judson FN, Murphy VL, et al.** Comparative study of ceftriaxone and spectinomycin in the treatment of uncomplicated gonorrhea in women. *Am J Med.* 1984;11:68–72.

10. **Moran JS.** Treating uncomplicated *Neisseria gonorrhoeae* infections: is the anatomic site of infection important? *Sex Transm Dis.* 1995;24:39–46.

11. **Wan WL, Farkas GC, May WN, Robin JB.** The clinical characteristics and course of adult gonococcal conjunctivitis. *Am J Ophthalmol.* 1986;102:575–83.

12. **Ross JDC.** Systemic gonococcal infection. *Genitourin Med.* 1996;72:404–7.

13. **Wise CM, Morris CR, Wasilauskas BL, Salzer WL.** Gonococcal arthritis in an era of increasing penicillin resistance. *Arch Intern Med.* 1994;154:2690–5.

14. **Morello JA, Bohnhoff M.** Serovars and serum resistance of *Neisseria gonorrhoeae* from disseminated and uncomplicated infections. *J Infect Dis.* 1989;160:1012–7.

15. **Curtis AH.** A cause of adhesions in the right upper quadrant. *JAMA.* 1930;94:1221–2.

16. **Fitz-Hugh T.** Acute gonococcal perihepatitis of the right upper quadrant in women. *JAMA.* 1934;102:2094–6.

17. **Jackman JD, Glamann BD.** Southwestern Internal Medicine Conference: gonococcal endocarditis: twenty-five year experience. *Am J Med Sci.* 1991;301:221–30.

18. **Jephcot AE.** Microbiological diagnosis of gonorrhea. *Genitourin Med.* 1997;73:245–52.

19. **Schebke JR, Zajackowski ME.** Comparison of DNA probe (Gen-Probe) with culture for the detection of *Neisseria gonorrhoeae* in an urban STD programme. *Genitourin Med.* 1996;72:108–10.

20. **Buimer M, van Doornum GJJ, Ching S, et al.** Detection of *Chlamydia trachomatis* and *Neisseria gonorrhoeae* by ligase chain reaction-based assays with clinical specimens from various sites: implications for diagnostic testing and screening. *J Clin Microbiol.* 1996;34:2395–2400.

21. **Stary A, Ching SF, Teodorowicz L, Lee H.** Comparison of ligase chain reaction and culture for detection of *Neisseria gonorrhoeae* in genital and extragenital specimens. *J Clin Microbiol.* 1997;35:239–42.

22. **Smith KR, Ching S, Ohhashi Y, et al.** Evaluation of ligase chain reaction for use with urine for identification of *Neisseria gonorrhoeae* in females attending a sexually transmitted disease clinic. *J Clin Microbiol.* 1995;33:455–7.

23. **Ching S, Lee H, Hook EW, et al.** Ligase chain reaction for detection of *Neisseria gonorrhoeae* in urogenital swabs. *J Clin Microbiol.* 1995;33:3111–4.

24. **Mahony JB, Luinstra KE, Tyndall M, et al.** Multiplex PCR for detection of *Chlamydia trachomatis* and *Neisseria gonorrhoeae* in genitourinary specimens. *Chlamydia trachomatis* and *Neisseria gonorrhoeae*. *J Clin Microbiol.* 1995;33:3049–53.

25. **Bassiri M, Mardh PA, Domeika M.** Multiplex AMPLICOR PCR screening for *Chlamydia trachomatis* and *Neisseria gonorrhoeae* in women attending non-sexually transmitted disease clinics. *J Clin Microbiol.* 1997;35:2556–2560.

25a. **Sparling PF, Handsfeld HH.** *Neisseria gonorrhoeae.* In Mandell GL, Bennett JE, Dolin R (eds). *Principles and Practices of Infectious Diseases,* 5th ed. Philadelphia: Churchill-Livingston; 2000:2242–58.

26. **Moran SJ, Levine WC.** Drugs of choice for the treatment of uncomplicated gonococcal infections. *Clin Infect Dis.* 1995;2(Suppl1):S47–S65.

27. **Bignell C.** Antibiotic treatment of gonorrhoea—clinical evidence for choice. *Genitourin Med.* 1996;72:315–20.

28. **Ison CA.** Antimicrobial agents and gonorrhoea: therapeutic choice, resistance, and susceptibility testing. *Genitourin Med.* 1996;72:253–7.

29. **Lind I.** Antimicrobial resistance in *Neisseria gonorrhoeae. Clin Infect Dis.* 1997;24(Suppl 1):S93–S7.

30. **Center for Disease Control and Prevention.** 1998 guidelines for treatment of sexually transmitted diseases. *MMWR Morb Mortal Wkly Rep.* 1998;47 RR1:59–69.

31. **Washington EA, Browner WS, Korenbrot CC.** Cost-effectiveness of combined treatment for endocervical gonorrhea. Considering co-infection with *Chlamydia trachomatis. JAMA.* 1987;257:2056–60.

32. **Peterman TA, Zaidi AA, Lieb S, Wroten JE.** Incubating syphilis in patients treated for gonorrhea: a comparison of treatment regimens. *J Infect Dis.* 1994;170:689–92.

33. **Haizlip J, Isbey SF, Hamilton HA, et al.** Time required for elimination of *Neisseria gonorrhoeae* from the urogenital tract in men with symptomatic urethritis: comparison of oral and intramuscular single-dose therapy. *Sex Transm Dis.* 1995;22:145–8.

34. **Carne CA.** Epidemiological treatment and tests of cure in gonococcal infection: evidence for value. *Genitourin Med.* 1997;73:12–5.

35. **Sanchez J, Gottuzzo E, Escamilla J, et al.** Sexually transmitted infections in female sex workers: reduction by condom use but not by a limited periodic examination program. *Sex Transm Dis.* 1998;25:82–9.

36. **McNagny SE, Parker RM, Zenilman JM, Lewis JS.** Urinary leukocyte esterase test: a screening method for the detection of asymptomatic chlamydial and gonococcal infections in men. *J Infect Dis.* 1992;165:573–6.

37. **O'Brien SF, Bell TA, Farrow JA.** Use of a leukocyte esterase dipstick to detect *Chlamydia trachomatis* and *Neisseria gonorrhoeae* urethritis in asymptomatic adolescent male detainees. *Am J Public Health.* 1988;78:1583–4.

38. **Schebke JR, Sadler R, Sutton M, Hook EW.** Positive screening tests for gonorrhea and chlamydial infection fail to lead consistently to treatment of patients attending a sexually transmitted disease clinic. *Sex Transm Dis.* 1997;24:181–4.

39. **Rice RJ, Roberts PL, Handsfield HH, Holmes KK.** Sociodemographic distribution of gonorrhea incidence: implications for prevention and behavioral research. *Am J Public Health.* 1991;81:1252–8.

40. **Mertz KJ, Levine WC, Mosure DJ, et al.** Screening women for gonorrhea: demographic screening criteria for general clinical use. *Am J Public Health.* 1997;87:1535–8.

41. **Holmes KK, Johnson DW, Kvale PA, et al.** Impact of gonorrhea control program, including selective mass treatment, in female sex workers. *J Infect Dis.* 1996;174(Suppl 2):S230–S9.

42. **Blake MS, Wetzler LM.** Vaccines for gonorrhea: where are we on the curve? *Trends Microbiol.* 1995;3:469–74.

43. **Schachter J.** Chlamydial infections. *N Engl J Med.* 1978;298:428–548.

44. **Jones RB.** Chlamydial diseases. In Mandell GL, Bennett JE, Dolin R (eds). *Principles and Practices of Infectious Diseases*, 4th ed. Philadelphia: Churchill-Livingston; 1995:1676–9.

45. **Martin DH.** Chlamydial infections. *Med Clinic North Am.* 1990;74:1367–87.

46. **Washington AE, Katz P.** Cost and payment source for pelvic inflammatory disease: trends and projections, 1983 through 2000. *JAMA.* 1991;266:2565–9.

47. **Weinstock H, Dean D, Bolan G.** *Chlamydia trachomatis* infections. *Infect Dis Clin North Am.* 1994;8:797–819.

48. **Stamm WE.** Diagnosis of *Chlamydia trachomatis* genitourinary infections. *Ann Intern Med.* 1988;108:710–7.

49. **Stamm WE, Koutsky LA, Benedetti JK, et al.** *Chlamydia trachomatis* urethral infections in men. *Ann Intern Med.* 1984;100:47–51.

50. **Holmes KK, Handsfield H, Wang SP, et al.** Etiology of nongonococcal urethritis. *N Engl J Med.* 1975;292:1199–1205.

51. **Mc Cutchan JA.** Epidemiology of venereal urethritis: comparison of gonorrhea and nongonococcal urethritis. *Rev Infect Dis.* 1984;6:669–88.

52. **Martin DH, Mroczkowski TF, Dalu ZA, et al.** A controlled trial of a single dose of azithromycin for the treatment of chlamydial urethritis and cervicitis. *N Engl J Med.* 1992;327:921–5.

53. **Brunham RC, Paavonen J, Stevens CE, et al.** Mucopurulent cervicitis—the ignored counterpart in women of urethritis in men. *N Engl J Med.* 1984;311:1–6.

54. **Cates W, Wasserheit JN.** Genital chlamydial infections: epidemiology and reproductive sequelae. *Am J Obstet Gynecol.* 1991;164:1771–81.

55. **Robinson AJ, Ridgway GL.** Modern diagnosis and management of genital *Chlamydia trachomatis* infection. *Br J Hosp Med.* 1996;55:388–93.

56. **Taylor-Robinson D, Thomas BJ.** Laboratory techniques for the diagnosis of chlamydial infections. *Genitourin Med.* 1991;67:256–66.

57. **Schachter J.** DFA, EIA, PCR, LCR and other technologies: what tests should be used for diagnosis of chlamydia infections? *Immunol Invest.* 1997;26:157–61.

58. **Shafer MA, Schachter J, Moncada J, et al.** Evaluation of urine-based screening strategies to detect *Chlamydia trachomatis* among sexually active asymptomatic young males. *JAMA.* 1993;270:2065–70.

59. **Chernesky MA, Lee H, Schachter J, et al.** Diagnosis of *Chlamydia trachomatis* urethral infection in symptomatic and asymptomatic men by testing first-void urine in a ligase chain reaction assay. *J Infect Dis.* 1994;170:1308–11.

60. **Sellors JW, Mahony JB, Jang D, et al.** Comparison of cervical, urethral, and urine specimens for the detection of *Chlamydia trachomatis* in women. *J Infect Dis.* 1991; 164:205–8.

61. **Schachter J, Moncada J, Whidden R, et al.** Noninvasive tests for diagnosis of *Chlamydia trachomatis* infection: application of ligase chain reaction to first-catch urine specimens of women. *J Infect Dis.* 1995;172:1411–4.

62. **Lee HH, Chernesky MA, Schachter J, et al.** Diagnosis of *Chlamydia trachomatis* genitourinary infection by ligase chain reaction assay of urine. *Lancet.* 1995;345:213–6.

63. **Ridgway GL, Mumtaz G, Robinson AJ, et al.** Comparison of the ligase chain reaction with cell culture for the diagnosis of *Chlamydia trachomatis* infection in women. *J Clin Pathol.* 1996;49:116–9.

64. **Gaydos CA, Crotchfelt KA, Howell MR, et al.** Molecular amplification assays to detect chlamydial infections in urine specimens from high school female students and to monitor the persistence of chlamydial DNA after therapy. *J Infect Dis.* 1998;177: 417–24.

65. **Andrews WW, Lee HH, Roden WJ, Mott CW.** Detection of genitourinary tract *Chlamydia trachomatis* infection in pregnant women by ligase chain reaction assay. *Obstet Gynecol.* 1997;89:556–60.

66. **Stamm WE, Hicks CB, Martin DH, et al.** Azithromycin for the empirical treatment of the nongonococcal urethritis syndrome in men: a randomized double-blind study. *JAMA.* 1995;274:545–9.

67. **Magid D, Douglas JM, Schwartz S.** Doxycycline compared with azithromycin for treating women with genital *Chlamydia trachomatis* infections: an incremental cost-effectiveness analysis. *Ann Intern Med.* 1996;124:389–99.

68. **Scholes D, Stergachis A, Heidrich FE, et al.** Prevention of pelvic inflammatory disease by screening for cervical chlamydial infection. *N Engl J Med.* 1996;334: 1362–1401.

69. **Cohen I, Vielle JC, Calkins BM.** Improved pregnancy outcome following successful treatment of chlamydial infection. *JAMA.* 1990;263:3160–3.

70. **Corey L, Adams HG, Brown ZA, Holmes KK.** Genital herpes simplex virus infections: clinical manifestations, course and complications. *Ann Intern Med.* 1983;98: 958–72.

71. **Johnson RE, Nahmics AJ, Magder LS.** A seroepidemiology survey of the prevalence of herpes simplex virus type 2 infection in the United States. *N Engl J Med.* 1989; 321:8–12.

72. **Frenkel LM, Garratty EM, Ping Shen J, et al.** Clinical reactivation of herpes simplex virus type 2 infection in seropositive pregnant women with no history of genital herpes. *Ann Intern Med.* 1993;118:414–8.

73. **Kulhanijian JA, Soroushi V, Au DS, et al.** Identification of women at unsuspected risk of primary infection with herpes simplex virus type 2 during pregnancy. *N Engl J Med.* 1992;326:916–20.

74. **Koutsky LA, Stevens CE, Holmes KK, et al.** Underdiagnosis of genital herpes by current clinical and viral-isolation procedures. *N Engl J Med.* 1992;326:1533–9.

75. **Mertz GJ, Benedetti J, Ashley R, et al.** Risk factors for the sexual transmission of genital herpes. *Ann Intern Med.* 1992;116:197–202.

76. **Bryson Y, Dillon M, Bernstein DI, et al.** Risk of acquisition of genital herpes simplex virus type 2 in sex partners of persons with genital herpes: a prospective couple study. *J Infect Dis.* 1993;167:942–6.

77. **Mertz GJ.** Epidemiology of genital herpes infections. *Infect Dis Clin North Am.* 1993;7: 825–39.

78. **Sacks SL.** Frequency and duration of patient-observed recurrent genital herpes simplex virus infection: characterization of the nonlesional prodrome. *J Infect Dis.* 1984;150:873–7.

79. **Benedetti J, Corey L, Ashley R.** Recurrence rates in genital herpes after symptomatic first-episode infection. *Ann Intern Med.* 1994;121:857–864.

80. **Koelle DM, Benedetti J, Langenberg A, Corey L.** Asymptomatic reactivation of herpes simplex virus in women after the first episode of genital herpes. *Ann Intern Med.* 1992;116:433–7.

81. **Hirsch MS.** Herpes simplex virus. In Mandell GL, Bennett JE, Dolin R (eds). *Principles and Practice of Infectious Diseases,* 4th ed. Philadelphia: Churchill-Livingston; 1995: 1336–45.

82. **Nahass GT, Goldstein BA, Zhu WY, et al.** Comparison of Tzanck smear, viral culture, and DNA diagnostic methods in detection of herpes simplex and varicella-zoster infection. *JAMA.* 1992;268:2541–4.

83. **DiCarlo RP, Armentor BS, Martin DH.** Chancroid epidemiology in New Orleans men. *J Infect Dis.* 1995;172:446–52.

84. **Mertz GJ, Critchlow CW, Benedetti J, et al.** Double-blind placebo-controlled trial of oral acyclovir in first-episode genital herpes simplex virus infection. *JAMA.* 1984;252: 1147–51.

85. **Whitley RJ, Gnann JW.** Acyclovir: a decade later. *N Engl J Med.* 1992;327:782–9.

86. **Spruance SL, Tyring SK, DeGregorio B, et al.** A large-scale, placebo-controlled, dose-ranging trial of peroral valaciclovir for episodic treatment of recurrent herpes genitalis. *Arch Intern Med.* 1996;156:1729–35.

87. **Sacks SL, Aoki FY, Diaz-Mitoma F, et al.** Patient-initiated, twice-daily oral famciclovir for early recurrent genital herpes. *JAMA.* 1996;276:44–9.

88. **Goldberg LH, Kaufman R, Kurtz TO, et al.** Long-term suppression of recurrent genital herpes with acyclovir. *Arch Dermatol.* 1993;129:582–7.

89. **Wald A, Zeh J, Barnum G, et al.** Suppression of subclinical shedding of herpes simplex virus type 2 with acyclovir. *Ann Intern Med.* 1996;124:8–15.

90. **Tramont EC.** *Treponema pallidum.* In Mandel GL, Bennett JE, Dolin R (eds) *Principles and Practice of Infectious Diseases,* 4th ed. Philadelphia: Churchill-Livingston; 1995: 2117–33.

91. **Hutchinson CM, Hook EW.** Syphilis in adults. *Med Clin North Am.* 1990;74: 1389–1416.

92. **Gordon SM, Eaton ME, George R, et al.** The response of symptomatic neurosyphilis to high-doseintravenous penicillin in patients with human immunodeficiency virus infection. *N Engl J Med.* 1994;331:1469–73.

93. **Hook EW, Marra CM.** Acquired syphilis in adults. *N Engl J Med.* 1992;326:1060–9.

94. **Simon RP.** Neurosyphilis. *Arch Neurol.* 1985;42:606–13.

95. **Lukehart SA, Hook EW, Baker-Zander SA, et al.** Invasion of the central nervous system by *Treponema pallidum*: implications for diagnosis and treatment. *Ann Intern Med.* 1988;109:855–62.

96. **Katz DA, Berger JR, Duncan RC.** Neurosyphilis: a comparative study of the effects of infection with human immunodeficiency virus. *Arch Neurol.* 1993;50:243–9.

97. **Johns DR, Tierney M, Felsenstein D.** Alteration in the natural history of neurosyphilis by concurrent infection with the human immunodeficiency virus. *N Engl J Med.* 1987;316:1569–72.

98. **Orle KA, Gates CA, Martin DH, et al.** Simultaneous PCR detection of *Haemophilius ducreyi, Treponema pallidum,* and herpes simplex virus types 1 and 2 from genital ulcers. *J Clin Microbiol.* 1996;34:49–54.

99. **Jethwa HS, Schmitz JL, Dallabetta G, et al.** Comparison of molecular and microscopic techniques for detection of *Treponema pallidum* in genital ulcers. *J Clin Microbiol.* 1995;33:180–3.

100. **Romanowski B, Sutherland R, Fick GH, et al.** Serologic response to treatment of infectious syphilis. *Ann Intern Med.* 1991;114:1005–9.

101. **Hart G.** Syphilis tests in diagnostic and therapeutic decision making. *Ann Intern Med.* 1986;104:368–76.

102. **Brown ST, Zaidi A, Larsen SA, Reynolds GH.** Serological response to syphilis treatment. *JAMA.* 1985;253:1296–9.

103. **Hand WL.** *Haemophilus* species (including chancroid). In Mandell GL, Bennett JE, Dolin R (eds). *Principles and Practice of Infectious Diseases*, 4th ed. Philadelphia: Churchill Livingston; 1995:2045–50.

104. **Schmid GP, Sanders LL, Blount JH, Alexander ER.** Chancroid in the United States. Reestablishment of an old disease. *JAMA.* 1987;258:3265–8.

105. **Hammond GW, Slutchuck M, Scatliff J, et al.** Epidemiological, clinical, laboratory, and therapeutic features of an urban outbreak of chancroid in North America. *Rev Infect Dis.* 1980;2:867–79.

106. **Strakosch EA, Kendell HW, Craig RM, Schwemlein GX.** Clinical and laboratory investigation of 370 cases of chancroid. *J Invest Dermatol.* 1945;6:95–107.

107. **Dangor Y, Ballard RC, Exposto FL, et al.** Accuracy of clinical diagnosis of genital ulcer disease. *Sex Transm Dis.* 1990;17:184–9.

108. **DiCarlo RP, Martin DH.** The clinical diagnosis of genital ulcer disease in men. *Clin Infect Dis.* 1997;25:292–8.

109. **Dillon SM, Cummings M, Rajagopalan S, McCormack WC.** Prospective analysis of genital ulcer disease in Brooklyn, New York. *Clin Infect Dis.* 1997;24:945–50.

110. **Hawkes S, West B, Wilson S, et al.** Asymptomatic carriage of *Haemophilus ducreyi* confirmed by the polymerase chain reaction. *Genitourin Med.* 1995;71:224–7.

111. **Beck-Sague CM, Cordts JR, Brown K, et al.** Laboratory diagnosis of sexually transmitted diseases in facilities within the United States. Results of a national survey. *Sex Transm Dis.* 1996;23:342–9.

112. **Jones CC, Rosen T.** Cultural diagnosis of chancroid. *Arch Dermatol.* 1991;127:1823–7.

113. **Orle KA, Gates CA, Martin DH, Body BA, Weiss JB.** Simultaneous PCR detection of *Haemophilus ducreyi, Treponema pallidum*, and herpes simplex virus types 1 and 2 from genital ulcers. *J Clin Microbiol.* 1996;34:49–54.

114. **Morse SA, Trees DL, Htun Y, et al.** Comparison of clinical diagnosis and standard laboratory and molecular methods for the diagnosis of genital ulcer disease in Lesotho: association with human immunodeficiency virus infection. *J Infect Dis.* 1997;175:583–9.

115. **Centers for Disease Control and Prevention.** Summary of notifiable diseases, United States, 1997. *MMWR Morb Mortal Wkly Rep.* 1997;46:1–6.

116. **Dangor Y, Ballard RC, Miller SD, Koornhof HJ.** Treatment of chancroid. Antimicrob Agents Chemother 1990;34:1308–11.

117. **Ernst AA, Marvez-Valls E, Martin DH.** Incision and drainage versus aspiration of fluctuant buboes in the Emergency Department during an epidemic of chancroid. *Sex Transm Dis.* 1995;22:217–20.

15

Pelvic Inflammatory Disease

Robert F. Flora, MD

Pelvic inflammatory disease (PID) is caused by an infection that ascends from the vagina or cervix into the upper genital tract. One or more sites in the upper genital tract can be involved, including the endometrium (endometritis), fallopian tubes (salpingitis), ovaries (oophoritis), myometrium (myometritis), serosa and broad ligament (parametritis), and pelvic peritoneum (peritonitis). Because of the inflammatory process, adherence of intra-abdominal pelvic organs and collection of pus can lead to the development of a tuboovarian complex or abscess. Involvement of the serosa of the appendix or liver can lead to a periappendicits or perihepatitis, respectively.

Clinically, the terms *salpingitis* and *PID* are used synonymously. *Salpingitis* refers to an inflammatory process that occurs in the fallopian tube. However, Jacobson and Westrom (1) showed that only two thirds of women with the clinical diagnosis of PID had laparoscopic evidence of a tubal infection. Aside from the acute problems that PID causes, it can have other sequelae, such as ectopic pregnancies, infertility, and chronic pelvic pain. In the past, the term *chronic PID* was used to describe patients with these sequelae, but this term has been largely abandoned.

Epidemiology

Unlike some sexually transmitted diseases (STDs), the reporting of PID is not mandatory. Additionally, an estimated 60% of PID can be subclinical (2).

Thus, accurate estimates of its prevalence are difficult to make. Rein and coworkers (3) used 3 years of insurance claims information and national survey data to estimate the direct and indirect medical cost of PID in the United States. They estimated that 1.76 million visits for acute PID and its sequelae were made annually from 1993 to 1995. Acute PID accounted for 1.2 million of these as either inpatient, outpatient, or STD-clinic visits. Among the sequelae of PID, chronic pelvic pain was responsible for 300,000 visits, ectopic pregnancies for 145,000 visits, and infertility for 78,000 visits. In 1998 dollars, the annual total direct cost attributable to PID was estimated at $1.62 to $1.88 billion dollars (3). This is much lower than the 1994 Institute of Medicine estimate of $3.12 billion dollars (4) or the 2000 projection by Washington and Katz (5) of $9 billion. The difference may be due to several factors, including a decrease in cases of PID and gonorrhea; better and more widespread screening for *Chlamydia*, switching from inpatient to outpatient management, and better data sources (3,6). From 1980 to 1998, a decrease in hospitalizations for ectopic pregnancies and PID was observed. Additionally, initial visits to physician offices by women 15 to 44 years of age dropped from more than 400,000 per year to approximately 250,000 per year (7). Regardless of this decrease, PID and its sequelae still have a profound effect on health care and its related costs.

Etiology

The infectious process in PID is polymicrobial and due to many different organisms (8). The spread of these organisms occurs through their progress from the vagina and endocervix through the cervical canal and into the upper genital tract. Four factors could contribute to this spread, including uterine instrumentation, hormonal changes during menses, retrograde menstruation, and virulence factors associated with specific organisms (9). The microbial etiology of PID is difficult to evaluate because of numerous factors, including difficulty in culturing from the upper-tract genitalia other than through a surgical approach, contamination by vaginal flora, differences in laboratory methods, and the difficulty in making a clinical diagnosis of PID. In their long-term study, Jossens and coworkers (10) determined that either *Neisseria gonorrhoeae* or *Chlamydia trachomatis* were identified in 65% of cases of PID (i.e., STD-related PID). In 30% of their cases, only anaerobic or facultative bacteria were isolated (i.e., non–STD-related PID). However, these anaerobic and facultative bacteria also were frequently recovered when an STD-causing organism was identified. These other organisms included *Gardnerella vaginalis*, *Escherichia coli*, and *Haemophilus influenzae* and species of *Prevotella*, *Bacteroides*, *Peptostreptococcus*, *Peptococcus*, and *Streptococcus*. *Mycoplasma hominis*, *Ureaplasma ure-*

alyticum, and *Trichomonas vaginalis* also have been isolated from the fallopian tubes. Additionally, bacterial vaginosis is believed to shift the vaginal flora to an anaerobic state and to increase the risk of PID (2,9,11).

The STDs caused by *N. gonorrheae* and *C. trachomatis* account for most PID cases. Both of these diseases start as a cervicitis, which can ascend the reproductive tract and lead to PID. Approximately 70% of such infections are asymptomatic; if not treated, 20% to 40% of these evolve to PID. The number of cases of chlamydial infection has been increasing every year. In 1998, the rate was 382.2 cases per 100,000 population. This increase is felt to have been the result of better screening practices, which can reduce the incidence of PID by 60% (7,12). Since the late 1970s, infections with *N. gonorrhoeae* have been decreasing steadily; however, an increase was noted between 1997 and 1998, from 119 to 131 cases per 100,000 population (5). If left untreated, 10% to 40% of these cases evolve to PID. Approximatey half of all gonococcal infections are asymptomatic (7,13).

Risk Factors

Several demographic and social risk factors have been linked with the development of PID, including young age, lower socioeconomic status, and a single or divorced marital status. No correlation has been reported for urban compared with rural residence. Risk factors associated with the acquisition of an STD also are associated with progression to PID, including sexual-partner characteristics, infectivity rates, duration of infection, and sociocultural environment. Use of barrier contraceptive methods and oral contraceptives decreases the risk of PID; however, the use of oral contraceptives is associated with an increased diagnosis of chlamydial cervicitis. Use of an intrauterine device (IUD) is associated with an increase in non–STD-related PID. Health care-seeking behavior decreases the risk of PID when it leads to prompt evaluation, compliance with treatment, and treatment of the patient's partner. Douching, smoking, and menses also are associated with an increased risk of PID. Substance abuse has been associated with an increased risk of STD but not with an increased risk of developing PID (9,14). Jossens and coworkers (10) studied factors that are more likely to be associated with an STD-related PID than with a non–STD-related PID. Patients with PID were more likely to have STD-related pelvic inflammatory infection if they 1) were black, 2) used no contraception, 3) had a prior history of gonorrhea as an STD, 4) had a previous pelvic inflammatory infection with gonorrhea, 5) presented with a history of pain of less than 3-days' duration, or 6) had two or more sexual partners in the previous 30 days or three or more partners in the previous 60 days. Factors that increased the likelihood of a non-STD-related pelvic inflammatory infection included current IUD use, a history of IUD use, and pelvic surgery in the previous 30 days. Multivariate analysis, performed to adjust for confounding factors, showed black race as a risk factor for STD-associated PID and current IUD use as a risk factor for non-STD-related PID. Douching was not shown to increase the likelihood of one type of PID over the other (10).

Diagnosis

The diagnosis of PID is difficult to make. The presentation of PID is severe in approximately 4% of cases, mild to moderate in 36%, and subclinical in 60% (2). Although, laparoscopy is considered the "gold standard" for the diagnosis of PID, most diagnoses are made clinically because of its high cost and limited availability. Furthermore, in a study of 813 women with clinical diagnoses of PID, only 532 (65%) had the disease confirmed on laparoscopy. Other conditions (e.g., appendicitis, endometriosis, ectopic pregnancy) were found. This incongruity was confirmed recently by Molander and coworkers (15) who confirmed PID in only 61% of their patients with clinically suspected PID. They managed their laparoscopically confirmed cases of PID with irrigation, lysis of adhesions, and drainage and irrigation of pyosalpinx and tuboovarian complexes (1,15).

The Centers for Disease Control and Prevention (CDC) 1998 Guidelines state that no single factor or combination of history, physical, or laboratory factors has adequate sensitivity and specificity to make the diagnosis of acute PID (16). Table 15.1 lists tests or procedures that may assist in the diagnosis and management of acute PID. A white blood cell count is not a reliable indicator of PID because half of all women with the disease may have no leukocytosis. The erythrocyte sedimentation rate (ESR) has a moderately high

Table 15.1   Possible Evaluative Tools in the Diagnosis and Management of Pelvic Inflammatory Disease

Pregnancy test	"Wet prep" to evaluate for bacterial vaginosis
White blood cell count	Culdocentesis
Erythrocyte sedimentation rate	Endometrial biopsy
C-reactive protein	Ultrasound
Gram stain (if cervical discharge is present)	CT or MRI
Cervical screening test or cultures for gonorrhea and chlamydia	Laparoscopy

CT = computed tomography; MRI = magnetic resonance imaging.
Republished with permission from (16).

sensitivity but a low specificity for PID. Acute-phase reactants, such as C-reactive protein, are only slightly more sensitive than ESR. A pregnancy test should be obtained to rule out an ectopic pregnancy. Cervical cultures for gonorrhea and chlamydia and a Gram stain of cervical discharge are helpful and should be obtained; however, these procedures can yield false-positive results even when an upper-tract infection with the identified organism exists and is documented. Ideally, cultures also should be obtained for the sexual partners of patients with PID. A culdocentesis can be helpful if purulent peritoneal fluid is found. An endometrial biopsy can confirm the presence of endometritis. Ultrasonography is helpful in identifying a tuboovarian complex, free peritoneal fluid, and hydrosalpinx or pyosalpinx.

Because of the difficulty in diagnosing PID and the severity of its sequelae if it is not diagnosed, a low threshold for diagnosis and treatment is recommended. The minimum criteria for empirical PID treatment comprise the following (16):

- Lower abdominal tenderness
- Adnexal tenderness
- Cervical tenderness on motion

Additional criteria that support the diagnosis include the following:

- Oral temperature >101°F (>38.3°C)
- Abnormal cervical or vaginal discharge
- Increased ESR
- Increased C-reactive protein
- Laboratory documentation of cervical infection with *N. gonorrhoeae* or *C. trachomatis*

Definitive criteria can include the following:

- Endometritis on endometrial biopsy
- Thickened, fluid-filled tubes with or without free pelvic fluid or tuboovarian complex that is confirmed by radiologic imaging
- Laparoscopic findings consistent with PID

Treatment

Ideally, treating lower genital tract infections of *N. gonorrhoeae* or *C. trachomatis* or of bacterial vaginosis prevents most cases of PID. However, no quality overall screening programs for PID exist in the United States. Additionally, because many lower-tract infections are asymptomatic, cases of acute PID do occur. Thus, once an acute upper-tract process occurs, the treatment of PID should be directed toward the treatment of a polymicrobial infection. Coverage should include *N. gonorrhoeae*, *C. trachomatis*, anaerobic bacteria, facultative bacteria, and streptococci. Figure 15.1 shows an algorithm for the care of a patient with PID. As previously mentioned, the threshold for treatment should be low. Treatment should be started as soon as possible to decrease the incidence of long-term sequelae. Treatment can be conducted on either an outpatient or an inpatient basis. A steadily decreasing trend was seen between 1981 to 1997 in the hospitalization of women 15 to 44 years of age who had PID (7). Approximately 20% to 25% of patients with acute PID are hospitalized (17). Multiple factors come into play when deciding on outpatient versus inpatient management; however, the CDC's 1998 guidelines have listed the following criteria for hospitalization with parenteral therapy (16):

- Inability to exclude the risk of a surgical emergency, such as appendicitis
- Pregnancy
- Lack of clinical response to oral therapy
- Inability to adhere to or tolerate oral therapy
- Severe illness, nausea, vomiting, and/or high fever
- Tuboovarian abscess or complex
- Immunodeficiency

For hospitalized patients who receive parenteral therapy, at least 24 hours of clinical improvement should occur before considering a switch from parenteral to oral therapy. For patients with tuboovarian abscesses or complexes, at least 24 hours of inpatient observation is recommended before considering home-based parenteral treatment.

Outpatient Oral Therapy

Outpatient oral treatments for PID are shown in Table 15.2. If no response is noted after 72 hours, parenteral therapy should be instituted. Other, alternative oral therapies are available; however, not enough data were available for the CDC to include them in their 1998 guidelines.

Parenteral Therapy

Parenteral therapy for PID is usually begun on an inpatient basis. After 24 hours of clinical improvement, transition to oral therapy can be considered. Table 15.3 shows both the parenteral and oral regimens to be used.

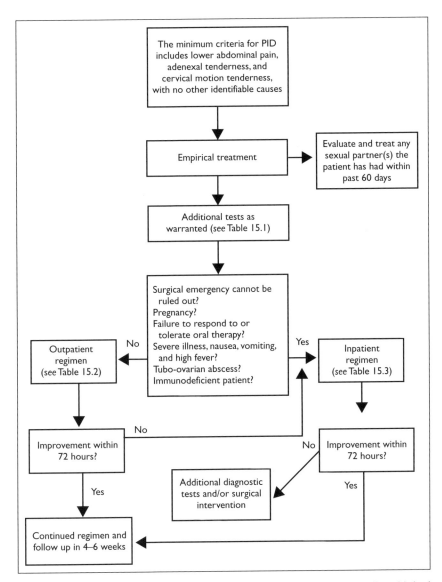

Figure 15.1 Algorithm for the treatment of pelvic inflammatory disease. (Republished with permission from the Centers for Disease Control and Prevention. 1998 Guidelines for treatment of sexually transmitted diseases. MMWR Morb Mortal Wkly Rep. 1998;47(RR-1):60–86.

In Regimen A in Table 15.3, the bioavailability of intravenous and oral doxycycline are equivalent, but the intravenous route can cause discomfort. Thus, doxycycline should be given orally whenever possible. Doxycycline

Table 15.2   Outpatient Regimens for the Treatment of Pelvic Inflammatory Disease

Regimen A
Ofloxacin 400 mg bid PO for 14 days
  and
Metronidazole 500 mg bid PO for 14 days

Regimen B
Doxycycline 100 mg bid PO for 14 days
  and one of the following:
Ceftriaxone 250 mg IM as a single dose*
  or
Cefoxitin 2 g IM + probenecid 1 g PO as a single dose

IM = intramuscularly; PO = orally.
* Cefotaxime may be used.
Republished with permission from (16).

should be continued for a total of 14 days. Other second- or third-generation cephalosporins (e.g., ceftizoxime, cefotaxime, ceftriaxone) can be substituted for cefotetan or cefoxitin, but the anaerobic coverage they provide may not be as thorough.

Regimen B in Table 15.3 combines gentamicin and clindamycin. Both of these agents are given every eight hours. After 24 hours of clinical improvement, parenteral therapy may be replaced by oral therapy with either doxycycline at 100 mg twice per day or clindamycin at 450 mg four times per day. A total of 14 days of therapy should be given. In cases of a tuboovarian abscess, oral clindamycin may be preferred over doxycycline because it provides better anaerobic coverage.

Alternative parenteral regimens for PID are shown in Table 15.4. These regimens are supported by at least one clinical trial and provide broad-spectrum coverage. A switch to oral therapy can be considered after 24 hours of clinical improvement, with continuation to 14 days of total therapy.

Follow-Up and Management of Sexual Partners

The cure rates are excellent with the aforementioned CDC regimens for PID. In the meta-analysis performed by Walker and coworkers (18), the inpatient regimens produced clinical cure rates of 92% to 94% and microbiologic cure rates of 97% to 100%. The outpatient regimen of cefoxitin and doxycycline produced a clinical cure rate of 95% and microbiologic cure rate of 91%. Ofloxacin produced clinical and microbiological cure rates of 95% and 100%, respectively.

Table 15.3   Inpatient Regimens for the Treatment of Pelvic Inflammatory Disease

Regimen A

Cefotetan 2 g IV every 12 hours or cefoxitin 2 g IV every 6 hours + doxycycline 100 mg IV
   or PO every 12 hours
   and after 24 hours of clinical improvement:
Doxycycline 100 mg PO for a total treatment of 14 days

Regimen B

Clindamycin 900 mg IV every 8 hours
   and
Gentamicin IV or IM with a loading dose of 2 mg/kg body weight followed by maintenance
   dose of 1.5 mg/kg every 8 hours
   And one of the following after 24 hours of clinical improvement:
Doxycycline 100 mg PO for a total treatment of 14 days
   or
Clindamycin 450 mg qid PO for a total treatment of 14 days (especially in cases of a tuboovarian abscess)

IM = intramuscularly; IV = intravenously; PO = orally.
Republished with permission from (16).

Clinical improvement should be noted within 3 days after the start of therapy. Patients whose treatment begins with an outpatient regimen should be evaluated within 72 hours. Follow-up rescreening tests for gonorrhea and chlamydia can be repeated from 4 to 6 weeks after the end of therapy. A 1-month interval after completion of therapy is needed for follow-up tests with polymerase chain reaction or ligase chain reaction technology (16).

Sexual partners who have had contact with the affected patient within 60 days of the onset of PID symptoms should be evaluated and treated empirically, even if the partners are asymptomatic. Interestingly, 13% of male partners found to have urethral gonorrhea were asymptomatic (17). Treatment for both gonorrheal and chlamydial infection should be given. Table 15.5 shows the recommended treatment for sexual partners who have these conditions. In this manner, the risk of reinfection can be decreased. Follow-up rescreening also may be helpful.

Tuboovarian Abscess or Complex

Tuboovarian abscess or complex is a major complication of an acute pelvic infection. It can occur in up to 34% of patients hospitalized with PID (2). Because of the inflammatory reaction that results from the infection, the fallopian tube and ovary agglutinate and become a complex with walled-off

Table 15.4   Alternative Inpatient Regimens for the Treatment of Pelvic Inflammatory Disease

Ofloxacin 400 mg IV every 12 hours + metronidazole 500 mg IV every 8 hours
   or
Ampicillin/sulbactam 3 g IV every 6 hours + doxycycline 100 mg IV or PO every 12 hours
   or
Ciprofloxacin 200 mg IV every 12 hours + doxycycline 100 mg IV or PO every 12 hours +
   metronidazole 500 mg IV every 8 hours

IV = intravenously; PO = orally.
Republished with permission from (16).

Table 15.5   Dual Treatment for Sexual Partners of Patients with Pelvic Inflammatory Disease

Cefixime 400 mg PO as a single dose
   or
Ceftriaxone 125 mg IM as a single dose
   or
Ciprofloxacin 500 mg PO as a single dose
   or
Ofloxacin 400 mg PO as a single dose
   And one of the following:
Azithromycin 1 g PO as a single dose
   or
Doxycycline 100 mg bid PO for 7 days

IM = intramuscularly; PO = orally.
Republished with permission from (16).

pus. Other intraperitoneal organs, including bowel and omentum, also may become involved.

More than two thirds of tuboovarian abscesses are unilateral. Early IUDs were associated with tuboovarian abscesses. The risk of abscess was believed to be related to the multifilament tail attached to the IUD (19). However, newer IUDs with monofilament tails have not been shown to be associated with an increased risk of PID, except in the first 21 days after insertion (20). After 5 months of IUD use, the risk of PID is not increased in women at low risk as compared with controls (21). Prophylaxis with doxycycline has not been shown to decrease this risk (22). Cultures for *N. gonorrhoeae* and *Chlamydia* species are recommended before insertion of the IUD. Also, when IUD users have a new sexual partner, they are encouraged to be seen for counseling about the risk of PID and continued IUD use.

Organisms shown to be involved in tuboovarian abscess are predominantly anaerobic and facultative aerobic organisms. *N. gonorrhoeae* and *C. trachomatis* can be isolated in cases of tuboovarian abscess or complex, but the absence of *N. gonorrhoeae* and *C. trachomatis* does not exclude their involvement in initiating the infection. The anaerobic state in the abscess can inhibit the growth and viability of *N. gonorrhoeae*. *Actinomyces israelii* is an organism that has been associated with tuboovarian abscesses and IUD use (2,16,23,24).

Treatment is initially antibiotic based. Between 3% and 5% of patients require initial surgical intervention. Response to antibiotics occurs in 60% to 70% of patients. Thirty percent require surgical intervention with either drainage or removal of the IUD. Treatment (specifically clindamycin) that is aimed at anaerobes has a reported success rate of 86%. It is recommended that 7 days of parenteral antibiotic therapy with clindamycin-gentamicin be given, with oral clindamycin given afterward to complete 14 days of therapy. A minimum of 24 hours of inpatient parenteral therapy is recommended before switching to home parenteral therapy. If an inpatient regimen of cefoxitin-cefotetan plus doxycycline was begun before the discovery of a tuboovarian abscess and if a clinical response is noted, then there is no need to change to clindamycin-gentamicin. No difference in the need for surgery was noted with either regimen. If *Enterococcus* species is suspected or if the patient is septic, then triple antibiotic therapy with ampicillin, clindamycin (or metronidazole), and gentamicin should be used. Because most tuboovarian abscesses are unilateral, surgery does not necessarily require extirpation of an unaffected uterus or opposite adnexa. Drainage alone can be successful. If a patient who uses an IUD is discovered to have a tuboovarian abscess, then parenteral therapy should be instituted at least 24 hours before removing the IUD. Rupture of an abscess causes a generalized peritonitis and is a surgical emergency. Prompt intervention is required. The mortality from rupture ranges from 3% to 8% (2,16,25-28).

Long-Term Sequelae

The long-term sequelae of PID are considered to be chronic pelvic pain, infertility, and ectopic pregnancies. Rein and coworkers (3) estimated that the 1998 PID-attributable costs of chronic pelvic pain, ectopic pregnancy, and infertility were $166 million, $295 million, and $360 million, respectively. More than 500,000 health care visits per year were attributed to the three sequelae of PID (3).

Westrom and coworkers (27) estimated that among women with acute PID, 20% have infertility, 9% have ectopic pregnancies, and 18% have chronic pelvic pain. According to the 1991 COC guidelines, after just one episode of

PID, 11% of women become infertile; after two and three bouts of PID, the incidence of infertility increases to 34% and 54%, respectively. The risk of ectopic pregnancy is increased sevenfold after having PID (9). Immediate treatment after symptom onset is paramount in preventing these problems. Hillis and coworkers (28) showed a lower incidence of infertility if treatment was begun before 3 days of symptoms had occurred.

Summary

Pelvic inflammatory disease has profound short- and long-term effects on patients and society. The prevention of ascending infections by treating infections in the lower genital tract is the best method of decreasing PID. If PID symptoms develop, prompt treatment with one of the CDC-recommended regimens has an excellent outcome and can prevent long-term sequelae.

REFERENCES

1. **Jacobson L, Westrom L.** Objectivized diagnosis of pelvic inflammatory disease: diagnostic and prognostic value of routine laparoscopy. *Am J Obstet Gynecol* 1969; 105:1088–98.

2. **Westrom L, Escenbach D.** Pelvic inflammatory disease. In Holmes KK, Sparling PD, Mardh P-A, et al. (eds). *Sexually Transmitted Diseases*, 3rd ed. New York: McGraw-Hill; 1999:783–803.

3. **Rein DB, Kassler WJ, Irwin KL, et al.** Direct medical cost of pelvic inflammatory disease and its sequelae: decreasing but still substantial. *Obstet Gynecol* 2000;95: 397–402.

4. **Siegel JE.** Estimates of the economic burden of STD: review of the lterature with updates. In Eng TR, Butler WT (eds). *Institute of Medicine: The Hidden Epidemic*. Washington DC: National Academy Press; 1997:330–56.

5. **Washington AE, Katz P.** Cost of and payment source for pelvic inflammatory disease: trends and projections, 1983-2000. *JAMA* 1991;266:2565–9.

6. **Centers for Disease Control and Prevention.** Gonorrhea–United States, 1998. *MMWR Morbid Mortal Wkly Rep.* 2000;49:538–42.

7. **Centers for Disease Control and Prevention.** *Sexually Transmitted Disease Surveillance 1998.* Atlanta: U.S. Department of Health and Human Services, Division of STD Prevention, CDC. 1999:39–47.

8. **Eschenbach DA, Buchanan RM, Pollock HM, et al.** Polymicrobial etiology of acute pelvic inflammatory disease. *N Engl J Med* 1975;292:166–71.

9. **Center for Disease Control and Prevention.** Pelvic inflammatory disease: guidelines for prevention and management. *MMWR Morbid Mortal Wkly Rep* 1991;40(RR-5):1–25.

10. **Jossens MO, Schachter J, Sweet RL.** Risk factors associated with pelvic inflammatory disease of differing microbial etiologies. *Obstet Gynecol* 1994;83:989–97.

11. **Sweet RL.** Gynecologic conditions and bacterial vaginosis: implications for the non-pregnant patient. *Infect Dis Obstet Gynecol* 2000;8:184–90.

12. **Stamm WE.** *Chlamydia trachomatis* infections of the adult. In Holmes KK, Sparling PD, Mardh P-A, et al. (eds). *Sexually Transmitted Diseases*, 3rd ed. New York: McGraw-Hill; 1999:407–22.

13. **Hook EW, Handsfield HH.** Gonococcal infections in the adult. In Holmes KK, Sparling PD, Mardh P-A, et al. (eds). *Sexually Transmitted Diseases*, 3rd ed. New York: McGraw-Hill; 1999:451–63.

14. **Padian NS, Washington AE.** Risk factors for pelvic inflammatory disease and associated sequelae. In Landers DV, Sweet RL (eds). *Pelvic Inflammatory Disease*. New York: Springer; 1997:21–9.

15. **Molander P, Cacciatore B, Sjoberg J, et al.** Laparoscopic management of suspected acute pelvic inflammatory disease. *J Am Assoc Gynecol Laparosc.* 2000;7:107–10.

16. **Centers for Disease Control and Prevention.** 1998 Guidelines for treatment of sexually transmitted diseases. *MMWR Morbid Mortal Wkly Rep.* 1998;47(RR-1):60–86.

17. **Sweet RL.** Treatment of acute pelvic inflammatory disease. In Landers DV, Sweet RL (eds). *Pelvic Inflammatory Disease*. New York: Springer; 1997:76–93.

18. **Walker CK, Kahn JG, Washington AE, et al.** Pelvic inflammatory disease: meta-analysis of antimicrobial regimen efficacy. *J Infect Dis.* 1993;168:969–78.

19. **Potts DM, Champion CB, Kozuh-Novak M, et al.** IUDs and PID: a comparative trial of strings versus stringless devices. *Adv Contracept.* 1991;7:231–40.

20. **Farley TMM, Rosenberg MJ, Rowe PJ, et al.** Intrauterine devices and pelvic inflammatory disease: an international perspective. *Lancet.* 1992;339:785–8.

21. **Lee NC, Rubin GL, Borucki R.** The intrauterine device and pelvic inflammatory disease revisited: new results from the Women's Health Study. *Obstet Gynecol.* 1998;72:1–6.

22. **Walsh TL, Bernstein GS, Grimes DA, et al.** Effect of prophylactic antibiotics on morbidity associated with IUD insertion: results of a private randomized controlled trial. *Contraception.* 1990;42:141–58.

23. **Landers DV.** Tubo-ovarian abcess complicating pelvic inflammatory disease. In Landers DV, Sweet RL (eds). *Pelvic Inflammatory Disease*. New York: Springer; 1997:94–106.

24. **Sweet RL, Gibbs RS.** Pelvic abscess. In Sweet RL, Gibbs RS (eds). *Infectious Diseases of the Female Genital Tract*. Baltimore: Williams & Wilkins; 1985:161–80.

25. **American College of Obstetricians and Gynecologists.** *Antibiotics and Gynecologic Infections* (ACOG Educational Bulletin 237). Washington DC: American College of Obstetricians and Gynecologists; 1997.

26. **Droegemueller W.** Upper genital tract infections. In Droegemueller W, Herbst AL, Mishell DR, Stenchever MA (eds). *Comprehensive Gynecology*. St. Louis: CV Mosby; 1987:635.

27. **Westrom L, Joesoef R, Reynolds G, et al.** Pelvic inflammatory disease and fertility: a cohort study of 1844 women with laparoscopically verified disease and 657 control women with normal laparoscopic results. *Sex Transm Dis* 1992;19:185–92.

28. **Hillis SD, Joesoef R, Marchbanks PA, et al.** Delayed care of pelvic inflammatory disease as a risk factor for impaired fertility. *Am J Obstet Gynecol* 1993;168:1503–9.

16

Vaginitis and Cervicitis

J.D. Sobel, MD

Vaginitis

Vaginal symptoms are extremely common, and vaginal discharge is among the 25 most common reasons for consulting a physician in private office practice in the United States (1). Vaginitis is not found in all women with vaginal symptoms but is found in some form in approximately 40% of such women (Table 16.1). It is found in more than one fourth of women attending sexually transmitted disease (STD) clinics.

Bacterial Vaginosis

Epidemiology

Bacterial vaginosis is the most common cause of vaginitis in women of child-bearing age and has been diagnosed in 17% to 19% of women who seek gynecologic care in family practice or in student health care settings (2). It also has been observed in 16% to 29% of pregnant women, and its prevalence increases considerably among symptomatic women in STD clinics, reaching a range of 24% to 37%. Although *Gardnerella vaginalis* has been found in 10% to 31% of virgin adolescent girls, it is still found significantly more often among sexually active women, reaching a prevalence of 50% to 60% in some populations at risk for infection.

Evaluation of epidemiologic factors has revealed few clues to the cause of bacterial vaginosis. The use of intrauterine devices, intravaginal pessaries,

Table 16.1 Causes of Vaginitis in Adult Women

Infectious Vaginitis

Common
Bacterial vaginosis (40%–50%)
Vulvovaginal candidiasis (20%–25%)
Trichomonal vaginitis (15%–20%)

Less Common
Atrophic vaginitis with second-degree bacterial infection
Foreign body with second-degree infection
Desquamative inflammatory vaginitis (clindamycin responsive)
Streptococcal vaginitis (group A)
Ulcerative vaginitis associated with *Staphylococcus aureus* and toxic shock syndrome
Idiopathic vulvovaginal ulceration associated with HIV

Noninfectious Vaginitis
Chemicals and/or irritants
Allergy, hypersensitivity, and contact dermatitis (lichen simplex)
Trauma
Atrophic vaginitis
Postpuerperal atrophic vaginitis
Desquamative inflammatory vaginitis (steroid responsive)
Erosive lichen planus
Collagen vascular disease, Behçets disease, and pemphigus syndromes
Idiopathic

---

and douches was found to be more common in women with bacterial vaginosis. Bacterial vaginosis is significantly more common in blacks and lesbians.

Pathogenesis

Bacterial vaginosis is the result of massive overgrowth of mixed flora, including peptostreptococci, *Bacteroides*, *G. vaginalis*, *Mobiluncus*, and genital mycoplasmas (3). There is little inflammation, and the disorder represents a disturbance of the vaginal microbial ecosystem rather than a true infection of tissues. The overgrowth of mixed flora is associated with a loss of the normal *Lactobacillus*-dominated vaginal flora. No single bacterial species is responsible for bacterial vaginosis. Experimental studies of human volunteers and animals indicate that inoculation of the vagina with individual species of bacteria associated with bacterial vaginosis (e.g., *G. vaginalis*) rarely results in the disease. Two factors support the role of mixed flora in the transmission of bacterial vaginosis: 1) the higher prevalence of bacterial vaginosis among sexually active young women than among sexually inexperienced women, and 2) the observation that bacterial vaginosis-associated microorganisms are isolated more often from the urethras of male partners of women with bacterial vaginosis (2).

The cause of the overgrowth of anaerobes, *Gardnerella*, mycoplasmas, and *Mobiluncus* that results in bacterial vaginosis is unknown. Theories include increased substrate availability, increased pH, and loss of the restraining effects of the predominant *Lactobacillus* flora of the vagina. Eschenbach and coworkers (4) reported that normal women are colonized by H_2O_2-producing strains of lactobacilli, whereas women with bacterial vaginosis have reduced numbers of lactobacilli and the species that are present lack the ability to produce H_2O_2 (4). The H_2O_2 produced by lactobacilli may inhibit the pathogens associated with bacterial vaginosis, either directly through the toxicity of H_2O_2 or as a result of the production of H_2O_2-halide complexes in the presence of natural cervical peroxidase.

Accompanying the bacterial overgrowth in bacterial vaginosis is the increased production of amines by anaerobes, which is facilitated by microbial decarboxylases. Amines in the presence of an increased vaginal pH volatilize to produce the typical fishy odor of bacterial vaginosis, which is also produced when 10% potassium hydroxide (KOH) is added to vaginal secretions in the disease. Trimethylamine is the dominant abnormal amine in bacterial vaginosis. It is likely that bacterial polyamines together with the organic acids found in the vagina in bacterial vaginosis (acetic and succinic acid) are cytotoxic, resulting in exfoliation of vaginal epithelial cells and creating the vaginal discharge that occurs in the disease. *G. vaginalis* attaches avidly to exfoliated epithelial cells, especially at the alkaline pH found in bacterial vaginosis. The adherence of *Gardnerella* organisms results in formation of the clue cells that are pathognomonic for bacterial vaginosis (Fig. 16.1).

Clinical Features

As many as 50% of women with bacterial vaginosis may be asymptomatic (2). An abnormal malodorous vaginal discharge (mentioned earlier and often described as fishy) is usually detected, often appearing after unprotected coitus, and is infrequently profuse. Examination reveals a nonviscous, grayish-white, adherent discharge. Pruritus, dysuria, and dyspareunia are rare.

Bacterial vaginosis has largely been considered to be only a nuisance; however, considerable evidence now exists of serious obstetric and gynecologic complications of bacterial vaginosis, including asymptomatic bacterial vaginosis diagnosed by Gram stain. Obstetric complications include chorioamnionitis, preterm labor, prematurity, and postpartum fever (5). Gynecologic sequelae include post-abortion fever, post-hysterectomy fever, cuff infection, and chronic mast cell endometritis. Although untreated bacterial vaginosis has been reported to be associated with cervical inflammation and low-grade dysplasia, confirmatory studies of this are needed (6).

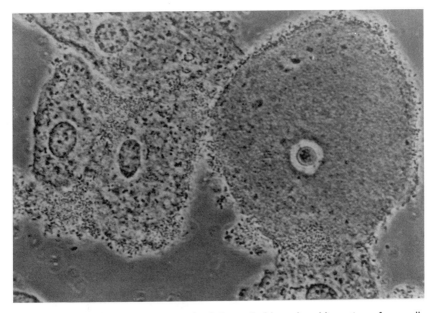

Figure 16.1   High-power micrograph of clue cells. Note the obliteration of normally sharp cell margins by adherent coccobacilliary organisms that obscure the cell membrane.

Diagnosis

Signs and symptoms are unreliable indicators in the diagnosis of bacterial vaginosis (Table 16.2). The clinical diagnosis can be made reliably in the presence of at least three of the following objective criteria: 1) an adherent, white, nonfloccular, homogenous discharge; 2) a positive amine test, with release of fishy odor on addition of 10% KOH to vaginal secretions; 3) a vaginal pH >4.5; and 4) the presence of clue cells on light microscopy, which is the most reliable predictor. These clinical signs are simple and reliable, and tests for them are easy to perform. Clue cells are exfoliated vaginal squamous epithelial cells covered with *G. vaginalis*, giving the cells a granular or stippled appearance with a characteristic loss of clearly defined cell borders. At least 20% of observed epithelial cells should be clue cells for this finding to be of diagnostic significance. Occasionally, epithelial cells covered exclusively with the curved gram-negative rods of *Mobiluncus* can be demonstrated. The offensive fishy odor of the disease may be apparent during the physical examination or may become apparent only during the amine test. A Gram stain of vaginal secretions is extremely valuable in making the diagnosis, with a sensitivity of 93% and specificity of 70% (2).

Table 16.2   Diagnostic Features of Infectious Vaginitis

	Normal	*Candida* Vaginitis	Bacterial Vaginosis	Trichomonas Vaginitis
Symptoms	None or physiologic leukorrhea	Vulvar pruritus, soreness, increased discharge, dysuria, dyspareunia	Moderate malodorous discharge	Profuse purulent discharge, offensive odor, pruritus, dyspareunia
Discharge				
Amount	Variable, scant to moderate	Scant to moderate	Moderate	Profuse
Color	Clear or white	White	White and/or gray	Yellow
Consistency	Floccular non-homogeneous	Clumped but variable	Homogeneous, uniformly coating walls	Homogeneous
"Bubbles"	Absent	Absent	Present	Present
Appearance of vulva and vagina	Normal	Introital and vulvar erythema, edema and occasional pustules, vaginal erythma	No inflammation	Erythema and swelling of vulvar and vaginal epithelium (strawberry cervix)
pH of vaginal fluid	<4.5	<4.5	>4.7	5.0–6.0
Amine test (10% KOH)	Negative	Negative	Positive	Occasionally present
Saline microscopy	Normal epithelial cell; lactobacilli predominate	Normal flora, blastospores (yeast); 40%–50% pseudohyphae	Clue cells and coccobacillary flora predominate; absence of leukocytes and motile curved rods	PMNLs; motile trichomonads (80%-90%); no clue cells; abnormal flora
10% KOH microscopy	Negative	Positive (60%–90%)	Negative (except in mixed infections)	Negative

KOH = potassium hydroxide; PMNLs = polymorphonuclear leukocytes.

Although cultures for *G. vaginalis* are positive in almost all cases of bacterial vaginosis, the organism also may be detected in 50% to 60% of women who do not meet the diagnostic criteria for the disease (2). Accordingly, vaginal culture has no part in the diagnosis of bacterial vaginosis.

Management

Poor efficacy has been observed in the treatment of bacterial vaginosis with triple sulfa creams, erythromycin, tetracycline, acetic acid gel, and providone–iodine vaginal douches (7).

Only moderate cure rates of bacterial vaginosis have been obtained with ampicillin (mean 66%) and amoxicillin (2). The most successful oral therapy remains metronidazole. Most studies that used multiple divided-dose regimens of metronidazole at 800 to 1200 mg/d for 1 week achieved clinical cure rates in excess of 90% immediately and of approximately 80% at 4 weeks (7). Although single-dose therapy with 2 g of metronidazole achieves similar immediate clinical response rates, higher recurrence rates have been reported with this regimen. The beneficial effect of metronidazole results predominantly from its antianaerobic activity and because *G. vaginalis* is susceptible to the hydroxymetabolites of metronidazole. Although *Mycoplasma hominis* is resistant to metronidazole, the organisms usually are not detected at follow-up visits of successfully treated patients. Similarly, *Mobiluncus curtisii* is resistant to metronidazole but usually disappears after therapy.

Topical therapy with 2% clindamycin (once daily for 7 days) or metronidazole gel 0.75% (once daily for 5 days) has been shown to be as effective as oral metronidazole in eliminating bacterial vaginosis without the side effects of the oral drug.

In the past, asymptomatic bacterial vaginosis was not treated, especially because patients often improve spontaneously over several months. However, the growing evidence linking asymptomatic bacterial vaginosis with numerous obstetric and gynecologic complications that involve the upper reproductive tract has prompted a reassessment of this policy, especially with the availability of convenient topical therapies (5,8). Asymptomatic bacterial vaginosis should be treated before pregnancy, in women with cervical abnormalities, and before elective gynecologic surgery. Routine screening and treatment for asymptomatic bacterial vaginosis in pregnancy remains controversial pending the outcome of studies that prove that treating the disease reduces preterm delivery and prematurity (9). Some controlled studies have shown that treatment of bacterial vaginosis with topical clindamycin and oral metronidazole may reduce preterm labor and prematurity, but only in women with a past history of preterm labor. At present, this category of women seems most suited for screening (9).

Despite indirect evidence of its sexual transmission, no study has documented reduced recurrence rates of bacterial vaginosis in women whose partners have been treated with a variety of regimens, including metronidazole. Accordingly, most clinicians do not routinely treat the male partners of affected women.

After treatment with oral metronidazole, symptoms of bacterial vaginosis recur within 3 months in approximately 30% of patients who initially respond (2). The reasons for such recurrence are unclear and include the possibility of reinfection but more likely reflect vaginal relapse, with failure to eradicate the offending organisms and concurrent failure of the normally protective *Lactobacillus*-dominant vaginal flora to reestablish itself. Management of symptoms of acute bacterial vaginosis during relapse includes treatment with oral or vaginal metronidazole or topical clindamycin, usually prescribed for a longer (10- to 14-day) period than the initial treatment regimen. Maintenance regimens of antibiotic therapy have been largely disappointing, and new approaches to treating bacterial vaginosis include recolonization with exogenous *Lactobacillus* using selected bacteria-containing suppositories.

Prevention

Because the pathogenesis of bacterial vaginosis is obscure, measures for its prevention have not been forthcoming. Although the disease is not typically sexually transmitted, barrier contraception may reduce its occurrence. Avoidance of douching is recommended.

Trichomoniasis

Epidemiology

Studies estimate that 2 to 3 million American women contract trichomoniasis annually, with a worldwide distribution of approximately 180 million cases of the disease each year (2). The prevalence of trichomoniasis correlates with the overall level of sexual activity of the specific group of women being studied, with the disease diagnosed in approximately 5% of women in family-planning clinics, 13% to 25% of women who attend gynecology clinics, 50% to 75% of prostitutes, and 7% to 35% of women in STD clinics. Recent surveys indicate a decline in the incidence of trichomoniasis in many industrialized countries.

Pathophysiology

Sexual transmission is the dominant method of introduction of *Trichomonas vaginalis* into the vagina (2). The organism was found in 70% of urethral cultures of men who had had sexual contact with infected women within the previous 48 hours (11). Women with trichomoniasis also show a high prevalence of gonorrhea, with both diseases significantly associated with the use of non-barrier methods of contraception.

Recurrent trichomoniasis is common and indicative of a lack of significant protective immunity. Nevertheless, an immune response to *T. vaginalis* does develop, as indicated by low titers of serum antibody, but is insufficient for diagnostic serology. Antitrichomonal IgA has been detected in vaginal secretions, but a protective role for it has not been defined. Delayed hypersensitivity in natural infection with *T. vaginalis* also can be demonstrated. The predominant host-defense response is provided by the numerous polymorphonuclear leukocytes (PMNLs) that respond to chemotactic substances released by trichomonads and are capable of killing *T. vaginalis* without ingesting it. *T. vaginalis* destroys epithelial cells by direct cell contact and cytotoxicity. The periurethral and Skene's glands are infected in most patients, and *T. vaginalis* organisms can be seen in the urine specimens of some infected individuals.

Clinical Features

The severity of *Trichomonas* infection in women ranges from an asymptomatic carrier state to severe acute inflammatory disease (10,11).

A vaginal discharge, usually foul smelling, is reported by 50% to 75% of women with diagnosed trichomoniasis; however, the discharge is not always malodorous. Pruritus occurs in 25% to 50% of patients and is often severe. Other infrequent symptoms include dyspareunia, dysuria, and rarely frequency of micturition. Lower abdominal pain occurs in fewer than 10% of patients and should alert the physician to the possibility of concomitant salinities caused by other organisms. Symptoms of acute trichomoniasis often appear during or immediately after menstruation. Although its duration is controversial, the incubation period has been estimated to range from 3 to 28 days (10,11).

Physical findings in trichomoniasis represent a spectrum that varies with the severity of disease. Vulvar findings may be absent but are typically characterized in severe cases by diffuse vulvar erythema (10%–33%), edema, and a profuse purulent vaginal discharge (11). The discharge is often described as being yellow-green and frothy but is often grayish white. A frothy discharge is seen in a minority of patients with trichomoniasis and is more commonly seen in bacterial vaginosis.

The vaginal walls in trichomoniasis are erythematous and, in severe cases, may have a granular appearance. Punctate hemorrhages (colpitis macularis) of the cervix may give its surface a strawberry-like appearance that, although apparent to the naked eye in only 1% to 2% of patients, is found in 45% patients on colposcopy (11).

The clinical course of trichomoniasis in pregnancy is identical to that in the nonpregnant state; when untreated, the disease is associated with premature rupture of membranes and prematurity. Trichomoniasis is reported to facilitate transmission of HIV.

Diagnosis

None of the clinical features of *Trichomonas* vaginitis is sufficiently specific to allow a diagnosis of trichomonal infection based on signs and symptoms alone (*see* Table 16.2) (10). A definitive diagnosis requires demonstration of the organism. The vaginal pH is markedly increased, almost always above 5.0, and sometimes as much as 6.0. On saline microscopy, an increase in PMNLs is almost invariably present. The ovoid trichomonal parasites are slightly larger than PMNLs and are best recognized by their motility. A wet mount is positive in only 40% to 80% of cases. The Gram stain is of little value because of its inability to differentiate PMNLs from nonmotile trichomonads, and the use of Giemsa, Acridine Orange, and other stains has no advantage over saline preparation. Although trichomonads are often seen on Pap smears, this method has a sensitivity of only 60% to 70% when compared with saline preparation microscopy, and false-positive results have been reported.

Several equivalent culture methods for *T. vaginalis* are available, and growth is usually detected within 48 hours. Culture is now recognized as the most sensitive method for detecting the presence of trichomonads (95% sensitivity) and should be considered in patients with vaginitis in whom one finds an increased pH, PMNL excess, absence of motile trichomonads, and absence of clue cells. Several new rapid-diagnosis kits that use DNA probes or the polymerase chain reaction test are under investigation, as are kits designed for patient self-diagnosis.

Management

Treatment for trichomoniasis remains based on the 5-nitroimidazole group of drugs (metronidazole, tinidazole, and ornidazole), all of which have similar efficacy (7). Oral therapy is preferred to topical vaginal therapy because of the frequency of infection of the urethra and periurethral glands, which provide sources for the endogenous recurrence of infection.

Treatment consists of oral metronidazole 500 mg twice daily for 7 days, which produces a cure rate of 95%. Similar results have been obtained with a single dose of oral metronidazole 2 g, which produced cure rates of 82% to 88%. The latter cure rate increases to >90% when sexual partners are treated simultaneously (7). The advantages of single-dose therapy include better patient compliance, a lower total dose, a shorter period of alcohol avoidance, and possibly decreased subsequent *Candida* vaginitis.

The 5-nitroimidazoles are not in themselves trichomonacidal, but low-redox proteins reduce the nitro group of these drugs, resulting in the formation of highly cytotoxic products within the infecting organisms. Aerobic conditions interfere with this reduction process and decrease the antianaerobic activity of the 5-nitroimidazoles. Most strains of *T. vaginalis* are highly susceptible to metronidazole, which has a minimal inhibitory concentration of 1 μg/mL against this organism.

Patients who do not respond to an initial 7-day course of treatment often respond to an additional standard 7-day course of therapy. Some patients are refractory to repeated courses of therapy even when compliance is assured and sexual partners are known to have been treated. If reinfection is excluded, these rare patients may have strains of *T. vaginalis* that are resistant to metronidazole, which can be confirmed *in vitro*. Increased doses of metronidazole and a longer duration of therapy are necessary to cure these refractory cases of the disease; patients should be given maximum tolerated doses of oral metronidazole of 2–4 g/day for 10 to 14 days. Rarely, intravenous metronidazole in doses as high as 2–4 g/d may be necessary, with careful monitoring for drug toxicity. Considerable success has been observed in the treatment of resistant trichomonal infections with oral tinidazole; however, this drug is not readily available, and the optimal dose to be used is unknown. Most investigators use high-dose tinidazole at 1–4 g/d for 14 days. Rare patients who do not respond to nitroimidazoles can be treated with topical paromomycin.

Side effects of metronidazole include an unpleasant or metallic taste, nausea (10%), transient neutropenia (7.5%), and a disulfiram-like effect when alcohol is ingested (7). Caution should be taken when 5-nitroimidazoles are used in patients taking warfarin. Long-term and high-dose therapy increases the risk of neutropenia and peripheral neuropathy. In experimental studies, metronidazole has been shown to be mutagenic for certain bacteria, indicating a carcinogenic potential; however, cohort studies have not established an increase in cancer morbidity with this drug. Thus, the risk of short-term, low-dose metronidazole treatment is extremely small. Superinfection with *Candida* is by no means uncommon.

Treatment of trichomoniasis in pregnancy gives unsatisfactory results (7). Metronidazole readily crosses the placenta, and because of concern for teratogenicity some consider it prudent to avoid the use of this drug in the first trimester of pregnancy. However, because considerable human and animal data support the safety of metronidazole in pregnancy, investigators have become more comfortable using it throughout pregnancy. Topical clotrimazole and povidone–iodine jelly offer minimal benefit in trichomoniasis.

Prevention

Sexual transmission of trichomonads is prevented efficiently by the use of barrier contraception. Spermicidal agents such as nonoxynol-9 also reduce transmission. However, reinfection of women is common and, therefore, mandates treatment with metronidazole of all sexual partners of the patient, preferably simultaneously.

Vulvovaginal Candidiasis

Epidemiology

Data from the United Kingdom reveal a sharp increase in the incidence in vulvovaginal candidiasis in that country. In the United States, *Candida* is now the second most common cause of vaginal infection (1,12). It is estimated that 75% of women experience at least one episode of vulvovaginal candidiasis during their childbearing years, and approximately 40% to 50% experience a second attack. A small subpopulation of women, of undetermined magnitude but probably constituting less than 5% of adult women, suffers from repeated, recurrent, often intractable episodes of *Candida* vaginitis (12).

Point-prevalence studies indicate that *Candida* is isolated from the genital tract of approximately 20% of asymptomatic, healthy women of childbearing age (12). The natural history of asymptomatic colonization is unknown; however, animal and human studies suggest that vaginal carriage continues for several months and perhaps for years. Several factors are associated with increased rates of asymptomatic vaginal colonization with *Candida*, including pregnancy (30%–40%), use of oral contraceptives, uncontrolled diabetes mellitus, and frequent visits to sexually transmitted disease (STD) clinics (Table 16.3). The rarity of isolating *Candida* from premenarchal girls, the lower prevalence of postmenopausal *Candida* vaginitis, and the possible association of vulvovaginal candidiasis with hormone-replacement therapy emphasize the hormonal dependence of this condition.

Table 16.3   Host Factors Associated with Increased Asymptomatic Vaginal Colonization with *Candida* and *Candida* Vaginitis

Genetic
Blood-group antigen and/or secretor status

Acquired
Biological
  Pregnancy
  Uncontrolled diabetes mellitus
  Corticosteroid and/or immunosuppressive therapy
  Antimicrobial therapy (systemic, topical)
  HIV infection
Behavioral (Sexual)
  Oral contraceptives
  Intrauterine device or contraceptive sponge
  Nonoxynol-9 spermicide
  Receptive oral sex
  Coital frequency (?)

Pathogenesis

Infecting Organisms

Between 85% and 90% of yeasts isolated from the vagina are strains of *Candida albicans*. The remainder belong to other species, the most common of which are *C. glabrata* and *C. tropicalis*. Non-*albicans Candida* species are capable of inducing vaginitis and are often more resistant to conventional therapy than is *C. albicans*. Some surveys indicate an increase in vulvovaginal candidiasis caused by non-*albicans Candida* species, particularly *C. glabrata* (12,13).

Germination of *Candida* enhances colonization and facilitates tissue invasion by the organism. Factors that enhance or facilitate germination (e.g., estrogen therapy, pregnancy) tend to precipitate symptomatic vaginitis, whereas measures that inhibit germination (e.g., bacterial flora, local mucosal cell-mediated immunity) may prevent acute vaginitis in women who are asymptomatic carriers of yeasts.

Candida organisms gain access to the vaginal lumen and secretions predominantly from the adjacent perianal area. This finding is borne out by epidemiologic typing studies. *Candida* vaginitis is seen predominantly in women of childbearing age, and only in the minority of cases can a precipitating factor be identified to explain the transformation from asymptomatic carriage of *Candida* organisms to symptomatic vaginitis in individual patients.

Host Factors

Host factors associated with increased asymptomatic vaginal *Candida* colonization and *Candida* vaginitis are shown in Table 16.3. During pregnancy, the vagina is more susceptible to vaginal infection, resulting in higher incidences of vaginal colonization and vaginitis and lower cure rates of infection. The clinical attack rate is the highest in the third trimester, but symptomatic recurrences are also common throughout pregnancy. The high levels of reproductive hormones during pregnancy result in a higher glycogen content in the vaginal environment and provide an excellent carbon source for the growth and germination of *Candida*. A more likely mechanism for susceptibility to infection is that estrogens enhance vaginal epithelial cell avidity for the adherence of *Candida*. Furthermore, a yeast cytosol receptor or binding system for female reproductive hormones has been documented. These hormones also enhance yeast mycelial formation. Several studies have shown increased vulvovaginal candidiasis associated with oral contraceptive use (14) and uncontrolled diabetes mellitus. Glucose tolerance tests have been recommended for women with recurrent vulvovaginal candidiasis, but their yield is low and such testing is not justified in otherwise healthy premenopausal women.

Symptomatic vulvovaginal candidiasis is often observed during or after courses of systemic antibiotic therapy. Antibiotics are responsible for approximately 20% of sporadic *Candida* vaginitis episodes (15). Although all antimicrobial agents can causing this complication, broad-spectrum antibiotics such as tetracycline and the beta-lactams are chiefly responsible for it and are thought to act by eliminating the normal protective vaginal bacterial flora. The dose and duration of antibiotic therapy further influence the risk of developing *Candida* vaginitis. The natural flora of the vagina provides a colonization-resistance mechanism and prevents *Candida* from germinating. *Lactobacillus* species have been singled out as providing this protective function (16). The interaction between *Lactobacillus* and *Candida* includes competition for nutrients, steric interference with *Candida* adherence, and elaboration of bacteriocins that inhibit yeast proliferation and germination.

Other factors that contribute to an increased incidence of *Candida* vaginitis include the use of tight, poorly ventilated clothing and nylon underclothing, which increases perineal moisture and temperature. Chemical contact, local allergy, and hypersensitivity reactions also may predispose to symptomatic *Candida* vaginitis by altering the local superficial vulvovaginal environment and facilitating tissue invasion by *Candida* organisms.

Candida may cause cell damage and resulting inflammation by direct hyphal invasion of epithelial tissue. It is possible that proteases and other hydrolytic enzymes of the organism facilitate its cell penetration with resultant inflammation, mucosal swelling, erythema, and exfoliation of vaginal epithelial cells. The characteristic nonhomogenous vaginal discharge of vaginal candidiasis consists of a conglomerate of hyphal elements and exfoliated nonviable epithelial cells, with few PMNLs. *Candida* also may induce symptoms by hypersensitivity or allergic reaction, particularly in women with idiopathic recurrent vulvovaginal candidiasis (*see* discussion of allergic vaginitis in the following section) (16).

Pathogenesis of Recurrent and Chronic Candida Vaginitis

Careful evaluation of women with recurrent vaginitis usually fails to reveal any precipitating or causal mechanism for such disease (17). In the past, investigators attributed recurring episodes of *Candida* vaginitis to repeated fungal reinoculation of the vagina from a persistent intestinal source, or to sexual transmission of the infecting organism.

The *intestinal reservoir theory* for the recurrence of *Candida* vaginitis is based on the report of *Candida* having been recovered from rectal cultures in almost 100% of women with vulvovaginal candidiasis. Furthermore, typing of simultaneously obtained vaginal and rectal isolates almost invariably reveals identical strains of the organism. This theory has been criticized in the past few years because of a lower concordance between rectal and vaginal culture results in patients with recurrent vulvovaginal candidiasis. Moreover, long-term therapy with oral nonabsorbable nystatin is ineffective in preventing recurrences.

Although sexual transmissions of *Candida* organisms occurs via vaginal intercourse and orogenital contact, the role of sexual reintroduction of yeast as a cause for recurrent vulvovaginal candidiasis is doubtful. Recurrent vulvovaginal candidiasis frequently occurs in celibate women, whereas only the minority of male partners of women with recurrent vulvovaginal candidiasis have been colonized with *Candida*. Although most studies aimed at treating male partners of infected women have not reduced the frequency of recurrent episodes of vaginitis, Spinillo and coworkers (18) achieved reduction in recurrent vulvovaginal candidiasis by treating the colonized male partners of such patients.

Vaginal relapse implies incomplete eradication or clearance of *Candida* from the vagina with antimycotic therapy. According to this concept, *Candida* organisms persist in small numbers in the vagina, causing their continued carriage. When host environmental conditions permit, the colonizing organisms increase in number and undergo mycelial transformation, resulting in a new clinical episode of infection.

Whether recurrence is caused by vaginal reinfection or relapse, women with recurrent vulvovaginal candidiasis differ from those with infrequent episodes of such infection in their inability to tolerate small numbers of *Candida* reintroduced into or persisting in the vagina. On the basis of typing of organisms, women with recurrent and infrequent infection are found to have the same distribution frequency of *Candida* strains as are women without symptoms.

Host factors responsible for frequent episodes of vulvovaginal candidiasis are not delineated clearly, and more than one mechanism may be at work. Patients who experience frequent reinfection show no evidence of complement, phagocytic cells, or immunoglobulin deficiency. Recurrent vulvovaginal candidiasis is rarely caused by antimicrobial drug resistance (19). Current theories about the pathogenesis of recurrent vulvovaginal candidiasis include qualitative and quantitative deficiency of the normal protective vaginal bacterial flora and an acquired, often-transient, antigen-specific deficiency in T-lymphocyte function that similarly permits unchecked yeast proliferation (17,20). Another theory is that of an acquired acute hypersensitivity reaction to *Candida* antigen that is accompanied by increased vaginal titers of *Candida* antigen–specific IgE. This theory has a clinical basis in that patients with recurrent vulvovaginal candidiasis often present with severe vulvar manifestations of the disease (rash, erythema, swelling, and pruritus) with minimal exudative vaginal changes, little discharge, and lower organism titers. Allergic responses to *Candida* have been reported to involve the male genitalia immediately after coitus with *Candida*-infected female genitalia and are characterized by the acute onset of erythema, edema, severe pruritus, and irritation of the penis (17). As yet, only a minority of women with recurrent vulvovaginal candidiasis have been shown to have increased *Candida*-specific vaginal IgE. Limited studies have found that the use of *Candida*-antigen desensitization helps reduce the frequency of recurrent episodes of vaginitis.

Women who are seropositive for HIV have higher vaginal colonization rates with *Candida* than do seronegative women, but the attack rate of symptomatic vulvovaginal candidiasis in the two groups seems similar. Reports of severe recurrent vulvovaginal candidiasis are largely unsubstantiated. Recurrent vulvovaginal candidiasis in the absence of other risk factors for HIV infection is not an indication for giving an HIV test (12).

Clinical Features

The most frequent symptom of vulvovaginal candidiasis is vulvar pruritus, because vaginal discharge is not invariably present and is often minimal (12). Although typically described as having a cottage cheese–like character, the discharge may vary from watery to homogenously thick. Vaginal soreness, irritation, vulvar burning, dyspareunia, and external dysuria are commonly present. Odor, if present, is minimal and nonoffensive. Examination frequently reveals erythema and swelling of the labia and vulva, often with discrete pustulopapular peripheral lesions (Fig. 16.2). The cervix is normal, and vaginal mucosal erythema with an adherent whitish discharge is present. Characteristically, symptoms are worst during the week before the onset of menses and are somewhat relieved with the onset of menstrual flow.

Diagnosis

The relative lack of specificity of symptoms and signs of vulvovaginal candidiasis precludes a diagnosis that is based only on history and physical examination. Most patients with symptomatic vulvovaginal candidiasis may be diagnosed readily on the basis of a simple microscopic examination of vaginal secretions (Fig. 16.3). A wet mount or saline preparation has a sensitivity of 40% to 60%. The 10% KOH preparation is even more sensitive in diagnosing the presence of germinated yeast. A normal vaginal pH (4.0–4.5) is found in *Candida* vaginitis; a pH finding higher than 4.5 suggests the possibility of bacterial vaginosis, trichomoniasis, or a mixed infection (12).

Although routine fungal cultures are unnecessary in patients who test negative for *Candida* by microscopy, cultures should be obtained in patients who have the highest predicted positive culture yield (i.e., those with a past history of confirmed *Candida* vaginitis and/or multiple signs and symptoms of vulvovaginitis) and when it is important to confirm the diagnosis and avoid empirical therapy. The Pap smear is unreliable, being positive in only approximately

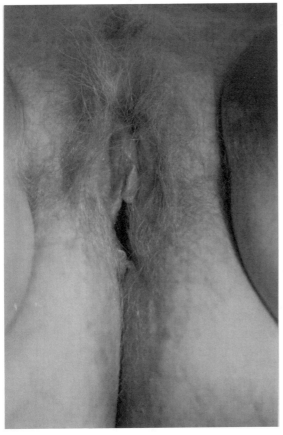

Figure 16.2 *Candida* vulvo-vaginitis. Note erythema and edema of labia and vestibule, with inflammatory reaction extending into perianal and intergluteal area.

25% of cases of vulvovaginal candidiasis. There is no reliable serologic technique for the diagnosis of symptomatic *Candida* vaginitis.

Management

Topical Agents for Acute Candida Vaginitis

Antimycotic agents are available for local use as creams, vaginal tablets, suppositories, and coated tampons (Table 16.4). There is little evidence to suggest that the formulation of a topical antimycotic influences its clinical efficacy in vulvovaginal candidiasis (21). Extensive vulvar inflammation dictates local vulvar application of a topical cream preparation.

The average mycologic cure rate of 7- and 14-day courses of nystatin in vulvovaginal candidiasis is approximately 75% to 80%. Azoles seem to

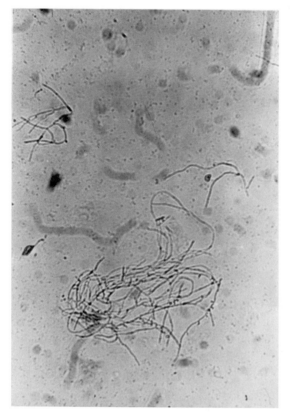

Figure 16.3 Low-power 10% potassium hydroxide preparation that reveals a clump of *C. albicans* organisms forming hyphae.

achieve slightly higher clinical mycologic cure rates (~85% to 90%) than do polyenes (nystatin). Although many studies have compared the clinical efficacy of the various azoles, there is little evidence that any one azole agent is superior to the others (21).

Topical azoles are remarkably free of local and systemic side effects; nevertheless, the initial application of topical agents is not infrequently accompanied by local burning and discomfort.

There has been a major trend toward shorter courses of treatment of vulvovaginal candidiasis with progressively higher doses of antifungal agents, culminating in highly effective single-dose topical regimens. However, although short-course regimens are effective for mild and moderate vaginitis, cure rates for severe and complicated vaginitis are lower.

Oral systemic azoles available for the treatment of vulvovaginal candidiasis include ketoconazole (400 mg bid for 5 days), itraconazole (200 mg/d for 3 days or bid for 1 day), and fluconazole (150-mg single dose) (22). All of these

Table 16.4   Therapy for Vaginal Candidiasis: Topical Agents

Drug	Formulation	Dosage Regimen
Butoconazole	2% cream	5 g for days
Clotrimazole	1% cream	5 g for 7–14 days
	100-mg vaginal tablet	1 tablet for 7 days
	100-mg vaginal tablet	2 tablets for 3 days
	500-mg vaginal tablet	1 tablet, single dose
Miconazole	2% cream	5 g for 7 days
	100-mg vaginal suppository	1 suppository for 7 days
	200-mg vaginal suppository	1 suppository for 3 days
	1200-mg vaginal suppository	1 suppository, single dose
Econazole	150-mg vaginal tablet	1 tablet for 3 days
Fenticonazole	2% cream	5 g for 7 days
Tioconazole	2% cream	5 g for 3 days
	6.5% cream	5 g, single dose
Terconazole	0.4% cream	5 g for 7 days
	0.8% cream	5 g for 3 days
	80-mg vaginal suppository	80 mg for 3 days
Nystatin	100,000-U vaginal tablet	1 tablet for 14 days

Table 16.5   Classification of Vulvovaginal Candidiasis

Complicated	Uncomplicated
Non-*albicans* Candida	*Candida albicans*
Resistant *C. albicans* (rare)	Infrequent episodes
History of recurrent VVC	Vaginitis mild to moderate
Severe VVC	Normal host
Abnormal host (e.g. uncontrolled diabetes, pregnant patient, immunocompromised patient)	

VVC = vulvovaginal candidiasis.

oral regimens achieve clinical cure rates in excess of 80%; however, only flu-conazole is approved for use in the United States. Women generally prefer oral treatment regimens for vulvovaginal candidiasis because of their convenience and lack of local side effects. None of the systemic regimens should be prescribed during pregnancy, and these regimens carry the potential for systemic side effects and toxicity. In particular, hepatotoxicity with ketoconazole precludes its widespread use in vulvovaginal candidiasis (21).

Vulvovaginal candidiasis is classified as either uncomplicated or complicated based on its likelihood of being cured clinically and mycologically with short-course therapy (Table 16.5). Uncomplicated vulvovaginal candidiasis, which by far represents the most common form of vaginitis seen clinically, is caused by highly sensitive strains of *C. albicans* and, when of mild to moderate severity, responds well to all topical or oral antimycotic therapy (including single-dose therapy), with cure rates exceeding 90% (23). In contrast, patients with complicated vulvovaginal candidiasis have either an organism, host factor, or severity of infection that dictates more intensive and prolonged treatment that lasts 7 to 14 days. Most infections with non-*albicans* species of *Candida* respond to conventional topical or oral antifungal agents provided they are administered for a sufficient period. Vaginitis caused by *C. glabrata* often fails to respond to azoles and may require treatment with vaginal capsules of boric acid at 600 mg/d for 14 days (24).

Treatment of Recurrent Vulvovaginal Candidiasis

The management of recurrent vulvovaginal candidiasis is directed at its control rather than its cure, and requires long-term maintenance therapy with a suppressive prophylactic regimen. The clinician should first confirm the diagnosis of recurrent vulvovaginal candidiasis. Uncontrolled diabetes must be controlled, and the use of corticosteroids and other immunosuppressive agents should be discontinued when possible. Unfortunately, no underlying or predisposing factor can be identified in most women with recurrent vulvovaginal candidiasis. Because of the chronicity of therapy for recurrent vulvovaginal candidiasis, the convenience of oral treatment is apparent; the best suppressive prophylaxis has been achieved with weekly fluconazole orally at a dose of 100 mg. An effective topical prophylactic regimen consists of weekly vaginal suppositories of clotrimazole in a dose of 500 mg (12,23).

Prevention

In women with confirmed recurrent vulvovaginal candidiasis that has been linked to frequent courses of systemic antibiotic therapy, prophylactic antimycotic therapy is justified. A useful regimen is fluconazole at 100 mg once weekly for the duration of antibiotic therapy. No other dietary or alternative method has stood the test of time in preventing vulvovaginal candidiasis. Women prone to vulvovaginal candidiasis should avoid the use of oral contraceptives, intrauterine devices, and the contraceptive sponge.

Atrophic Vaginitis

Clinically significant atrophic vaginitis is quite rare, and most women with mild to moderate atrophy from atrophic vaginitis are asymptomatic. Because of reduced endogenous estrogen production, the epithelium becomes thin and lacking in glycogen, which contributes to a reduction in lactic acid production and an increase in vaginal pH. This change in the environment encourages the overgrowth of nonacidophilic coliform organisms and the disappearance of *Lactobacillus* organisms. Despite these major but usually gradual changes, symptoms are rare, especially in the absence of coitus.

With advanced atrophy, symptoms of atrophic vaginitis include vaginal soreness, dyspareunia, and occasional spotting or discharge. Burning is a frequent complaint and is often precipitated by intercourse. The vaginal mucosa is thin, with diffuse redness, occasional petechiae, or ecchymoses with few or no vaginal folds. Vulvar atrophy also may be apparent. A serosanguineous, thick, or watery vaginal discharge may be present, and the pH of vaginal secretions ranges from 5.5 to 7.0. The wet smear frequently shows increased PMNLs associated with small, round epithelial cells. These parabasal cells represent immature squamous epithelial cells that have not been exposed to sufficient estrogen. The *Lactobacillus*-dominated flora of the vagina is replaced by a mixed flora of gram-negative rods. Bacteriologic cultures in these patients are not unnecessary and can be misleading.

The treatment of atrophic vaginitis, especially in the absence of systemic symptoms, consists primarily of topical application of vaginal estrogen. Nightly use of half or all the contents of an applicator for 1 to 2 weeks is usually sufficient to alleviate atrophic vaginitis.

Table 16.6   Differential Diagnosis of Vulvar Inflammation

Noninfectious Causes	Infectious Causes
Diffuse	*Diffuse*
Atopic dermatitis	Candidiasis
Allergy/hypersensitivity (e.g., azoles, latex, nickel)	Trichomoniasis
Chemicals (e.g., chlorine, betadyne, parobens, detergents)	Bacterial cellulitis (rare)
Trauma	Fournier's gangrene (rare)
Drug-related (e.g., topical 5-fluorouracil)	*Focal*
Idiopathic vestibulitis	Bartholin's abscess
Erosive lichen planus	Folliculitis
Lichen sclerosus	Herpes simplex
Crohn's disease	Herpes zoster
Other (e.g., minipads)	HIV idiopathic ulceration
Focal	LGV
Behçets syndrome	Syphilis
Pemphigus	Chancroid
Idiopathic vestibulitis (vestibular adenitis)	
Lichen sclerosus	
Psoriasis	

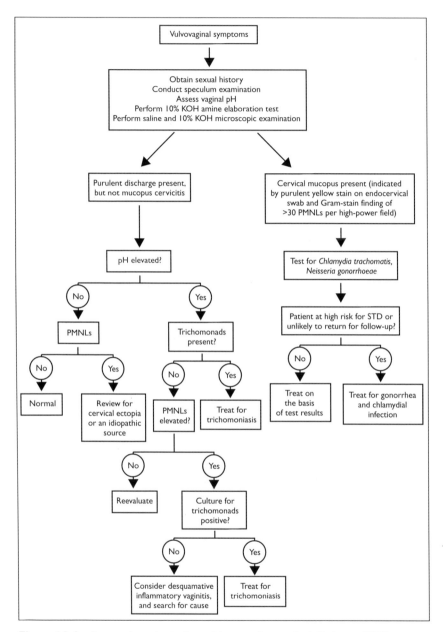

Figure 16.4   Approach to the patient with a purulent vaginal discharge. KOH = potassium hydroxide; PMNLs = polymorphonuclear leukocytes; STD = sexually transmitted disease.

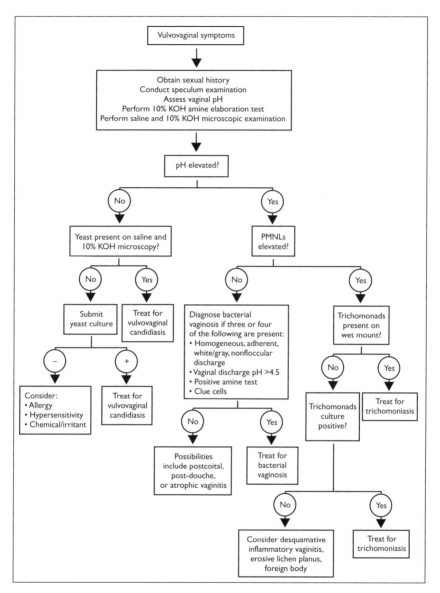

Figure 16.5 Algorithm for the management of the patient with vulvovaginal symptoms. KOH = potassium hydroxide; PMNLs = polymorphonuclear leukocytes.

Noninfectious Vaginitis and Vulvitis

Women often present with acute or chronic vulvovaginal symptoms of noninfectious etiology. Theses symptoms are indistinguishable from those of infectious syndromes but are most commonly confused with those of acute *Candida*

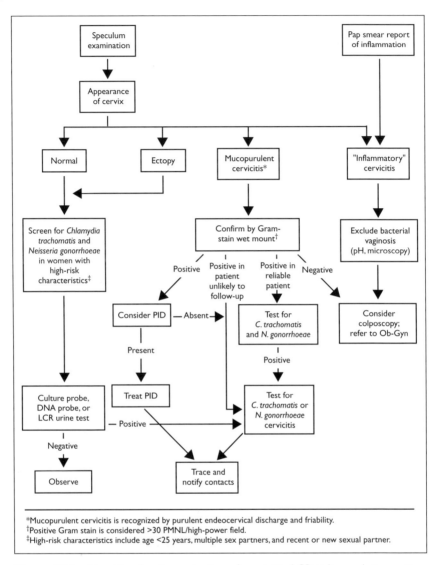

*Mucopurulent cervicitis is recognized by purulent endocervical discharge and friability.
†Positive Gram stain is considered >30 PMNL/high-power field.
‡High-risk characteristics include age <25 years, multiple sex partners, and recent or new sexual partner.

Figure 16.6 Algorithm for the evaluation of cervicitis. LCR = ligase-chain reaction; PID = pelvic inflammatory disease; PMNLs = polymorphonuclear leukocytes.

vaginitis (e.g., pruritus, irritation, burning, soreness, variable discharge). Noninfectious causes of vaginitis and vulvitis include physical irritants (e.g., minipads), chemical irritants (e.g., spermicides, Betadine, topical antimycotics, soaps and perfumes, topical 5-flurouracil), and allergens responsible for immunologic acute and chronic hypersensitivity reactions, including contact dermatitis (e.g., latex condoms, antimycotic creams) (Table 16.6). There is an enormous list of topical factors that are responsible for local inflammatory reactions and symptoms, and many more have yet to be defined. Depending on the site of contact, symptoms may be vaginal or vulvar. A noninfectious mechanism may coexist with or follow an infectious process and should be considered when 1) the three common infectious causes of vulvovaginal symptoms, as well as hormone deficiency, are excluded, 2) the vaginal pH and saline content are normal, and 3) KOH microscopy and a yeast culture are negative. Unfortunately, given the anticipated 20% colonization rates in normal asymptomatic women, a positive yeast culture sometimes reflects the presence of an "innocent bystander" organism rather than the cause of a patient's vulvovaginal symptoms. The only logical way of establishing the role of *Candida* in this context is to treat the patient with an oral antifungal agent and assess the clinical response.

Once a local chemical, irritant, or allergic reaction is suspected as the cause of vaginitis and/or vulvitis, a detailed inquiry into possible causal factors is essential. Offending agents or behaviors should be eliminated whenever possible, including the avoidance of chemical irritants and allergens (e.g., soaps, detergents). The immediate management of severe vulvovaginal symptoms of noninfectious etiology should not rely on topical corticosteroids, which are rarely the solution to such symptoms; moreover, high-potency steroid creams often cause intense burning. Local relief measures include sodium bicarbonate sitz baths and oral antihistamines.

The diagnosis and management of vaginitis are summarized in Figures 16.4, 16.5, and 16.6.

REFERENCES

1. **Kent HL**. Epidemiology of vaginitis. *Am J Obstet Gynecol*. 1991;165:1168–76.

2. **Holmes KK**. Lower genital tract infections in women: cystitis, urethritis, vulvovaginitis, and cervicitis. In Holmes KK, Mardh P-A, Sparling PF, et al. (eds). *Sexually Transmitted Diseases*, 2nd ed. New York: McGraw Hill; 1990.

3. **Hill GB**. Microbiology of bacterial vaginosis. *Am J Obstet Gynecol*. 1969;169:450–4.

4. **Eschenbach DA, Davick PR, Williams BL, et al.** Prevalence of hydrogen peroxide producing *Lactobacillus* species in normal women and women with bacterial vaginosis. *J Clin Microbiol*. 1989;27:251–6.

5. **Hillier SL, Krohn MA, Cassen E, et al.** The role of bacterial vaginosis and vaginal bacteria in amniotic fluid infection in women in preterm labor with intact fetal membranes. *Clin Infect Dis*. 1995;20(Suppl 2):276–8.

6. **Platz-Christensen JJ, Sundstrom F, Larsson PG**. Bacterial vaginosis and cervical intraepithelial neoplasia. *Acta Obstet Gynecol Scand*. 1994;73:586–8.

7. **Centers for Disease Control and Prevention**. 1998 Sexually transmitted diseases treatment guidelines. *MMWR Morbid Mortal Wkly Rep*. 1998;47:75–9.

8. **Hillier SL, Nugent RP, Eschenbach DA, et al.** Association between bacterial vaginosis and preterm delivery of a low-birth-weight infant. *N Engl J Med.* 1995;333: 1737–42.

9. **Hauth JC, Goldenberg RL, Andrews WW, et al.** Reduced incidence of preterm delivery with metronidazole and erythromycin in women with bacterial vaginosis. *N Engl J Med.* 1995;333:1732–6.

10. **Spence MR, Hollander DH, Smith J, et al.** The clinical and laboratory diagnosis of *Trichomonas vaginalis* infection. *Sex Transm Dis.* 1980;7:168–71.

11. **Wolner-Hanssen P, Krieger JN, Stevens CE, et al.** Clinical manifestations of vaginal trichomoniasis. *JAMA.* 1989;261:571–6.

12. **Sobel JD.** Candidal vulvovaginitis. *Clin Obstet Gynecol.* 1993;36:153–65.

13. **Spinillo A, Capuzzo E, Egbe TO, et al.** *Torulopsis glabrata* vaginitis. *Obstet Gynecol.* 1995;85:993–8.

14. **Foxman B.** Epidemiology of vulvovaginal candidiasis: risk factors. *Am J Public Health.* 1996;80:329–31.

15. **Spinillo A, et al.** Effect of antibiotic use on the prevalence of symptomatic vulvovaginal candidiasis. *Am J Obstet Gynecol.* 1999;180:14–7.

16. **Hooton TM, Roberts PL, Stamm WF.** Effects of recent sexual activity and use of a diaphragm on the vaginal microflora. *Clin Infect Dis.* 1994;19:274–8.

17. **Fidel PL Jr, Sobel JD.** Immunopathogenesis of recurrent vulvovaginal candidiasis. *Rev Clin Microbiol.* 1996;9:335–48.

18. **Spinillo A, Carrato L, Pizzoli G.** Recurrent vulvovaginal candidiasis: results of a cohort study of sexual transmission and intestinal reservoir. *J Reprod Med.* 1992;37: 353–357.

19. **Lynch ME, Sobel JD.** Comparative *in vitro* activity of antimycotic agents against pathogenic yeast isolates. *J Med Vet Mycol.* 1994;32:267–74.

20. **Fidel PL Jr, Lynch ME, Redondo-Lopez V, et al.** Systemic cell-mediated immune reactivity in women with recurrent vulvovaginal candidiasis. *J Infect Dis.* 1993;168: 1458–65.

21. **Reef S, Levine WC, McNeil MM, et al.** Treatment options for vulvovaginal candidiasis, background paper for development of 1993 STD treatment recommendations. *Clin Infect Dis.* 1995;20(Suppl 1):580–90.

22. **Sobel JD, Brooker D, Stein GE, et al.** Single oral dose fluconazole compared with clotrimazole in topical therapy of *Candida* vaginitis: Fluconazole Vaginitis Study Group. *Am J Obstet Gynecol.* 1955;172:1263–8.

23. **Sobel JD, Faro S, Force R, et al.** Vulvovaginal candidiasis: epidemiologic, diagnostic, and therapeutic considerations. *Am J Obstet Gynecol.* 1998;178:203–11.

24. **Sobel JD, Chaim W.** Treatment of *Candida glabrata* vaginitis: a retrospective review of boric acid therapy. *Clin Infect Dis.* 1997;24:649–52.

17

Human Papillomavirus

Denise J. Signs, MD, MS
William Bonnez, MD

Papillomaviruses cause tumors of the stratified squamous epithelia of the skin and mucous membranes in vertebrates, including humans. For a long time, wart virus was thought to be a unique virus, but many different human papillomavirus (HPV) genotypes have been recognized since the 1970s. More than 80 genotypes of HPV have been fully characterized; when partially characterized isolates are included, the number exceeds 150 and continues to grow. These viruses can be arranged into three groups according to the anatomical areas they infect and the diseases they cause (Table 17.1). The first group consists of the cutaneous HPVs, which are responsible for warts found on the hands, feet, and face. The second group consists of HPVs that are responsible for a rare disease of the skin: epidermodysplasia verruciformis. Patients with this disease have flat papules distributed over the trunk, face, and proximal extremities. In sun-exposed areas of the skin, these lesions are prone to evolve into squamous cell carcinomas by early adulthood. Mucosal or genital HPVs comprise the third and largest group of these viruses. They are found in the lower genitalia and anus and in the upper respiratory mucous membranes. Mucosal or genital HPVs, which are the focus of this chapter, are responsible for benign (e.g., warts, condylomas), premalignant (e.g., intraepithelial lesions and/or neoplasias), and malignant (e.g., squamous cell carcinomas) tumors (1). However, most HPV infections are asymptomatic, subclinical, or unrecognized.

A clinician should be able to recognize the diseases associated with HPV infection, to use appropriate diagnostic testing and treatment options for these diseases, and to advise patients about their proper personal care.

Table 17.1   Human Papillomavirus Types and Disease Association

HPV Group	Diseases	Common HPV Types*
Cutaneous	Deep plantar warts	1, 2
	Common warts	2, 1
	Flat warts	3, 10
Epidermodysplasia verruciformis	Epidermodysplasia verruciformis	2, 3, 10, **5**, **8**, 9, 12, **14**, 15, **17**
Mucosal or genital	Anogenital warts	6, 11
	Recurrent respiratory papillomatosis	11, 6
	Intraepithelial neoplasia[†]	
	Low grade	6, 11
	High grade	**16, 18**
	Cervical carcinoma	**16, 18**

HPV = human papillomavirus
* HPV types that have a high risk of oncogenicity are indicated in bold.
[†] Variants of intraepithelial neoplasia have been described, including squamous cell carcinoma in situ, bowenoid papulosis, Bowen's disease, and erythroplasia of Queyrat.

Epidemiology

The vast majority of genital HPV infections are transmitted through direct contact during vaginal, anal, or oral sex (2). The description in very young children of genital warts that are associated with cutaneous HPVs indicates the possibility of nonsexual transmission, including autoinoculation (3,4). Juvenile-onset recurrent respiratory papillomatosis is probably acquired by passage at the time of delivery through an infected birth canal (5).

Every year, an estimated one million U.S. citizens develop genital HPV infection, which makes this disease the most commonly acquired viral sexually transmitted disease in the United States (6). Most HPV infections seem to be transient; however, there is suspicion that as many as 40% to 50% of sexually active men and women have or have had genital HPV infection.

Approximately two thirds of sexual partners of patients with genital warts eventually develop genital HPV infections on follow-ups of up to 2 years (2). The incubation period is typically 4 to 6 weeks but can be considerably longer, possibly lasting for years (7). The incidence of genital warts is estimated to be 1%, and the prevalence seems to be rising. From 1966 to 1984, the number of physician office visits for genital HPV infection increased sixfold (8).

There is strong evidence that HPV is necessary for the development of virtually all cervical cancers. For example, in a worldwide survey of cervical cancers, the prevalence of HPV was 99.7%, consisting predominantly of types 16, 18, 31, or 45 (9). The higher the histologic grade of intraepithelial neoplasia, the more often are oncogenic types of HPV present. In prospective studies, the development of high-grade lesions is always preceded by infection with oncogenic types of HPV. Furthermore, no other epidemiologic factor is as highly associated with the development of high-grade cervical lesions as is the presence of HPV. Moreover, strong epidemiologic arguments now exist for implicating HPV in the development of anal cancer (10). HPVs also are incriminated as the cause of at least a fraction of other epithelial cancers of the lower genital, upper respiratory, and upper digestive tracts. Substantial costs are associated with screening for cervical cancer, but morbidity and mortality from this disease can be substantial. For example, cervical cancer is the third most commonly diagnosed cancer in women worldwide and is the second most common such cancer in the developing world (11).

Pathogenesis

Papillomaviruses are small, circular, double-stranded, nonenveloped DNA viruses that cause various proliferative diseases in the squamous stratified epithelia they infect. Because papillomaviruses cannot be grown readily in tissue culture or in animal models, the study and diagnosis of HPV rely largely on molecular technology (12).

Human papillomaviruses are host specific and do not have an animal reservoir. Table 17.1 illustrates the tissue tropism of different HPVs (13). The HPVs also have different oncogenic potentials. Among genital HPVs, types 16 and 18 have frequent association with malignant lesions; types 31, 33, 35, and 45 are less frequently associated with malignant lesions; and types 6 and 11 are rarely associated with malignancy (14).

The replication and expression of HPV DNA depend on epithelial differentiation. The early stage of viral infection is not well known but presumably begins with the infection of a keratinocyte stem cell in the basal layer of the epithelium. The infected cell divides, and a normally nondividing daughter cell pushes upward. As it transits the epithelium, this daughter cell differentiates, triggering virus replication. The daughter cell then senesces and is ultimately shed as a cornified shell that contains virus particles.

The histology of a benign HPV lesion is characterized by a deepening of the rete ridges (papillomatosis) in the affected area of skin and a hyperproliferation of the layers above the basal cells, causing acanthosis, parakeratosis, and hyperkeratosis. A distinctive histologic feature of the lesion may be the presence of koilocytes. These cells, which appear in the upper stratum spinosum, are large and contain one or two enlarged hyperchromatic nuclei that are surrounded by a well-demarcated clear space that pushes the cytoplasm of the cell to the periphery. For the cytologist, koilocytes are the hallmark of HPV infection (15). Malignant and premalignant HPV-infected lesions are characterized by proliferation of the basal cell layer, with the presence of normal and abnormal mitoses (dyskaryosis) and cells with high nuclear-to-cytoplasm ratios. When this process is contained by the basal membrane, it is called intraepithelial neoplasia (the cytologic equivalent is called a squamous intraepithelial lesion [SIL]). Breakage of the basal membrane signals an invasive squamous cell carcinoma.

A series of molecular events must take place from the onset of HPV infection to the development of cancer. Foremost among these is the interaction of two viral proteins (E6 and E7) with two important cellular proteins (p53 and the retinoblastoma protein) that control cell division and have tumor-suppressor properties (16). Further events, including viral integration, DNA methylation, and chromosomal rearrangements are also required for a cell to become malignant. Epidemiologic evidence shows that smoking is also a cofactor in the transformation to malignancy. Consequently, HPV is necessary but not sufficient for malignancy. Furthermore, the oncogenic process is not instantaneous. Although the prevalence of latent HPV infection is approximately 40%, it culminates in cancer in less than 1% of women (17). Typically, an average of approximately 10 years must pass from the detection of an HPV infection to that of cancer (range 24 months to 19 years) (18,19). This variability may be explained by differences in genetic factors, HPV viral load, immune responses, and HPV variants (17).

Immunosuppressed and immunodeficient patients (e.g., renal allograft recipients, patients treated with corticosteroids, patients with HIV infection) are prone to have extensive lesions and low rates of spontaneous regression of lesions when infected with HPV (20–22). Furthermore, they also are known to develop squamous cell carcinomas in sun-exposed areas of their skin (especially renal allograft recipients) and cervical or anal intraepithelial neoplasias. This is consistent with the higher rate of persistent infection with high-risk oncogenic HPVs in HIV-seropositive women (20%) compared with that of HIV-seronegative women (3%) (23).

Clinical Manifestations and Natural History

An HPV-induced wart on the external genitalia may present as a firm, well-circumscribed, slightly keratotic, exophytic papule with a jagged surface contour that resembles a cockscomb or mulberry. This is the typical condyloma acuminatum (24). These lesions usually measure from 2 to 8 mm in diameter but sometimes can be considerably larger or can grow to confluency. Another clinical presentation is that of a smaller, sessile, smooth papule with slightly overhanging edges. Small flat papules may be encountered, particularly on mucosal surfaces.

In circumcised men, most HPV-induced warts are found on the penile shaft. The glans, scrotum, or the urethral meatus are rarely involved. When warts are present, the foreskin is often involved on its occluded surface. In women, warts are distributed over the entire vulva. Most patients have from 1 to 10 warts, with an average total wart surface area of 0.5 to 1.0 cm^2. The perianal region is more commonly involved in women than in heterosexual men. However, receptive anal intercourse, a practice that is becoming more frequent in young women, carries a higher risk of perianal and intra-anal warts. Surprisingly, HPV DNA in women is found more often in the anus than in the cervix. Warts occasionally may be found in the oral cavity.

On the internal mucosal surfaces, warts may appear as small papillomas. However, on the cervix, they appear as single, large, flat papules that turn white after the application of 3% to 5 % acetic acid. This "aceto-whitening" may aid in the identification of subclinical lesions (i.e., lesions that would otherwise not be detected with the naked eye).

Cervical intraepithelial neoplasia (CIN) typically appears as "aceto-white" macules or flat papules. The borders, light reflection, punctation, shape of blood vessels, and surface contour of lesions help in differentiating condyloma from CIN of different grades. All CINs and cervical condylomas are located within the transitional zone, i.e., the area of the glandular epithelium that is replaced by the squamous epithelium with sexual maturation and aging.

Most HPV infections are not clinically recognizable and, even when associated with clinical disease, are symptomatic in only a minority of patients. In addition to the sight or feel of the lesions, the patient may report discomfort, itching, bleeding, discharge, and dyspareunia. When the diagnosis is established, the greatest burden is usually psychological.

The natural history of anogenital warts is poorly defined; however, most patients experience spontaneous regression of their lesions over time. Rates of spontaneous regression (observed on an average of 2 months in the placebo arm of reported randomized studies) are approximately 7% and 12% for men and women, respectively.

The grade of CIN or SIL influences the probability of complete regression or progression to a higher grade of disease or to cancer. For example, it is estimated that at 2-year follow-up, low-grade SIL will have regressed in 47% of cases (25). In contrast, 21.00% and 0.15% of the lesions of low-grade SIL will have progressed over the same period to high-grade SIL and cancer, respectively.

HIV infection affects the natural history of anogenital HPV disease. An increase in HIV load or a decrease in the number of CD4 T cells is associated with an increase in the frequency of detection of HPV DNA, especially with high-risk oncogenic genotypes of the virus. These changes are paralleled by an increase in the rates of cervical and anal intraepithelial neoplasias and of anal cancer (10).

Diagnosis

The diagnosis of anogenital warts is made clinically. In addition to the anogenital area, the examination includes the oral cavity. An anoscopic examination also is indicated if anorectal symptoms are present, perianal warts are seen, or the patient engages in receptive anal intercourse. The application of 3% to 5% acetic acid (or white vinegar) for 1 to 3 minutes facilitates the detection of small lesions, particularly on mucosal surfaces. This is done by wrapping the genitalia in soaked gauzes or by swabbing the vaginal, cervical, or anal surfaces. Magnifying optics, consisting either of a loupe (of at least 3× magnifying power) or a colposcope, are extremely helpful for the proper identification of lesions; however, these tools are not indispensable and should not be used to search for subclinical infections.

Many conditions may mimic warts. The most common is molluscum contagiosum, a poxvirus infection. Molluscum contagiosum manifests as small, sessile, dome-shaped, waxy-appearing papules that often have a tell-tale central umbilication. Noninfectious, normal but exaggerated pearly papules around the glans corona or in the introitus (hirsutoid papillomatosis) may be confusing. The location and the more lissome nature of these structures help the diagnosis. Condylomata lata of syphilis should be easy to distinguish from HPV-induced warts. They are flat-topped, large, moist papules. Referral and/or lesion biopsy should be considered, particularly when the patient is immunodeficient, the diagnosis is uncertain, and the lesions are pigmented, persistent, or rapidly changing.

Women who present with anogenital warts should be offered screening for cervical cancer with a Pap smear, which also offers an opportunity to inspect the vagina and cervix. In the general population, a Pap smear should be performed when the patient becomes sexually active or when she reaches her 18th birthday (26). If the smear is normal, two more normal annual Pap smears should be obtained before changing the screening interval to every 3 to 5 years if the patient is compliant. Annual Pap smears are recommended so long as the patient has anogenital warts or if the patient is immunodeficient. Screening at twice this frequency has been proposed for HIV-infected patients who, because of sexual behavior or severity of immunosuppression, may be at a higher risk for cervical cancer. The variability of Pap smear sensitivity (30%–87%) and specificity (86%–100%) creates the need for repeat testing and alternative confirmatory methods (15). The role of cytologic screening for anal cancer in the HIV-infected population remains to be defined (22).

The results of the Pap smear usually are reported according to the Bethesda classification system, which was implemented in 1988 to offer a way of assessing the quality of cervical samples used for the smear and to provide a simple classification system of the squamous cell abnormalities associated with HPV infection (27). Diagnostic categories include carcinoma, low-grade SIL (LSIL), and high-grade SIL (HSIL). HSIL typically corresponds to CIN grades 2 and 3. Patients with HSIL should be referred for colposcopy and biopsy. LSIL is the cytologic correlate of both cervical condyloma and CIN grade 1. An additional category (atypical squamous cells of unknown significance, or ASCUS) was created for abnormal smears that did not match the criteria for LSIL, HSIL, or carcinoma. The optimal triage strategy for patients with ASCUS and LSIL (from whom are obtained more than 90% of the Pap smears with squamous abnormalities) is still undefined and may range from the costly combination of colposcopy and biopsy to simple observation with repeated Pap smears every 4 to 6 months for 2 years (until three consecutive negative results are obtained). The choice may be guided by the patient's age, history, and compliance; by additional communication with the pathologist; and by the availability of HPV DNA testing and quantitation (17).

The Hybrid Capture II assay (Digene Corp.) is the only FDA-approved test for detecting HPV DNA in clinical specimens. This liquid-phase assay is based on the binding of HPV DNA in a specimen to a panel of immobilized RNA probes. The DNA-RNA complexes are recognized by a labeled antibody, with the intensity of the labeling measured through a chemiluminescence reaction. The assay is quantitative and reveals DNA of most of the genital HPV genotypes. Two groups of probes can be used independently, either to test only for the presence of high-risk oncogenic HPVs or for both high- and low-risk oncogenic HPVs. The quality of the Pap smear can be improved by using a liquid collection system for cervical cells (ThinPrep) (27). This technology allows a single cytologic specimen to be processed both as a Pap smear and for the Hybrid Capture II assay. In the United States, the use of HPV DNA testing has not yet been endorsed by professional societies or by public health organizations; however, the Hybrid Capture II assay is expected to be recommended to aid in the triage of ASCUS patients. Only those patients infected with high-risk oncogenic types of HPV will then be referred for colposcopy and biopsy (28,29). Assays for HPV based on the polymerase chain reaction test are investigational, and no serologic assay for HPV is available for clinical use.

The sexual partners of patients with anogenital warts should be examined for the same disease and other sexually transmitted diseases. Only symptomatic sexual partners of women with abnormal Pap smears should be examined (26).

Treatment

No single highly effective treatment exists for HPV infections. Consequently, the currently available treatment options for anogenital warts are aimed at eradicating the disease rather than the infection or any subclinical disease. Removing anogenital warts by any means is desirable for cosmetic reasons and to alleviate the physical and psychological symptoms they may produce. Whether these treatments affect the contagiousness of HPV infection or the very low but increased risk of malignancy is uncertain (30). The benefits of treating anogenital warts have to be balanced against the financial costs, risks of adverse reactions, the imperfect efficacy of the treatment, and the background rate of spontaneous regression of disease. In practice, most patients with anogenital warts are treated, but simple observation may be a valid option, especially after repeated treatment failures.

The main modalities available to treat anogenital warts are either physical or chemical (26,31,32), and all the physical methods can be applied to the pregnant patient. Cryotherapy is one of the most popular physical methods for treating anogenital warts, during which liquid nitrogen is applied to the lesion via spray, probe, or swab. Freezing causes a severe but transient pain that can be blunted by the prior application of EMLA cream (lidocaine and prilocaine). As many as six or more treatments may be needed to obtain the 50% to 100% complete response rates reported in the literature. Long-term side-effects are uncommon. Electrosurgery, which is available in different modalities (e.g., electrocautery, electrodessication, fulguration, electrocoagulation), may be more effective than cryotherapy but is also more prone to cause scarring. Excision using scissors or a scalpel performed under local anesthesia can be a effective and well-tolerated approach to eradicating sparse lesions. Laser surgery is costly, and the results are not necessarily superior to those of other methods and are strongly operator dependent. Furthermore, laser surgery requires either local or general anesthesia.

Chemical treatment modalities for anogenital warts are also diverse; however, with the exception of acid treatment, they should not be used during pregnancy. Podophyllin (podophyllum resin, USP), ordinarily used as a 25% solution in benzoin, has been available for over half a century. This resin extract from the rhizome of the American mandrake (*Podophyllum peltatum*) inhibits cell division by preventing formation of the mitotic spindle. It is a toxic compound and should be administered by a health practitioner once a week for up to six treatments. Ingestion or extensive application of podophyllin can be fatal, and its application on healthy skin is to be avoided because it causes severe inflammation and even necrosis. Podophyllin therapy is not a very effective treatment for anogenital warts, and its potency varies from one batch to another. Complete response rates range from 20% to 40%, and recurrences are common. The main advantage of podophyllin is its low cost.

Podophyllotoxin (Podofilox), a lignan, is the most active component of podophyllin but is not as toxic. It is available as a 0.5% solution (Condylox9) for self-application twice daily on each of three consecutive days, a treatment that is repeated in weekly cycles up to a maximum of four such cycles. Complete response rates range from 45% to 60%. To avoid the frequent recurrence of warts, treatment with podophyllotoxin may be continued once daily on three consecutive days per week for up to 8 weeks.

Gynecologists who treat anogenital warts favor trichloroacetic and bichloroacetic acids. They are used as 10% to 90% solutions applied directly to the warts. During this procedure, the surrounding skin must be protected with a cream because the treatment is painful and may cause ulceration. However, acid therapy is inexpensive and, in women, seems to be as effective as cryotherapy for anogenital warts. Furthermore, it can be used during pregnancy.

Interferons have been the best-studied therapeutic agents for anogenital warts. Unfortunately, their efficacy is modest and largely limited to the intralesional route of administration, which essentially limits the benefit of this treatment to the individual lesion that receives an interferon injection. Recently, imiquimod (an imidazoquinoline amine derivative) has been marketed as a 5% topical cream (Aldara) for the self-treatment of genital warts. This compound is an inducer of interferon and other cytokines. When applied every other day for a total of three times per week for a period of up to 16 weeks, topical treatment with Aldara produced a complete response rate of 50% (72% in women and 33% in men) compared with a 14% rate with placebo. The recurrence rate of warts was low (10%) in the 12 weeks after the end of therapy (33). The treatment causes local inflammation with itching, burning, and erosions. Nonetheless, it is a well-accepted and convenient, albeit relatively expensive, treatment for anogenital warts.

5-Fluorouracil is a pyrimidine antagonist available as a 5% cream (Efudex) that has been used mainly for treating vaginal or penile intrameatal warts. Pain, ulceration, and allergic reactions limit its use. Cidofovir (Vistide), an acyclic nucleotide analog with anti–herpes virus activity, seems to be effective against anogenital warts when delivered intralesionally.

Table 17.2 summarizes the treatment recommendations made by Centers for Disease Control and Prevention (CDC) for anogenital warts. Choices among different options may be further guided by their availability and by patient preference, cost, convenience, and clinical circumstances (32). After successful treatment, a 3-month follow-up may be offered to detect recurrences. When warts persist, regular follow-up is advisable. In the absence of any data, it seems reasonable to model this follow-up on the schedule proposed for cervical cancer screening. The management of intraepithelial neoplasias and cancers should be reserved for the specialist.

Patient Education

Public and health education in schools have disseminated an awareness of the risk of the sexual transmission of HIV and about the traditional causes of gen-

Table 17.2 CDC Treatment Recommendations for External Genital Warts

Disease	Treatment Delivery	Treatments
External genital warts	Patient applied	Podofilox 0.5 % solution or gel
		Imiquimod 5% cream (Aldara)
	Provider applied	
	First line	Cryotherapy
		Podophyllin resin 10%–25%
		TCA or BCA 80%–90%
		Surgical removal
	Second line	Intralesional interferon
		Laser surgery
Cervical warts		Refer to expert
Vaginal warts	Provider applied	Cryotherapy
		TCA or BCA 80%–90%
		Podophyllin 10%–25%
Urethral meatus warts	Provider applied	Cryotherapy
		Podophyllin 10%–25%
Anal warts	Provider applied	Cryotherapy
		TCA or BCA 80%–90%
		Surgical removal
Oral warts	Provider applied	Cryotherapy
		Surgical removal

BCA = bichloroacetic acid; TCA = trichloroacetic acid.

ital discharge and ulcers; however, the public remains largely uniformed about genital HPV disease. Table 17.3 summarizes the principal issues that should be discussed with the patient who presents with genital warts or an abnormal Pap smear. The goal is not only to educate but also to engage the trust of the patient so that proper follow-up and screening can be provided. The Web sites of the CDC (www.cdc.gov/nchstp/dstd/dstdp.html) and that of the American Social Health Association (ASHA) (www.ashastd.org) offer excellent resources for patients, including links to patient support groups. Both organizations also operate hotlines (CDC: 800-227-8922, Monday to Friday from 8 AM to 11 PM; ASHA: 877-478-5868, Monday to Friday from 2 PM to 7 PM).

Most HPV diseases seem to be caused by a relapse of clinical or subclinical disease rather than by primary or secondary infection, and the efficacy of condoms in preventing HPV diseases is controversial (34–36). However, HPV infection may occur much earlier than the disease, and indirect evidence suggests that condoms may have a protective role against such infection (37). At present, the best argument for the use of condoms is that at it reduces the risk of transmission of other sexually transmitted diseases. Consequently, the use of condoms should be encouraged in the nonmonogamous, sexually active patient.

Table 17.3 Patient Education on Human Papillomavirus

- Genital HPV infections are extremely common, possibly affecting up to 50%–80% of the population at some point during life.
- A single sexual encounter is sufficient for transmission; however, for most patients, the infection is harmless, unrecognized, and does not cause disease.
- Because disease may be delayed until long after the infection, a diagnosis of HPV infection does not necessarily mean that a sexual partner has cheated.
- HPV infections are contagious even in the absence of visible lesions.
- Most HPV diseases resolve spontaneously over time.
- Many different types of HPV can infect the genitalia, but only a subgroup causes lesions that may evolve into cancer. This subgroup of HPVs is typically not encountered in genital warts.
- Because smoking may contribute to the risk of cervical cancer, smoking cessation is encouraged.
- Virtually all cervical cancers are caused by HPV infection; however, the vast majority of women do not develop cervical or other genital cancers because of HPV infection. Furthermore, these cancers take several years to grow and can be detected by regular screening.
- Screening for cervical cancer should be performed with regularly scheduled Pap smears. Women who cease to be sexually active (e.g., older women) or who are lesbians should undergo Pap smear screening.
- Most abnormal Pap smears do not indicate cervical cancer.
- Pap smears are not perfect detection tools; their regular repetition ensures their screening efficiency. When necessary, they can be complemented by HPV testing.
- Having genital warts during pregnancy carries only a very small risk for the baby to develop recurrent respiratory papillomatosis.
- HPV infections are contagious. Although condoms may help reduce that risk, they cannot be relied on for complete protection. Female partners of patients with genital warts should be reminded about cervical cancer screening.

HPV = human papillomavirus.

REFERENCES

1. **Koutsky LA, Galloway DA, Holmes KK.** Epidemiology of genital human papillomavirus infection. *Epidemiol Rev.* 1988;10:122–63.
2. **Oriel JD.** Natural history of genital warts. *Br J Vener Dis.* 1971;47:1–13.
3. **Obalek S, Jablonska S, Orth G.** Anogenital warts in children. *Clin Dermatol.* 1997;15:369–76.
4. **Fairley CK, Gay NJ, Forbes A, et al.** Hand-genital transmission of genital warts? An analysis of prevalence data. *Epidem Infect.* 1995;115:169–76.
5. **Green GE, Bauman NM, Smith RJ.** Pathogenesis and treatment of juvenile onset recurrent respiratory papillomatosis. *Otolaryngol Clin North Am.* 2000;33:187–207.
6. **Centers for Disease Control and Prevention.** *Division of STD/HIV Prevention 1992 Annual Report.* Atlanta: US Department of Health and Human Services, Public Health Service, Centers for Disease Control and Prevention; 1993.
7. **Barrett TJ, Silbar JD, McGinley JP.** Genital warts: a venereal disease. *JAMA.* 1954;154:333–4.
8. **Becker TM, Blount JF, Guinan ME.** Trends in genital herpes infections among private practitioners in the United States, 1966–1981. *JAMA.* 1985;253:1601–3.

9. **Walboomers JM, Jacobs MV, Manos MM, et al.** Human papillomavirus is a necessary cause of invasive cervical cancer worldwide. *J Pathol.* 1999;189:12–9.

10. **Frisch M, Glimelius B, van den Brule AJC, et al.** Sexually transmitted infection as a cause of anal cancer. *N Engl J Med.* 1997;337:1350–8.

11. **Parkin DM, Pisani P, Ferlay J.** Global cancer statistics. *Cancer J Clin.* 1999;49:33–64.

12. **Lörincz AT.** Molecular methods for the detection of human papillomavirus infection. *Obstet Gynecol Clin North Am.* 1996;23:707–30.

13. **de Villiers EM.** Human pathogenic papillomavirus types: an update. *Curr Top Microbiol Immunol.* 1994;79:328–37.

14. **Lorincz AT, Reid R, Jenson AB, et al.** Human papillomavirus infection of the cervix: relative risk associations of 15 common anogenital types. *Obstet Gynecol.* 1992;79: 328–37.

15. **Nanda K, McCrory DC, Myers ER, et al.** Accuracy of the Papanicolaou test in screening for and follow-up of cervical cytologic abnormalities: a systematic review. *Ann Intern Med.* 2000;132:810–9.

16. **zur Hausen H.** Papillomaviruses causing cancer: evasion from host-cell control in early events in carcinogenesis. *J Natl Cancer Inst.* 2000;92:690–8.

17. **Johnston C.** Quantitative tests for human papillomavirus. *Lancet.* 2000;355:2179–80.

18. **Koutsky L.** Epidemiology of genital human papillomavirus infection. *Am J Med.* 1997;102:3–8.

19. **Ylitalo N, Sorensen P, Josefsson AM, et al.** Consistent high viral load of human papillomavirus 16 and risk of cervical carcinoma in situ: a nested case-control study. *Lancet.* 2000;355:2194–8.

20. **McGregor JM, Proby CM, Leigh IM.** Virus infection and cancer risk in transplant recipients. *Trends Microbiol.* 1996;4:2–3.

21. **Ellerbrock TV, Chiasson MA, Bush TJ, et al.** Incidence of cervical squamous intraepithelial lesions in HIV-infected women. *JAMA.* 2000;283:1031–7.

22. **Volberding P.** Looking behind: time for anal cancer screening. *Am J Med.* 2000;108: 674–5.

23. **Sun X-W, Kuhn L, Ellerbrock TV, et al.** Human papillomavirus infection in women infected with the human immunodeficiency virus. *N Engl J Med.* 1997;337:1343–9.

24. **Jablonska S, Majewski S.** Human papillomavirus infection in women. Special aspects of infectious diseases in women. *Clin Dermatol.* 1997;15:67–79.

25. **Melnikow J, Nuovo J, Willan AR, et al.** Natural history of cervical squamous intraepithelial lesions: a meta-analysis. *Obstet Gynecol.* 1998;92(Part 2):727–35.

26. **Anonymous.** 1998 guidelines for the treatment of sexually transmitted diseases. *MMWR Morb Mortal Wkly Rep.* 1998;47(RR-1):1–116. (http://www.cdc.gov/nchstp/dstd/dstdp.html).

27. **Walsh JM.** Cervical cancer: developments in screening and evaluation of the abnormal Pap smear. *West J Med.* 1998;169:304–10.

28. **Ledger WJ, Jeremias J, Witkin SS.** Testing for high-risk human papillomavirus types will become a standard of clinical care. *Am J Obstet Gynecol.* 2000;182:860–5.

29. **Manos MM, Kinney WK, Hurley LB, et al.** Identifying women with cervical neoplasia: using human papillomavirus DNA testing for equivocal Papanicolaou results. *JAMA.* 1999;281:1605–10.

30. **Friis S, Kjaer SK, Frisch M, et al.** Cervical intraepithelial neoplasia, anogenital can-

cer, and other cancer types in women after hospitalization for condylomata acuminata. *J Infect Dis.* 1997;175:743–8.

31. **Beutner KR, Wiley DJ, Douglas JM, et al.** Genital warts and their treatment. *Clin Infect Dis.* 1998;28(Suppl 1):S37–S56.

32. **Beutner KR, Reitano MV, Richwald GA, Wiley DJ.** External genital warts–Report of the American Medical Association Consensus Conference. *Clin Infect Dis.* 1998;27:796–806.

33. **Beutner KR, Spruance SL, Hougham AJ, et al.** Treatment of genital warts with an immune-response modifier (imiquimod). *J Am Acad Dermatol.* 1998;38:230–9.

34. **Krebs H-B, Helmkamp BF.** Treatment failure of genital condylomata acuminata in women: role of the male sexual partner. *Am J Obstet Gynecol.* 1991;165:660–3.

35. **Ward BG, Thomas IL.** Randomized prospective intervention study of human cervical wart virus infection. *Aust N Z J Obstet Gynaecol.* 1994;34:182–5.

36. **Wen LM, Estcourt CS, Simpson JM, Mindel A.** Risk factors for the acquisition of genital warts: are condoms protective? *Sex Trans Infect* 1999;75:312–6.

37. **Young TK, McNicol P, Beauvais J.** Factors associated with human papillomavirus infection detected by polymerase chain reaction among urban Canadian aboriginal and non-aboriginal women. *Sex Trans Dis* 1997;24:293–8.

18

Pharyngotonsillitis, Peritonsillar, Retropharyngeal, and Parapharyngeal Abscesses, and Epiglottitis

Itzhak Brook, MD, MSc

Pharyngotonsillitis

Definition

Pharyngotonsillitis (PT) is characterized by the presence of increased redness and an exudate or ulceration in the pharynx or tonsil or a membrane that covers the tonsils. Because the pharynx is served by lymphoid tissues of Waldeyer's ring, an infection can spread to include various parts of the ring, such as the nasopharynx, uvula, soft palate, tonsils, adenoids, and cervical lymph glands (1,2). Based on its extent, the infection can be called pharyngitis, tonsillitis, tonsillopharyngitis, or nasopharyngitis. Furthermore, any of these illnesses can be acute, subacute, or recurrent.

Etiology

The finding of PT generally requires the consideration of infection with group A β-hemolytic streptococci (GABHS); however, numerous other bacteria, viruses, other infectious agents, and noninfectious causes should be considered sources of PT (1). Recognizing the causative agent(s) and choosing appropriate therapy are of the utmost importance in ensuring a rapid recovery and for preventing complications.

The different agents that cause PT and the characteristic clinical features they produce are shown in Table 18.1. The occurrence of a particular etio-

Table 18.1   Infectious Agents of Pharyngotonsillitis

Organism	Clinical Lesions	Clinical Frequency
Bacteria		
Aerobic		
Groups A, B, C, and G streptococci	Er, Ex, F, P	A
Streptococcus pneumoniae	E	C
Staphylococcus aureus	Er, Ex, F	C
Neisseria gonorrhoeae	Er, Ex	C
Neisseria meningitidis	Er, Ex	C
Corynebacterium diphtheriae	Er, Ex	C
Corynebacterium haemolyticum	Er, Ex	C
Arcanobacterium haemolyticum	Er, Ex	C
Bordetella pertussis	Er, Ex	C
Haemophilus influenzae	Er, Ex	C
Haemophilus parainfluenzae	Er, Ex	C
Salmonella typhi	Er	C
Francisella tularensis	Er, Ex	C
Yersinia pseudotuberculosis	Er	C
Treponema pallidum	Er, F	C
Mycobacterium spp.	Er	C
Anaerobic		
Peptostreptococcus spp.	Er, E	C
Actinomyces spp.	Er, U	C
Pigmented *Prevotella* and *Porphyromonas* spp.	Er, Ex, U	B
Bacteroides spp.	Er, Ex, U	C
Mycoplasma		
Mycoplasma pneumoniae	Er, Ex, F	B
Mycoplasma hominis	Er, Ex	C
Viruses and Chlamydia		
Adenovirus	Er, Ex, F	A
Enteroviruses (e.g., poliovirus, echovirus, coxsackie virus)	Er, Ex, U	A
Parainfluenza virus types 1–4	Er	A
Epstein–Barr virus	Er, Ex, F	B
Herpesvirus hominis	Er, Ex, U	C
Respiratory syncytial virus	Er	C
Influenza virus A and B	Er	A
Cytomegalovirus	Er	C
Rheovirus	Er	C
Measles virus	Er, P	C
Rubella virus	P	C
Rhinovirus	Er	C
Chlamydia trachomatis and *C. pneumoniae*	Er	C
Fungi		
Candida spp.	Er, Ex	B
Parasites		
Toxoplasma gondii	Er	C
Rickettsia		
Coxiella burnetii	Er	C

A = most frequent (>66% of cases); B = frequent (33%–66% of cases); C = uncommon (<33% of cases);
Er = erythematous; Ex = exudative; F = follicular; U = ulcerative; P = petechial.

logic agent depends on numerous variables, including environmental conditions (e.g., season, geographic location, exposure) and individual variables (e.g., age, host resistance, immunity). The most prevalent agents responsible for PT are GABHS, adenoviruses, influenza and parainfluenza viruses, Epstein–Barr virus, and enteroviruses. However, the precise cause is generally not determined, and the role of some potential pathogens is uncertain.

Recent studies have suggested that interactions between various organisms, including GABHS, other aerobic and anaerobic bacteria, and viruses, may occur during PT. Some of these interactions may be synergistic (e.g., the relationship between Epstein–Barr virus and anaerobic bacteria) (3), thus enhancing the virulence of some pathogens. Others may be antagonistic (e.g., the relationship between GABHS and certain "interfering" α-hemolytic streptococci) (4). Furthermore, β-lactamase–producing bacteria (BLPB) can protect themselves and other bacteria from β-lactam antibiotics (5).

Aerobic Bacteria

Infection with GABHS is the most common bacterial cause of PT. It is an endemic infection, peaks in late winter and early spring, is rare in children younger than 2 years of age, and generally occurs in children 5 to 11 years of age. However, people of all ages are susceptible. Non-GABHS organisms are more often obtained from adults than from children with PT. Crowded settings are a risk factor for the transmission of the organisms responsible for PT.

Infection with GABHS can have numerous, potentially suppurative and nonsuppurative, complications. Suppurative complications include peritonsillar abscess, retropharyngeal cellulitis and abscess, cervical adenitis, otitis media, mastoiditis, sinusitis, and bacteremia. Nonsuppurative complications include acute rheumatic fever, acute glomerulonephritis, scarlet fever, and toxin-mediated streptococcal shock syndrome.

Because of the potential for serious suppurative and nonsuppurative sequelae of GABHS infection, these organisms are the best known cause of sore throat (1); however, group B, C, and G β-hemolytic streptococci also occasionally are responsible for pharyngitis (6–11). PT caused by all types of streptococci generally has an identical clinical presentation, characterized by exudation, petechiae, and follicles (11). Streptococcal tonsillitis can be a serious illness because of the occurrence of rheumatic fever and the increased virulence of GABHS noted in recent years (10). Increased numbers of cases of streptococcal sepsis and toxic shock syndrome have been observed in the past decade. Streptococci also can be involved in suppurative complications of tonsillitis, such as peritonsillar and retropharyngeal abscesses.

Less common causes of PT are described in the ensuing discussion. *Streptococcus pneumoniae* can be involved in PT that can either subside or spread to other sites. *Corynebacterium diphtheriae* and *C. haemolyticum* cause an early exudative PT with a thick, grayish-green membrane that may be difficult to dislodge and often leaves a bleeding surface when removed. The infection can spread to the throat, palate, and larynx. *C. haemolyticum* produces a lethal systemic exotoxin (1). The incidence of PT caused by *Arcanobacterium haemolyticum* is from 2.5% to 10% and occurs mainly in individuals 15 to 18 years of age (12). Approximately half of affected patients have a scarlatiniform rash.

Neisseria gonorrhoeae is commonly present in homosexual men and also can be detected in adolescents with pharyngitis. PT infection caused by this organism is often asymptomatic but may result in bacteremia and can persist after treatment. *N. meningitidis* can cause symptomatic or asymptomatic PT that can be a prodrome of septicemia or meningitis.

Nontypable *Haemophilus influenzae* and *H. parainfluenzae* can be recovered from inflamed tonsils. These organisms can cause invasive disease in infants and elderly persons, as well as acute epiglottitis, otitis media, and sinusitis.

The role of *Staphylococcus aureus* in PT is unclear. *S. aureus* is often recovered from chronically inflamed tonsils and peritonsillar abscesses and can produce β-lactamase, which may interfere with the eradication of GABHS (5).

Rare causes of PT are *Francisella tularensis, Treponema pallidum, Mycobacterium* species, and *Toxoplasma gondii.*

Mycoplasma

Both *Mycoplasma pneumoniae* and *M. hominis* can cause PT, usually as a manifestation of a generalized infection. The prevalence of *Mycoplasma* infection increases with age.

Anaerobic Bacteria

The anaerobic organisms that have been implicated in PT are species of *Actinomyces, Fusobacterium,* and pigmented *Prevotella* and *Porphyromonas* (13). Several observations support the role of anaerobic bacteria in acute PT, including the following:

- Anaerobes outnumber their aerobic counterparts in the oral flora in a 100-to-1 ratio (14).
- Anaerobes (e.g., *Fusobacterium* species and spirochetes) are predominant in tonsillar or retropharyngeal abscesses (15) and cause Vincent's angina (16).
- Encapsulated, pigmented *Prevotella* and *Porphyromonas* species have been isolated in greater numbers from acutely inflamed tonsils than from normal tonsils (17) and were recovered from the cores of recurrently inflamed, non–GABHS-infected tonsils (18).
- Patients with non–GABHS tonsillitis (e.g., those with infectious mononucleosis) responded to antibiotics directed only against anaerobes (metronidozole) (3).

- Increased serum levels of antibodies to *Prevotella intermedia* and *Fusobacterium nucleatum* have been found in patients with recurrent non–GABHS tonsillitis (13) and in those with peritonsillar cellulitis and abscess (19).

Viruses and Chlamydia

The viruses known to cause PT are adenoviruses, parainfluenza viruses, enteroviruses (e.g., coxsackie A virus), Epstein–Barr virus, herpes simplex viruses, respiratory syncytial virus, and cytomegalovirus (1). *Chlamydia pneumoniae* may cause pharyngitis, which often accompanies pneumonia or bronchitis. *Chlamydia trachomatis* has been associated with nasopharyngeal infections and pneumonia in infants and with PT in individuals who have engaged in fellatio.

Clinical Manifestations

Generally of sudden onset, PT exhibits fever, sore throat, nausea, vomiting, headache, and, rarely, abdominal pain. Redness of the throat and tonsils is observed at an early stage, and the cervical lymph glands become enlarged. The clinical manifestations may vary with different etiologic agents (*see* Table 18.1) but are rarely specific to a particular agent. Erythema is common to most agents, but the occurrence of ulceration, petechiae, exudation, or follicles is variable (2). The common features of PT caused by specific etiologic agents are exudative pharyngitis in GABHS infection, ulcerative lesions in enterovirus infection, and membranous pharyngitis in *C. diphtheriae* infection. Petechiae often can be seen in GABHS, Epstein–Barr virus, measles virus, and rubella virus infections.

Viral PT is generally self-limited (lasting 4 to 10 days) and associated with the presence of nasal secretions. Bacterial illness lasts longer if untreated. The unique features of anaerobic tonsillitis or PT are the enlargement and ulceration of the tonsils in association with a fetid or foul odor and the presence of fusiform bacilli, spirochetes, and other organisms seen with Gram stain (16).

Diagnosis

Clinical Evaluation

Commonly, antimicrobial therapy is indicated only for PT that is caused by GABHS; therefore, it must be determined clinically whether the infection is due to this organism. Patients with acute PT caused by GABHS are between 5 and 11 years of age, present with infection during late winter and early spring, and generally have a sudden onset of sore throat, fever, and pain on swallowing (11). Younger members of this group typically have nausea, vomiting, abdominal pain, and headache and may have a PT exudate and/or cervical lymphadenitis (1). Palatal petechiae, a scarlatiniform rash, and a red, swollen uvula may be present (2). However, these findings are not specific for GABHS infection and can occur with other organisms, including viruses.

Laboratory Evaluation

Testing for the presence of GABHS should be considered when the clinical picture suggests that GABHS is present, that potential contact with a documented case of GABHS infection has occurred, or that the prevalence of GABHS infection in the community is high. Testing is not recommended in asymptomatic individuals at the conclusion of therapy. Scoring systems for predicting GABHS infection are accurate only in up to 80% of cases (11,20).

Throat culture (with a specimen obtained by throat swabbing of both tonsillar surfaces and the posterior pharyngeal wall and plated on sheep blood agar media) is the standard laboratory test for the diagnosis of PT. Incubation under anaerobic conditions and the use of selective media can increase the recovery rate of pathogens (21,22). A single throat culture has a sensitivity of 90% to 95% for GABHS in the pharynx. False-negative results can occur in patients who have received antibiotics. Identifying GABHS by direct growth may take 24 to 48 hours. Reexamination of culture plates at 48 hours is advisable (23). Use of a Bacitracin disk provides presumptive identification through the absence of growth (24,25). Attempts to identify β-hemolytic streptococci other than those of group A may be worthwhile in older individuals (7–9). Commercial kits that contain group-specific antisera are available for identifying the specific group to which a streptococcal pathogen belongs (26).

More than 10 colonies of GABHS per plate are considered to represent a true infection as opposed to a colonization. However, using the number of colonies of GABHS on the plate as an indicator for the presence of true infection may fail to yield reliable results, because there is an overlap between carriers and infected individuals (26).

An increase in the titer of antistreptococcal O (ASO) antibody after 3 to 6 weeks can provide retrospective evidence for GABHS infection and can assist in differentiating between such infection and the carrier state (1). Determining the ASO titer is indicated when there is a need to prove the occurrence of GABHS infection.

Rapid methods of identification for GABHS take 10 to 60 minutes. Although more expensive than routine culture, they allow the rapid initiation of therapy and the reduction of morbidity (27–30). However, these rapid methods have a 5% to 15% rate of false-negative results (31). Consequently, it is recommended that a bacterial culture be performed in instances in which a rapid streptococcal test result is negative.

Other pathogens should be identified in specific situations, either when no GABHS is found or when a search for other organisms is warranted. Because many of the other PT-causing pathogens are part of the normal pharyngeal flora, interpreting the findings in such cases is difficult.

Attempts to identify corynebacteria should be made whenever a membrane is present in the throat. Cultures should be obtained from beneath the membrane using a special moisture-reducing transport medium. A Loeffler's slant, sodium tellurite plate, and blood agar plate all should be inoculated (26). Corynebacteria also may be identified by the fluorescent-antibody technique.

Both viral culture methods and rapid tests for some viruses (e.g., respiratory syncytial virus) are available. A heterophil slide test or other rapid tests for infectious mononucleosis can provide a specific diagnosis.

Treatment

Many antimicrobial agents are available for treating PT caused by GABHS (26); however, the recommended optimal treatment for GABHS infection is penicillin administered three times daily for 10 days (Tables 18.2 and 18.3). Oral penicillin-VK is used more often than is intramuscular benzathine penicillin-G (20). However, intramuscular penicillin can be given to ensure compliance or as initial therapy to patients who cannot tolerate oral medication.

Many antimicrobial agents have been used to treat GABHS tonsillitis successfully. An alternative to penicillin is amoxicillin, which is as active against GABHS but has characteristics that give it a theoretical advantage (e.g., a more reliable absorption, higher blood-level yields, a longer plasma half-life, lower protein binding). Furthermore, oral liquid amoxicillin gives better compliance than oral penicillin (because of its more pleasing taste). However, amoxicillin should not be used in patients suspected of having infectious mononucleosis, in whom it can produce a skin rash.

Alternative agents for treating acute GABHS tonsillitis are the macrolides. However, in countries in which these drugs have had extensive use, GABHS resistance to them has increased, reaching as high as 70% (33). The current level of resistance of GABHS to macrolides in the United States is 5% to 10%; therefore, it is advisable to limit the use of macrolides to patients with true allergy to penicillins. Compliance with the newer macrolides (clarithromycin and azithromycin) is better than that with erythromycin because of their longer half-lives and fewer adverse gastrointestinal side effects.

All generations of oral cephalosporins have been found to be as effective as penicillin (or more so) for treating acute GABHS tonsillitis (34). The clinical failure rate with penicillin is 10% to 15%, and cephalosporins fail in 5% to 8% of cases. The greater efficacy of the cephalosporins against GABHS may be due to their activity against aerobic BLPB such as *S. aureus* and *Haemophilus* species. Another possible reason for the greater efficacy of the cephalosporins

Table 18.2   Ten-Day Oral-Antibiotic Treatment Course for Acute Pharyngotonsillitis Caused by Group A Beta-Hemolytic Streptococci

Generic Name	Dosage Pediatric (mg/kg/d)	Dosage Adult (mg/dose)	Frequency (hours)
Penicillin-V	25–50	250	q 6–8
Amoxicillin	25–50	250	q 8
Cephalexin*	25–50	250	q 6–8
Cefadroxyl*	30	500	q 12
Cefaclor*	40	250	q 8
Cefuroxime-axetil*	30	250	q 12
Cefpodoxime-proxetil*	10	500	q 12
Cefprozil*	30	250	q 12
Cefixime	8	400	q 24
Ceftibuten	9	400	q 24
Erythromycin estolate[§]	40	250	q 8–12
Azithromycin[†]	12	250[‡]	q 24
Clarithromycin	15	500	q 12
Amoxicillin-clavulanate[¶]	45	875	q 12
Clindamycin[¶]	20–40	150	q 6–8

* Also effective against aerobic beta-lactamase–producing bacteria.
[†] Also effective against aerobic and anaerobic beta-lactamase–producing bacteria.
[‡] First-day dose is 500 mg.
[§] For *Corynebacterium diphtheriae*.
[¶] Duration of therapy is 5 days.

Table 18.3   Oral Antimicrobials in Treatment of Tonsillitis Caused by Group A Beta-Hemolytic Streptococci*

	Acute	Recurrent or Chronic	Carrier State
First-line therapy	Penicillin or amoxicillin	Clindamycin or amoxicillin–clavulanate	Clindamycin or penicillin + rifampin
Second-line therapy	Cephalosporins[†], clindamycin, amoxicillin–clavulanate, or macrolides[‡]	Metronidazole + macrolide or penicillin + rifampin	

* For dosages and length of therapy, see Table 18.2.
[†] All generations.
[‡] GABHS may be resistant.

is that the nonpathogenic α-hemolytic streptococci that compete with GABHS and help to eliminate them are more resistant to cephalosporins than they are to penicillin (35,36). Therefore, these streptococci are more likely to survive cephalosporin therapy.

The duration of therapy for acute tonsillitis with antimicrobial agents other than penicillin has not been determined in large, comparative, controlled studies. However, certain new agents have been administered in short courses of 5 or more days (37). Until a large number of comparative studies are performed, it is safe to use the same 10-day duration of therapy as with penicillin (*see* Tables 18.2 and 18.3). Early initiation of antimicrobial therapy results in faster resolution of signs and symptoms of disease (26–28). However, the spontaneous disappearance of fever and other symptoms occurs generally within 3 to 4 days after their onset even without antimicrobial therapy (37). Furthermore, acute rheumatic fever can be prevented even when therapy is postponed for up to 9 days (37).

When *C. diphtheriae* infection is suspected, erythromycin is the drug of choice (penicillin or rifampin are alternatives). Supportive therapy of PT includes giving antipyretic and analgesic agents (e.g., aspirin, acetaminophen) and ensuring proper hydration of the patient.

Recurrent and Chronic Tonsillitis

Studies have documented bacteriologic failure rates of 25% or more in penicillin-treated patients with acute GABHS tonsillitis and even higher rates in retreatment (38). Although approximately half of all patients who harbor GABHS after therapy may be carriers, the remainder still may show signs of infection and may represent true cases of clinical failure (39). The greater failure rates with penicillin have necessitated the consideration of alternative therapies for patients in whom penicillin therapy has failed.

Carriers harbor GABHS but have no immune response to these organisms (39). During the winter and spring, up to 20% of asymptomatic school-age children may be carriers of GABHS. They are less likely to spread these organisms and to suffer from complications of GABHS infection.

Carriers of GABHS generally do not require antimicrobial therapy (39,40). Exceptions include those who may spread the infection and those who have had a complication (e.g., rheumatic fever). It is often difficult to differentiate a carrier of GABHS from an infected individual. Antimicrobial agents that are effective in eradicating the carrier state are clindamycin and penicillin plus rifampin (*see* Table 18.3) (39).

Penicillin failure in eradicating PT caused by GABHS can have any of several explanations (Table 18.4). These include noncompliance with a 10-day course of therapy, existence of the carrier state (40), reinfection, bacterial internalization (41), bacterial interference (42), and penicillin tolerance (42). Another explanation is that repeated penicillin administration shifts the balance among the oral microflora, with the selection of β-lactamase–producing strains

Table 18.4   Possible Reasons for Antibiotic Failure or Relapse in Tonsillitis Caused by Group A Beta-Hemolytic Streptococci

Presence of beta-lactamase–producing oral microflora
Resistance (e.g., erythromycin) or tolerance (e.g., penicillin) to antibiotic
Inadequate bacterial interference or production of bacteriocins by oral flora (generally by alpha-hemolytic streptococci)
Bacterial internalization
Inappropriate dose, duration of therapy, or choice of antibiotic
Poor compliance with taking medication
Reacquisition from close contact or a fomite
Carrier state, not disease

of *S. aureus*, *Haemophilus* species, *Moraxella catarrhalis*, *Fusobacterium* species, pigmented *Prevotella* and *Porphyromonas* species, and *Bacteroides* species (5).

That BLPB were recovered more often from patients treated with penicillin and from their household contacts suggests a possible transfer of these organisms within families (43). The organisms persisted in the oral flora of more than a quarter of treated children for as long as 3 months after the initial finding. The recovery rate of BLPB infection in the community is highest during the winter season and in persons who have had recent antimicrobial therapy (44).

It is possible that BLPB protects GABHS from penicillin by inactivating the antibiotic (5). Such organisms, present in a localized soft-tissue infection, could degrade penicillin in the area of the infection, thereby protecting not only themselves but also penicillin-susceptible pathogens such as GABHS. Thus, penicillin therapy directed against a susceptible pathogen might be rendered ineffective.

An increase in the *in vitro* resistance of GABHS to penicillin was observed when GABHS was inoculated with *S. aureus*, *Haemophilus* species, and pigmented *Prevotella* and *Porphyromonas* species. (5). *Bacteroides* species protected a penicillin–sensitive GABHS from penicillin therapy in mice (45); however, both clindamycin and the combination of penicillin and clavulanic acid (a β-lactamase inhibitor), which are active against both GABHS and anaerobic Gram-negative bacilli, were effective in eradicating the infection.

Considerable clinical data support the role of BLPB in the failure of recurrent streptococcal tonsillitis to respond to penicillin therapy. Also supporting this theory is a correlation between colonization with BLPB prior to the administration of penicillin therapy and failure to respond to penicillin. Approximately one quarter of individuals who respond to penicillin harbored BLPB before penicillin therapy was begun, whereas almost 70% of patients in whom penicillin had failed carried BLPB before therapy (36,46). If sufficient amounts of β-lactamase are excreted into the tonsillar tissue, streptococci would be surrounded by enough enzyme to shield them from β-lactam antibiotics. In other studies, aerobic and anaerobic BLPB were recovered from more than three fourths of tonsils removed from patients with recurrent GABHS tonsillitis (47–49), and β-lactamase activity was detected in extracts of tonsillar tissues (50).

Several clinical studies demonstrated the superiority of linocomycin, clindamycin (51) and amoxicillin-clavulanic acid (38) over penicillin. Antimicrobial agents are effective against aerobic as well as anaerobic BLPB and GABHS in eradicating recurrent tonsillar infection. However, no studies have shown these agents to be superior to penicillin in treating acute tonsillitis. Other drugs that may be effective in treating recurrent tonsillitis are either the combination of penicillin plus rifampin or a macrolide (e.g., erythromycin) plus metronidazole (*see* Table 18.3).

Peritonsillar, Retropharyngeal, and Lateral Pharyngeal Abscesses

Peritonsillar, retropharyngeal, and lateral pharyngeal abscesses are deep neck infections that generally result from the contiguous spread of infection from local sites. They share some clinical features but have distinct manifestations and complications (Table 18.5). All three types of abscess are potentially life threatening if not recognized early.

Etiology

Most deep abscesses are caused by polymicrobial infections; the average number of isolates from such lesions is 5 (range 1–10) (52–57). Predominant anaerobic organisms recovered in peritonsillar (56–58), lateral pharyngeal (55,58), and retropharyngeal (54,58) abscesses are *Prevotella, Porphyromonas, Fusobacterium,* and *Peptostreptococcus* species; aerobic organisms are group A streptococci (e.g., *S. pyogenes*), *S. aureus,* and *H. influenzae.* Anaerobic bacteria can be isolated from most abscesses, whereas *S. pyogenes* is isolated in only approximately one third of cases (53–56). More than two thirds of deep neck abscesses contain BLPB (53–55). *Fusobacterium necrophorum* is especially associated with deep neck infections that cause septic thrombophlebitis of great vessels and metastatic abscesses (Lemierre's syndrome) (59,60). Rarely, *Mycobacterium tuberculosis* (61), atypical mycobacteria, or *Coccidioides immitis* (62)

Table 18.5 Clinical Features of Peritonsillar, Retropharyngeal, and Pharyngeal Abscesses

Abscess Type	Age	Sites of Origin	Location	Clinical Findings	Complications/ Extension Site	Management
Peritonsillar abscess	Adolescents, adults	Tonsillitis	Tonsillar capsule and space below superior constrictor muscle	Swelling on one tonsil, displacement of the uvula, trismus, muffled voice	Spontaneous rupture and aspiration, spread to pterygomaxillary space	Antibiotic, surgical drainage
Retropharyngeal abscess	Usually <4 years	Pharyngitis, trauma, dental infection	Between posterior pharynx and prevertebral fascia	Unilateral posterior pharyngeal bulging, hyperextension of the neck, drooling, respiratory distress	Spontaneous rupture and aspiration, spread to posterior mediastinum and/or parapharyngeal space	Antibiotics, surgical drainage, artificial airway
Lateral pharyngeal abscess	Older children, adolescents, adults	Tonsillitis, otitis media, mastoiditis, parotitis, dental manipulation	Anterior and posterior pharyngomaxillary space	Anterior compartment: swelling of parotid area, trismus, prolapse of the tonsil/tonsillar fossa. Posterior compartment: septicemia; minimal pain or trismus	Carotid erosion; airway obstruction; spread intracranially, to lung, to mediastinum; septicemia	Antibiotics, surgical drainage, artificial airway

is isolated. Specimens should be collected during surgical drainage and should be transported, inoculated, and incubated to optimize the recovery of aerobic and anaerobic organisms.

Antimicrobial Therapy

The recovery of BLPB from most abscesses mandates the use of antimicrobial agents effective against these organisms. BLPB include *Prevotella, Fusobacterium, Haemophilus,* and *Staphylococcus* species. Antimicrobial agents with expected efficacy include cefoxitin, a carbapenem (e.g., imipenem, meropenem), the combination of penicillin (e.g., ticarcillin) and a β-lactamase inhibitor (e.g., clavulanate), chloramphenicol, or clindamycin (Table 18.6). The duration of therapy varies from 7 to 21 days and can be reduced in the presence of adequate drainage. Antimicrobial therapy can abort abscess formation if given at an early stage of infection. However, when pus has formed, antimicrobial therapy is effective only in conjunction with adequate surgical drainage.

Peritonsillar Abscess (Quinsy)

Peritonsillar abscess is the most common deep head and neck infection. It generally occurs in adolescents and adults as a complication of repeated episodes of bacterial tonsillitis; it can occur infrequently as a secondary complication of viral infection, such as infectious mononucleosis. The most common location is the superior pole of the tonsil.

Table 18.6   Antimicrobial Agents with Expected Efficacy in Treatment of Oropharyngeal Abscesses*

Cefoxitin (from 1 g every 8 hours to 2 g every 4 hours IM or IV)

Cefotetan (1–3 g every 12 hours IV)

Clindamycin (0.30–0.45 g every 6 hours PO or 600–900 mg every 8 hours IV or IM)

Metronidazole (7.5 mg/kg every 6 hours; maximum 4 g/d IV or PO) plus β-lactam–resistant penicillin (e.g., oxacillin 1–2 g every 4 hours IV or IM)

A carbapenem (e.g., imipenem 0.5 g every 6 hours IV, meropenem 0.5–1.0 g every 8 hours IV)

A combination of a penicillin (e.g., amoxicillin 875 mg every 12 hours PO, ampicillin 1.5–3.0 g every 6 hours IV, piperacillin 3.375 g every 6 hours IV) and a beta-lactamase inhibitor (e.g., clavulanate, sulbactam, tazobactam)

Chloramphenicol (50 mg/kg IV)

IM = intramuscularly; IV = intravenously; PO = orally.
* Adult dosages.

Clinical Manifestations

A peritonsillar abscess is often preceded by acute PT; either an afebrile interval of a few days can occur or fever from the primary infection can persist. Quinsy is usually unilateral. The patient can be apprehensive and pale, and his or her temperature and pulse rate rise (often after a rigor). There is difficulty in swallowing and/or speaking. Pain increases in severity, radiates to the ear, and causes trismus resulting from spasm of the pterygoid muscle. The breath has a foul odor, and saliva may dribble from the mouth. The tonsil is swollen and inflamed, but the soft palate does not bulge. The uvula is edematous and is pushed toward the opposite side. The involved tonsil is usually hidden by the swelling but can have some mucopurulent secretions on it surface. Ipsilateral cervical lymph nodes are enlarged and tender. When the peritonsillar abscess has developed, there is acute pain on one side of the throat and considerable constitutional disturbance. If not reversed by antibiotic therapy or surgical drainage, the abscess can leak slowly or burst, possibly leading to aspiration.

Treatment

The treatment of choice for a peritonsillar abscess is needle aspiration of the abscess under topical anesthesia combined with the administration of parenteral antimicrobial therapy. The antimicrobial agents used in this treatment have been discussed previously (*see* Table 18.6). Emergency tonsillectomy is also an option. Patients with peritonsillar abscess and a history of recurrent tonsillitis should be considered for tonsillectomy after the acute episode subsides (63).

Retropharyngeal Abscess

A retropharyngeal abscess often follows bacterial pharyngitis or nasopharyngitis. Rarely is it an extension of vertebral osteomyelitis, the result of a wound infection after a penetrating injury of the posterior pharynx, or a complication of endoscopy, a dental procedure, or other medical or surgical trauma.

Clinical Manifestations

The patient with a retropharyngeal abscess generally suffers first from acute pharyngitis or nasopharyngitis with a high fever of sudden onset, difficulty in swallowing, and associated drooling, dysphagia, dyspnea, and neck pain and hyperextension. Usually, anterior bulging of the posterior pharyngeal wall is observed, often to one side of the midline. Nasal obstruction can follow, and signs of difficulty in breathing can dominate the clinical picture (*see* Table 18.5). Cervical lymphadenopathy is often present (64).

The oropharynx can be examined carefully only in a cooperative patient. Using indirect (mirror) hypopharyngeal inspection and digital palpation, the patient should be examined in the Trendelenburg position; adequate suction equipment should be available in the event that the abscess ruptures.

A lateral radiograph of the nasopharynx and neck may reveal the retropharyngeal mass. Chest radiography can identify extension into the mediastinum. Computed tomography with contrast medium may distinguish neck cellulitis from deep neck abscess and may identify the extension of an abscess and any involvement of vascular structures.

The differential diagnosis of retropharyngeal abscess includes cervical osteomyelitis, meningitis, Pott's disease, and calcified tendonitis of the longus colli muscle.

Treatment

Drainage of a retropharyngeal abscess and the intravenous administration of antimicrobial agents are needed (65). The agents used in this therapy have been discussed previously (*see* Table 18.6). Most abscesses can be evacuated by peroral incision and suction. External incision is rarely required but is often needed when the abscess is longitudinally extensive or when fever persists after peroral drainage. Tracheostomy may be needed when the risk of airway obstruction is great. Complications of a retropharyngeal abscess include aspiration, extension of infection to the side of the neck, and dissection into the posterior mediastinum. Death can occur from aspiration, obstruction of the airway, erosion into major blood vessels, or extension to the mediastinum.

Lateral Pharyngeal Abscess

Involvement of the lateral pharyngeal (anterior and posterior pharyngomaxillary) space determines the clinical manifestations and complications of abscesses in these locations.

Clinical Manifestations

Infection of the lateral pharyngeal space can be the result of tonsillitis, pharyngitis, otitis media, mastoiditis (Bezold's abscess), parotitis, or dental infections (usually of the mastication space).

Infection in the anterior compartment usually is accompanied by high fever, chills, tender swelling below the angle of the mandible, induration and erythema of the side of the neck, and trismus. Most patients are acutely ill and have odynophagia, dysphagia, and mild dyspnea. A bulge in the lateral pharyngeal wall can be seen, but the tonsil size is normal. Torticollis toward the side of the abscess (due to muscle spasm) is often seen, as is cervical lymphadenitis. The classic triad of pharyngomaxillary abscess occurs only in anterior-compartment syndrome and consists of 1) prolapse of the tonsils and tonsillar fossa, 2) trismus, and 3) swelling of the parotid area. Signs of septicemia, with minimal pain or trismus, characterize infection in the posterior compartment. Swelling can be overlooked because it is deep behind the palatopharyngeal arch. Indirect laryngoscopy can reveal ipsilateral obliteration of the pyriform sinus. A tender, high cervical mass can be palpated.

The most frequent complications of infection in the posterior compartment include the following (64,66):

- Respiratory distress
- Laryngeal edema
- Airway obstruction
- Septicemia
- Pneumonia
- Septic thrombosis of the internal jugular vein with metastatic abscesses (Lemierre's syndrome)
- Intracranial extension (causing meningitis, brain abscess, and cavernous and lateral sinus thrombosis)
- Erosion of the carotid artery

Carotid artery erosion can cause bleeding from the external auditory canal. Additionally, abscess dissection through the junction of the cartilaginous external canal and bone can cause suppurative otorrhea. Extension of infection inferiorly along the carotid sheath or posteriorly into the retropharyngeal space can lead to mediastinitis. Computed tomography or magnetic resonance imaging can delineate the affected structures and any vascular complications.

Treatment

Drainage of the lateral neck in conjunction with appropriate high-dose intravenous antimicrobial therapy is needed for treating a lateral pharyngeal abscess. The antimicrobial agents used in this treatment have been discussed previously (*see* Table 18.6). An external excision below the angle of the jaw is preferred because it provides access to the carotid artery, which should be ligated in case of arterial erosion. Surgical drainage is best performed after the infection has been localized, unless a hemorrhage or respiratory obstruction necessitates earlier intervention. Tracheostomy may be required prophylactically. Airway obstruction caused by laryngeal edema can develop abruptly.

Epiglottitis

Epiglottitis (or supraglottitis) is usually a bacterial infection of the supraglottic area that primarily affects the epiglottis but can also affect the arytenoids and the aryepiglottic areas. Swelling of the epiglottis can cause laryngeal obstruction. Epiglottitis is most common in children under 5 years of age and is characterized by several upper respiratory tract infections that may progress rapidly to fatal obstruction.

Etiology

Viral infection can precede bacterial epiglottitis. Edema of the supraglottic structures, which can obstruct the airway, then progresses rapidly. Rarely, infection spreads to the paraglottic space. Infection can be associated with transient bacteremia (in up to 90% in patients with *H. influenzae* type b). Circulatory collapse is unusual and is caused by hypoxia and dehydration. Pulmonary edema occurs in approximately one quarter of patients due to negative intrathoracic pressure generated with obstruction of the extrathoracic airway.

Epiglottis is generally caused by encapsulated bacteria (67,68). It has been postulated that a viral respiratory tract infection permits local invasiveness of an organism that previously colonized the airway asymptomatically. *H. influenzae* type b was the predominant cause of epiglottitis before infants were universally immunized against it (67,68), and epiglottitis with bacteremia caused by other organisms was uncommon. The incidence of epiglottitis has fallen dramatically in the past decade (69). The organisms now recovered are *S. pneumoniae*, *S. aureus*, nontypeable *H. influenzae*, *H. parainfluenzae*, and β-hemolytic streptococci (groups A, B, and C) (70).

Clinical Manifestations

The diagnosis of epiglottitis is suspected on the basis of signs of upper airway obstruction (e.g., inspiratory stridor, hoarseness, barking cough, retractions) (71). In the young child, acute epiglottitis is a fulminant illness characterized by high fever of acute onset, dyspnea, rapidly progressive respiratory obstruction (within hours), and prostration. Aphonia, drooling, and respiratory distress accompany stridor. In an older child, sore throat and dysphagia generally are followed rapidly by progressive respiratory distress and the sensation of suffocation. Cough and hoarseness usually are not present. The child appears toxic but sits still with his or her chin up, neck hyperextended, hands extended behind the body in a tripod position, mouth open, and tongue protruding. Progression of epiglottitis to a shock-like condition characterized by cyanosis, pallor, and impaired consciousness can occur rapidly.

Diagnosis

In a cooperative patient who willingly opens his or her mouth, epiglottitis can be diagnosed by visualizing a cherry-red, swollen epiglottis arising at the base of the tongue. If the diagnosis is suspected, indirect visualization by laryngoscopy should be performed urgently in a controlled setting by skilled individuals who have the facility and intention to perform intubation (or tracheostomy if necessary) (72,73). Differentiation among causes of infectious upper airway obstruction is facilitated by careful attention to the history of the patient's illness, physical findings, and the context of the illness in the family and community. Life-saving management depends on accurate diagnosis. A lateral neck radiograph can be made before examination in cases of suspected epiglottitis if the child's clinical state is favorable; this can be done rapidly and without agitating the child in the presence of individuals who are skilled and prepared for resuscitation. If the clinical presentation suggests epiglottitis, visualization of the epiglottitis and intubation should not be delayed by radiography. A lateral neck film shows a thickening of the epiglottis (thumb sign) and aryepiglottic folds in the presence of an apparently normal laryngeal ventricle and subglottic airway.

Both blood and epiglottis swab cultures (taken at the time of intubation) usually yield positive results when *H. influenzae* type b is the etiologic organism. Gram stain and culture of an epiglottis swab specimen can confirm other bacterial causes. Blood cultures are variably positive.

Treatment

Maintenance of adequate respiratory exchange is of primary importance in cases of epiglottitis and requires careful observation and monitoring of the patient for signs of increasing obstruction or fatigue. Complete airway obstruction is the major risk in acute epiglottitis. An artificial airway should be secured, preferably by nasotracheal intubation or, in extreme cases, by cricothyrotomy (74); tracheostomy is rarely required. Establishing an artificial airway is best done in the operating room under halothane anesthesia. Oxygen should be given until intubation is complete, and the child should be kept calm in a parent's arms. In addition to establishing an airway, antimicrobial therapy is required. Cefuroxime 200 mg/kg/d or ceftriaxone 100 mg/kg/d are appropriate for initial therapy. Improvement in respiratory distress is immediate after an artificial airway is secured. Fever and toxicity subside over 24 to 72 hours, and extubation is usually accomplished within 72 hours (75).

Prevention

When *H. influenzae* type b is the agent responsible for epiglottitis, a 4-day course of rifampin (20 mg/kg/d in a single dose; 600 mg maximum) should be administered prophylactically to all household contacts of the patient if anyone in the household is younger than 4 years of age and has not been immunized completely (the patient also should receive a 4-day course of rifampin after completing his or her initial course of antimicrobial therapy). All contacts of the patient should be instructed about the signs and symptoms of *H. influenzae* infection, because it can occur, albeit rarely, in older individuals. Immunization of all children with conjugated *H. influenzae* type b polysaccharide vaccine reduces the incidences of *H. influenzae* epiglottitis.

REFERENCES

1. **Bisno AL.** Acute pharyngitis: etiology and diagnosis. *Pediatrics.* 1996; 97(Suppl): 949–54.

2. **Tsevat J, Kotagal UR.** Management of sore throats in children: a cost-effectiveness analysis. *Postgrad Med J.* 1999;75:141–4.

3. **Brook I, Leavy F.** Immune response to *Fusobacterium nucleatum* and *Prevotella melaninogenica* in patients with infectious mononucleosis. *J Med Microbiol.* 1996;44:131–4.

4. **Brook I.** Bacterial interference. *Crit Rev Microbiol.* 1999;25:155–72.

5. **Brook I.** The role of β-lactamase–producing bacteria in the persistence of streptococcal tonsillar infection. *Rev Infect Dis.* 1984;6:601–7.

6. **Cimolai N, Elford RW, Bryan L, et al.** Do the β-hemolytic non–group A streptococci cause pharyngitis? *Rev Infect Dis.* 1988;10:587–601.

7. **Turner JC, Hayden GF, Kiselica D, et al.** Association of group C β-hemolytic streptococci with endemic pharyngitis among college students. *JAMA.* 1990;264:2644–7.

8. **Turner JC, Hayden FG, Lobo MC, et al.** Epidemiologic evidence for Lancefield group C β-hemolytic streptococci as a cause of exudative pharyngitis in college students. *J Clin Microbiol.* 1997;35:1–4.

9. **Gerber MA, Randolph MF, Martin NJ, et al.** Community-wide outbreak of group G streptococcal pharyngitis. *Pediatrics.* 1991;87:598–603.

10. **Davies HD, McGreer A, Schwartz B, et al.** Invasive group A streptococcal infections in Ontario, Canada. *N Engl J Med.* 1996;335:547–54.

11. **Chowdhury MN, Kambal AM, al-Eissa YA, et al.** Non-group A streptococci: Are they pathogens in the throat? *J R Soc Health.* 1997;117:160–3.

12. **Mackenzie A, Fuite LA, Chan FT, et al.** Incidence and pathogenicity of *Arcanobacterium haemolyticum* during a 2-year study in Ottawa. *Clin Infect Dis.* 1995;21:177–81.

13. **Brook I, Foote PA Jr, Stote J, Johnson W:** Immune response to *Prevotella intermedia* in patients with recurrent nonstreptococcal tonsillitis. *Ann Otolol Rhinol Laryngol.* 1993; 102:113–6.

14. **Rosbery T.** *Microorganisms Indigenous to Man.* New York: McGraw-Hill; 1962.

15. **Brook I, Frazier EH, Thompson DH.** Aerobic and anaerobic bacteriology of peritonsillar abscess. *Laryngoscope.* 1991;101:289–92.

16. **Kaplan D.** Acute necrotizing ulcerative tonsillitis and gingivitis (Vincent's infections). *Ann Emerg Med.* 1981;10:593–5.

17. **Brook I, Foote PA.** Microbiology of "normal" tonsils. *Ann Otol Rhinol Laryngol.* 1990; 99:980–3.

18. **Brook I, Yocum P.** Comparison of the microbiology of Group A streptococcal and non–Group A streptococcal tonsillitis. *Ann Otol Rhino Laryngol.* 1988;97:243–6.

19. **Brook I, Foote PA, Slots J.** Immune response to anaerobic bacteria in patients with peritonsillar cellulitis and abscess. *Acta Otolaryngol.* 1996;116:888–9.

20. **Breese BB.** A simple scorecard for the tentative diagnosis of streptococcal pharyngitis. *Am J Dis Child.* 1977;131:514–7.

21. **Roddey OF Jr, Clegg HW, Martin ES, et al.** Comparison of throat culture methods for the recovery of group A streptococci in a pediatric office setting. *JAMA.* 1995;274:1863–5.

22. **Pacifico L, Ranucci A, Ravagnan G, Chiesa C.** Relative value of selective group A streptococcal agar incubated under different atmospheres. *J Clin Microbiol.* 1995;33:2480–2.

23. **Kellogg JA.** Suitability of throat culture procedures for detection of group A streptococci and as reference standards for evaluation of streptococcal antigen detection kits. *J Clin Microbiol.* 1990;28:165–9.

24. **Ederer GM, Herrmann MM, Bruce R, et al.** Rapid extraction method with pronase for grouping β-hemolytic streptococci. *Appl Microbiol.* 1972;23:285–8.

25. **Murray PR, Wold AD, Hall MM, Washington JA II.** Bacitracin differentiation for presumptive identification of group A β-hemolytic streptococci: comparison of primary and purified plate testing. *J Pediatr.* 1976;89:576–9.

26. **Pichiahero ME.** Group A beta-hemolytic streptococcal infections. *Pediatr Rev.* 1998:19:291–302.

27. **Randolph MF, Gerber MA, DeMeo KK, Wright L.** Effect of antibiotic therapy on the clinical course of streptococcal pharyngitis. *J Pediatr.* 1985;106:870–5.

28. **Krober MS, Bass JW, Michels GN.** Streptococcal pharyngitis: placebo-controlled double-blind evaluation of clinical response to penicillin therapy. *JAMA.* 1985;253:1271–4.

29. **Holbrook T.** Rapid strep tests in the pediatric clinical setting. *J Pediatr Nurs.* 1998;13:131–3.

30. **Lieu TA, Fleisher GR, Schwartz JS.** Clinical evaluation of a latex agglutination test for streptococcal pharyngitis: performance and impact on treatment rates. *Pediatr Infect Dis J.* 1988;7:847–54.

31. **Gerber MA.** Comparison of throat cultures and rapid strep tests for diagnosis of streptococcal pharyngitis. *Pediatr Infect Dis.* 1989;8:820–4.

32. **Denny FW, Wannamaker LW, Brink WR, et al.** Prevention of rheumatic fever: Treatment of the preceding streptococci infection. *JAMA.* 1950;143:151–3.

33. **Seppala H, Klaukka T, Vuopio-Varkila J, et al.** The effect of changes in the consumption of macrolide antibiotics on erythromycin resistance in group A streptococci in Finland. *N Engl J Med.* 1997;337:441–6.

34. **Pichichero ME, Margolis PA.** A comparison of cephalosporins and penicillins in the treatment of group A β-hemolytic streptococcal pharyngitis: a meta-analysis supporting the concept of microbial copathogenicity. *Pediatr Infect Dis J.* 1991;10:275–281.

35. **Brook I, Gilmore JD.** Evaluation of bacterial interference and β-lactamase production in the management of experimental infection with group A β-hemolytic streptococci. *Antimicrob Agents Chemother* 1993;37:1452–5.

36. **Brook I, Gober EA.** Role of bacterial interference and β–lactamase–producing bacteria in the failure of penicillin to eradicate group A streptococcal pharyngotonsillitis. *Arch Otolaryngol Head Neck Surg.* 1995;121:1405–9.

37. **Pichichero ME, Cohen R.** Shortened course of antibiotic therapy for acute otitis media, sinusitis, and tonsillopharyngitis. *Pediatr Infect Dis J.* 1997;16:680–95.

38. **Kaplan EL, Johnson DR.** Eradication of group A streptococci from the upper respiratory tract by amoxicillin with clavulanate after oral penicillin V treatment failure. *J Pediatr.* 1988;113:400–3.

39. **Tanz RR, Poncher JR, Croydon KE, et al.** Clindamycin treatment of chronic pharyngeal carriage of group A streptococci. *J Pediatr.* 1991;119:123–8.

40. **Kaplan EL, Gastanaduy AS, Huwe BB.** The role of the carrier in treatment failures after antibiotic therapy for group A streptococci in the upper respiratory tract. *J Lab Clin Med.* 1981;98:326–35.

41. **Neeman R, Keller N, Barzilai A, et al.** Prevalence of internalisation-associated gene, prtF1, among persisting group A streptococcus strains isolated from asymptomatic carriers. *Lancet.* 1998;352:1974–7.

42. **Grahn E, Holm SE, Roos K.** Penicillin tolerance in β–streptococci isolated from patients with tonsilitis. *Scand J Infect Dis.* 1987;19:421–6.

43. **Brook I, Gober AE.** Emergence of β–lactamase–producing aerobic and anaerobic bacteria in the oropharynx of children following penicillin chemotherapy. *Clin Pediatr.* 1984;23:338–41.

44. **Brook I, Gober AE.** Monthly changes in the rate of recovery of penicillin-resistant organisms from children. *Pediatr Infect Dis J.* 1997;16:255–7.

45. **Brook I, Pazzaglia G, Coolbaugh JC, et al.** *In vivo* protection of Group A β–hemolytic streptococci from penicillin by β–lactamase–producing *Bacteroides* species. *J Antimicrob Chemother.* 1983;12:599-606.

46. **Brook I.** Role of β-lactamase–producing bacteria in penicillin failure to eradicate group A streptococci. *Pediatr Infect Dis.* 1985;4:491–495.

47. **Brook I, Yocum P, Friedman EM.** Aerobic and anaerobic bacteria in tonsils of children with recurrent tonsillitis. *Ann Otol Rhinol Laryngol.* 1981;90:261–3.

48. **Tuner K, Nord CE.** β-Lactamase–producing anaerobic bacteria in recurrent tonsillitis. *J Antimicrob Chemother.* 1982;10:153–6.

49. **Rajasuo A, Jousimies-Somer H, Savolainen S, et al.** Bacteriologic findings in tonsillitis and pericoronitis. *Clin Infect Dis.* 1996;23:51–60.

50. **Brook I, Yocum P.** Quantitative measurement of β-lactamase level in tonsils of children with recurrent tonsillitis. *Acta Otolaryngol Scand.* 1984;98:446–60.

51. **Brook I, Hirokawa R.** Treatment of patients with a history of recurrent tonsillitis due to group A β-hemolytic streptococci. *Clin Pediatr.* 1985;24:331–5.

52. **Finegold SM.** *Anaerobic Bacteria in Human Disease.* New York: Academic Press; 1977.

53. **Brook I, Frazier EH, Thompson DH.** Aerobic and anaerobic bacteriology of peritonsillar abscess. *Laryngoscope.* 1991;101:289–92.

54. **Brook I.** Microbiology of retropharyngeal abscesses in children. *Am J Dis Child.* 1987;141:202–4.

55. **Brook I.** Microbiology of abscesses of the head and neck in children. *Am Otol Rhinol Laryngol.* 1987;96:429–33.

56. **Jokipii AMM, Jokipii L, Sipila P, et al.** Semiquantitative culture results and pathogenic significance of obligate anaerobes in peritonsillar abscesses. *J Clin Microbiol.* 1988;26:957–61.

57. **Mitchelmore IJ, Prior AJ, Montgomery PQ, Tabaqchali S.** Microbiological features and pathogenesis of peritonsillar abscesses. *Eur J Clin Microbiol Infect Dis.* 1995;14: 870–7.

58. **Asmar BI.** Bacteriology of retropharyngeal abscess in children. *Pediatr Infect Dis J.* 1990;9:595–6.

59. **Hughes CE, Spear RK, Shinabarger CE, et al.** Septic pulmonary emboli complicating mastoiditis: Lemierre's syndrome. *Clin Infect Dis.* 1994;18:633–5.

60. **Golpe R, Marin B, Alonso M.** Lemierre's syndrome (necrobacillosis). *Postgrad Med J.* 1999;75:141–4.

61. **Mathur NN, Bais AS.** Tubercular retropharyngeal abscess in early childhood. *Indian J Pediatr.* 1997;64:898–901.

62. **Barratt GE, Koopmann CF, Coulthard SW.** Retropharyngeal abscess: a 10-year experience. *Laryngoscope.* 1984;94:455–63.

63. **Friedman NR, Mitchell RB, Pereira KD, et al.** Peritonsillar abscess in early childhood: presentation and management. *Arch Otolaryngol Head Neck Surg.* 1997;123:630–2.

64. **Blomquist IK, Bayer AS.** Life-threatening deep fascial space infections of the head and neck. *Infect Dis Clin North Am.* 1988;2:237–64.

65. **Gidley PW, Ghorayeb BY, Stiernberg CM.** Contemporary management of deep neck space infections. *Otolaryngol Head Neck Surg.* 1997;116:16–22.

66. **Chen MK, Wen YS, Chang CC, et al.** Predisposing factors of life-threatening deep neck infection: logistic regression analysis of 214 cases. *J Otolaryngol.* 1998;27:141–4.

67. **Brilli RJ, Benzing G, Cotcamp DH.** Epiglottitis in infants less than two years of age. *Pediatr Emerg Care.* 1989;5:16–21.

68. **Losek JD, Dewitz-Zink BA, Melzer-Lange M, et al.** Epiglottitis: comparison of signs and symptoms in children less than 2 years old and older. *Ann Emerg Med.* 1990;19:99–102.

69. **Garpenholt O, Hugosson S, Fredlund H, et al.** Epiglottitis in Sweden before and after introduction of vaccination against *Haemophilus influenzae* type b. *Pediatr Infect Dis J.* 1999;18:490–3.

70. **Solomon P, Weisbrod M, Irish JC, Gullane PJ.** Adult epiglottitis: the Toronto Hospital experience. *J Otolaryngol.* 1998;27:332–6.

71. **Skolnik NS.** Treatment of croup: a critical review. *Am J Dis Child.* 1989;143:1045–9.

72. **Baugh R, Gilmore BB.** Infectious croup: a critical review. *Otolaryngol Head Neck Surg.* 1986;95:40–6.

73. **Custer JR.** Croup and related disorders. *Pediatr Rev.* 1993;14:19–29.

74. **Park KW, Darvish A, Lowenstein E.** Airway management for adult patients with acute epiglottitis: a 12-year experience at an academic medical center (1984–1995). *Anesthesiology.* 1998;88:254–61.0

75. **Damm M, Eckel HE, Jungehulsing M, Roth B.** Management of acute inflammatory childhood stridor. *Otolaryngol Head Neck Surg.* 1999;121:633–8.

19

Sinusitis and Otitis

David H. Canaday, MD

Robert A. Salata, MD

Sinusitis

Sinusitis, an inflammatory disorder of the mucosal lining of the paranasal sinuses, is a common infection in both children and adults. Most cases complicate the common cold or other upper respiratory infections (URI), with
occasional cases associated with dental infection (maxillary sinuses). An understanding of the epidemiology, pathophysiology, microbiology, and clinical
manifestations of sinusitis is essential for its early diagnosis and effective treatment, and to prevent life-threatening complications or chronic sequelae.

Etiology

The paranasal sinuses are air-filled cavities lined with ciliated pseudocolum-
nar epithelial tissue. They are connected indirectly with the nasal cavity
through small ostia that drain into this cavity. The frontal, anterior ethmoidal,
and maxillary sinuses open into the middle meatus, whereas the posterior ethmoidal and sphenoid sinuses open into the superior meatus.

The paranasal sinuses are generally considered to be sterile. Microorganisms frequently find access to the paranasal sinuses, since the upper respiratory tract, the oropharynx, and certain parts of the ears and eyes are
anatomically adjacent to these sinuses and are usually heavily populated with
colonizing flora. Patent ostia and normal mucociliary function are the keys to
maintaining aeration and mucosal defenses of the sinuses. The cilia of the epithelium of the paranasal sinuses, contiguous with the nasal cavity, beat to-

ward the ostia and clear the sinuses. Secretory immunoglobulins and an intact epithelium serve as additional barriers to infection. Conditions that impair ostial patency, mucociliary function, epithelial integrity, or normal immune defenses are the major factors predisposing to sinusitis (Table 19.1).

Clinical Manifestations

Most cases of acute, community-acquired sinusitis are superimposed on an existing viral URI, and their clinical features reflect a dual infection. Acute sinusitis complicates approximately 0.5% to 2% of URI (1). Eighty-seven percent of patients with the common cold have some sinus cavity disease. In children, the most common symptoms of acute sinusitis are cough (80%), nasal discharge (76%), and fever (63%). In adults, purulent nasal discharge and facial pain are the major manifestations, with fever occurring in less than 20% of cases. One of the most consistent features of acute sinusitis is the occurrence of cold symptoms persisting either for more than a week or longer than the usual course for the individual patient. Other reported symptoms are postnasal drainage, pain with mastication, hyposmia, nasal congestion, and worsening pain on leaning

Table 19.1   Risk Factors That Predispose to Sinusitis

Obstruction of the Sinus Ostia
Viral upper respiratory infection
Allergic rhinitis
Rhinitis medicamentosa
Anatomical abnormalities (e.g., deviated nasal septum, polyp, tumor, foreign body)

Impaired Mucociliary Function or Disrupted Epithelial Integrity
Viral upper respiratory infection
Cold or dry air
Chemicals, drugs, and smoke
Cystic fibrosis or ciliary dysmotility syndromes

Immune Defects
IgA deficiency
IgG_{2a} or IgG_4 subclass deficiency
Neutropenia
AIDS
Corticosteroids or cytotoxic drugs

Increased Microbial Invasion
Odontogenic infections
Nasotracheal intubation
Head trauma
Swimming or diving
Cocaine sniffing

forward. From 5% to 10% of cases of acute maxillary sinusitis have a dental origin. Acute sinusitis has a duration of 4 weeks or less.

Headaches or a sensation of pressure are prominent features of frontal sinusitis, since a branch of the ophthalmic division of the trigeminal nerve supplies this area of the head. The superior alveolar nerves supply both the molar teeth and the mucosa of the maxillary sinus. Toothache can occur with maxillary sinusitis. Severe, intractable headache is seen with sphenoid sinusitis, and can mimic ophthalmic migraine or trigeminal neuralgia. Depressed mental status, clinical signs of meningeal irritation, and palsies of structures served by the third, fourth, and fifth cranial nerves suggest the extension of infection to the cavernous sinus. Edema of the eyelids and excessive tearing are prominent features of ethmoidal sinusitis. Retro-orbital pain and proptosis indicate orbital extension of sinus infection.

Subacute sinusitis (lasting from 1 to 3 months) and chronic sinusitis (lasting more than 3 months) generally present with symptoms that are less severe but more protracted than those of acute sinusitis. Fatigue and malaise are more prominent than local nasal or sinus symptoms. Frequently, patients with chronic sinusitis have a dental cause of infection. Fungal sinusitis is often a more chronic condition that more often presents with pressure-related symptoms. Nasal polyps are commonly encountered in chronic maxillary sinusitis. Chronic sinusitis may mimic asthma, allergic rhinitis, or chronic bronchitis.

Diagnosis

Most cases of sinusitis are caused by bacterial infection (2,3). Sinus aspiration is the most accurate diagnostic method. The results of nasal swab cultures correlate with those of sinus aspirate cultures in less than 65% of cases. The microbiology of sinusitis depends on the chronicity of infection, on whether the infection was acquired from the community or was nosocomial, and on the patient's age and underlying status (Table 19.2).

The diagnosis of sinusitis is most often based on clinical presentation. It is often a challenge to distinguish infectious from allergic and other noninfectious sources of the condition. An allergic etiology can usually be identified from a history of paroxysmal sneezing, allergen exposure, itching eyes, and similar prior occurrences.

Transillumination of the sinuses may be a helpful bedside diagnostic procedure for sinusitis. The finding of complete sinus opacity is highly suggestive of infection, whereas normal light transmission indicates the absence of infection.

Radiologic evaluation is a common, noninvasive diagnostic modality for sinusitis (Fig. 19.1). Abnormal radiologic findings of complete sinus opacification, an air–fluid level, or mucosal thickening (> 4 mm in children, > 5 mm in adults) are indicative of infection as established by sinus aspiration in 75% of

Table 19.2   Microbiology of Acute Community-Acquired Maxillary Sinusitis

Organism	Mean Percentage of Cases (Range)	
	Adults	Children
Bacteria		
Streptococcus pneumoniae	31 (20–35)	36
Haemophilus influenzae (unencapsulated)	21 (6–26)	23
S. pneumoniae and H. influenzae	5 (1–9)	—
Anaerobes	6 (0–10)	—
S. aureus	4 (0–8)	—
S. pyogenes	2 (1–3)	2
Moraxella catarrhalis	2	19
Gram-negative bacilli	9 (0–24)	2
Viruses		
Rhinovirus	15	—
Influenza virus	5	—
Parainfluenza virus	3	2
Adenovirus	—	2

Adapted from Gwaltney JM Jr. Acute community-acquired sinusitis. *Clin Infect Dis.* 1996;23:1209–23.

cases, whereas a normal radiograph correlates with a negative aspirate in 80% of cases (4). Radiology is less useful in cases of chronic sinusitis because of persistent abnormalities, and in infants under 12 months of age because of redundant sinus mucosa and asymmetry of sinus development. Limited-view computed tomography (CT), a very sensitive means of diagnosing sinus abnormalities, is recommended over plain sinus radiography because of similar cost (*see* Fig. 19.1). CT scanning has a role in chronic sinusitis in helping to differentiate bacterial from fungal disease, with bone destruction sometimes seen in the latter.

Sinus aspiration is considered the gold standard procedure for the diagnosis of sinusitis. The maxillary sinus can be easily accessed intranasally below the inferior turbinate. The frontal sinus can be approached below the rim of the eye. Table 19.3 summarizes the indications for sinus aspiration. Quantitative cultures can be useful in distinguishing true infection from colonization.

Most cases of sinus infection are of bacterial origin. The predominant common organisms are *Streptococcus pneumoniae* and *Haemophilus influenzae*, which together are responsible for more than 50% of cases of acute maxillary sinusitis in both children and adults. In children, *Moraxella catarrhalis* is another common pathogen. Recovery of anaerobes in acute sinusitis should prompt an investigation for an odontogenic source of infection. Anaerobes are also more commonly encountered in cases of chronic sinusitis. *Staphylococcus aureus*, although a common nasal colonist, is an uncommon cause of community ac-

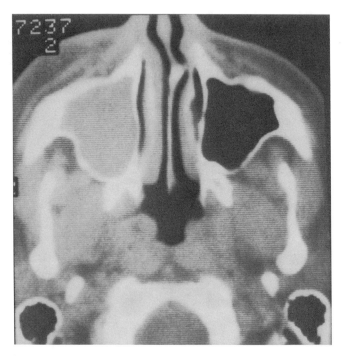

Figure 19.1   Computed tomography scan of sinusitis that shows opacification of the right maxillary sinus.

quired maxillary sinusitis. However, *S. aureus* and streptococci are major pathogens in sphenoid sinusitis. The sinuses also have been reported to serve as reservoirs of *S. aureus* in cases of toxic shock syndrome.

Viruses can be isolated in approximately 15% of cases of sinusitis. The most common viral isolate is rhinovirus. Viruses are thought to be the major agents predisposing to bacterial sinusitis, but the temporal delay between URI and bacterial sinusitis may account for the low viral culture rate seen at the time of presentation with sinusitis.

Nosocomial sinusitis is commonly polymicrobial and caused by gram-negative bacilli or *S. aureus*, and less frequently by anaerobes. Predisposing factors include the presence of nasopharyngeal or nasogastric tubes, nasal packing, nasal cranial fractures, prior antibiotic use, corticosteroid therapy, and mechanical ventilation.

Fungal sinusitis is rare among cases of community-acquired disease. It is usually seen in debilitated patients. *Aspergillus* is the most common fungal pathogen, and it can infect in a noninvasive or invasive manner. The noninvasive infection, more often seen in immunocompetent individuals, includes al-

Table 19.3   Indications for Sinus Aspiration

Severe symptomatology or toxicity
Failure of appropriate and adequate antimicrobial therapy
Evidence for suppurative complications
Immunocompromised hosts
Nosocomial sinusitis
Diagnostic uncertainty (FUO in patient with sinus opacification and no other source)

FUO = fever of unknown origin.

lergic aspergillosis and rarely mycetoma. Invasive *Aspergillus* occurs primarily in immunocompromised or HIV-infected patients.

Rhinocerebral mucormycosis is a fulminant fungal infection occurring in debilitated and immunocompromised patients. It is often observed in individuals with uncontrolled diabetes with ketoacidosis, profoundly dehydrated children, and persistently neutropenic patients (especially those with lymphoreticular malignancy). Mucormycosis begins in the nose and can rapidly spread by way of the sinuses to the orbits or central nervous system. The diagnosis is suspected in acutely febrile patients with a blackened nasal discharge and eschar on the palate and nasal mucosa, cranial nerve findings, or altered mental status.

Certain patients are predisposed to sinus infection with specific organisms. Patients with cystic fibrosis, for example, are predisposed to sinus infection with *Pseudomonas aeruginosa* and *S. aureus*. Immunocompromised patients with nosocomial sinusitis have a higher rate of polymicrobial infection with gram-negative bacteria such as *Escherichia coli*, *Pseudomonas* species, and *Serratia* species.

Treatment

The goals of therapy for sinus infection are to eradicate infection, restore or improve sinus function, provide symptomatic relief, and prevent suppurative complications. Empiric treatment for sinus infection should target the most common infections in the patient's age and cultural/environmental group, while also taking into consideration the duration of the infection. The specific bacterial resistance patterns in each community and hospital should also be taken into account. Until recently, ampicillin was the mainstay of treatment for sinus infection. With the increase in beta-lactamase–producing strains of *Haemophilus* and *Moraxella*, other agents can be considered. Increasing emergence of resistant *S. pneumoniae* is also of concern. Ideal oral agents that cover all three of these more-resistant pathogens are unavailable. Antibiotics to consider include amoxicillin–clavulanate, cefuroxime axetil, new macrolides, and fluoroquinolones that have enhanced pneumococcal activity. Trimethoprim–sulfamethoxazole (TMP-SMX), which is recommended for penicillin-allergic patients, is a poor substitute because of increasing resistance (Table 19.4). The local incidence of resistant *S. pneumoniae* should be taken into consideration when selecting a first-line antimicrobial agent for treating sinus infection.

Antibiotic therapy for nosocomial sinusitis should be guided by the results of Gram stain and culture of sinus aspirates. Empiric therapy should include broad-spectrum coverage of aerobic gram-negative bacilli, *S. aureus*, and anaerobes such as *Bacteroides* or *Fusobacterium* until microbiological data are available.

Chronic sinusitis may require surgical intervention in up to half of cases (5). A course of antibiotic therapy and sinus irrigation can be attempted with success in up to 58% of cases. Acute exacerbation of infection in patients with chronic sinusitis is treated as described above for acute sinusitis. In a case series, functional endoscopic sinus surgery was shown to provide moderate to complete relief of symptoms in 80% to 90% of patients (6).

Rhinocerebral mucormycosis is treated with aggressive surgical debridement and systemic antifungal therapy.

Other supportive therapy includes the use of decongestants, irrigation, and glucocorticoids (7). Decongestants are useful in conjunction with antibiotic therapy for acute disease. Antihistamines are contraindicated in the management of acute sinusitis because they may interfere with clearance of purulent secretions by promoting mucosal dryness. Irrigation of the nasal cavity has been shown to provide symptomatic relief. Glucocorticoids have not been shown to be of any notable benefit in treating acute sinusitis, although they may have a selective role in chronic or recurrent sinusitis when a patient would otherwise be considered for surgery.

Table 19.4   Treatment of Acute Sinusitis or Otitis Media*

Drug	Dosage	Pediatric Dosage
Amoxicillin	500 mg tid or 875 mg bid	40–100 mg/kg/d
Amoxicillin–clavulanate	875 mg bid	40–100 mg/kg/d
Cefuroxime	250 mg bid	30 mg/kg/d
Cefpodoxime	100–400 mg bid	10 mg/kg/d for otitis
Clarithromycin	250–500 mg bid	7.5 mg/kg bid, up to 500 mg bid
Azithromycin[†]	500 mg on day 1, then 250 mg qd for 4 days	10 mg/kg on day 1, then 5 mg/kg/d for 4 days
Levofloxacin	500 mg qd	—
Trimethoprim–sulfamethoxazole[‡]	1 double-strength dose bid	5 mL liquid per 10-kg dose bid

* Duration of therapy for all of these agents (except azithromycin) is 10–14 days.
[†] Not approved for sinusitis.
[‡] Not recommended when drug resistance is >20% in the community.

Prevention

There are no effective methods for specifically preventing sinusitis. However, prevention of URI is helpful. Prophylactic use of antimicrobial agents to prevent recurrence promotes the emergence of resistant flora. Treatment should be undertaken on an early and aggressive basis to avoid complications or chronic disease. Surgical correction of anatomic sinus ostial abnormalities, promotion of good dental hygiene, and control of allergic manifestations are several important preventive measures.

Otitis Media

Otitis media is an inflammatory disorder of the middle ear. The presence of fluid in the middle ear accompanied by signs or symptoms of illness define acute otitis media. Otitis media can also be recurrent or occur with chronic effusion. Chronic suppurative otitis media is a chronic middle ear infection with perforation of the tympanic membrane and mastoid involvement.

Etiology

Otitis media in children seems to be related to dysfunction of the eustachian tubes. Infants are more predisposed to ear infections because their eustachian tubes are shorter, wider, lie more horizontally, and have a less developed musculature than those of older children (8).

The usual sequence of infection in otitis media in children and adults begins with an antecedent viral infection or allergic episode that causes increased secretion. The eustachian tube becomes blocked and the middle ear accumulates fluid, which becomes secondarily infected with flora that normally colonize the nasopharynx.

Risk factors that have been associated with a greater rate of middle ear infection in children include attendance at large group daycare facilities, a genetic familial predisposition, living in developing countries, hostile climatic environments (e.g., Inuits), acquired immune deficiency syndrome (AIDS), and anatomic abnormalities such as cleft palate. The highest incidence of otitis media occurs in children 6 to 24 months old (9). Only 23% of children have not had an episode of otitis media by 2 years of age.

Clinical Manifestations

Otitis media occurs primarily in children, although it occasionally occurs in adults, with a clinical presentation and microbiology similar to that which occurs in children. The treatment is also very similar (12,13).

Acute otitis media is characterized by signs and symptoms of rapid onset. These include, fever, otalgia (indicated by pulling of the ear by young children), irritability of recent onset, hearing loss, headache, lethargy, anorexia, or vomiting. Other, less common symptoms include vertigo, tinnitus, and nystagmus (10).

Chronic otitis media can occur with persistent effusion or perforation. Persistent effusion can lead to a hearing loss of up to 25 dB when fluid is present in the middle ear (11). This may be a significant problem when a child is in the critical period of language development. If there is perforation, it is usually associated with some degree of mastoid infection. Mastoiditis begins with acute otitis media leading to localized erythema, swelling, and tenderness.

Diagnosis

Physical examination is the most important means of establishing the diagnosis of acute otitis media. The normal tympanic membrane is in a neutral position and is gray, mobile, and translucent. Evidence of a fluid-filled, acutely inflamed middle ear includes bulging, redness, and lack of mobility of the tympanic membrane (Fig. 19.2). Otorrhea—a purulent discharge either through perforation or a tympanostomy tube—is also diagnostic of acute otitis media.

Diagnosis of acute otitis media by sampling of middle ear fluid should be considered for patients who are severely ill or toxic on presentation, for newborn infants, in association with a potential or confirmed suppurative complication, in cases of a known immunologic defect, and in cases of continued toxicity with failure of multiple days of appropriate antibiotic therapy. Sampling of the fluid is a simple and safe procedure, but should be reserved for otolaryngologists, pediatricians, or other clinicians with experience in this procedure.

The microbiology of acute otitis media most commonly includes *S. pneumoniae* (29%), *H. influenzae* (23%), *M. catarrhalis* (13%), and others (17%), with the balance (18%) consisting of cases of culture negative disease (Table 19.5). In chronic otitis, cultures are commonly negative (24%) or grow other organisms such as *S. aureus, P. aeruginosa, Streptococcus pyogenes,* or fungi (44%). In acute otitis media, at least 30% of isolates of *H. influenzae* and 80% of isolates of *M. catarrhalis* are beta-lactamase producers. When appropriate cultures are performed, viruses can be isolated in up to one quarter of cases of acute otitis media.

Treatment

Most experts agree that patients with signs and symptoms of otitis media should be given antibiotic therapy (*see* Table 19.4). There is no definitive stan-

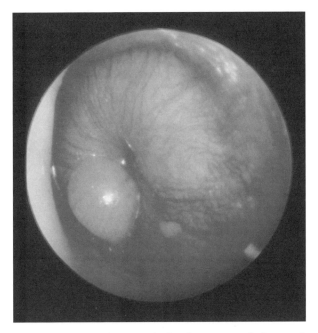

Figure 19.2   A tympanic membrane with the characteristic bulging and erythema of acute otitis media. (Courtesy of Dr. Richard A. Chole.)

dard length of treatment, but most patients are treated for 10 days; however, a 5-day course of azithromycin should be adequate because of its long half-life. Amoxicillin is the initial drug of choice for healthy, non-newborn and immunocompetent patients. TMP-SMX or erythromycin–SMX are good choices for penicillin-allergic patients. Newer macrolides, such as azithromycin, could be considered for patients allergic to sulfa drugs. If the patient is known to be infected with *H. influenzae* or *M. catarrhalis*, both of which may be associated with higher levels of beta-lactamase production, amoxicillin–clavulanate, TMP-SMX, or oral cephalosporins such as cefuroxime or cefixime could be given. The local incidence of resistant *S. pneumoniae* should be taken into consideration when selecting a first-line antimicrobial agent.

If a patient is initially given amoxicillin and does not respond adequately or worsens, and if severe toxicity exists, consideration should be given to a diagnostic tympanocentesis. Existing antibiotic therapy should be changed to an agent effective against beta-lactamase–producing organisms, such as a cephalosporin or amoxicillin/ clavulanate.

Use of decongestants or antihistamines for treating otitis media with effusion has theoretical benefits, but these have not been borne out in clinical trials.

Table 19.5   Microbiology of Acute and Chronic Otitis Media*

Organism	Acute Otitis Media (% of cases)	Chronic Otitis Media (% of cases)
Streptococcus pneumoniae	29	8
Haemophilus influenzae[†]	23	13
Moraxella catarrhalis	13	9
Streptococcus pyogenes	4	1
Staphylococcus aureus	2	3
Pseudomonas aeruginosa	2	4
No growth	18	25
Others	9	36

* 4375 aspirates from infants and children with acute and chronic otitis media were studied at the Pittsburgh Otitis Media Research Center during 1983–1986.
†Unencapsulated.
Data from Bluestone CD. In Mandel GL, Bennett JE, Dolin R (eds). *The Ear and Mastoid Infections,* 4th edition. New York: Churchill Livingston; 1995:441–448.

Chemoprophylaxis is an option that can be considered for patients with three documented episodes of otitis media in a 6-month period; two infections in the first year of life; or one infection in the first 6 months of life, accompanied by a family history of frequent ear infections. Amoxicillin or sulfonamide at half standard therapeutic dosage (once per day) is commonly chosen for prophylaxis. The most important times for providing chemoprophylaxis are during the peak periods of URI in the fall, winter, and early spring. Another approach is to begin prophylaxis at the onset of symptoms of URI. Antibiotic prophylaxis has been shown to be at least as effective at preventing new infections as ventilating tubes are.

Placement of ventilating tubes (tympanostomy tubes) is another option, especially for patients with persistent effusion or chronic infection. Such tube placement is one of the most common surgical procedures performed in children. The hearing attenuation that often accompanies middle ear effusion is relieved after ventilating tubes are placed. Other indications for tube placement include effusion for at least 3 months with signs of hearing loss, unresponsiveness to medical therapy, and recurrent otitis media for which chemoprophylaxis fails. Adenoidectomy can also be considered for children whose adenoids are thought to cause significant eustachian tube dysfunction.

Prevention

In children with recurrent otitis media, vaccination with pneumococcal and influenza vaccines may be reasonable. Pneumococcal vaccine may elicit an inadequate immunologic response in children less than 2 years of age. Newer protein-conjugated pneumococcal vaccines are under development, and should have increased efficacy in younger children.

Removal of a child with frequent URI from a large daycare setting may help decrease the incidence of predisposing infection and therefore of otitis media. It has been shown that daycare settings with six or fewer children have a lower incidence of URI. Parents should also be counseled about measures that may reduce otitis, such as breast feeding and limiting exposure to tobacco smoke. Feeding infants by bottle-propping is associated with an increased incidence of otitis and should be avoided.

Otitis Externa

Otitis externa represents infection of the external auditory canal. The disease can be subdivided into the four categories of acute localized, acute diffuse, chronic, and invasive otitis externa.

Etiology

Otitis externa is a soft tissue infection resembling this type of infection at other sites. The major difference is the anatomic limitation on the swelling of inflamed tissues in the external auditory canal. The ear canal is also a site where desquamating skin can build up. This, combined with a warm moist environment, can constitute a favorable milieu for bacterial invasion if macerated skin is present. Humid climates, warm weather, and use of a hearing aid are several factors predisposing to otitis externa. Interestingly, overaggressive cleansing of the ear canal also can predispose to infection.

Otitis externa usually results from infection by the flora that colonize the skin of the auditory canal (as at other skin sites), with a predominance of *Staphylococcus epidermidis, S. aureus, Corynebacterium* species, and occasionally of anaerobes. The pathogens that cause otitis media are not normally part of the flora of the external canal when the tympanic membrane is intact.

Clinical Manifestations and Diagnosis

There are four major clinical manifestations of otitis externa. Acute localized otitis externa is caused primarily by *S. aureus* infection at a hair follicle in the ear canal. Group A *Streptococcus* can cause erysipelas in the ear canal. In this localized infection, pain is often severe, and hemorrhagic bullae may be present in the canal and even over the tympanic membrane. Adenopathy of the draining lymph nodes may be present. The diagnosis is established by physical examination, and the drainage fluid should be cultured if resistant flora are considered likely to be present.

Swimmer's ear is the classic presentation of acute diffuse otitis externa (Fig. 19.3). It usually occurs in hot and humid weather. The major clinical symptoms include a painful, pruritic ear and tenderness to palpation. Fullness and hearing loss are common with edema of the canal. Physical examination shows the lining of the auditory canal to be diffusely erythematous. Gram-negative bacilli, mainly *P. aeruginosa*, are the major pathogens of swimmer's ear, with *S. aureus* also encountered.

Fungal otitis externa can be responsible for up to 10% of cases of the disease. It occurs most commonly in patients with chronic ear canal moisture or those receiving long-term topical antibiotic therapy. A past medical history of diabetes mellitus or immunocompromise may be present. The patient usually has pruritus and thick otorrhea. The physical examination commonly shows growth of fungal appearance of various colors, which may have the appearance of a mold. *Aspergillus* causes 80% to 90% of fungal otitis externa, with *Candida* species the next most common pathogens. Fungal cultures should be obtained.

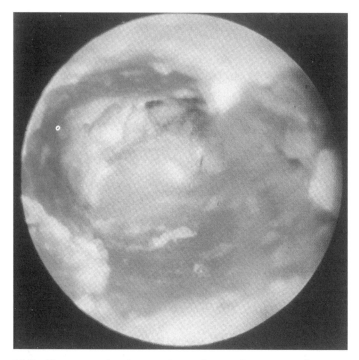

Figure 19.3   The ear canal and tympanic membrane of a patient with acute otitis externa. (Courtesy of Dr. Richard A. Chole.)

Chronic otitis externa is most often due to chronic drainage from the middle ear in patients with draining suppurative otitis media. Clinically, patients with chronic otitis externa will complain of pruritus as well as middle ear manifestations.

Malignant or invasive otitis externa is a severe local infection that spreads into the adjacent tissues, including blood vessels and bone. There is usually drainage from the ear canal accompanied by severe pain and tenderness to palpation. Diabetic individuals, immunocompromised hosts including AIDS patients, and the debilitated elderly are groups at risk. Malignant otitis externa can be life threatening if there is spread into the temporal bone and subsequent involvement of the sphenoid sinus, meninges, and brain. Facial paralysis and cranial nerves IX, X, and XII can be affected. CT scanning or magnetic resonance imaging are useful for evaluating the extent of infection. *P. aeruginosa* is the most likely pathogen.

Treatment

The treatment of acute localized otitis externa includes local application of heat and systemic antibiotic therapy (14). Incision and drainage may be needed to relieve severe pain. An ear wick can be inserted if the ear canal is occluded.

For acute diffuse otitis externa, local care is paramount (15). Gentle removal of debris with hypertonic saline (3%) and cleansing with alcohol (70%–95%), hydrogen peroxide, or dilute acetic acid can be undertaken. Inflammation can be reduced through the administration of steroid-containing ear drops or irrigation with Burrow's solution for several days. Antibacterial topical eardrops containing neomycin and polymyxin are the mainstays of treatment. The otic antibiotics are fairly acidic. For some patients, the use of otic antibiotics will be so painful that compliance decreases. Ophthalmic antibiotics or steroid and antibiotic preparations can be used. The ophthalmic solutions have a more favorable pH. Adequate analgesic medication is important for patient comfort and to promote adherence to medical treatment. Nonsteroidal anti-inflammatory drugs or even opioids are often necessary for analgesia. Systemic antibiotic therapy can be included if there are signs of significant tissue involvement.

Fungal otitis externa is most commonly treated with topical antifungal ear drops, local cleansing, and acidifying local agents.

If chronic otitis is caused by a draining middle ear infection, treatment should be targeted at the middle ear infection. Other cases of chronic otitis will probably require frequent cleansing and debridement, and should be referred to an otolaryngologist.

Malignant otitis externa is a potentially life-threatening condition that in most cases initially requires inpatient treatment. Systemic intravenous therapy should include the combination of an antipseudomonal antibiotic such as piperacillin or ceftazidime with an aminoglycoside or ciprofloxacin for 4 to 6 weeks. Local care should include cleansing of the ear canal and instillation of a topical steroid as well as an antipseudomonal antibiotic.

A number of reasons exist for referring a patient with otitis externa to an otolaryngologist. These include unresponsiveness to medical treatment, signs or symptoms suggesting a necrotizing infection (malignant otitis externa), or for help in ruling out a neoplasm.

Prevention

Water-impermeable ear plugs may be effective for people who are prone to frequent infections after water sports. Drying of the ear canals with a blow dryer after exposure to water, followed by swabbing with 70% alcohol, can help prevent infection. Other possibilities for nonswimmers include prophylactic use of 3% boric acid in 70% alcohol every other day. Regular care and evaluation by an otolaryngologist are sometimes necessary.

REFERENCES

1. **Berg O, Carefelt C, Rystedt G, Anggard A.** Occurrence of asymptomatic sinusitis in common cold and other acute ENT infections. *Rhinology.* 1986;24:223–5.

2. **Antila J, Suonpaa J, Lehtonen OP.** Bacteriological evaluation of 194 adult patients with acute frontal sinusitis and findings of simultaneous maxillary sinusitis. *Acta Otolaryngol Suppl.* 1997;529:162–4.

3. **Penttila M, Savolainen S, Kiukaanniemi H, et al.** Bacterial findings in acute maxillary sinusitis: European study. *Acta Otolaryngol Suppl.* 1997;529:165–8.

4. **Gwaltney JM Jr, Sydnor Jr, Sande MA.** Etiology and antimicrobial treatment of acute sinusitis. *Ann Otol Rhinol Laryngol.* 1981;90(Suppl 3):68–71.

5. **Kennedy DW, Senior BA.** Endoscopic sinus surgery: a review. *Prim Care.* 1998;25: 703–20.

6. **Hartog B, van Benthem PP, Prins LC, Hordijk GJ.** Efficacy of sinus irrigation versus sinus irrigation followed by functional endoscopic sinus surgery. *Ann Otol Rhinol Laryngol.* 1997;106:759–66.

7. **Low DE, Desrosiers M, McSherry J, et al.** A practical guide for the diagnosis and treatment of acute sinusitis. *CMAJ.* 1997;15:S1–S14.

8. **Klein JO.** Otitis media. *Clin Infect Dis.* 1994;19:823–33.

9. **Teele DW, Klein JO, Rosner B.** Epidemiology of otitis media during the first seven years of life in children in greater Boston: a prospective cohort study. *J Infect Dis.* 1989;160:83–94.

10. **Berman S.** Otitis media in children. *N Engl J Med.* 1995;332:1560–5.

11. **Fria TJ, Cantekin EI, Eichler JA.** Hearing acuity of children with effusion. *Arch Otolaryngol.* 1985;111:10–16.

12. **Celin SE, Bluestone CD, Stephenson J, et al.** Bacteriology of acute otitis media in adults. *JAMA.* 1991;266:2249–52.

13. **Schwartz LE, RB Brown.** Purulent otitis media in adults. *Arch Intern Med.* 1992;152: 2301–4.

14. **el-Silimy O, Sharnuby M.** Malignant external otitis: management policy. *J Laryngol Otol.* 1992;106:5–6.

15. **Clayton MI, Osborne JE, Rutherford D, Rivron RP.** A double-blind, randomized, prospective trial of a topical antiseptic versus a topical antibiotic in the treatment of otorrhoea. *Clin Otolaryngol.* 1990;15:7–10.

20

Acute Bronchitis and Acute Exacerbations of Chronic Bronchitis

Richard B. Kohler, MD
James S. Tan, MD

ACUTE BRONCHITIS

Definition

Most primary care physicians have a particular illness in mind when they diagnose *acute bronchitis*, but what seems intuitive becomes complicated when one tries to formulate a definition for this disorder (1–5). There are many definitions of acute bronchitis in the literature. Most physicians would probably agree with Badham, who in 1808 described acute bronchitis as an inflammation of the mucous membranes of the bronchi (5). However, clinicians must infer inflammation because they do not view the bronchial mucosa directly when managing patients with acute bronchitis. In a retrospective review of charts of patients coded with the diagnoses of acute bronchitis and upper respiratory infection, Dunlay and Reinhardt (1) sought to learn how practicing physicians implicitly define acute bronchitis. They found that all patients with a diagnosis of acute bronchitis complained of cough but that this was also true for most patients with upper respiratory infection. Most of the acute bronchitis patients' coughs were productive but some were not, whereas the opposite was true of patients with upper respiratory infection. Purulent sputum was much more likely to occur in the acute bronchitis group but was absent in some cases; furthermore, a small proportion of the upper respiratory infection group complained of producing purulent sputum. Lung examination was usually normal in patients with upper respiratory infection but was also normal in approximately half of the patients with acute bronchitis.

Patients with pneumonia often have associated inflammation of the bronchial mucous membranes, but most physicians who choose the term *acute bronchitis* intend to infer the absence of pneumonia. Many studies of acute bronchitis have required that pneumonia be ruled out by chest radiography (6–8); however, in many this has not been a requirement (9–13).

Most physicians probably seek to differentiate the bronchitis-like illness seen in patients who have chronic obstructive pulmonary disease (COPD) from that seen in basically healthy patients. Thus, patients with chronic pulmonary diseases are excluded from many studies of acute bronchitis (6,11,13,15–19). The term *acute* also is defined variously as bronchitis that lasts less than 30 days (11) or 14 days or less (1,6,20).

This chapter cites findings from many studies, with no uniform definition of acute bronchitis used by all. Generally, however, patients in these studies had an illness that was acute, usually lasting 14 days or less at the time of presentation for study, often (but not always) with a productive cough as the dominant symptom. Upper respiratory symptoms such as sore throat were often present but did not dominate the clinical picture. Pneumonia was generally assumed to be absent, but radiologic proof of its absence was not always provided. Chronic pulmonary disease was excluded to prevent confounding from chronic inflammation of the bronchial mucous membranes. In nearly every case, the authors of the studies cited inferred that the cause of bronchial symptoms was an infectious agent. The discussion that follows focuses on acute bronchitis in adults.

Etiology

Noninfectious insults can inflame the bronchial mucosa and produce symptoms that resemble those of infectious acute bronchitis. These insults include thermal and chemical injuries (21) and injuries from environmental pollutants (22,23), medicines (24), and various systemic conditions (25). This section focuses on infectious causes of acute bronchitis.

Viruses

Influenza Virus
A bronchoscopic study confirmed that patients with otherwise uncomplicated influenza virus infection have gross mucosal injection and edema and show microscopic evidence of epithelial cellular injury and associated inflammatory changes (26). Cough usually accompanies the flu-like illness associated with

influenza virus infections. In one study, 8% of patients with a clinical diagnosis classified as bronchitis/tracheitis/laryngitis complex had serologic evidence of influenza virus infection (27). In three studies of college students with bronchitis, influenza virus was isolated or seroconversion was demonstrated in five of 12 (42%), nine of 63 (14%), and 12 of 139 (9%) subjects with acute bronchitis (28–30). Thus, influenza virus clearly can cause bronchitis, and clinicians may recognize the illness as acute bronchitis.

Respiratory Syncytial Virus

Of 893 elderly patients admitted to a Stockholm hospital with a lower respiratory infection, seroconversion for respiratory syncytial virus (RSV) occurred in 18 patients, six of whom had acute bronchitis (31). In a nursing home population of 52 patients with respiratory illnesses associated with seroconversion for RSV, 11 patients had a syndrome diagnosed as acute bronchitis (32). Three of 139 (2%) college students with bronchitis demonstrated seroconversion (28). Clearly, RSV can cause the syndrome of acute bronchitis.

Rhinovirus

Bronchial mucosal biopsies from patients with experimental rhinovirus infections show an increase in submucosal lymphocytes, epithelial eosinophils, and histamine responsiveness (33). Among 16 healthy individuals infected experimentally with rhinoviruses by small-particle aerosol, two developed wheezing and many developed coughs associated with chest pain (34). Seroconversion for rhinovirus was documented in seven of 19 individuals who presented with the bronchitis/tracheitis/laryngitis complex (27). Rhinoviruses were the second most frequent viruses implicated by isolation or seroconversion from institutionalized elderly subjects with respiratory infections. Seventy-one percent of those with rhinovirus infections complained of cough, which was productive in 21% (35). Thus, rhinoviruses can cause cough and inflammation of the bronchial mucosa. It is not clear how often physicians classify these infections as acute bronchitis versus upper respiratory infection.

Parainfluenza Virus

Parainfluenza viruses were isolated from a small number of institutionalized elderly patients with respiratory syndromes, and seroconversion was documented in others (35). Most patients infected with parainfluenza virus type 1 complained of cough, whereas those infected with the type 2 virus did not. It is not clear from the description of these patients whether their physicians would have made the diagnosis of acute bronchitis or another disease. Seroconversion for parainfluenza virus did not occur among 893 elderly patients with acute lower respiratory illnesses admitted to a Stockholm hospital (28) nor among a smaller group of university, military, and industrial personnel with the bronchitis/tracheitis/laryngitis complex (27). Thus, in adults, parainfluenza viruses can cause an acute respiratory illness associated with coughing, but it is not clear how often physicians would diagnose this as acute bronchitis.

Adenovirus

Adenoviruses can cause a syndrome that includes a prominent bronchitic component in the absence of pneumonia (36). However, adenoviruses probably are relatively uncommon causes of acute bronchitis, at least in adults (27,28). In one study of bronchitis in college students, seroconversion for adenovirus was documented in 2% (30).

Herpes Simplex Virus

Herpes simplex virus (HSV) can be isolated from the bronchial tree of hospitalized patients with tracheobronchitis (37), and bronchoesophageal fistula has been described as a complication of herpetic bronchitis (38). So far, most patients described as having bronchial HSV infections have been immunosuppressed, burned, or already intubated. In one study of respiratory diseases, HSVs were isolated about as often from the respiratory samples of controls as from sick patients (34). Whether HSV causes acute bronchitis in otherwise healthy individuals is unclear.

Coronavirus

Coronaviruses clearly can cause the common cold. In one study of coronavirus infections, approximately half of the infected patients complained of cough (39). Whether this was due to bronchial mucosal inflammation is not known. It is also not clear whether any of these patients had a diagnosis of acute bronchitis as opposed to one of upper respiratory infection. The evidence linking coronavirus with acute bronchitis is currently tenuous.

Summary

Of the respiratory viruses, influenza virus, RSV, and rhinovirus cause acute bronchitis with reasonable frequency. Adenovirus and parainfluenza virus can cause coughing associated with respiratory illnesses and probably can cause acute bronchitis syndrome; however, this is apparently not common in adults. HSV can cause bronchitis in selected patient populations, but it remains to be shown whether this virus is an important cause of acute bronchitis in relatively healthy adults. The case for coronaviruses as a cause of acute bronchitis is currently weak.

Bacteria

Mycoplasma pneumoniae

Studies of university students suggest that *Mycoplasma pneumoniae* causes from 3% to 17% of cases of bronchitis that is severe enough to warrant a clinic visit

(27–30,40). Confounding the interpretation of these studies is a subsequent report that up to 13.5% of subjectively healthy individuals carried *M. pneumoniae* in their throats during periods of prevalent *M. pneumoniae* disease (41). Thus, studies attempting to attribute causation of acute bronchitis to this organism ideally should include matched healthy controls. In a study of 893 elderly patients with various symptoms of lower respiratory infection, none demonstrated seroconversion for *M. pneumoniae*. The evidence supports a role for *M. pneumoniae* as a significant cause of acute bronchitis (especially in young adults), but this evidence is not overwhelming.

Chlamydia pneumoniae

Chlamydia pneumoniae was proposed to cause bronchitis in university students when isolated from the nasopharynx of two of 63 students presenting to the student health service (30). In a subsequent report of students with respiratory illnesses, seroconversion for *C. pneumoniae* occurred in 4%, 2%, and 18% with acute bronchitis during three study periods (42). *C. pneumoniae* can be carried chronically and asymptomatically: The organism was isolated from 11 of 234 (4.7%) subjectively healthy adults who presented to a travel clinic (43) and was found by polymerase chain reaction in the nasopharynx of two of 104 medical personnel who could not recall having a respiratory illness within the 3 months before the study in which the organism was found (44). Prolonged asymptomatic carriage of *C. pneumoniae* after acute respiratory illnesses is also well documented (45). As with *M. pneumoniae*, the existence of an asymptomatic carriage state raises doubts about the evidence available so far for *C. pneumoniae* as a cause of acute bronchitis. It seems likely that *C. pneumoniae* does cause acute bronchitis, but further studies with appropriate controls are needed to prove this.

Bordetella pertussis

Serologic evidence suggests that *Bordetella pertussis* can cause a bronchitis-like illness in adults (46–48). Limited data from culture and polymerase chain reaction bolster this claim (49–52). The illness is dominated by prolonged cough, sometimes with an associated whoop. Serologic studies suggest that *B. pertussis* may actually be fairly common (20%–25%) among young adults with prolonged acute bronchitis (47,48); however, these data must be interpreted cautiously because many serologic diagnoses were based on a single high titer of antibody.

Streptococcus pneumoniae

Healthy adults may carry *Streptococcus pneumoniae* in the nasopharynx. In a 1931 family study largely involving adults, 21% of the population carried *S.*

pneumoniae on a chronic basis and another 52% carried it periodically or transiently (53). More recently, a longitudinal study of four healthy adult populations found the average pneumococcal carriage rate to be 19% when children lived in the house. Adult carriage rates were higher (18%–25%) when children under 6 years of age were present but lower (2%) when the children were over 12 years of age. Among adults not exposed to children in the home, the carriage rate was 6% among community dwellers and 35% and 10%, respectively, among men and women institutionalized on a psychiatric ward (54). Summarizing previous studies, the investigators who reported these findings also reported carriage rates in adults that ranged from 5% to 59% (54); these rates are similar to those summarized by others (55,56). Thus, the growth of *S. pneumoniae* from the sputum of adults with acute bronchitis does not prove cause.

S. pneumoniae was grown from the sputum of 11% of 488 and 7% of 221 patients, respectively, in two trials that compared antibiotics in treating acute bronchitis (6,7). Brickfield and coworkers (20) isolated *S. pneumoniae* from the sputum of one of 52 (2%) patients in an antibiotic trial. The investigators in these studies regarded *S. pneumoniae* as a true pathogen. In the absence of appropriate controls, however, this conclusion must be regarded as suspect.

On the basis of microbiologic evidence, it remains unclear whether *S. pneumoniae* can cause acute bronchitis in adults with basically healthy airways.

Haemophilus influenzae

As with *M. pneumoniae*, *C. pneumoniae*, and *S. pneumoniae*, *H. influenzae* can be isolated from the oropharyngeal secretions of healthy adults, ranging from 5% to 80% (56,57). Thus, attributing *H. influenzae* as a cause of acute bronchitis on the basis of its growth from expectorated sputum should result from studies that include suitable controls. Unfortunately, such studies are lacking. Musher and coworkers (58) reported 14 adults who had febrile respiratory illnesses, purulent respiratory secretions, abundant gram-negative coccobacilli on sputum gram stain, no infiltrates on chest radiography, and growth of *H. influenzae* from sputum. Most had COPD, but three did not (all three were otherwise debilitated). In four antibiotic trials, *H. influenzae* was alleged to be the cause of 2%, 8%, 18%, and 13% of acute bronchitis cases in adults (6–8,20). However, controls were not included in any of these studies.

As is true for *S. pneumoniae*, whether *H. influenzae* can cause acute bronchitis in otherwise healthy adults remains unclear.

Other Bacteria

Some authors have stated that acute bronchitis can be caused, primarily or secondarily, by other bacteria, including *Moraxella catarrhalis*, *H. parainfluenzae*,

Staphylococcus aureus, and *Klebsiella pneumoniae*. They support these claims by citing the presence of abundant polymorphonuclear leukocytes and the relative absence of squamous epithelial cells in microscopically evaluated specimens of sputum from which these organisms were isolated (7,8,59). However, all of these species of bacteria can be present in the oropharynx of healthy people (56).

Macfarlane and coworkers (60) performed detailed studies on a subset of adults with lower respiratory tract infections, most of whom (88%) had normal chest radiographs. The studies included semiquantitative sputum cultures, pneumococcal antigen detection in sputum and urine, and acute and convalescent serum testing for influenza viruses, respiratory syncytial viruses, adenoviruses, *Chlamydia*, *Coxiella burnetii*, and *M. pneumoniae*. No pathogens were identified in 56% of the patients. Causes attributed on the basis of these tests were *Streptococcus pneumoniae* in 30% of cases (largely by antigen detection), influenza virus in 8%, RSV in 2%, *M. catarrhalis* in 2%, *H. parainfluenzae* in 1%, *Staphylococcus aureus* in 1%, *Pseudomonas aeruginosa* in 0.5%, *Mycobacterium malmoense* in 0.5%, *Mycoplasma pneumoniae* in 0.5%, *Coxiella burnetii* in 0.5%, adenovirus in 0.5%, and rhinovirus in 0.5%.

Boldy and coworkers (61) performed culture and serologic studies on patients who were thought to have acute bronchitis. No pathogen could be identified during 71% of the 42 episodes studied. In 12 patients, the pathogens identified were rhinovirus in four, influenza virus in three, *M. pneumoniae* in three, *H. influenzae* in one, and adenovirus in one. In addition, *M. catarrhalis* and *S. pneumoniae* were each grown once from patients with viral isolates.

Fungi

Aspergillus species can cause bronchitis in immunocompromised patients (62,63). Cases in immunocompetent individuals have not been reported.

Summary

In most cases, studies of the microbial causes of acute bronchitis in adults fail to recognize a pathogen either culturally or serologically. When a pathogen is recognized, it is usually a virus. Attempts to associate particular species with acute bronchitis are complicated by the presence in healthy individuals of most of the putative bacterial causes of the disease and some of its allegedly causative viral species. This is particularly true not only of *S. pneumoniae*, *H. influenzae*, *M. catarrhalis*, and *C. pneumoniae* but also of *M. pneumoniae*.

Because there is no clear evidence that these bacteria play a role in causing acute bronchitis, the findings in placebo-controlled studies of empirical antibiotic therapy for this disease are instructive (*see* section on Treatment below).

Risk Factors

Because respiratory viruses can cause bronchitis, living with infected household members and working closely with children are likely to be risk factors for contracting acute bronchitis (mostly resulting from how these microbes are spread). Patients with asthma may be at increased risk for presenting to physicians with acute bronchitis (16,64).

Clinical Manifestations

Given the uncertainties in diagnosing acute bronchitis, its reported clinical manifestations vary according to the definition used. A problem with most clinical studies is that they do not require chest radiography, justified by the authors as appropriate because this is how acute bronchitis is diagnosed in clinical practice. In most clinical studies, a common problem is that the authors have not required chest radiographs to exclude pneumonia. Thus, patients were included on the basis of a clinical syndrome and physical examination findings and those with pneumonia may have contaminated the findings of these studies.

On average, patients in clinical diagnostic studies of acute bronchitis waited 10 days with their symptoms before presenting to a physician (range 2–35 days) (61). Patients in the 20- to 60-year age group tended to wait longer than both their younger and older counterparts. Studies in the United Kingdom showed a consistent seasonal variation in the acute bronchitis attack rate, ranging from highs of 140 to 170 per 100,000 individuals in January and February to lows of 25 to 40 in late August (65). Attack rates were highest in people aged 0 to 4 years and those over 64. Those aged 15 to 44 years were least likely to have bronchitis diagnosed.

Coughing, essentially by definition, was present in all patients with acute bronchitis (Fig. 20.1) (1,61,66). Many physicians are willing to diagnose acute bronchitis in the presence of a cough that is not productive, and this happened in 10% to 30% of cases in the three series described here (1,61,65). The main reasons for consulting the physician were cough (90%), difficulty in sleeping (primarily due to coughing) (61%), a general feeling of illness (56%), worrying about a more serious illness (particularly pneumonia) either by the patient (56%) or by someone else (47%), shortness of breath (47%), inability to work (38%), and other reasons (19%) (66). Patients often complained of other respiratory symptoms, such as nasal congestion (approximately half), rhinorrhea (half or more), sore throat (approximately half), headache (approximately half), and feverishness (approximately one third) (1,61,66). Verheij and coworkers (66) found that, at baseline, 35% of patients felt sick enough to

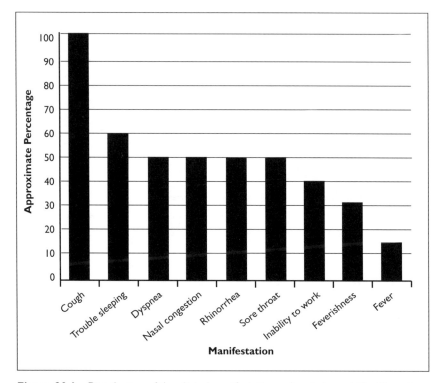

Figure 20.1   Distribution of the clinical manifestations of acute bronchitis. (Data from references 1, 61, and 66.)

have stopped daily work activities and that 33% were spending extra time in bed. Sixty-nine percent of patients reported at least some limitation in their normal physical activities. Asthmatic individuals with acute bronchitis may develop an exacerbation of their asthma. In one careful prospective evaluation of a cohort of asthmatic subjects, 44% of all asthma exacerbations were associated with a viral respiratory tract infection (67). On physical examination, the lungs of the patients were abnormal in 40% to 70% of cases (61,66). Rhonchi were the most commonly reported finding, occurring in 68% of patients in one study (66); wheezes occurred in 18% to 43% (61,66). Crackles were reported in 24% to 33%. Although approximately one third of patients in two other studies reported feverishness, fever was documented on examination in only 12% to 20% (1,8).

At 1 and 2 weeks, 30% and 13% of patients in one study reported ongoing frequent coughing (Fig. 20.2); 53% and 28%, respectively, reported ongoing productive coughing (66). At 2 weeks, 34% of patients continued to report dyspnea, 27% nasal congestion, 13% sore throat, and 5% feverishness. In one

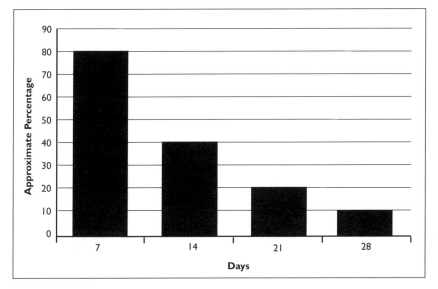

Figure 20.2   Percentage of patients with acute bronchitis who are still coughing after presenting for care. (Data from Williamson HA. A randomized, controlled trial of doxycycline in the treatment of acute bronchitis. *J Fam Pract.* 1984;19:481–6.)

antibiotic trial in which the final assessment was made between 10 and 45 days after presentation, 47% of patients reported continued symptoms, usually cough (7). In a trial of oral albuterol for acute cough syndrome (68), the mean duration of cough was 10 days and the range was 1 to 28 days. Thus, many patients with acute bronchitis continue to complain of cough for 2 weeks after presentation, and coughing even at 28 days is not uncommon.

Leukocytosis was documented in only 22% of patients in whom the white blood cell count was examined (61).

Pulmonary function testing shows diminished airflow in some patients with acute bronchitis. In one study of acute bronchitis that excluded patients known to have asthma, 11 of 33 patients had a forced expiratory volume in 1 second (FEV1) of less than 80% of the predicted normal value at the time of their presentation (16). Those with lower FEV1 values at study entry missed more days of work on average than those with normal values, but the cough duration, likelihood of being smokers, and overall health ratings of the two groups did not differ during the 14 days of observation.

Hallett and Jacobs (64) suggested that a history of recurrent acute bronchitis may be a marker for underlying asthma. They found that, among 46 consecutive patients with at least two physician-diagnosed episodes of acute bronchitis within the previous 5 years, 15 patients (33%) met American Thoracic Society spirometric criteria for asthma and 15 of the remaining 31 had an abnormal methacholine challenge test.

Documented progression of acute bronchitis to pneumonia is apparently rare. Only one instance (61) is noted in the previously mentioned studies.

Diagnosis

Perhaps the major diagnostic task for a clinician who is entertaining a diagnosis of acute bronchitis is to differentiate it from pneumonia. As noted later in this chapter, treatments for acute bronchitis (as opposed to those for pneumonia) have little or no beneficial effect.

Can acute bronchitis be distinguished from pneumonia on clinical grounds alone? Metlay and coworkers (69) reviewed the English-language literature to determine the accuracy of the clinical examination in patients with community-acquired pneumonia. The chest radiograph–the "gold standard"–is imperfect for this purpose. Albaum coworkers (70) presented the initial chest film of patients suspected of having community-acquired pneumonia to two staff radiologists. Among the 282 patients whose initial pulmonary radiographs were evaluated, there was disagreement between the two staff radiologists about whether an infiltrate was present in 21%. With this imperfection in mind, chest radiography is still used in studies to differentiate pneumonia from other illnesses, including acute bronchitis.

Examiners often disagree about the chest findings on physical examination in cases of acute bronchitis (71,72). Spiteri and coworkers (72) asked 24 members of the British Royal College of Physicians to examine patients, with four physicians assigned to each of four patients. The four physicians were in complete agreement only 55% of the time. The extent of agreement was greatest for percussion note, wheezing, and pleural rub; least for whispering pectoriloquy, tactile vocal fremitus, and tracheal displacement; and intermediate for crackles and bronchial breathing.

With chest radiography as the diagnostic gold standard, the likelihood of pneumonia in all patients who present to physicians' offices with acute cough in one study was 2.6% (73). In an emergency department study confined only to patients whose physicians ordered a chest radiograph to rule out pneumonia, it was present in 38% (74).

Metlay and coworkers (69) found that no individual historical factor sufficiently reduced the odds of pneumonia so as to exclude this diagnosis. A possible exception is a history of asthma, which in one study reduced the odds of pneumonia by a factor of 0.1. Likewise, there was no individual historical finding that sufficiently raised the odds of pneumonia so as to confirm the diagnosis without a chest film. For example, in a study by Diehr and coworkers

(73), a history of fever had a likelihood ratio of 2.1. Given the pretest probability of pneumonia in their patient population of 0.026, the presence of fever raised the probability only to 0.055 (5.5%). Rhinorrhea had a negative likelihood of 2.4, thus raising the likelihood that pneumonia was absent from 97.6% to 99.6%.

Regarding the physical examination, Gennis and coworkers (74) found that if the patient's temperature was less than 37.8°C, the heart rate less 100 bpm, and the respiratory rate less than 30 breaths per minute, then the negative likelihood of pneumonia was 0.18. In other words, these findings decreased the likelihood of pneumonia to 18% of its prevalence in the reference population. During the trial, in which 38% of patients suspected of having pneumonia had an abnormal chest radiograph, normal vital signs reduced the likelihood of pneumonia to 7%. When asymmetric respiration was noted, pneumonia was always present; however, asymmetric respiration was present in only 4% of patients with pneumonia. Other findings, such as egophony and dullness to percussion increased the likelihood of pneumonia by a factor of 2.2 from its prevalence in the reference population. However, given the low prevalence of pneumonia in the overall study population, these findings had only a modest effect on the estimated probability of pneumonia. All four studies reviewed by Metlay and coworkers (69) supported the conclusion that neither the presence nor the absence of crackles on examination would be sufficient to rule in or rule out the diagnosis of pneumonia. For example, with a prevalence of pneumonia of 5% in the target population, the absence of crackles reduced the probability of pneumonia to only 3%, whereas the presence of crackles raised the probability to only 10%.

Metlay and coworkers (69) also examined the value of prediction algorithms in diagnosing pneumonia. In one study in which the prevalence of pneumonia was 7%, a physician's judgment that a patient did not need chest radiography reduced the probability of pneumonia to 2%, and these judgments outperformed all prediction rules produced by earlier studies. However, when the physician judged that the patient did *not* need a chest radiograph to diagnose pneumonia, the probability of pneumonia increased to only 13%.

Metlay and coworkers (69) drew three main conclusions from their review:
1. Physicians frequently disagree about the presence or absence of individual findings on chest examinations in patients with respiratory illnesses.
2. Individual symptoms and signs have inadequate diagnostic performance characteristics to rule in or rule out the diagnosis of pneumonia.
3. The decision rules that use the presence or absence of several symptoms and signs to modify the probability of pneumonia are available but may not increase or decrease the probability of pneumonia sufficiently to displace the use of chest radiography. (A possible exception

is the *normal vital signs* rule of Gennis and coworkers (74), which, if applied, would reduce the ordering of chest radiography by approximately 40%. However, even this helpful rule would have missed 38% of patients who were subsequently shown to have pneumonia via chest radiography.)

Thus, if diagnostic certainty is needed to differentiate acute bronchitis from pneumonia, within the limits of the interpretation accuracy of the chest radiograph itself, then chest radiography should be performed to include or exclude pneumonia. This might be the case if a strategy is chosen of not treating acute bronchitis with antibiotics.

Treatment

Antibiotics

Most physicians prescribe antibiotics to treat adults with acute bronchitis (1,17,61,75,76). In a recent analysis of data from the National Ambulatory Medical Care Survey, bronchitis was the reason for 11% of all antibiotics prescribed and was the second-ranked reason for prescribing antibiotics in the ambulatory setting (77). The antibiotic prescription rate was 66%, and antibiotics were more likely to be prescribed for bronchitis in 1994 (70% likelihood) than in 1980 (59% likelihood) (76). A recent comparison of antibiotic prescription rates for bronchitis in a staff-model health maintenance organization (HMO) versus a fee-for-service multispecialty clinic revealed no difference in these rates, which were 82% and 73%, respectively (78). However, the antibiotics prescribed by the HMO were more likely to be narrow-spectrum, low-cost choices than were those prescribed in the fee-for-service practice.

Given the uncertainty about the role of antibiotic-susceptible microbes as causes of acute bronchitis, we must review the results of placebo-controlled trials of antibiotic therapy to determine whether this liberal use of antibiotics for acute bronchitis is appropriate.

Doxycycline compared with placebo failed to produce a benefit in adolescents and adults with acute purulent cough when assessed on the seventh day of treatment (79). The parameters that were evaluated included daytime cough, nighttime cough, production of yellow sputum, and number of days away from work. The patients were queried at 6 months, and there were no differences in morbidity except that fewer patients in the doxycycline group had developed upper respiratory illnesses. In a later, similar, but smaller trial, doxycycline again failed to produce overall benefits in acute bronchitis compared with placebo (14).

Trimethoprim–sulfamethoxazole (TMP-SMX) produced measurably better outcomes than did placebo for patients with acute productive cough (9).

These results are remarkable because the number of patients studied was small (34 in the antibiotic-treatment group and 33 in the placebo group, of whom 13 dropped out of the study). Patients kept daily symptom diaries. One-tailed *t* tests and a multivariate analysis were performed. Outcomes were better in the antibiotic group for cough resolution, fever, and need for antihistamine/decongestant medications. Chest radiographs were not made; thus, it is possible that some of these patients had pneumonia.

Erythromycin was compared with placebo in two trials. In the first (20), pneumonia was excluded by chest radiography in all patients. Participants kept daily symptom diaries, with the final analysis being made on day 8 of treatment. Of 140 statistical comparisons made, 10 yielded statistically significant differences, with six favoring erythromycin and four favoring placebo. There was no statistically significant difference in overall outcomes, with resolution or improvement in 81% of the erythromycin recipients and in 58% of the placebo recipients. The power of this study was quite limited; there were only 27 patients in the erythromycin arm and 25 in the placebo arm. In the second erythromycin trial (10) (which was approximately the same size as the first), patients again kept daily symptom diaries and followed multiple parameters. Many statistical analyses were again performed. For those parameters in which one arm was favored over the other, the patients who were given erythromycin fared better than those who were given placebo between days 6 and 10, showing less sputum production, diminished cold symptoms, better general health, and lower mean symptom score. On day 10, however, there were no differences in the proportions of patients in the two groups with cough or sore throat; however, fewer erythromycin recipients complained of congestion. Thus, in these two underpowered erythromycin trials, erythromycin seemed to produce measurable, albeit limited, benefits when compared with placebo.

Orr and coworkers (80) systematically analyzed the trials cited above and one other trial. They concluded that these trials were inconclusive and recommended further trials of erythromycin and TMP-SMX in treating acute bronchitis.

Subsequently, doxycycline was again compared with placebo in a multicenter trial of patients with acute cough and purulent sputum (12). Chest films were not required; some of these patients may have had pneumonia. Numerous statistical analyses were performed because the patients recorded daily observations of many symptoms. The doxycycline recipients scored statistically significantly better on days 4 through 8 for daytime cough frequency and on days 5 through 7 for less impairment of daily activities. There were no significant differences after day 7 for duration of nighttime cough, presence of productive cough, feeling ill, or impairment of daily activities. In a subgroup analysis, the study investigators found that individuals over 54 years of age or those who coughed frequently at study entry were most likely to benefit from doxycycline.

Gonzales and Sande (81), following the study described in the preceding paragraph, urged physicians not to prescribe antibiotics for acute bronchitis, citing the following factors as reasons to support their recommendation: 1) the weaknesses in those trials that showed benefits of antibiotic use in bronchitis, 2) the minimal benefits in those trials that reported benefits, and 3) the emergence of antibiotic resistance.

An even more recent trial compared erythromycin with placebo (13). Again, however, the trial was relatively small, with 49 patients in the erythromycin arm and 42 in the placebo arm. Erythromycin recipients missed fewer days of work (2.16 and 0.80, respectively) over the 18 study days. There were no outcome differences for cough frequency, use of cough medicine, general feeling of well being, or feeling of chest congestion. More erythromycin recipients (36%) reported side effects than did placebo recipients (15%).

A recent meta-analysis (82) of the trials cited above focused on specific outcomes: the proportion of subjects reporting a productive cough on days 7 to 11, the proportion who had not improved clinically at reexamination, and the proportion who reported side effects. Antibiotic treatment was no better than placebo when the resolution of cough at days 7 to 11 was assessed (relative risk [RR] 0.85, 95% confidence interval [CI] 0.73–1.00). The proportion of subjects who had not improved clinically at days 7 to 11 was similar in the antibiotic and placebo groups (RR 0.62, 95% CI 0.36–1.09). The placebo recipients were just as likely as were the antibiotic recipients to report side effects. The authors noted a "near miss" for the first two parameters assessed and concluded that, given the relatively small numbers of patients studied up to the time of their analysis, larger and better designed prospective randomized trials are needed to determine whether antibiotics produce benefits in acute bronchitis.

To summarize the effects of antibiotics in acute bronchitis, it is still not known whether they produce benefits. If they do, the benefits are small and difficult to measure. However, physicians who decide not to use antibiotics to treat acute bronchitis still face the problem of not knowing whether their patients have acute bronchitis or pneumonia. As noted earlier, the history and physical examination are quite imperfect in distinguishing the two diagnoses. The following process might be considered; however, it also should be subject to prospective study:

1. Patients suspected of having acute bronchitis without fever, tachycardia, or hypotension, or some overt sign of more significant intrathoracic disease (e.g., definite dullness to percussion, markedly decreased breath sounds, unequal expansion of the two sides of the chest) should not receive antibiotics.

2. All other patients should undergo chest radiography to rule out pneumonia.

3. Patients thought to have acute bronchitis after review of the chest radiograph should not receive antibiotics.

Bronchodilators

In Kentucky, bronchodilators were prescribed to 17% of patients with acute bronchitis (17). Oral and inhaled bronchodilators have been compared with placebo and other treatments for acute bronchitis. Melbye and coworkers (83) compared fenoterol with placebo for the ability to relieve symptoms of cough and dyspnea. Patients with a history of asthma or a baseline FEV1 less than 60% of the predicted value were excluded. There were 37 patients in the fenoterol group and 36 in the placebo group. Although the fenoterol group reported a smaller number of nearly every symptom studied, the differences did not reach statistical significance except for sputum production. FEV1 improved to a greater extent in the fenoterol group.

Hueston (84) compared oral albuterol with erythromycin in adults with acute productive cough. Identical-appearing liquid preparations of each medication were used. At day 7, fewer of the 20 albuterol recipients complained of persistent cough and productive cough than did the 22 erythromycin recipients. There was no difference between the two groups in improvement in overall well being, number of work days missed, or frequency of use of other medications for symptomatic relief.

In another study, Hueston (11) compared inhaled albuterol with placebo. Patients with known asthma and COPD were excluded. The study was designed to enroll 132 patients, but was suspended when a statistically significant end point was reached with only 46 patients. At 7 days, fewer albuterol than placebo recipients were still coughing (61% and 91%, respectively). The proportion of subjects with productive or nighttime cough did not differ in the two treatment groups.

Littenberg and coworkers (68) compared oral albuterol with placebo in adults with an acute cough of less than 4-weeks' duration. They excluded patients with known asthma or COPD. There was no significant difference between albuterol-treated and control subjects in any measure of efficacy.

In summary, the evidence that bronchodilators provide symptomatic relief in acute bronchitis remains controversial.

Antitussives

Cough is often the major symptom of acute bronchitis. Codeine has been used as an antitussive since 1838 (85). Irwin and Curley (86) reviewed studies of cough therapies and concluded that codeine and dextromethorphan are effective antitussives. Following this review, Eccles and coworkers (87) compared the efficacy of codeine and placebo syrups for cough associated with upper respiratory infection. Cough severity was assessed after the first dose of therapy in the laboratory and subsequently by the subjects in their homes. Cough frequency decreased dramatically in both the codeine and placebo groups in the laboratory phase of the study, with no difference seen between the two groups. During the home phase of the study, no differences were noted in cough relief between the codeine and placebo groups. The authors concluded that codeine did not work better than the sugar-syrup vehicle in this trial.

Guiafenesin failed to show an antitussive effect in young adults with natural colds (88), although it did seem to reduce the sputum thickness in those patients with a productive cough. Irwin and Curley (86) likewise concluded that guiafenesin does not reduce coughing.

Summary

If antibiotics produce any benefits in acute bronchitis, they are small and difficult to measure. Much larger trials than those performed to date are needed to clarify this issue and to detect particular subgroups that would benefit from their use. Pneumonia must be excluded, however, if one adopts the policy of not using antibiotics for acute bronchitis. Normal vital signs make pneumonia unlikely. Chest radiographs to exclude pneumonia may be warranted to minimize antibiotic use in the current era of selection of resistant pathogens. Antitussives are also controversial. The most recent evidence suggests that they provide little benefit over a sugar-syrup placebo. Counseling and observation seem to be warranted for most patients with acute bronchitis. An overall strategy for managing suspected acute bronchitis is outlined in Figure 20.3.

Prevention and Future Directions

Influenza and diphtheria immunization should decrease the risk for acute bronchitis. As noted above, the frequency of antibiotic use for acute bronchitis warrants large-scale trials designed to test antibiotic efficacy.

ACUTE EXACERBATIONS OF CHRONIC BRONCHITIS

Definition

In practical terms, chronic bronchitis may be defined as a chronic productive cough without a medically discernible cause that is present for more than half the year for at least two sequential years (89). When patients with chronic bronchitis develop increased cough production, sputum production, sputum purulence, and dyspnea, they are said to have an acute exacerbation of chronic bronchitis (90). Often, a more formal definition is used, in which two of these three elements are present (91). Implicit in this definition is that

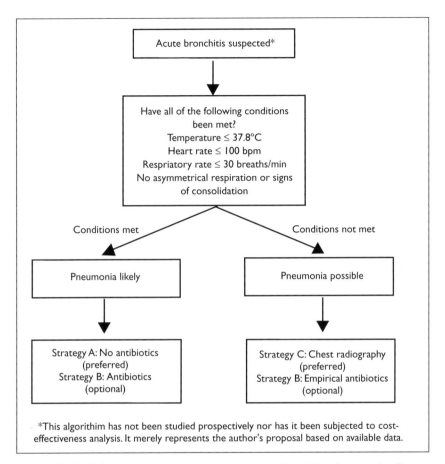

Figure 20.3 illustration contents:

Acute bronchitis suspected*

Have all of the following conditions been met?
Temperature ≤ 37.8°C
Heart rate ≤ 100 bpm
Respiratory rate ≤ 30 breaths/min
No asymmetrical respiration or signs of consolidation

Conditions met → Pneumonia likely
Conditions not met → Pneumonia possible

Pneumonia likely:
Strategy A: No antibiotics (preferred)
Strategy B: Antibiotics (optional)

Pneumonia possible:
Strategy C: Chest radiography (preferred)
Strategy B: Empirical antibiotics (optional)

*This algorithim has not been studied prospectively nor has it been subjected to cost-effectiveness analysis. It merely represents the author's proposal based on available data.

Figure 20.3 Strategies for managing suspected acute bronchitis. Strategy A = Patient is unlikely to have pneumonia, expected benefits of antibiotics are minimal, and selective pressure for antibiotic resistance should be minimized. Strategy B = Small benefits from antibiotics are possible, but there is increased public risk concerning antibiotic-resistant bacteria. Strategy C = Increased radiation exposure and higher cost are exchanged for the decrease in antibiotic use. Strategy D = Less expensive in the short term, less radiation exposure, and less time consuming for the patient; however, there is increased public risk concerning antibiotic-resistant bacteria.

no easily documented cause of these symptoms, particularly pneumonia, is present (92).

Chronic bronchitis occurs in 3% to 7% of the middle-aged to elderly population in most parts of the world, with higher prevalence rates sometimes reported (93). Together, acute bronchitis and acute exacerbations of chronic bronchitis account for approximately 14 million physician visits per year in the United States (92).

Etiology and Risk Factors

Factors proposed as possible causes of exacerbations of chronic bronchitis include infection (possibly by viruses, bacteria, or a mixture of both), irritation, and allergic reaction to environmental pollutants or allergens (94).

It has been difficult to prove that acute exacerbations of chronic bronchitis are caused by infection. Individuals with stable chronic bronchitis (i.e., not in a state of exacerbation) may harbor bacteria such as *H. influenzae* and *S. pneumoniae* in their bronchial secretions. Lees and McNaught (95) and Laurenzi and coworkers (96) compared patients with stable chronic bronchitis with controls for the presence of bacteria in bronchoscopically obtained bronchial cultures. *H. influenzae*, *S. pneumoniae*, and other bacteria were absent from the bronchial secretions of the controls but were present in most of those of patients with chronic bronchitis. Gump and coworkers (97) closely followed 25 patients with chronic bronchitis over a 5-year period both serologically and culturally. Only 34% of exacerbations could be associated with an infectious agent. Neither *S. pneumoniae* nor *H. influenzae* was present more often in the sputum of patients in exacerbation than during periods of remission. Quantitative sputum cultures showed greater numbers of *S. pneumoniae* in sputum during exacerbations, but this was not true for *H. influenzae*. Fagon and coworkers (98) performed fiberoptic bronchoscopy in 54 patients who required mechanical ventilation for hypercapneic exacerbations of chronic bronchitis. They sampled with a protected specimen brush before antibiotic therapy was administered. Bacteria were isolated from only half the patients. Monso and coworkers (99) performed bronchoscopy with protected specimen brushing followed by culture in 40 outpatients with stable COPD and in 29 outpatients with exacerbated disease. Cultures from 25% of the patients with stable disease and 52% of those with exacerbations grew bacteria, mainly *H. influenzae* and *S. pneumoniae* but also occasionally *M. catarrhalis* and gram-negative bacilli. Bacterial concentrations tended to be higher in patients with exacerbations. Thus, bacterial infection probably does play a role in acute exacerbations of chronic bronchitis but most likely only in the minority of such episodes.

Clinical Manifestations

The reported clinical manifestations in exacerbations of chronic bronchitis depend on how *exacerbation* is defined. Ball and coworkers (94) described findings in 471 patients who were diagnosed as having acute exacerbations of chronic bronchitis by 127 British practitioners using no predefined criteria for this diagnosis. The most common symptom was increased sputum production (77%). Other symptoms were mucopurulent or purulent sputum (66%), a moderate to severe increase in breathlessness (45%), and fever (12%). Sixty-nine percent of the patients met the definition for acute exacerbation of chronic bronchitis, which requires having two of the following three elements: increased dyspnea, increased sputum production, and sputum purulence. The reported number of previous exacerbations in the preceding year was less than three in 37% of patients, three to four in 31%, and more than four in 32%. Thirteen percent returned within 4 weeks with the same symptoms, of whom 2% required hospitalization. Having a history of cardiopulmonary disease plus more than four exacerbations in the previous year predicted return within 4 weeks with a specificity of 47% and sensitivity of 75%. Receiving antibiotics did not decrease the likelihood of return within 4 weeks. In a 1-year longitudinal study of patients with chronic bronchitis, exacerbations lasted an average of approximately 14 days (90). In 10% of patients, exacerbations lasted at least 25 days.

Diagnosis

Exacerbations of chronic bronchitis are diagnosed on the basis of the patient's history. Corroboration of the history of sputum purulence involves gross inspection of the sputum. Deteriorating arterial blood gas findings can substantiate a history of worsening dyspnea. Chest radiography can exclude pneumonia if it is suspected.

Treatment

In the study by Ball and coworkers (94) discussed above, most patients received antibiotic therapy.

Given the uncertainty about the role of bacteria in the exacerbations of chronic bronchitis, placebo-controlled antibiotic trials are important to define the role of these drugs in the routine management of these exacerbations. Saint and coworkers (100) performed a meta-analysis of trials published through May 1994 that enrolled patients having an exacerbation of COPD, used an antibiotic in the treatment group and placebo in the control group, and provided sufficient data to calculate an effect size. Nine trials met these criteria; they were reported between 1957 and 1992 and used the following antibiotics: oxytetracycline (three trials), tetracycline (two trials), chloramphenicol (one trial), ampicillin (one trial), and amoxicillin (one trial). The ninth trial permitted a choice among TMP-SMX, amoxicillin, and doxycycline. The meta-analysis showed a small, statistically significant effect of antibiotic therapy on clinical and spirometric outcomes. The increment in peak expiratory flow rate of the antibiotic over the placebo recipients was 10.75 L/min. It seems likely that a subset of patients might benefit from antibiotics but that most patients would not. Unfortunately, it is still impossible to discern before instituting treatment who is most likely to benefit.

In treating acute exacerbations of chronic bronchitis, no particular antibiotic has shown a clear advantage over others. Given the small benefit size of antibiotics compared with placebo (at least among the antibiotics tested to date), real differences between antibiotics may be difficult to detect. Theoretically, in the face of tetracycline-, sulfonamide-, and penicillin-resistant *S. pneumoniae* and ampicillin-resistant *H. influenzae*, newer drugs (e.g., levofloxacin, moxifloxacin, gatifloxacin, amoxicillin–clavulanate) might work better than tetracycline or amoxicillin. Unless future trials demonstrate a clear advantage for the newer and usually more expensive antibiotics, the relatively inexpensive ones (e.g., tetracycline, amoxicillin, TMP-SMX) should be used. Hopefully, future antibiotic trials will be conducted because of the increasing resistance of isolates of *S. pneumoniae* and *H. influenzae* to the older antibiotics (Table 20.1).

Patients with exacerbations of advanced lung disease may require mechanical ventilatory support. Generally, a combination of an inhaled beta-agonist with an anticholinergic drug is used to treat acute exacerbations of chronic bronchitis. Corticosteroids seem to hasten recovery (101). Oxygen therapy may be needed to keep the patient's oxygen saturation above 90%.

Table 20.1   Treatment of Bronchitis

Clinical Syndrome	Common Etiologic Agents (usually viral)	First-Line Treatments	Second-Line Treatments
Acute bronchitis	*H. influenzae*	None*	Erythromycin 500 mg qid†
Acute exacerbations of chronic bronchitis	*S. pneumoniae*	Doxycycline 100 mg qd‡ or amoxicillin 500 mg tid‡	Levofloxacin 500 mg qd or moxifloxacin 400 mg qd or gatifloxacin 400 mg qd or amoxicillin–clavulanate 875 mg bid

*Antibiotics seem to have little or no benefit in clinical outcomes in acute bronchitis.
† Erythromycin demonstrated minor benefits in some but not all placebo-controlled trials. Side effects may have outweighed the slight benefits. It is difficult to justify more expensive drugs for acute bronchitis because they have not been compared with placebo in clinical trials for this diagnosis.
‡ Theoretically, in the face of tetracycline- and penicillin-resistant *Streptococcus pneumoniae* and ampicillin-resistant *Haemophilus influenzae*, the second-line treatments listed above might work better. In the face of the relatively small treatment effect shown in placebo-controlled trials to date (and until future trials show benefits of the more expensive drugs), the use of these older, less-expensive drugs is recommended.

Prevention and Future Directions

Annual influenza immunization and at least one pneumococcal polysaccharide immunization repeated every 5 to 10 years are recommended for all patients with chronic lung disease (101). Smoking cessation diminishes the decline of FEV1 with time; however, whether it decreases the frequency of exacerbations is not known.

REFERENCES

1. **Dunlay J, Reinhardt R.** Clinical features and treatment of acute bronchitis. *J Fam Pract*. 1984;18: 719–22.

2. **Hahn DL.** Acute asthmatic bronchitis: a new twist to an old problem. *J Fam Practice*. 1994;39: 431–435.

3. **Kaufman D.** Treating acute bronchitis. *J Fam Pract*. 1996;43: 527.

4. **Leiner S.** Acute bronchitis in adults: commonly diagnosed but poorly defined. *Nurse Pract*. 1997;22: 104–17.

5. **Oeffinger KC, Snell LM, Foster BM, et al.** Diagnosis of acute bronchitis in adults: a national survey of family physicians. *J Fam Pract*. 1997;45: 402–9.

6. **Dere WH, Farlow D, Therasse DG, et al.** Loracarbef versus amoxicillin/clavulanate in the treatment of acute purulent bacterial bronchitis. *Clin Ther*. 1992;14: 166–77.

7. **Adam D.** Clarithromycin in the treatment of respiratory tract infections. *Infection*. 1993;21: 265–71.

8. **Henry D, Ruoff G, Rhudy J, et al.** Effectiveness of short-course therapy (5 days) with cefuroxime axetil in treatment of secondary bacterial infections of acute bronchitis. *Antimicrob Agents Chemother*. 1995;39: 2528–34.

9. **Franks P, Gleiner JA.** The treatment of acute bronchitis with trimethoprim and sulfamethoxazole. *J Fam Pract*. 1984;19: 185–90.

10. **Dunlay J, Reinhardt R, Roi LD.** A placebo-controlled, double-blind trial of erythromycin in adults with acute bronchitis. *J Fam Pract*. 1987;25: 137–41.

11. **Hueston WJ.** Albuterol delivered by metered-dose inhaler to treat acute bronchitis. *J Fam Pract*. 1994;39: 437–40.

12. **Verheij T, Hermans J, Kaptein A, Julder J.** Acute bronchitis: course of symptoms and restrictions in patients' daily activities. *Scand J Prim Health Care*. 1995;13: 8–12.

13. **King DE, Williams WC, Bishop L, Shecter A.** Effectiveness of erythromycin in the treatment of acute bronchitis. *J Fam Pract*. 1996;42: 601–5.

14. **Williamson HA.** A randomized, controlled trial of doxycycline in the treatment of acute bronchitis. *J Fam Pract*. 1984;19: 481–6.

15. **Williamson HA Jr.** Pulmonary function tests in acute bronchitis: evidence for reversible airway obstruction. *J Fam Pract*. 1987;25: 251–6.

16. **Williamson HA Jr, Schultz P.** An association between acute bronchitis and asthma. *J Fam Pract*. 1987;24: 35–8.

17. **Mainous AG III, Zoorob RJ, Hueston WJ.** Current management of acute bronchitis in ambulatory care: the use of antibiotics and bronchodilators. *Arch Fam Med*. 1996: 5: 79–83.

18. **MacKay DN.** Treatment of acute bronchitis in adults without underlying lung disease. *J Gen Intern Med.* 1996;11: 557–62.

19. **Brown RB, Aklilu Y.** Acute bronchitis: to treat or not to treat. *J Respir Dis.* 1997;18: 886–91.

20. **Brickfield FX, Carter WH, Johnson RE.** Erythromycin in the treatment of acute bronchitis in a community practice. *J Fam Pract.* 1986;23: 119–22.

21. **Monafo WW.** Initial management of burns. *N Engl J Med.* 1996;335: 1581–6.

22. **Baxter PJ, Ing R, Falk H, Pliaytis B.** Mount St. Helens eruptions: the acute respiratory effects of volcanic ash in a North American Community. *Arch Environ Health.* 1983;38: 138–41.

23. **Choudhury AH, Gordian ME, Morris SS.** Associations between respiratory illness and PM10 air pollution. *Arch Environ Health.* 1997;52: 113–17.

24. **Reynolds RD, Smith RM.** Nebulized bacteriostatic saline as a cause of bronchitis. *J Fam Pract.* 1995;40: 35–40.

25. **Osmanski JP, Fraire AE, Schaefer OP.** Necrotizing tracheobronchitis with progressive airflow obstruction associated with paraneoplastic pemphigus. *Chest.* 1997;112: 1704–7.

26. **Walsh JJ, Dietlin LF, Low FN, Mogabgab WJ.** Bronchotracheal response in human influenza. *Arch Intern Med.* 1961;108: 98–110.

27. **Mogabgab WJ.** Acute respiratory illnesses in university (1962–1966) and military and industrial (1962–1963) populations. *Am Rev Respir Dis.* 1968;98: 359–79.

28. **Thom DH, Grayston JT, Wang S, et al.** *Chlamydia pneumoniae* strain TWAR, *Mycoplasma pneumoniae*, and viral infections in acute respiratory disease in a university student health clinic population. *Am J Epidemiol.* 1990;132: 248–256.

29. **Evans AS, Brobst M.** Bronchitis, pneumonitis and pneumonia in University of Wisconsin students. *N Engl J Med.* 1961;265: 401–9.

30. **Grayston JT, Kuo CC, Wang SP, Altman J.** A new *Chlamydia psittaci* strain, TWAR, isolated in acute respiratory tract infections. *N Engl J Med.* 1986;315: 161–8.

31. **Fransen H, Sterner G, Forsgren M, et al.** Acute lower respiratory illness in elderly patients with respiratory syncytial virus infection. *Acta Med Scand.* 1967;182: 323–330.

32. **Agius G, Dindinaud G, Biggar RG, et al.** An epidemic of respiratory syncytial virus in elderly people: clinical and serological findings. *J Med Virol.* 1990;30: 117–27.

33. **Bardin PG, Fraenkel DJ, Sanderson G, et al.** Lower airways inflammatory response during rhinovirus colds. *Int Arch Allergy Immunol.* 1995;107: 127–9.

34. **Cate TR, Couch RB, Fleet WF, et al.** Production of tracheobronchitis in volunteers with rhinovirus in a small-particle aerosol. *Am J Epidemiol.* 1965;81: 95–105.

35. **Falsey AR, Treanor JJ, Betts RF, Walsh MD.** Viral respiratory infections in the institutionalized elderly: clinical and epidemiologic findings. *J Am Geriatr Soc.* 1992;40: 115–9.

36. **Dascomb HE, Hillman MR.** Clinical and laboratory studies in patients with respiratory disease caused by adenoviruses. *Am J Med.* 1956:161–74.

37. **Sherry MK, Klainer AS, Wolff M, Gerhand H.** Herpetic tracheobronchitis. *Ann Intern Med.* 1988;109: 229–33.

38. **Remy DP, Kuzmowych TV, Rohatgi PK, Ortega LG.** Herpetic bronchitis with a broncho-oesophageal fistula. *Thorax.* 1995;50: 906–7.

39. **Hendley JO, Fishburne HB, Gwaltney JM Jr.** Coronavirus infections in working adults. *Am Rev Respir Dis.* 1972;105: 805–811.

40. **Denny FW, Clyde WA, Glezen WP.** *Mycoplasma pneumoniae* disease: clinical spectrum, pathophysiology, epidemiology, and control. *J Infect Dis.* 1971;123: 74–92.

41. **Gnarpe J, Lundback A, Sundelof B, Gnarpe H.** Prevalence of *Mycoplasma pneumoniae* in subjectively healthy individuals. *Scand J Infect Dis.* 1992;24: 161–4.

42. **Grayston JT, Aldous MB, Easton A, et al.** Evidence that *Chlamydia pneumoniae* causes pneumonia and bronchitis. *J Infect Dis.* 1993;168: 1231–5.

43. **Hyman CL, Augenbraun MH, Roblin PM, et al.** Asymptomatic respiratory tract infection with *Chlamydia pneumoniae* TWAR. *J Clin Microbiol.* 1991;29: 2082–3.

44. **Gnarpe J, Gnarpe H, Sundelof B.** Endemic prevalence of *Chlamydia pneumoniae* in subjectively healthy persons. *Scand J Infect Dis.* 1991;23: 387–8.

45. **Hammerschlag MR, Chirgwin K, Roblin PM, et al.** Persistent infection with *Chlamydia pneumoniae* following acute respiratory illness. *Clin Infect Dis.* 1992;14: 178–82

46. **Maclean DW.** Adults with pertussis. *J R Coll Gen Pract.* 1982;32: 298–300

47. **Mink CM, Cherry JD, Christenson P, et al.** A search for *Bordetella pertussis* infection in univeristy students. *Clin Infect Dis.* 1992;14: 464–71.

48. **Wright SW, Edwards KM, Decker MD, Zeldin MH.** Pertussis infection in adults with persistent cough. *JAMA.* 1995;273: 1044–6.

49. **Addis DG, Davis JP, Meade BD, et al.** A pertussis outbreak in a Wisconsin nursing home. *J Infect Dis.* 1991;164: 704–10.

50. **Rosenthal S, Strebel P, Cassiday P, et al.** Pertussis infection among adults during the 1993 outbreak in Chicago. *J Infect Dis.* 1995;171: 1650–2.

51. **Smith S, Tilton RC.** Acute *Bordetella pertussis* infection in an adult. *J. Clin Microbiol.* 1996;34: 429–30.

52. **Dworkin MS, Spitters C, Kobayashi JM.** Pertussis in adults. *Ann Intern Med.* 1998;128: 1047.

53. **Webster LT, Hughes TP.** The epidemiology of pneumococcus infection. The incidence and spread of pneumococci in the nasal passages and throats of healthy persons. *J Exp Med.* 1931;53: 535–52.

54. **Hendley JO, Sande MA, Stewart PM, Gwaltney JM Jr.** Spread of Streptococcus pneumoniae in families. Part I: Carriage rates and distribution of type. *J Infect Dis.* 1975;132: 55–61.

55. **Austrian R, Bennett IL Jr.** Pneumococcal infections. In Wintrobe MM, Thorn GW, Adams RD, et al. (eds). *Harrison's Principles of Internal Medicine,* 7th ed. New York: McGraw Hill; 1974: 766–72.

56. **Youmans GP, Paterson PT, Somers HM (eds).** The indigenous microbiota of the human host. In *The Biologic and Clinical Basis of Infectious Diseases.* Philadelphia: WB Saunders; 1975: 81–96.

57. **Hirschmann JV, Everett ED.** *Haemophilus influenzae* infections in adults: report of nine cases and a review of the literature. *Medicine.* 1979;58: 80–94.

58. **Musher DM, Kubitschek KR, Crennan F, Baughn RE.** Pneumonia and acute febrile tracheobronchitis due to *Haemophilus influenzae.* *Ann Intern Med.* 1983;99: 444–50.

59. **Wood GM, Johnson BC, McCormack JG.** *Moraxella catarrhalis:* pathogenic significance in respiratory tract infections treated by community practitioners. *Clin Infect Dis.* 1996;22: 632–6.

60. **Macfarlane JT, Colville A, Guion A, et al.** Prospective study of aetiology and outcome of adult lower respiratory tract infections in the community. *Lancet.* 1993;341: 511–4.

61. **Boldy DAR, Skidmore SJ, Ayres JG.** Acute bronchitis in the community: clinical features, infective factors, changes in pulmonary function and bronchial reactivity to histamine. *Respir Med.* 1990;84: 377–85.

62. **Kuo PH, Lee LN, Yang PC, et al.** *Aspergillus* laryngotracheobronchitis presenting as stridor in a patient with peripheral T-cell lymphoma. *Thorax.* 1996;51: 869–70.

63. **Harari S, Schiraldi GF, De Juli E, Gronda E.** Relapsing *Aspergillus* bronchitis in a double lung transplant patient successfully treated with a new oral antimycotic agent. *Chest.* 1997;111: 835–36.

64. **Hallett JS, Jacobs RL.** Recurrent acute bronchitis: the association with undiagnosed bronchial asthma. *Ann Allergy.* 1985;55: 568–70.

65. **Ayres JG.** Seasonal pattern of acute bronchitis in general practice in the United Kingdom, 1976–1983. *Thorax.* 1986;41: 106–10.

66. **Verheij T, Hermans J, Kaptein A, Julder J.** Acute bronchitis: course of symptoms and restrictions in patients' daily activities. *Scand J Prim Health Care.* 1995;13: 8–12.

67. **Atmar RL, Guy E, Guntupalli KK, et al.** Respiratory tract viral infections in inner-city asthmatic adults. *Arch Intern Med.* 1998;158: 2453–9.

68. **Littenberg B, Wheeler M, Smith DS.** A randomized controlled trial of oral albuterol in acute cough. *J Fam Pract.* 1996;42: 49–53.

69. **Metlay JP, Kapoor WN, Fine MJ.** Does this patient have community-acquired pneumonia? Diagnosing pneumonia by history and physical examination. *JAMA.* 1997;278: 1440–5.

70. **Albaum MN, Hill LC, Murphy M, et al.** Interobserver reliability of the chest radiograph in community-acquired pneumonia. *Chest.* 1996;110: 343–50.

71. **Schilling RSF, Hughes JPW, Dingwall-Fordyce I.** Disagreement between observers in an epidemiological study of respiratory disease. *BMJ.* 1955;65–8.

72. **Spiteri MA, Cook DG, Clarke SW.** Reliability of eliciting physical signs in examination of the chest. *Lancet.* 1988;1: 873–5.

73. **Diehr P, Wood R, Bushyhead J, et al.** Prediction of pneumonia in outpatients with acute cough: a statistical approach. *J Chron Dis.* 1984;37: 215–25.

74. **Gennis P, Gallagher J, Falvo C, et al.** Clinical criteria for the detection of pneumonia in adults: guidelines for ordering chest roentgenograms in the emergency department. *J Emerg Med.* 1989;7: 263–8.

75. **Hueston WJ.** Antibiotics: neither cost effective nor "cough" effective. *J Fam Pract.* 1997;44: 261–5.

76. **Metlay JP, Stafford RS, Sinter DE.** National trends in the use of antibiotics by primary care physicians for adult patients with cough. *Arch Intern Med.* 1998;158: 1813–8.

77. **Gonzales R , Steiner JF, Sande MA.** Antibiotic prescribing for adults with colds, upper respiratory tract infections, and bronchitis by ambulatory care physicians. *JAMA.* 1997;278: 901–4.

78. **Hueston WJ, Mainous AG III, Brauer N, Mercuri J.** Evaluation and treatment of respiratory infections: Does managed care make a difference? *J Fam Pract.* 1997;44: 572–7.

79. **Stott N, West RR.** Randomized controlled trial of antibiotics in patients with cough and purulent sputum. *Br Med J.* 1976;2: 556–9.

80. **Orr WJ, Scherer K, Macdonald A, Moffatt M.**Randomized placebo-controlled trials of antibiotics for acute bronchitis: a critical review of the literature. *J Fam Pract.* 1993;36: 507–12.

81. **Gonzales R, Sande M.** What will it take to stop physicians from prescribing antibiotics in acute bronchitis? *Lancet.* 1995;345: 665–6.

82. **Fahey T, Stocks N, Thomas T.** Quantitative systematic review of randomized controlled trials comparing antibiotic with placebo for acute cough in adults. *BMJ.* 1998;316: 906–10.

83. **Melbye J, Aasebo U, Straume B.** Symptomatic effect of inhaled fenoterol in acute bronchitis: a placebo-controlled, double-blind study. *Fam Pract.* 1991;8: 216–22.

84. **Hueston WJ.** A comparison of albuterol and erythromycin for the treatment of acute bronchitis. *J Fam Pract.* 1991;33: 476–80

85. **Eddy N.** Codeine and its alternates for pain and cough relief. *Ann Intern Med.* 1969;71: 1209–12.

86. **Irwin RS, Curley FJ.** The treatment of cough: a comprehensive review. *Chest.* 1991;99: 1477–84.

87. **Eccles R, Morris S, Jawad M.** Lack of effect of codeine in the treatment of cough associated with acute upper respiratory tract infection. *J Clin Pharm Ther.* 1992;17: 175–80.

88. **Kuhn JJ, Hendley O, Adams F, et al.** Antitussive effect of guaiafenesin in young adults with natural colds. *Chest.* 1982;82: 713–8.

89. **Snider GL, Faling J, Rennard SI.** Chronic bronchitis and emphysema. In Murray JF, Nadel JA (eds). *Textbook of Respiratory Medicine,* 2nd ed. Philadelphia: WB Saunders; 1994: 1331–97.

90. **Grossman R, Mukherjee J, Vaughan D, et al.** A one-year community-based health economic study of ciprofloxacin vs. usual antibiotic treatment in acute exacerbations of chronic bronchitis: the Canadian Ciprofloxacin Health Economic Study Group. *Chest.* 1998;113: 131–41.

91. **Antonisen NR, Manfreda J, Warren CPW, et al.** Antibiotic therapy in exacerbations of chronic obstructive lung diseases. *Ann Intern Med.* 1987;106: 196–204.

92. **Grossman RF.** Guidelines for the treatment of acute exacerbations of chronic bronchitis. *Chest.* 1997;112(6S): 310–3S.

93. **Ball P, Make B.** Acute exacerbations of chronic bronchitis: an international comparison. *Chest.* 1998;113(3 Suppl): 199–204S.

94. **Ball P, Harris JM, Lowson D.** Acute infective exacerbations of chronic bronchitis. *Q J Med.* 1995;88: 61–8.

95. **Lees AW, McNaught.** Bacteriology of lower-respiratory-tract secretions, sputum, and upper respiratory tract secretions in "normals" and chronic bronchitics. *Lancet.* 1959: 2: 1112–5.

96. **Laurenzi GA, Potter RT, Kass EH.** Bacteriologic flora of the lower respiratory tract. *N Engl J Med.* 1961;265: 1273–8.

97. **Gump DW, Phillips CA, Forsyth BR, et al.** Role of infection in chronic bronchitis. *Am Rev Respir Dis.* 1976;113: 465–74.

98. **Fagon J-Y, Chastre J, Trouillet J-L, et al.** Characterization of distal bronchial microflora during acute exacerbation of chronic bronchitis. *Am Rev Respir Dis.* 1990;142: 1004–8.

99. **Monso E, Ruiz J, Rosell A, et al.** Bacterial infection in chronic obstructive pulmonary disease: a study of stable and exacerbated outpatients using the protected specimen brush. *Am J Respir Crit Care Med.* 1995;152: 1316–20.

100. **Saint S, Bent S, Vittinghoff E, Grady D.** Antibiotics in chronic obstructive pulmonary disease exacerbations. *JAMA.* 1995;273: 957–60.

101. **Niroumand M, Grossman RF.** Airway infection. *Infect Dis Clin North Am.* 1998;12: 671–88.

21

Community-Acquired Pneumonia

Thomas J. Marrie, MD

Definition

Pneumonia is a disease of the alveoli and respiratory bronchioles that is caused by an infectious agent. Pathologically, it is characterized by increased weight and replacement of the normal lung sponginess by induration (consolidation) (Fig. 21.1). This induration may involve most or all of a lobe (*see* Fig. 21.1), or it may be patchy and localized around bronchi, as with bronchopneumonia (Fig. 21.2). Microscopic examination can show dense alveolar infiltration with polymorphonuclear leukocytes (Fig. 21.3), as is found in patients with pneumonia that is caused by bacterial agents or those with interstitial inflammation usually associated with viral pneumonia (Fig. 21.4).

The clinical definition of pneumonia is a new opacity on chest radiography in the presence of at least two of the following symptoms and signs: cough, sputum, pleuritic chest pain, oral temperature above 38°C, crackles, and consolidation (i.e., dullness to percussion, bronchial breathing, egophony, and whispered pectoriloquy).

Epidemiology

Pneumonia is a common and often serious illness. It is the sixth-leading cause of death in the United States. Approximately 600,000 people are hospitalized with pneumonia each year, and the disease is responsible for 64 million days of restricted activity annually (1,2).

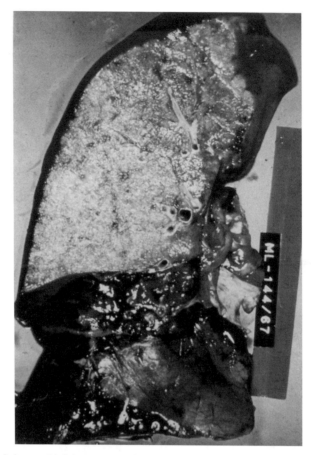

Figure 21.1 Lung with lobar pneumonia.

The rate of pneumonia is highest at the extremes of age. In a population-based study in a Finnish town, Koivula and coworkers (3) found that, among the population over 60 years of age, 14 per 1000 people per year developed pneumonia. Seventy-five percent of these cases were community-acquired pneumonia (CAP). In this study, independent risk factors for CAP were alcoholism (relative risk [RR] 9), asthma (RR 4.2), immunosuppression (RR 1.9), and age over 70 years versus age 60 to 69 years (RR 1.5).

For specific causes of pneumonia, the risk factors may differ from those for pneumonia as a whole. Thus, dementia, seizures, congestive heart failure, cerebrovascular disease, and chronic obstructive pulmonary disease were found to be risk factors for pneumococcal pneumonia (4). Among HIV-in-

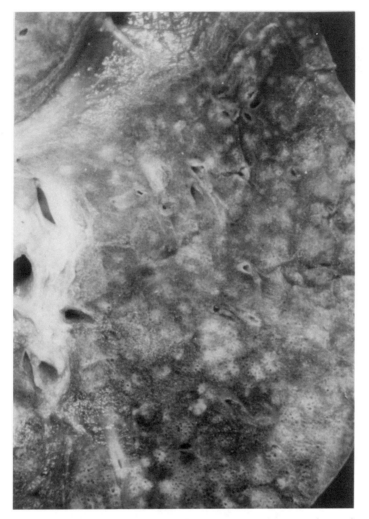

Figure 21.2 Lung with bronchopneumonia. The white areas represent the patchy consolidation commonly seen in bronchopneumonia.

fected patients, the rate of pneumococcal pneumonia is 41.8-fold greater than among non–HIV-infected people in the same age group (5). Risk factors for legionnaires' disease include male gender, tobacco smoking, diabetes, hematologic malignancy, cancer, end-stage renal disease, and HIV infection (6).

Major changes in both the host and microorganisms are reflected in epidemiologic changes of pneumonia (Table 21.1). Penicillin-resistant *Streptococcus*

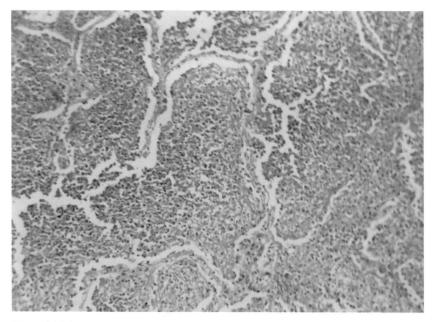

Figure 21.3 Lung tissue from a patient with pneumococcal pneumonia. Note the dense infiltration of the alveoli with inflammatory cells (magnification ×400).

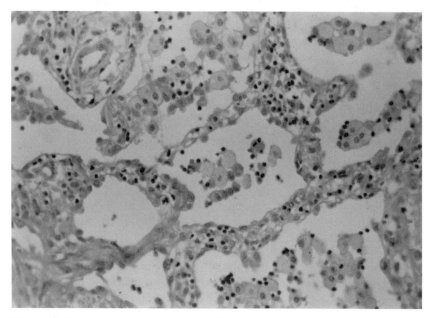

Figure 21.4 Lung tissue from a patient with cytomegalovirus pneumonia. Note the widening of the interstitium and desquamated cells in the alveoli (magnification ×450).

Table 21.1   Host and Microorganism Factors That Have Changed the Epidemiology of Community-Acquired Pneumonia

Host Factors

Increasing age of the population

Marked increase in number of nursing home residents

Increase in number of immunocompromised persons living in the community (e.g., organ-transplant recipients, HIV-infected persons, those receiving immunosuppressive treatment for a variety of diseases)

Microorganism Factors

Newly discovered microorganisms that cause pneumonia (e.g., hantavirus, *Chlamydia pneumoniae*).

Increasing *Streptococcus pneumoniae* resistance to antimicrobial drugs (e.g., penicillin, macrolide, multidrug)

pneumoniae (PRSP) is now a fact of life in most North American communities. Many PRSP isolates are resistant to three or more antibiotic classes (multidrug resistance). In a recent study, 14% of bacteremic *S. pneumoniae* isolates were resistant to penicillin, 12% to ceftazidime, and 24% to trimethoprim–sulfamethoxazole (5). In a study by Butler and coworkers (7), 740 *S. pneumoniae* isolates were collected from sterile sites during 1993 and 1994. Twenty-five percent of the isolates were resistant to more than one antibiotic (3.5% were resistant to erythromycin and 5% were resistant to clarithromycin) (7). This is probably a harbinger for the future because, in Madrid in 1992, 15.2% of *S. pneumoniae* isolates were resistant to erythromycin (8). Fortunately, it is possible to predict who is likely to have pneumonia caused by PRSP. Previous use of β-lactam antibiotics, alcoholism, noninvasive disease, age under 5 years or over 65 years, and immunosuppression are risk factors for PRSP pneumonia (9,10).

The rate of pneumonia shows a seasonal variation. Both attack and mortality rates are highest in the winter months (11), which is probably due to an interaction between influenza viruses and *S. pneumoniae*. In a squirrel monkey model, infection with influenza A virus before inoculation with *S. pneumoniae* led to a 75% mortality rate compared with no mortality for infection with influenza virus alone (12).

Etiology

In studies reporting the cause of CAP and in evaluations of individual patients, it is wise to categorize the cause of the pneumonia as definite, probable, or possible (13) (Table 21.2).

Table 21.2   Causes of Pneumonia

Definite
Pathogen recovered from blood, pleural fluid, or lung tissue
Isolation of *Legionella* species or *Mycobacterium tuberculosis* from sputum
Positive urinary antigen test for *Legionella* species
Fourfold or greater rise in antibody titers between acute and convalescent serum samples

Probable
Isolation from a purulent sputum specimen of the following organisms in which a morphologically compatible organism was seen on Gram stain in moderate or large numbers:
  Staphylococcus aureus
  Streptococcus pneumoniae
  Haemophilus influenzae
  Moraxella catarrhalis
  Pseudomonas aeruginosa

Possible
Gram stain of sputum showing a predominance of the following organisms:
  Gram-positive diplococci (*S. pneumoniae*)
  Gram-positive cocci in clusters (*S. aureus*)
  Gram-negative coccobacilli (*H. influenzae*)
Isolation of a pathogen from a purulent sputum specimen in the absence of a compatible gram stain
High single or static antibody titers against the following organisms
  Legionella pneumophila (titer ≥ 1:1024)
  Mycoplasma pneumoniae (titer ≥ 1:64)

Republished with permission from Marston BJ, Plouffe JF, File TM Jr, et al. Incidence of community-acquired pneumonia requiring hospitalization: results of a population based active surveillance study in Ohio. *Arch Intern Med.* 1997;157:1709–18.

More than 100 different microbiological agents can cause pneumonia. Fortunately, only a few organisms predominate: *S. pneumoniae, Haemophilus influenzae, Chlamydia pneumoniae, Mycoplasma pneumoniae, Staphylococcus aureus,* and to a lesser extent *Legionella pneumophila.* The rank order of various pathogens does differ in certain clinical situations. For example, in pneumonia treated on an ambulatory basis, *M. pneumoniae* is the most common etiologic agent (14–18). Table 21.3 shows the frequency of various microbial agents in 439 patients with ambulatory pneumonia.

It is likely that *S. pneumoniae* causes more than the reported figure of 5% of cases of ambulatory pneumonia, because many patients in the studies that gave rise to this figure did not have sputum or blood cultures done.

The cause of pneumonia among patients who require hospital admission for treatment has been studied in many countries (13,19–25). Because some studies did not test for all causes, it is difficult to know the exact frequency with which each etiologic agent causes pneumonia. A study that used sero-

Table 21.3   Causes of Pneumonia in 439 Patients Treated on an Ambulatory Basis

Agent	Number	Percentage
Mycoplasma pneumoniae	104	24.0
Influenza A virus	31	7.0
Streptococcus pneumoniae	23	5.0
Haemophilus influenzae	10	2.3
Coxiella burnetii	8	1.8
Adenovirus	6	1.4
Legionella species	5	1.1
Unknown etiology	211	48.0
Chlamydia pneumoniae*	16	10.7

Data from references 14–18.
* Data from one study only.

Table 21.4   Most Common Causes of Community-Acquired Pneumonia That Required Hospital Admission

Organism	Percentage
Streptococcus pneumoniae	30%–50%
Chlamydia pneumoniae	15%
"Aspiration"	10%
Haemophilus influenzae	7%
Staphylococcus aureus	2%–5%
Legionella species	2%–7%
Aerobic gram negative bacilli	4%
Pneumocystis carinii	3%
Mycoplasma pneumoniae	5%–10%
Moraxella catarrhalis	1%
Mycobacterium tuberculosis	1%

Data from references 13 and 18–27.

logic methods to diagnose pneumococcal pneumonia found that this agent accounted for 50% of all cases of pneumonia (23). Table 21.4 shows the rank order of the most common causes of CAP that require hospital admission. Viruses are not included in this table, but respiratory syncytial virus and influenza A and B viruses are important in the pathogenesis of CAP. From 10% to 15% of cases of CAP are preceded by infection with these viruses. In some instances, the virus causes the pneumonia (*see* Chapter 27 for further discussion of viral pneumonia.)

Aspiration pneumonia is underdiagnosed. Features that suggest aspiration are altered level of consciousness, seizures, impaired gag reflex, alcohol intoxication, and advanced Parkinson's or Alzheimer's diseases.

Pneumocystis carinii remains an important cause of pneumonia among HIV-infected people. Mundy and coworkers (21) studied 385 patients who were admitted to Johns Hopkins Hospital with pneumonia over a 1-year period. One hundred and eighty were HIV infected, and 48 of these (26.7%) had *P. carinii* pneumonia.

Clues to the cause of pneumonia can be obtained from historical data and from the clinical setting (Table 21.5).

Clinical Manifestations

Fever, cough (which may produce purulent or rust-colored sputum or may be nonproductive), pleuritic chest pain, chills, rigors, and shortness of breath are classic manifestations of pneumonia. Not infrequently, headache, nausea, vomiting, diarrhea, myalgia, and arthralgia also are reported. The frequency with which these symptoms are seen in patients with pneumonia is given in Table 21.6. The physical signs associated with pneumonia are tachypnea, dullness to percussion, increased tactile and vocal fremitus, egophony, whispered pectoriloquy, crackles, and pleural friction rub. Unfortunately, symptoms and signs are, in most cases, neither sufficiently sensitive nor specific to make a diagnosis of pneumonia clinically without radiographic confirmation (26). A chest radiograph is necessary to substantiate the clinical diagnosis.

The clinical presentation of pneumonia changes with age. Metlay and coworkers (27) found that with increasing age, patients with pneumonia had fewer symptoms. Thus, those over 75 years of age with pneumonia had an average of 3.3 fewer symptoms than did pneumonia patients aged 18 through 44 years.

The severity of illness in patients with CAP encompasses a considerable clinical spectrum. In any age group, patients may be mildly to severely ill. It is useful for clinicians to have a method to categorize the severity of illness in their pneumonia patients. One simple system categorizes patients as having severe pneumonia if they have two or more of the following findings: respiratory rate over 30 breaths per min, a diastolic blood pressure below 60 mm Hg, and a blood urea nitrogen above 7 mmol/L (28). Patients with all three of these findings had a mortality rate that was 16-fold greater than those who did not have such findings (29).

Fine and coworkers (30) described a more complex system for scoring illness severity. Using this system, points are assigned for 20 different items (Table 21.7). These points are then totaled to place a patient into one of five risk strata for mortality. Patients in Class I are those under 50 years of age who have no comorbidity or abnormal findings on physical examination. The mortality rate for this group of patients in the study was 0.1%. Class II (<70 points) has a mortality rate of 0.6%, Class III (71–90 points) 2.8%, Class

Table 21.5   Clues to the Cause of Pneumonia from the Medical History or Clinical Setting

Feature	Possible Etiologic Agents
Occupational History	
Health care workers	*Mycobacterium tuberculosis*, acute HIV seroconversion with pneumonia (if recent needlestick injury from an HIV-positive patient)
Veterinarian, farmer, abattoir worker	*Coxiella burnetii*
Host Factors	
Diabetic ketoacidosis	*Streptococcus pneumoniae, Staphylococcus aureus*
Alcoholism	*S. pneumoniae, Klebsiella pneumoniae, S. aureus*
Chronic obstructive lung disease	*S. pneumoniae, Haemophilus influenzae, Moraxella catarrhalis*
Recipient of a solid organ transplant (pneumonia occurring >3 months after transplant)	*S. pneumoniae, H. influenzae, Legionella* species, *Pneumocystis carinii*, cytomegalovirus, *Strongyloides stercoralis*
Sickle cell disease	*S. pneumoniae*
HIV infection and CD4 count of <200 cells /µL	*S. pneumoniae, P. carinii, H. influenzae, Cryptococcus neoformans, M. tuberculosis, Rhodococcus equi*
Environmental Factors	
Exposure to contaminated air conditioning units, cooling towers, hot tub, recent stay in a hotel, exposure to grocery store mist machine, or visit to or recent stay in a hospital with contaminated drinking water	*Legionella pneumophila*
Pneumonia develops after wind storm in an area of endemicity	*Coccidioides immitis*
Outbreak of pneumonia occurs in a shelter for homeless men or in a prison	*S. pneumoniae, M. tuberculosis*
Outbreak of pneumonia occurs in a military training camp	*S. pneumoniae, Chlamydia pneumoniae,* adenovirus
Outbreak of pneumonia in a nursing home	*C. pneumonia, S. pneumoniae,* respiratory syncytial virus, influenza A virus
Animal Contact	
Exposure to infected parturient cats, cattle, sheep, or goats	*Coxiella burnetii*
Exposure to contaminated bat caves or excavation in areas of endemicity	*Histoplasma capsulatum*
Exposure to turkeys, chickens, ducks, or psittacine birds	*Chlamydia psittaci*
Exposure to rabbits	*Francisella tularensis*
Travel	
Travel to Thailand or other Southeast Asia countries	*Burkholderia pseudomallei (melioidosis)*
Immigration from countries with high endemic prevalence of tuberculosis	*M. tuberculosis*

Table 21.6   Frequency of Various Symptoms and Signs in 588 Patients Hospitalized with Community-Acquired Pneumonia

Symptom or Sign	Number	Percent
Cough	482	82
Productive cough	355	60
Fever	402	68
Anorexia	359	61
Chills	297	51
Pleuritic chest pain	232	39
Headache	171	29
Nausea	171	29
Myalgia	161	27
Vomiting	132	22
Sore throat	110	19
Arthralgia	92	16
Abdominal pain	71	12
Diarrhea	67	11
Temperature >37°C	458	78
Crackles	459	78
Rhonchi	199	34
Confusion	175	30
Consolidation	171	29

Republished with permission from Kauppinen MT, Herva E, Kujala P, et al. The etiology of community-acquired pneumonia among hospitalized patients during a Chlamydia pneumoniae epidemic in Finland. J Infect Dis. 1995; 172:1330–5.

IV (91–130 points) 8.2%, and Class V (>130 points) 29.2%. This scoring system can be used to help decide whether or not to admit a patient. Patients in Classes I and II can be treated on an ambulatory basis; those in classes IV and V should be admitted. Patients in Class III may require a period of observation in the emergency room before a decision is made about admission or discharge. Those who are improving can be sent home. Clearly, other factors (e.g., psychosocial factors) are also part of the site-of-care decision. All patients with pneumonia who are discharged from the emergency department should be given a follow-up telephone call at 48 hours. Those who have positive blood cultures or who are not improving should be reassessed. Fine and coworkers' scoring system looks complex but is easy to use. Printing the point tabulation on tear-off, adhesive-backed sheets that can be attached to the patient's record makes the system user friendly.

Diagnosis

Chest radiography (posteroanterior and lateral views) is needed to confirm the clinical impression that a patient has pneumonia. The extent of the re-

Table 21.7   Assigning Points in the Community-Acquired Pneumonia Severity-of-Illness Scoring System*

Patient Characteristics	Points
Demographic Factors	
Age	
Men	Age in years
Women	Age in years minus 10
Nursing home resident	10
Coexisting Illnesses	
Neoplastic disease[†]	30
Liver disease[‡]	20
Congestive heart failure[§]	10
Cerebrovascular disease[¶]	10
Renal disease[**]	10
Physical Examination Findings	
Altered mental status[††]	20
Respiratory rate >30 breaths/min	20
Systolic blood pressure <90 mm Hg	20
Temperature <35°C (95°F) or >40°C (104°F)	15
Pulse rate >125 bpm	10
Laboratory and Radiographic Findings	
Arterial pH <7.35	30
Blood urea nitrogen >30 mg/dL (11 mmol/L)	20
Sodium <130 mmol/L	20
Glucose >250 mg/dL (14 mmol/L)	10
Hematocrit <30%	10
Partial pressure of arterial oxygen <60 mm Hg	10
Pleural effusion	10

Republished with permission from Fine MJ, Auble TE, Yealy DM, et al. A prediction rule to identify low-risk patients with community-acquired pneumonia. *N Engl J Med.* 1997;336:243–50.

* Based on Pneumonia Patient Outcomes Research Team (PORT) cohort study data.

† Any cancer (except basal or squamous cell carcinoma of the skin) that is active at presentation or within 1 year of presentation for community-acquired pneumonia.

‡ Clinical or histologic cirrhosis or chronic active hepatitis.

§ Diagnosis documented by history or by findings on physical examination, chest radiograph, echocardiogram, multiple-gated acquisition scan, or left ventriculogram.

¶ Clinical diagnosis of stroke or transient ischemic attack or of stroke documented by magnetic resonance imaging or by computed tomography.

** History of chronic renal disease or abnormal blood urea nitrogen and creatinine concentrations documented in this medical record.

†† Stupor, coma, or disorientation as to person, place, or time that is not known to be chronic.

mainder of the diagnostic work-up depends on the severity of the pneumonia and the site of treatment (e.g., outpatient, hospital ward, hospital intensive care unit). Table 21.8 presents a suggested diagnostic work-up for patients

Table 21.8   Diagnostic Work-Up for Community-Acquired Pneumonia According to the Site of Treatment

Site of Treatment	Tests
Outpatient*	Complete blood count[†] Creatinine[‡] Oxygen saturation[†] Glucose[‡] Electrolytes[‡]
Hospital ward	Complete blood count[†] Blood urea nitrogen Creatinine[†] Electrolytes[†] Liver function tests Glucose[†] Blood cultures (two sets)[†] Oxygen saturation (arterial blood gases if patient has chronic obstructive pulmonary disease or if oxygen saturation <92%)[†] Sputum gram stain and culture[†] Electrocardiogram Urine for *Legionella* antigen Induced sputum for *Pneumocystis carinii* (based on history of possible or proven HIV disease in combination with a compatible chest radiograph) Acute and 2- and 6-week convalescent serum samples for antibody testing in patients in whom "atypical" pneumonia is suspected Thoracentesis if clinically significant pleural effusion is present (i.e., >1 cm of fluid on a lateral decubitus chest radiograph)
Hospital intensive care unit	Same as for hospital ward (if no sputum is available, use bronchoalveolar lavage and protected brush specimen to obtain material for culture)

* For patients seen in an office setting who have illness of mild severity and who are known to the attending physician, a chest radiograph is probably the only diagnostic work-up that is required.
[†] Essential tests.
[‡] All patients ≥55 years of age and/or those with comorbid illness should have these tests before being discharged from the emergency department.

with pneumonia. For patients who are mildly ill, are seen in an office setting, and are known to the attending physician, chest radiography is probably the only work-up procedure required.

Some authorities question the need for blood cultures from all patients with pneumonia who require hospital admission, because blood-culture yield is low (6%–10%) and the results rarely change management decisions (31). However, if a blood culture is positive, the cause of a particular case of pneumonia is certain, and therapy can modified if necessary. Furthermore, bacteremic pneumococcal pneumonia in patients younger than 45 years of age should prompt a test for HIV infection, because the rate of such infection in HIV-positive patients is 41.8-fold greater than in HIV-negative patients (5). In the current era of changing antimicrobial susceptibility of respiratory pathogens, susceptibility of invasive strains of these organisms can be used to guide empirical therapy.

Sputum Gram stain and culture are among the most controversial tests in all of medicine. Because sputum has to pass through a heavily colonized oral cavity, distinguishing colonization from infection can be problematic; consequently, a sputum culture result can be interpreted only in conjunction with a Gram stain. For example, a heavy growth of *S. pneumoniae* from a sputum specimen in conjunction with many polymorphonuclear leukocytes and a finding of only gram-positive diplococci on Gram staining is highly suggestive of pneumonia caused by *S. pneumoniae*. In contrast, a heavy growth of *Escherichia coli* from a sputum specimen that shows no gram-negative, rod-like bacteria on Gram staining is more suggestive of colonization. Sputum Gram stain and culture are recommended for patients who have not received antibiotic therapy before collection of the specimen, because the Gram stain can give a rapid (15 minutes to 1 hour) answer about the cause of a case of pneumonia. In addition to the results of the sputum culture, this allows antibiotic therapy to be directed toward a specific cause. Penicillin, for example, is still the drug of choice for pneumococcal pneumonia.

The urinary antigen test for *Legionella* is a rapid (4 hours), sensitive (70%), and specific (99%) test that detects antigen of *Legionella pneumophila* serogroup 1 in urine (32). Antigen excretion persists for 42 days on average but can last up to 1 year (33). This test probably should be done on all patients who have severe or rapidly progressive pneumonia.

Many causes of pneumonia are either best or only diagnosed through finding a fourfold or greater difference in antibody titer between acute and convalescent serum samples. These samples are usually obtained 2 weeks apart but, for some infections (e.g., *Legionella*), should be obtained 6 weeks apart. Also of frequent concern is the sensitivity of the method used to detect an increase in antibody titer. For example, the readily available complement fixation test is approximately four times less sensitive than an enzyme immunoassay test for the diagnosis of respiratory syncytial virus infection in adults.

In most instances, serologic identification of the cause of pneumonia does not help in the management of an individual patient. However, serologic tests are valuable as epidemiologic and public health tools. Although viral pneumonia can occasionally be clinically indistinguishable from bacterial pneumonia in nonimmunocompromised adults, a work-up for viral pneumonia is not routinely recommended. Exceptions to this include outbreaks of pneumonia among military recruits in a barracks (where adenoviral pneumonia is common). Furthermore, during the influenza season, an attending physician often has to decide whether or not to include a rapid antigen-detection test or culture for influenza virus.

Using the polymerase chain reaction method, it is now possible to detect the DNA of *M. pneumoniae*, *C. pneumoniae*, and *L. pneumophila* from material obtained with nasopharyngeal swabs (34). Because these microorganisms colonize only the oropharyngeal mucosa in patients with pneumonia, the presence of any of their DNA in the nasopharynx of a patient is evidence that that particular organism is the cause of the patient's pneumonia. However, this test is expensive and is unnecessary on a routine basis.

The diagnostic work-up should be more extensive in seriously ill patients than in those who are mildly to moderately ill, especially in the case of patients who require admission to an intensive care unit and assisted ventilation. Bronchoscopy with a protected bronchial brush to obtain a sample of lower respiratory tract secretions, or by bronchoalveolar lavage, should be performed in this group of patients if sputum is not available for culture. Specimens of respiratory secretions obtained in this manner should be subjected to quantitative culture. The diagnostic yield from these invasive tests is approximately 70% (35). In patients with lobar consolidation, fine-needle aspiration can be performed to obtain material for culture (36). Rarely, open-lung biopsy has to be performed to make a diagnosis (37).

Many patients who require hospital admission for pneumonia treatment are elderly and have comorbid illnesses. Additional testing is dictated by specific comorbidities, but all patients should have a complete blood count, blood urea nitrogen, creatinine, electrolytes, blood glucose, and liver function tests.

Treatment

In most instances, CAP treatment must be empirical because the cause of the pneumonia is usually unknown when treatment has to be initiated. Guidelines have been developed to help with the decision-making in this setting (38). These guidelines are based largely on expert opinion rather than on evidence from randomized clinical trials. Indeed, a recent study has shown that dividing patients who are to be treated on an ambulatory basis into those who are under 60 years of age and those who are over (as is suggested by the American Thoracic Society guidelines [38]) has no rational basis (39). In this study, older patients who were treated with macrolide antimicrobials—a treatment inconsistent with the ATS guidelines—showed a trend toward having a better outcome than did those treated according to the guidelines. More-recent guidelines for empirical antibiotic CAP therapy do not use age as a criterion for dividing patients who are to be treated on an ambulatory basis (40).

A major consideration in the choice of an antibiotic for empirical CAP therapy is whether PRSP are present in the community, because these organisms also may be resistant to macrolides and trimethoprim–sulfamethoxazole (5,7). The so-called respiratory quinolones are being advocated to treat CAP, because they have greater activity than ciprofloxacin against *S. pneumoniae* and because they are also active against PRSP. These agents include levofloxacin, sparfloxacin, grepafloxacin, moxifloxacin, and trovafloxacin. (Trovafloxacin, however, has been withdrawn from routine use because of hypersensitivity hepatitis.) Other antimicrobial agents, currently in clinical trials, include the fluoroquinolones gemifloxacin and gatifloxacin. These new fluoroquinolones are probably drugs of choice for patients who require hospital admission for CAP treatment. File and coworkers (41) studied 590 patients with CAP (both inpatients and outpatients) of whom 226 were treated with levofloxacin and 230 were treated with 1) intravenous ceftriaxone followed by oral cefuroxime, 2) oral cefuroxime alone, or 3) oral cefuroxime in conjunction with a macrolide or doxycycline if, in the opinion of the investigator, an atypical pathogen was likely. Clinical success at 5 to 7 days after treatment was begun was superior for the levofloxacin-treated group compared with the other group (96% and 90%, respectively; 95% confidence interval [CI] –0.7 to –1.3).

Table 21.9 provides an outline for empirical antibiotic CAP therapy. The guidelines shown in the table are a modified version of the recently published guidelines of the Infectious Diseases Society of America for antibiotic CAP treatment, which suggest using a respiratory fluoroquinolone for the treatment of pneumonia on an ambulatory basis if risk factors for PRSP are present (40). An extended-spectrum cephalosporin in combination with a macrolide, a respiratory fluoroquinolone alone, or the combination of a β-lactam drug, a β-lactamase inhibitor, and a macrolide are recommended as the antibiotics of choice for patients who require hospital admission for CAP treatment.

Because the respiratory fluoroquinolones as a class are active against most of the pathogens that cause CAP, use of one of these drugs allows single-drug therapy. There is concern, however, about emerging resistance to the fluoroquinolones, and the Drug-Resistant *Streptococcus pneumoniae* Therapeutic Working Group recommends that the use of the new fluoroquinolones be limited to 1) patients for whom therapy with a β-lactam drug plus a macrolide has failed, 2) patients who are allergic to alternative agents, and 3) patients who have a documented infection with highly drug-resistant pneumococci (e.g., an organism for which the minimum inhibitory concentration [MIC] of penicillin is 4 mg/L [43]). The working group also recommends that first-generation cephalosporins, ceftazidime, ceftizoxime, and ticarcillin not be used to treat hospitalized patients with pneumonia because of the high rate of resistance to these agents among penicillin-resistant pneumococci (42).

Because the respiratory fluoroquinolones are absorbed extremely well, these agents can be given orally throughout the course of therapy for patients who are not hypotensive and who can eat and drink. Ramirez and coworkers

Table 21.9   Antibiotic Therapy (First and Second Choices) for Community-Acquired Pneumonia When the Cause Is Unknown

Patient Treated on an Ambulatory Basis
Macrolide (erythromycin 500 mg q6h PO for 10 days, clarithromycin 500 mg bid PO for 10
   days, or azithromycin 500 mg PO once then 250 mg/d PO for 4 days)
Doxycycline 100 mg bid PO for 10 days (if risk factors for penicillin- or macrolide-resistant
   Streptococcus pneumoniae are present, consider a fluoroquinolone with enhanced activity
   against *S. pneumoniae**)
Patient Treated in a Hospital Ward
Fluoroquinolone with enhanced activity against *S. pneumoniae* (e.g., levofloxacin[†] 500 mg/d
   IV, sparfloxacin 400 mg as a single dose then 200 mg/d PO, moxifloxacin 400 mg/d PO,
   gatifloxacin 400 mg IV or PO)
An extended-spectrum cephalosporin (e.g., cefuroxime 750 mg q8h IV, ceftriaxone 1 g/d IV,
   cefotaxime 2 g q6h IV plus a macrolide (e.g., azithromycin 500 mg/d IV)
Patient Treated in an Intensive Care Unit
Azithromycin 1 g IV as a single dose then 500 mg/d IV *plus* ceftriaxone 1 g q12h IV or cefo-
   taxime 2 gm q6h IV (use ceftazidime, piperacillin, piperacillin–tazobactam, imipenem, or
   meropenem and ciprofloxacin if *Pseudomonas aeruginosa*[‡] is suspected)
Fluoroquinolone with enhanced activity against *S. pneumoniae* (not recommended as first
   choice because of lack of clinical trial data in the ICU setting)
Patient Treated in a Nursing Home
Amoxicillin–clavulanate 500 mg q8h PO
Fluoroquinolone with enhanced activity against *S. pneumoniae*
Ceftriaxone 1 g/d IM or IV or cefotaxime 500 mg IM q12h
Aspiration Pneumonia
Large-volume aspiration
   For previously healthy individuals, do not institute antibiotic therapy
Small-volume aspiration
   For pneumonia (poor dental hygiene) and suspected anaerobic infection, use clindamycin
   or penicillin
   For pneumonia in a nursing home or in elderly subjects at home, use fluoroquinolone with
   or without clindamycin, metronidazole, or a β-lactam/β-lactamase inhibitor

---

IM = intramuscularly; IV= intravenously; PO = orally.
* Risk factors for penicillin-resistant *S. pneumoniae* are previous use of β-lactam antibiotics, alcoholism,
age <5 years or >65 years. Risk factors for macrolide-resistant *S. pneumoniae* are age <5 years or nosocomial acquisition of infection.
† If creatinine clearance <50 mL/min, reduce levofloxacin dosage to 250 mg/d.
‡ Patients with structural lung disease such a bronchiectasis are at high risk for *P. aeruginosa* infection.
Modified from File TM Jr, Segretti J, Dunbar L, et al. A multicenter, randomized study comparing the efficacy and safety of intravenous and/or oral levofloxacin versus ceftriaxone and/or cefuroxime axetil in
treatment of adults with community-acquired pneumonia. *Antimicrob Agents Chemother.* 1997;41:1965–72.

(43) and Ramirez and Ahkee (44) have shown that patients with CAP who
are treated intravenously with antibiotics can have this treatment replaced by
oral antibiotic therapy when 1) the white blood cell count returns to normal,
2) there are two normal temperature recordings 16 hours apart, and 3) there is

subjective improvement in cough and shortness of breath. However, oral antibiotic therapy is generally considered sufficient for most patients who can eat and drink (45). Empirical antibiotic therapy should be replaced by pathogen-specific treatment once an etiologic agent has been identified (Table 21.10).

Pneumonia Caused by Penicillin-Resistant *Streptococcus pneumoniae*

The most appropriate treatment for patients with PRSP is unclear. It is known that this infection can be treated successfully with intravenous penicillin (46). It is also known that treatment with penicillin is unsuccessful if there is concomitant pneumococcal meningitis. In this setting, vancomycin and ceftriaxone are recommended. To effect the cure of pneumococcal pneumonia, concentrations of antibiotic must exceed the MIC of the causative strain of *S. pneumoniae* for at least 40% of the treatment period (47,48). The studies in which this has been found indicate that oral cefaclor and perhaps oral cefuroxime are unlikely to be effective against PRSP (48). Amoxicillin was the most effective oral β-lactam antibiotic for the treatment of PRSP in a study by Goldstein (49). Other options include the so-called *respiratory fluoroquinolones* (i.e., levofloxacin, moxifloxacin, gemifloxacin, and gatifloxacin).

Pneumonia Caused by Macrolide-Resistant *Streptococcus pneumoniae*

Apart from PRSP, macrolide-resistant *S. pneumoniae* is an issue in many communities. Because 50% of cases of ambulatory pneumonia are of unknown etiology and because there is less than 1% mortality among these patients, an increase in the mortality rate among outpatients with pneumonia treated with macrolides may not be detected unless large randomized controlled trials are performed. Other outcome measures that may be more readily apparent are 1) the failure of therapy resulting in hospitalization, and 2) a longer time to clinical resolution of the pneumonia than with more effective agents. Currently, approximately 2% of penicillin-susceptible *S. pneumoniae* isolates are resistant to macrolides, 12% of isolates with intermediate resistance to penicillin are resistant to macrolides, and 25% of isolates that are highly resistant to macrolides are resistant to penicillin (50). Macrolide susceptibility of *S. pneumoniae* is defined as an MIC of up to 0.5 mg/L. The mean MICs for strains that are resistant because they have a drug efflux mechanism (which accounts for 55% of the macrolide resistance in *S. pneumoniae*) is 10 mg/L. Modification of the target (ribosomal) site of a macrolide accounts for 45% of the resistance and results in MICs of 64 mg/L or greater (50). Ongoing studies are necessary to provide guidance about the best treatment for CAP that is caused by macrolide-resistant *S. pneumoniae*.

Table 21.10   Treatment of the Most Common Pathogens That Cause Community-Acquired Pneumonia

Agent	Treatments
Streptococcus pneumoniae	
Penicillin susceptible (MIC ≤ 0.1 mg/L)	Penicillin V 500 mg q6h PO or penicillin G 500,000 U q4h IV
	Doxycycline 100 mg bid PO for 10 days
	Clarithromycin 500 mg bid PO for 10 days
	Azithromycin 500 mg PO in a single dose then 250 mg/d PO for 4 days
Intermediate penicillin resistance (MIC 0.1–1.0 mg/L)	Penicillin G 3 MU q4h IV
	Ceftriaxone 1 g q12h IV
	Levofloxacin 500 mg/d IV if CrCl > 50 mL/min or 250 mg/d IV if CrCl <50 mL/min
	Amoxicillin–clavulanate 500 mg tid PO for 10 days
	Amoxicillin 500 mg tid PO for 10 days
High penicillin resistance (MIC ≥ 2.0 mg/L)	Vancomycin 1 g q12h plus ceftriaxone 2 g q12h IV if meningitis has complicated the pneumonia or levofloxacin 500 mg/d IV
Moraxella catarrhalis	Cefuroxime* 500 mg bid PO or 750 mg q8h IV
	Amoxicillin–clavulanate 500 mg q8h PO
Staphylococcus aureus†	
Methicillin susceptible S. aureus	Nafcillin or cloxacillin 2 g q4h IV
	Vancomycin 1 g q12h IV
Methicillin resistant S. aureus	Vancomycin 1 g q12h IV
Haemophilus influenzae	Cefuroxime** 500 mg bid PO
	Azithromycin 500 mg PO as a single dose then 250 mg/d PO for 4 days
	Amoxicillin–clavulanate 500 mg q8h PO
	Doxycycline 100 mg bid PO
Mycoplasma pneumoniae	Clarithromycin 500 mg bid PO for 14 days
	Azithromycin 500 mg as a single dose then 250 mg/d PO for 4 days
	Doxycycline 100 mg bid PO for 14 days
Legionella species	Levofloxacin 500 mg/d IV until clinical improvement is evident then PO therapy to complete a 21-day course‡ or moxifloxacin 400 mg/d PO or gatifloxacin 400 mg/d IV or PO
	Azithromycin 1 g IV as a single dose then 500 mg/d IV until clinical improvement is evident then 500 mg/d PO to complete a 14-day course‡
Chlamydia pneumoniae	Doxycycline 100 mg bid PO for 21 days
	Clarithromycin 500 mg/d PO for 14 days
	Azithromycin 500 mg as a single dose then 250 mg/d PO for 4 days
Anaerobes	Clindamycin or penicillin plus metronidazole
Pseudomonas aeruginosa	Aminoglycoside§ plus piperacillin or ticarcillin or mezlocillin or ceftazidime or imipenem or meropenem or ciprofloxacin

CrCl = creatinine clearance; IM = intramuscularly; IV= intravenously; MIC = minimum inhibitory concentration; MU = million units; PO = orally.

* Other second- or third-generation cephalosporins can substituted for cefuroxime.

† Always check for endocarditis in patients with *S. aureus* pneumonia

‡ Rifampin 600 mg/d PO may be added to this regimen for patients with severe infection.

§ Appropriate aminoglycosides include gentamicin, tobramycin, and amikacin.

Results of Clinical Trials

One of the reasons for the debate about empirical CAP treatment is the inadequacy of the clinical trials that have been done in this area. Most of these trials have enrolled small numbers of patients and do not reflect the spectrum of illness severity for these patients as seen in practice, usually because they have enrolled only mildly to moderately ill patients, which is reflected in the very low mortality rates and extremely high cure rates. However, two retrospective studies do suggest that there are differences in outcomes according to the initial empirical antibiotic regime chosen. Gleason and coworkers (51) reviewed the hospital records of 12,945 Medicare patients hospitalized for CAP treatment and found that initial therapy with a second-generation cephalosporin plus a macrolide, a nonpseudomonal third-generation cephalosporin plus a macrolide, or a fluoroquinolone alone was independently associated with a lower 30-day mortality than was treatment with a nonpseudomonal third-generation cephalosporin alone. Use of a combination β-lactam/β-lactamase inhibitor in conjunction with a macrolide or an aminoglycoside plus another agent was associated with increased 30-day mortality. Dudas and coworkers (52), in an observational study of 2963 patients, made essentially the same observations. Another issue in antimicrobial CAP treatment is the effect of a delay in initiating such therapy. Meehan and coworkers (53) conducted a retrospective, multicenter cohort study of patients over 65 years of age with CAP who presented to emergency departments. The authors used the Medicare National Claims history file from October 1, 1994, through September 30, 1995. Approximately 75% of patients received antibiotics within 8 hours of presentation and had a significantly lower 30-day mortality rate than patients who did not receive treatment within 8 hours.

Nursing Home–Acquired Pneumonia

Degelau and coworkers (54) found that the failure rate of treatment for pneumonia in the nursing home was high if a patient exhibited more than two of the following factors: respiratory rate above 30 breaths per min, temperature above 100.5°F, pulse rate above 90 bpm, feeding dependence, and mechanically altered diet. Nicolle and coworkers (55) noted that 70% of patients with nursing home–acquired pneumonia who were treated with ampicillin were cured compared with 93% of those treated with ceftriaxone. It would seem that treatment of nursing home–acquired pneumonia with one of the respiratory fluoroquinolones would be appropriate; however, data from randomized controlled trials are still lacking for this group of patients. Other appropriate therapies include amoxicillin or intramuscular ceftriaxone.

Duration of Treatment

It has been shown that in-hospital observation of low-risk patients is unnecessary after they are switched from intravenous to oral antibiotic therapy (56). Elimination of this practice usually reduces the hospital stay by 1 day.

The duration of antibiotic therapy for CAP has not been defined adequately, but 10 to 14 days of treatment is usually sufficient for most infections. However, legionnaires' disease should be treated for 21 days (32).

Other Aspects of Treatment

Patients with pneumonia and a pleural effusion should undergo chest radiography in the lateral decubitus position. If the effusion is found to be more than 1 cm wide, it should be aspirated. Subsequent management depends on the characteristics of the effusion fluid (57).

Other aspects of CAP treatment include the management of comorbid illnesses, which is beyond the scope of this chapter.

Follow-Up

Patients who respond to antibiotic treatment do not require repeat chest radiography while in the hospital; however, patients over 40 years of age and patients who smoke tobacco should undergo follow-up chest radiography to ensure that their pneumonia has resolved. In 2% of patients with CAP, this pneumonia is the presenting manifestation of cancer of the lung (58); 50% of these cancers are evident at the time of presentation, but the remaining 50% are detected only on a follow-up chest radiograph. The time for radiographic resolution of pneumonia depends on the age of the patient and the presence of chronic obstructive pulmonary disease (59). If the opacity has not resolved in 10 weeks, bronchoscopy should be performed.

Prevention

Yearly influenza vaccination of target populations (i.e., those over 65 years of age, nursing home residents, and those with cardiac or pulmonary disease) is associated with a 48% to 57% lower rate of hospitalization for pneumonia and influenza (60). An unexpected benefit of influenza vaccination is that the rate of hospitalization for congestive heart failure is reduced by 37% during influenza A epidemics (60).

Pneumococcal vaccine has been shown to be cost effective in patients over 65 years of age (61) and protective against bacteremic pneumococcal pneumonia (62).

Prevention of aspiration in patients at risk (i.e., after a stroke, with advanced Parkinson's disease, and with advanced Alzheimer's disease) is difficult (63). Head positioning, stimulation techniques, exercises to enhance the swallowing reflex, and oral feeding with pureed foods all can help to reduce the risk of aspiration (64).

Summary

The treatment of CAP is a challenge. A key element in successful treatment is an accurate assessment of illness severity. A pneumonia-specific severity-of-illness scoring system is now available to help with the admission decision. The diagnostic work-up and antimicrobial therapy should be tailored to the illness severity of the patient.

REFERENCES

1. **Dixon RE.** Economic costs of respiratory tract infections in the United States. *Am J Med.* 1985;78:45–51.

2. **National Centre for Health Statistics.** National Hospital Discharge Survey: Annual Summary, 1990. *Vital Health Stat.* 1992;13:1–225.

3. **Koivula I, Stenn M, Makela PH.** Risk factors for pneumonia in the elderly. *Am J Med.* 1994;96:313–20.

4. **Lipsky BA, Boyko EJ, Inui TS, et al.** Risk factors for acquiring pneumococcal infections. *Arch Intern Med.* 1986;146:2179–85.

5. **Plouffe JF, Breiman RE, Facklam RR, and the Franklin County Pneumonia Study Group.** Bacteremia with *Streptococcus pneumoniae*: implications for therapy and prevention. *JAMA.* 1996;275:194–8.

6. **Marston BJ, Lipman HB, Breiman RF.** Surveillance for legionnaires' disease: risk factors for morbidity and mortality. *Arch Intern Med.* 1994;154:2417–22.

7. **Butler JC, Hofmann J, Cetron MS, et al.** The continued emergence of drug-resistant *Streptococcus pneumoniae* in the United States: an update from the Centres for Disease Control and Prevention's surveillance system. *J Infect Dis.* 1996;174:986–93.

8. **Moreno S, Garcia-Leoni ME, Cercenado E, et al.** Infections caused by erythromycin-resistant *Streptococcus pneumoniae*: incidence, risk factors, and response to therapy in a prospective study. *Clin Infect Dis.* 1995;20:1195–200.

9. **Clavo-Sanchez AJ, Giron-Gonzalez JA, Lopez-Prieto D, et al.** Multivariate analysis of risk factors for infection due to penicillin-resistant and multidrug-resistant *Streptococcus pneumoniae*: a multicenter study. *Clin Infect Dis.* 1997;24:1052–9.

10. **Nava JM, Bella F, Garau J, et al.** Predictive factors for invasive disease due to penicillin-resistant *Streptococcus pneumoniae*: a population-based study. *Clin Infect Dis.* 1994;19:884–90.

11. **Flournoy DJ, Stalling FH, Catron TL.** Seasonal and monthly variation of *Streptococcus pneumoniae* and other pathogens in bacteremia (1961–1981). *Ecol Dis.* 1983;2:157–60.

12. **Berendt RF, Long GG, Walker JS.** Influenza alone and in sequence with pneumonia due to *Streptococcus pneumoniae* in the squirrel monkey. *J Infect Dis.* 1975;132:689–93.

13. **Marston BJ, Plouffe JF, File TM Jr, et al.** Incidence of community-acquired pneumonia requiring hospitalization: results of a population based active surveillance study in Ohio. *Arch Intern Med.* 1997;157:1709–18.

14. **Berntsson E, Lagergard T, Strannegard O, et al.** Etiology of community-acquired pneumonia in outpatients. *Eur J Clin Microbiol.* 1986;5:446–7.

15. **Marrie TJ, Peeling RW, Fine MJ, et al.** Ambulatory patients with community-acquired pneumonia: the frequency of atypical agents and clinical course. *Am J Med.* 1996;101:508–15.

16. **Erard PH, Moser F, Wenger A, et al.** Prospective study on community-acquired pneumonia diagnosed and followed up by private practitioner: abstracts of the 1991 Interscience Conference on Antimicrobial Agents and Chemotherapy. *American Society for Microbiology.* 1991:108:56A.

17. **Langille DB, Yates L, Marrie TJ.** Serological investigation of pneumonia as it presents to the physician's office. *Can Infect Dis.* 1993;4:328–32.

18. **Porath A, Schlaeffer F, Lieberman D.** The epidemiology of community-acquired pneumonia among hospitalized patients. *J Infect.* 1997;34:41–8.

19. **Burman LA, Trollfors B, Andersen B, et al.** Diagnosis of pneumonia by cultures, bacterial and viral antigen detection tests, and serology with special reference to antibodies against pneumococcal antigen. *J Infect Dis.* 1993;163:1087–93.

20. **Bohte R, van Furth R, van den Broek PJ.** Aetiology of community-acquired pneumonia: a prospective study among adults requiring admission to hospital. *Thorax.* 1995;50:543–7.

21. **Mundy LM, Aurwaeter PG, Oldach D, et al.** Community-acquired pneumonia: impact of immune status. *Am J Respir Crit Care Med.* 1995;152:1309–15.

22. **Marrie TJ, Durant H, Yates L.** Community-acquired pneumonia requiring hospitalization. *Rev Infect Dis.* 1989;11:586–99.

23. **Kauppinen MT, Herva E, Kujala P, et al.** The etiology of community-acquired pneumonia among hospitalized patients during a *Chlamydia pneumoniae* epidemic in Finland. *J Infect Dis.* 1995; 172:1330–5.

24. **Levy M, Dromer F, Brion N, et al.** Community-acquired pneumonia: importance of initial noninvasive bacteriologic and radiographic investigations. *Chest.* 1988;92:43–8.

25. **Fang G-D, Fine M, Orleff J, et al.** New and emerging etiologies for community-acquired pneumonia with implications for therapy. *Medicine.* 1990;69:307–16.

26. **Metlay JP, Kapoor WN, Fine MJ.** Does this patient have community-acquired pneumonia by history and physical examination? *JAMA.* 1997;278:1440–5.

27. **Metlay JP, Schulz R, Li Y-H, et al.** Influence of age on symptoms and presentation in patients with community-acquired pneumonia. *Arch Intern Med.* 1997;157:1453–9.

28. **British Thoracic Society Research Committee.** The aetiology, management, and outcome of severe community-acquired pneumonia in the intensive care unit. *Respir Med.* 1992;86:7–13.

29. **Karalis NC, Cursons RT, Cepulis S, et al.** Community-acquired pneumonia: aetiology and prognostic index evaluation. *Thorax.* 1991; 46:413–8.

30. **Fine MJ, Auble TE, Yealy DM, et al.** A prediction rule to identify low-risk patients with community-acquired pneumonia. *N Engl J Med.* 1997; 336:243–50.

31. **Chalasani NP, Valdecanas MAL, Gopal AK, et al.** Clinical utility of blood cultures in adult patients with community-acquired pneumonia without underlying risks. *Chest.* 1995;108:932–6.

32. **Stout JE, Yu VL.** Legionellosis. *N Engl J Med.* 1997;337:682–7.

33. **Koler RB, Winn WC Jr, Wheat LJ.** Onset and duration of antigen excretion in legionnaires' disease. *J Clin Microbiol.* 1984;20:605–7.

34. **Ramirez JA, Ahkee S, Tolentino A, et al.** Diagnosis of *Legionella pneumophila, Mycoplasma pneumoniae*, or *Chlamydia pneumoniae* lower respiratory tract infections using the polymerase chain reaction in nasopharyngeal swabs. *Diagn Microbiol Infect Dis.* 1996;24:7–14.

35. **Jimenez P, Saldias F, Meneses W, et al.** Diagnostic fiberoptic bronchoscopy in patients with community-acquired pneumonia: comparison between bronchoalveolar lavage and telescopic plugged catheter cultures. *Chest.* 1993;103:1023–7.

36. **Palmer DL, Davidson M, Lusk R.** Needle aspiration of the lung in complex pneumonias. *Chest.* 1980;78:16–21.

37. **Dunn IJ, Marrie TJ, Bhan V, Janegan DT.** The value of open lung biopsy in immunocompetent patients with community-acquired pneumonia requiring hospitalization. *Chest.* 1994;106:23–7.

38. **Neiderman MS, Bass JB Jr, Campbell GD, et al.** Guidelines for the initial management of community-acquired pneumonia, diagnosis, assessment of severity and initial antimicrobial therapy. *Am Rev Respir Dis.* 1993;148:1418–26.

39. **Gleason PR, Kapoor WN, Stone RA, et al.** Medical outcomes and antimicrobial costs with the use of the American Thoracic Society Guidelines for outpatients with community-acquired pneumonia. *JAMA.* 1997;278:32–9.

40. **Bartlett JG, Dowell SF, Mandell LA, et al.** Practice guidelines for the management of community-acquired pneumonia. *Clin Infect Dis.* 2000;31:347–82.

41. **File TM Jr, Segretti J, Dunbar L, et al.** A multicenter, randomized study comparing the efficacy and safety of intravenous and/or oral levofloxacin versus ceftriaxone and/or cefuroxime axetil in treatment of adults with community-acquired pneumonia. *Antimicrob Agents Chemother.* 1997;41:1965–72.

42. **Heffelfinger JD, Dowell SF, Jorgensen JH, et al.** Management of community-acquired pneumonia in the era of pneumococcal resistance: a report from the drug-resistant *Streptococcus pneumoniae* therapeutic working group. *Arch Intern Med.* 2000;160:1399–1408.

43. **Ramirez JA, Srinath L, Ahkee S, et al.** Early switch from intravenous to oral cephalosporins in treatment of hospitalized patients with community-acquired pneumonia. *Arch Intern Med.* 1995;155:1273–6.

44. **Ramirez JA, Ahkee S.** Early switch from intravenous antibiotics to oral clarithromycin in patients with community-acquired pneumonia. *Infect Med.* 1997;14:319–23.

45. **Chan R, Hemeryck L, O'Regan M, et al.** Oral versus intravenous antibiotics for community-acquired lower respiratory tract infection in a general hospital: open randomized controlled trial. *BMJ.* 1995; 310:1360–2.

46. **Pallares R, Linares J, Vadillo, et al.** Resistance to penicillin and cephalosporin and mortality from severe pneumococcal pneumonia in Barcelona, Spain. *N Engl J Med.* 1995;333:474–80.

47. **Craig WA.** Antimicrobial resistance issues of the future. *Diagn Microbiol Infect Dis.* 1996;25:213–7.

48. **Craig WA.** Pharmacokinetic/pharmacodynamic parameters: rationale for antibiotic dosing of mice and men. *Clin Infect Dis.* 1990;26:1–12..

49. **Goldstein FW.** Choice of an oral β-lactam antibiotic for infections due to penicillin resistant *Streptococcus pneumoniae. Scand J Infect Dis.* 1997;29:255–7.

50. **Low DE.** Resistance issues and treatment implications: *Pneumococcus, Staphylococcus aureus*, and gram-negative rods. *Infect Dis Clin North Am.* 1998;12:613–30.

51. **Gleason PP, Meehan TP, Fine JM, et al.** Associations between initial antimicrobial therapy and medical outcomes for hospitalized elderly patients with pneumonia. *Arch Intern Med.* 1999;159:2562–72.

52. **Dudas V, Hopefl A, Jacobs R, Guglielmo J.** Antimicrobial selection for hospitalized patients with presumed community-acquired pneumonia: a survey of nonteaching U.S. community hospitals. *Ann Pharmacother.* 2000;34:446–52.

53. **Meehan TP, Fine MJ, Krumholz HM, et al.** Quality of care, process, and outcomes in elderly patients with pneumonia. *JAMA.* 1997;278:2080–4.

54. **Degelau J, Guay D, Straub K, et al.** Effectiveness of oral antibiotic treatment in nursing home–acquired pneumonia. *J Am Geriatr Soc.* 1995;43:245–51

55. **Nicolle LE, Kirshen A, Boustcha B, Montgomery P.** Treatment of moderate-to-severe pneumonia in elderly, long-term care facility residents. *Infect Dis Clin Pract.* 1996;5:130–7.

56. **Rhew DC, Hackner D, Henderson L, et al.** The clinical benefit of in-hospital observation in "low risk" pneumonia patients after conversion from parenteral to oral antimicrobial therapy. *Chest.* 1998;113:142–6.

57. **Bryant RE, Salmon CJ.** Pleural empyema. *Clin Infect Dis.* 1996; 22:747–62.

58. **Marrie TJ.** Pneumonia and carcinoma of the lung. *J Infect.* 1994;29:45–52.

59. **Jay SJ, Johnson WG Jr, Pierce AK.** The radiographic resolution of *Streptococcus pneumoniae* pneumonia. *N Engl J Med.* 1975;293:791–4.

60. **Nichol KL, Margolis KL, Wuorenma J, von Sternberg T.** The efficacy and cost effectiveness of vaccination against influenza among elderly persons living in the community. *N Engl J Med.* 1994;331:778–84.

61. **Sisk JE, Moskowtiz AJ, Whang W, et al.** Cost-effectiveness of vaccination against pneumococcal bacteremia among elderly people. *JAMA.* 1997;278:1333–9.

62. **Fine MJ, Smith MA, Carson CA, et al.** Efficacy of pneumococcal vaccination in adults: a meta-analysis of randomized controlled trials. *Arch Intern Med.* 1994; 154:2666–77

63. **Holas MA, DePippo KL, Reading MJ.** Aspiration and relative risk of medical complications following stroke. *Arch Neurol.* 1994;51:1051–3

64. **Neuman S, Bartolome G, Buchholz D, Prosiegel M.** Swallowing therapy of neurological patients: correlation of outcome with pretreatment variables and therapeutic methods. *Dysphagia.* 1995;10:1–5.

22

Nosocomial Pneumonia

Stephen M. Seink, MD

Thomas M. File Jr., MD, MS

Nosocomial pneumonia (NP) is defined as pneumonia that was neither present nor incubating at the time of admission to the hospital. NP is the second most common nosocomial infection in the United States and is considered the most serious hospital-acquired infection because of its high morbidity and mortality. Crude mortality rates of up to 70% have been reported; however, the attributable mortality rate has been estimated to be 33% to 50% (1). NP increases hospital length of stay by an average of 7 to 9 days per patient; the cost of prolonged hospitalization for NP has been estimated to be $1.2 billion in the United States (2,3).

Epidemiology

Available data suggest that NP occurs at a rate of five to 10 cases per 1000 hospital admissions, with the incidence increasing by as much as six- to 20-fold in patients who are ventilated mechanically (1). The incidence of NP is much lower in community and small hospitals and among patients admitted to obstetric or psychiatric wards than it is in large tertiary centers and among patients admitted to medical or surgical wards (partly because of the underlying conditions that are more commonly associated with patients in these settings). Most cases of NP occur in intensive care units (ICUs) or in postsurgical recovery areas.

In mechanically ventilated patients, the risk of ventilator-associated pneumonia (VAP) is estimated to be 1% per day of ventilation; however, the rate of new cases decreases with prolonged length of stay. Because crude rates of VAP do not adjust for time of mechanical ventilation, using an index of cases per 1000 ventilator days is advocated. Rates of VAP per 1000 ventilator days range from 5 in pediatric ICU patients to 34 in patients with thermal injury (15 for medical and surgical ICU patients). Such rates may be biased by the overrepresentation of studies from tertiary teaching hospitals.

Pathogenesis and Risk Factors

The primary route of infection of the lower respiratory tract that is associated with hospital-acquired pneumonia involves the microaspiration of organisms that have colonized the oropharyngeal tract. Most healthy individuals are colonized by organisms with limited virulence; however, in hospitalized patients, oropharyngeal colonization with *Staphylococcus aureus* and enteric gram-negative bacilli increases with the severity of the underlying disease. Therefore, risk factors for the development of NP usually are associated with increased microbial colonization of upper airway secretions or an increased risk of aspiration. These factors generally can be categorized as being patient related, infection-control related, or intervention related (Table 22.1).

Table 22.1 Risk Factors for Nosocomial Pneumonia

Patient-Related Factors	Infection-Control Factors
Severe acute or chronic illnesses	Poor infection control practices
Coma	Not washing hands or changing gloves between
Malnutrition	patients
Prolonged hospitalization and/or preoperative period	Contaminated respiratory therapy devices and equipment
Hypotension	
Metabolic acidosis	
Cigarette smoking	**Intervention-Related Factors**
CNS dysfunction	Prolonged or complicated surgery (especially
COPD	thoracoabdominal procedures)
Diabetes mellitus	Endotracheal tubes
Alcoholism	Nasogastric tubes
Azotemia	Enteral feedings
Respiratory failure	Antacids and H_2-blockers
Advanced age	Prolonged and inappropriate use of antibiotics

CNS = central nervous system; COPD = chronic obstructive pulmonary disease.
Adapted from Campbell GD, Niederman MS, Broughton WA, et al. Hospital-acquired pneumonia in adults. Diagnosis, assessment of severity, initial antimicrobial therapy, and preventive strategies: a consensus statement. *Am J Respir Crit Care Med.* 1998;153:1711–25.

Patient-related risk factors for NP include age, severity of underlying illness, malnutrition, coma or other causes of impaired consciousness (e.g., sedating medications), prolonged hospitalization, and certain comorbid conditions (e.g., diabetes, heart disease, chronic obstructive pulmonary disease). Risk factors related to infection control include poor hand-washing practices, inappropriate use of gloves, and contaminated respiratory therapy devices and equipment. Therapeutic interventions that adversely affect host defenses and result in the direct inoculation of pathogens into the lower respiratory tract include the presence of endotracheal or nasogastric tubes. The most significant intervention-related risk factor for NP is mechanical ventilation; the risk of developing pneumonia increases with the duration of mechanical ventilation. Additional intervention-related risk factors include feeding by nasogastric tube, increased gastric volume or distention, and supine positioning of the patient. The role of the stomach may vary, with factors that include gastric pH, presence of ileus or upper gastrointestinal disease, use of antacid medications or enteric feeding, gastric reflux associated with the supine position, and the presence of a gastric or nasogastric tube. Migration of microorganisms from the stomach to the lungs may occur through various mechanisms (4). A nasogastric tube may act as a conduit for microorganisms to ascend into the nasopharynx. The nasogastric tube also may affect lower esophageal sphincter competence and thus allow the reflux of organisms from the stomach to the nasopharynx. This is most likely to occur when the patient is in the supine position. Once the nasopharynx becomes colonized, organisms may descend into the respiratory tract and cause lower respiratory tract disease.

Predictors of mortality for pneumonia include the Acute Physiology and Chronic Health Evaluation (APACHE) II score, the number of dysfunctional organs, nosocomial bacteremia, NP, the presence of an underlying fatal disease, and admission from another ICU (5).

Etiology

Numerous studies have evaluated pathogens associated with NP; however, variations in patient populations, the methods used to obtain and analyze specimens, and even the definitions used for NP have led to variable results. Additionally, the upper respiratory tract of hospitalized patients often is colonized by potentially pathogenic microorganisms; thus it is difficult to know which of the multiple organisms present in a respiratory specimen culture are colonizing organisms and which are true pathogens. Because aspiration of upper airway secretions is the most common route of entry for microorganisms into the lower airways, the etiology of NP often depends on the organisms colonizing the oropharynx (3).

In general, the pathogens associated with bacterial NP are gram-negative bacilli (especially *Klebsiella, Enterobacter, Serratia,* and *Pseudomonas* species) and *S. aureus.* However, recent studies have begun to show an increase in prevalence of gram-positive pathogens (e.g., non-*aureus Staphylococcus* species and *Streptococcus* species) as significant pathogens that contribute to bacterial NP. The microbiology identified in several studies of NP is shown in Table 22.2 (6–10). The predominant organisms observed in studies at larger, tertiary hospitals (where most patients are in an ICU and on a ventilator) have been gram-negative bacilli (particularly multidrug-resistant strains) and *S. aureus* (often methicillin-resistant *S. aureus* [MRSA]). In contrast, a study at a community hospital (where only a minority of patients were on mechanical ventilation) found a high prevalence of both *Streptococcus* and *Haemophilus* species. For practical purposes, the etiology of NP can be divided into early onset (<5 days in the hospital, for which *Streptococcus pneumoniae* remains a common pathogen) and late onset (>5 days in the hospital for which Enterobacteriaceae and *Pseudomonas* species are common pathogens) (Table 22.3).

Table 22.2   Bacteriology of Nosocomial Pneumonia: Prevalence of Etiologic Organisims

	Schaberg et al. (6)	Bartlett et al. (7)	Fagon et al. (8)	Schleupner et al. (9)	Fagon et al. (10)	Fagon et al. (10)
Hospital type	University	Veteran	Tertiary	General community (nontertiary)	31 ICUs	31 ICUs
Ventilated or nonventilated?	Mixed	Mixed	Ventilated	Mostly non-ventilated	Ventilated	Ventilated
Specimens	Sputum, TTA	TTA, Blood	PSB	Sputum, ETS, TTA	PSB, BAL	TTA
Bacteria						
Polymicrobial	NR	54%	40%	NR	25%	95%
Gram-negative bacilli	50%	46%	75%	15%	53%	>75%
Pneumococcus aeruginosa	17%	9%	31%	4%	27%	57%
Acinetobacter spp.	NR	0%	15%	NR	6%	11%
Haemophilus influenzae	6%	17%	10%	12%	9%	12%
Staphylococcus aureus	16%	25%	33%	5%	10%	40%
Streptococcus spp.	1%	31%	21%	20%	19%	28%
Legionella spp.	NR	NR	2%	NR	NR	NR

BAL = bronchoalveolar lavage; ETS = endotracheal aspirate; ICUs = intensive care units; NR = not reported; PSB = protected specimen brush; TTA = transtracheal aspirate.

Table 22.3   Bacteriology of Nosocomial Pneumonia Based on Disease Onset

Late-Onset Pneumonia (>5 days)	Early-Onset Pneumonia (<5 days)
Pneumococcus aeruginosa	Streptococcus pneumoniae
Enterobacter spp.	Haemophilus influenzae
Acinetobacter spp.	M. catarrhalis
Klebsiella pneumoniae	Staphylococcus aureus
Serratia marcescens	Enteric gram-negative bacilli*
Escherichia coli	
Other gram-negative bacilli	
Staphylococcus aureus (MRSA)	**Other**
	Anaerobic bacteria
	Legionella pneumophila
	Candida spp.

MRSA = methicillin-resistant *S. aureus*.
Adapted from Campbell GD, Niederman MS, Broughton WA, et al. Hospital-acquired pneumonia in adults. Diagnosis, assessment of severity, initial antimicrobial therapy, and preventive strategies: a consensus statement. *Am J Respir Crit Care Med.* 1998;153:1711–25.

The following specific organisms also are associated with the epidemiologic setting of NP:

- Anaerobes in association with abdominal surgery or following aspiration
- *S. aureus* in association with coma, head trauma, recent influenza infection, diabetes mellitus;
- *Legionella* species in association with corticosteroid use or presence of *Legionella* species in the hospital water supply
- *Aspergillus* species associated with construction

Diagnosis and Microbiological Studies

The standard clinical criteria often used to establish a diagnosis (or possible diagnosis) of NP include some combination of fever, leukocytosis, and purulent respiratory secretions in association with a new or progressive infiltrate on chest radiography. Unfortunately, these criteria do not provide a reliably accurate diagnosis of NP; rather, the definition they give is sensitive but not specific for NP, particularly in mechanically ventilated patients (in whom other conditions may cause fever and pulmonary infiltrates). When all four criteria (i.e., fever, leukocytosis, purulent respiratory secretions, and a new pulmonary infiltrate) are present, specificity improves but sensitivity drops to less than 50%, which is not clinically acceptable (15). Less than half of patients who have fever and pulmonary infiltrates have the diagnosis of bacterial pneumonia confirmed microbiologically. Other conditions that can mimic NP clinically include pulmonary infarction, adult respiratory distress syndrome, pulmonary edema with another infection site, pulmonary hemorrhage, vasculitis, malignancy, drug toxicity, radiation pneumonitis, and preexisting lung disease (e.g., fibrosing alveolitis).

Unfortunately, the techniques now used to obtain respiratory secretions for culture are not consistently helpful in diagnosing NP because it is difficult to obtain specimens that are not contaminated with upper respiratory tract organisms. Therefore, the value of examining expectorated sputum in patients with NP is limited and any interpretation of the microbiological results is challenging and must be performed with caution. Expectorated sputum is often contaminated with upper respiratory flora acquired by patients after hospitalization. Sputum (or endotracheal secretions) should be examined microscopically by Gram staining and screening for the appropriateness of the specimen (using cytologic criteria based on the presence of polymorphonuclear leukocytes and the absence of squamous cells). In the intubated patient, lower airway secretions usually are obtained easily with routine endotracheal aspiration. Cultures of endotracheal aspirates often are used for microbiological studies because health care workers can perform the aspiration procedure at the bedside with minimal training. Such cultures usually identify not only the pathogenic organisms that are found by invasive tests (suggesting a high level of sensitivity) but also the nonpathogenic organisms (reducing the positive predictive value of the procedure). Most studies have shown that when VAP is present, the etiologic pathogens usually are contained in the endotracheal aspirate, suggesting a high sensitivity of endotracheal aspiration even though additional colonizing organisms also may be present (15). Thus, the absence of a specific organism from nonquantitative endotracheal-aspiration cultures (assuming that the specimen is obtained while the patient is not receiving effective antibiotic therapy) is highly predictive against that organism as a pathogen. This information may allow the clinician to exclude certain pathogens and may be helpful when modifying antimicrobial therapy once cultures results are known.

A variety of quantitative culture methods that generally utilize invasive bronchoscopic methods have been developed to differentiate colonization from active pathogenicity and, thus, to define the presence of pneumonia and to identify more specifically the pathogenic organisms causing the disease. However, the sensitivity and specificity of invasive diagnostic techniques for determining the true microbiological identity of bacteria associated with NP are variable. The sensitivity of quantitative bronchoalveolar lavage (BAL) fluid cultures ranges from 40% to 90%, with a mean of approximately 70%

(15). The variability in sensitivity reflects the characteristics of the study population as well as the effect of previous antibiotic therapy (which reduces the rate of isolation). Most studies cite 10^4 colony-forming units (CFU) per milliliter as a positive result. The finding of an intracellular organism by BAL is highly specific and has a high positive predictive value (90%–100%). The sensitivity of the protected-specimen–brush (PSB) technique ranges from 33% to 100%, with a median of 67% and specificity of approximately 95% (15). Concerns about diagnostic accuracy and the lack of clinical outcome data have made it difficult to interpret the results of studies using BAL and the PSB technique. This is further complicated when the patient has received antimicrobial agents within the preceding few days. Several studies indicate that a change in antimicrobial therapy within 72 hours before obtaining a quantitative culture by invasive means reduces the accuracy of the culture results. Therefore, it is recommended that such tests be performed either before the use of antibiotics or after 72 hours of an existing antimicrobial regimen (16). Isolating organisms in a significant quantity ($>10^4$ CFU/mL for BAL; $>10^3$ CFU/mL for PSB) after 72 hours of antimicrobial therapy suggests that the treatment regimen is ineffectual.

Recently, the Health and Science Policy Committee of the American College of Chest Physicians assembled a panel of scientific experts to develop recommendations for assessing diagnostic tests for VAP based on a rigorous review of the literature (15). The panel, which included experienced methodologists to ensure that the review process was justified and unbiased, determined that there was insufficient high-level evidence to suggest that quantitative testing procedures produce better clinical outcomes than empirical treatment alone. However, one acknowledged benefit of quantitative culture is the reduced use of antibiotics, which may reduce the selective potential for resistance and adverse effects and may reduce the costs associated with overuse of broad-spectrum antimicrobials (10).

Although the sensitivity of blood culture is low, when it is positive it helps to distinguish between contaminants and the true infectious agent in NP cases.

Antimicrobial Management

Antimicrobial management of NP can be divided into empirical and pathogen-directed therapy. Certainly, once a pathogen is isolated from an appropriate specimen, direct therapy can be given on the basis of *in vitro*-susceptibility test results and other characteristics of the antimicrobial agent and host. However, the great majority of patients initially are treated empirically, and the choice of antimicrobial agent(s) should be based on local susceptibility patterns and the most likely pathogens. Clinicians should be aware of the most common bacterial pathogens in NP and their susceptibility patterns associated in the hospitals where they practice.

Generally, initial antimicrobial therapy for NP should be aimed at gram-negative bacteria (often including *Pseudomonas* species for patients with late-onset infection) and *S. aureus*. Although present practice patterns indicate a preference for combination therapy (e.g., a beta-lactam drug plus an aminoglycoside or fluoroquinolone) for NP, such practice is not supported conclusively by direct scientific evidence. The potential for additive or synergistic efficacy of two-drug therapy against gram-negative bacilli and the argument that combination therapy may reduce the emergence of resistance are two commonly cited reasons for the popularity of combination therapy for NP. However, there is little evidence that two agents with gram-negative activity offer better outcomes than a single effective agent for treating gram-negative pneumonia. Nevertheless, some have the opinion that empirical combination therapy be used for severe NP or in cases associated with a risk of resistant pathogens (e.g., prolonged ICU stay, previous use of antibiotics, steroid use) pending the results of appropriately obtained cultures. The rationale for this is based in part on the greater spectrum of antimicrobial activity that often can be achieved with combination therapy.

Available information suggests that the outcome of NP is improved when effective antimicrobial agents are given initially (11–14). The importance of providing early effective antimicrobial therapy for NP patients has been demonstrated in several recent investigations of VAP patients. These studies have shown that the mortality attributable to VAP was significantly greater among patients who received inadequate initial antimicrobial therapy (during the first 24 hours) than it was among patients who received adequate initial therapy (Table 22.4). Most clinical failures were associated with use of antimicrobial agents that were not effective for *Pseudomonas* species or MRSA. Prescribing an initial broad-spectrum antimicrobial regimen to cover all likely pathogens helps reduce the occurrence of inadequate treatment and may result in improved clinical outcomes. In settings in which multidrug-resistant

Table 22.4   Effect of Initial Antimicrobial Therapy for Ventilator-Associated Pneumonia

Study	Mortality (%)	
	Adequate Therapy	**Inadequate Therapy**
Luna (11)	38	91 ($p < 0.001$)
Alvarez-Lerma (12)	16	25 ($p < 0.039$)
Rello (13)	42	63 ($p < 0.060$)
Kollef (14)	33	61 ($p < 0.001$)

strains of pathogens are present, a combination of antimicrobial agents may allow a greater chance of early effective therapy. To avoid the emergence of antibiotic-resistant infections, however, a broad-spectrum treatment regimen should not be prolonged unnecessarily, unless such a decision is supported by appropriate culture data.

Monotherapy with several broad-spectrum beta-lactam drugs (including combinations of beta-lactam and beta-lactamase inhibitors) seems appropriate for most patients who are not at risk for resistant pathogens (Table 22.5). Some authorities recommend avoiding monotherapy with broad-spectrum cephalosporins because of concern about selecting resistant strains of extended-spectrum, beta-lactamase–producing organisms or about selecting vancomycin-resistant enterococci. When risks involving anaerobic organisms exist (e.g., in cases of witnessed aspiration, recent thoracoabdominal surgery, or impaired swallowing), agents such as beta-lactam/beta-lactamase inhibitor combinations or carbapenems are more appropriate. (Clindamycin can be added to a fluoroquinolone or aztreonam for penicillin-allergic patients.) If nosocomial legionellosis is a concern (i.e., if *Legionella* is known to be present in the water supply), a fluoroquinolone or macrolide should be used.

Initial therapy with combination agents may be more prudent for severely ill patients and for those at greater risk for drug-resistant pathogens. Such therapy could include an antipseudomonal beta-lactam drug plus an aminoglycoside or a fluoroquinolone (*see* Table 22.5). In the past, an aminoglycoside was most commonly used as the second agent; however, because of better penetration into the respiratory tract and potentially less toxicity, a fluoroquinolone now provides an appealing choice. The addition of vancomycin should be considered if the Gram stain reveals gram-positive organisms that are compatible with staphylococci and if MRSA are present in the patient's hospital setting.

There are no good data about duration of therapy; recommendations about this are based on expert opinion. Carefully controlled studies that document duration of therapy have not been reported. The presence of multilobar involvement, severe underlying disease, or necrotizing gram-negative pneumonia may be associated with delayed and often incomplete resolution. In these settings, it seems reasonable to continue antibiotic therapy for a minimum of 14 to 21 days to reduce the chance of relapse. By contrast, cure rates that exceed 95% have been noted for NP that is caused by methicillin-susceptible *S. aureus* or *Haemophilus*; for these pathogens, a 7-day course of therapy may be adequate. Substituting an oral antibiotic (as in the case of fluoroquinolone therapy) may be appropriate, provided that 1) the pathogen is susceptible to it *in vitro*, 2) clinical improvement has occurred, and 3) adequate absorption can be ensured.

Recently, Singh and coworkers (17) reported the use of a Clinical Pulmonary Infection Score to assist in the decision regarding duration of therapy

Table 22.5   Empirical Therapy for Nosocomial Pneumonia

Single-Drug Therapy*

Broad-spectrum beta-lactam/beta-lactamase inhibitor (e.g., ticarcillin–clavulanate, piperacillin–tazobactam)

or

Carbapenem (e.g., imipenem, meropenem)

or

Broad-spectrum cephalosporin (e.g., ceftazidime, cefepime)[†]

or

Fluoroquinolone (e.g., ciprofloxacin, trovafloxacin[‡], levofloxacin) with or without clindamycin[§]

Therapy for Severe Disease or in Patients at Risk for *Pseudomonas* or Resistant Organisms[¶]

Piperacillin or broad-spectrum beta-lactam/beta-lactamase inhibitor (e.g., ticarcillin–clavulanate, piperacillin–tazobactam)

or

Antipseudomonal cephalosporin (e.g., ceftazidime, cefepime)

or

Carbapenem (imipenem or meropenem)

plus

Aminoglycoside (gentamicin, tobramycin, amikacin) or fluoroquinolone (e.g., ciprofloxacin)[**]

Penicillin allergy: Fluoroquinolone plus clindamycin or vancomycin

---

* Most patients can be treated with monotherapy; see text for discussion.
† Ceftriaxone, cefotaxime if *Pseudomonas* species unlikely.
‡ Only for severe infections, per FDA advisory of June 1, 1999.
§ Alternative regimen that can be used in the penicillin-allergic patient.
¶ Risk factors are use of steroids and/or antibiotics, structural lung disease, and a prolonged stay in an intensive care unit.
** Consider adding vancomycin if Gram stain shows organisms compatible with *Staphylococcus* (especially methicillin-resistant *S. aureus* present in the hospital).

for ICU patients with pulmonary infiltrates. For patients with low scores, suggesting that these patients did not have pneumonia, therapy was discontinued after 3 days. Such an approach led to significantly lower microbial costs, antimicrobial resistance, and superinfection rates without adversely affecting the length of stay or mortality.

Prevention

The pathogenesis of NP usually requires two major processes: microbial colonization of upper airway secretions and aspiration of these secretions into the

Table 22.6   Prevention of Nosocomial Pneumonia

Prevention Type	Effective	Ineffective
Pharmacologic	Limiting stress-ulcer prophylaxis*	Aerosolized antibiotic prophylaxis[†]
	Oral rinsing with chlorhexidine*	Selective GI decontamination[†]
Nonpharmacologic	Hand washing*[†]	Routine change of ventilator circuits[†] or in-line suction catheter*
	Semirecumbency*	
	Avoiding gastric distention*	Dedicated, disposable suction catheter[†]
	Subglottic suctioning[†]	Daily change of heat and moisture exchangers[†]
		Chest physiology[†]

GI = gastrointestinal

* Supported by at least one randomized controlled investigation.

[†] Supported by at least two randomized controlled investigations.

Modified from Kollef MH. The prevention of ventilator-associated pneumonia. *N Engl J Med.* 1999;340:627–34.

lung. Therefore, strategies aimed at reducing the incidence of NP focus on reducing the amount of bacterial colonization or reducing the incidence of aspiration (18). Many different strategies for preventing NP have been evaluated (Table 22.6). The most effective methods that are supported by controlled studies include adequate hand-washing between patient contacts, maintaining semirecumbent patient positioning, avoiding gastric overdistention, continuous subglottic suctioning for patients on mechanical ventilation, limiting stress-ulcer prophylaxis, and using chlorhexidine oral rinses. Importantly, the use of aerosolized antibiotic prophylaxis and routine use of antimicrobial agents for selective digestive decontamination have not been found to be beneficial.

Isolating patients with resistant organisms (e.g., MRSA) can decrease the likelihood of transferring these pathogens between patients.

REFERENCES

1. **Campbell GD, Niederman MS, Broughton WA, et al.** Hospital-acquired pneumonia in adults. Diagnosis, assessment of severity, initial antimicrobial therapy, and preventive strategies: a consensus statement. *Am J Respir Crit Care Med.* 1998;153: 1711–25.

2. **Centers for Disease Control and Prevention.** Guidelines for prevention of nosocomial pneumonia. *MMWR Morbid Mortal Wkly Rep.* 1997;46(RR-1):1–79.

3. **Craven DE, Steger KA, LaForce FM.** Pneumonia. In Bennett JV, Brachman PS (eds). *Hospital Infections,* 4th ed. Philadelphia: Lippincott-Raven; 1998:487–509.

4. **Craven DE.** Nosocomial pneumonia: new concepts of an old disease. *Infect Control Hosp Epidemiol.* 9:57–58;1988.

5. **Fagon JY, Chastre J, Vuagnat A, et al.** Mortality risks for nosocomial infection in the ICU. *JAMA.* 1996;275:866–9.

6. **Schaberg DR, Culver DH, Gaynes RP.** Major trends in the microbial etiology of nosocomial infection. *Am J Med.* 1991;91:72–5S.

7. **Bartlett JG, O'Keefe P, Tally FP, et al.** Bacteriology of hospital-acquired pneumonia. *Arch Intern Med.* 1986;146:868–71.

8. **Fagon JY, Chastre J, Domart Y, et al.** Nosocomial pneumonia in patients receiving continuous mechanical ventilation: prospective analysis of 52 episodes with use of a protected specimen brush and quantitative culture techniques. *Am Rev Respir Dis.* 1989; 139:877–84.

9. **Schleupner CJ, Cobb DK.** A study of the etiologies and treatment of nosocomial pneumonia in a community-based teaching hospital [See comments] [Review]. *Infect Contr Hosp Epidemiol.* 1992;13:515–25.

10. **Fagon JY, Chastre J, Wolff M, Stephan F, et al.** Invasive and noninvasive strategies for management of suspected ventilator-associated pneumonia. *Ann Intern Med.* 2000;132:621–30.

11. **Luna CM, Vujacich P, Niederman MS, et al.** Impact of BAL data on the therapy and outcome of ventilator-associated pneumonia. *Chest.* 1997;111:676–85.

12. **Alvarez-Lerma F.** Modification of empiric antibiotic treatment in patients with pneumonia acquired in the intensive care unit: ICU-Acquired Pneumonia Study Group. *Intensive Care Med.* 1996;22:387–94.

13. **Rello J, Gallego M, Mariscal D, et al.** The value of routine microbial investigation in ventilator-associated pneumonia. *Am J Respir Crit Care Med.* 1997;156:196–200.

14. **Kollef MH, Ward S.** The influence of mini-BAL cultures on patient outcomes: implications for the antibiotic management of ventilator associated pneumonia. *Chest.* 1998;113:412–20.

15. **Grossman RF, Fein A.** Evidence-based assessment of diagnostic tests for ventilator-associated pneumonia: executive summary of the clinical practice guideline panel. *Chest.* 2000;117(Suppl 2):177–81S.

16. **Mayhall CG.** Nosocomial pneumonia: diagnosis and prevention. *Infect Dis Clin North Am.* 1997;11:427–57.

17. **Singh N, Rogers P, Atwood CW, et al.** Short course empiric antibiotic therapy for patients with pulmonary infiltrates in the intensive care unit. *Am J Respir Crit Care Med.* 2000;162:505–11.

18. **Kollef MH.** The prevention of ventilator-associated pneumonia. *N Engl J Med.* 1999;340:627–34.

23

Tuberculosis

Donald K. Maxwell, DO

Tuberculosis (TB), also known as the *consumption disease, wasting disease,* and *white plague,* is one of the most common infectious causes of death in the world. Each year, approximately 2 to 3 million people die from this disease worldwide. Although there has been an 8-year decline in TB in the United States, the disease remains a critical health issue owing to factors such as human immunodeficiency virus (HIV) infection, drug resistance, immigration, poverty, injection drug use, long-term care facilities, poorly managed TB programs, and widespread third-world prevalence (1,2). The objective of this chapter is to educate the clinician on the pathogenesis, clinical presentation, and treatment of latent TB infection (LTBI) and active TB.

As of 2002, it is estimated that one-third of the world is infected with TB. Each year nearly 1% of the world's population becomes infected with TB, and 8 million persons develop active TB. If left untreated, each person with active TB can infect from 10 to 15 individuals each year. Although it is estimated that 10 to 15 million individuals in the United States are currently infected with TB, there has been a progressive decline in active TB since 1992 (1,3,4).

Since 1953, the United States surveillance program for TB has recorded the reduction of TB by approximately 6% per year up to 1986. Between 1986 and 1992, there was an increase in the number of TB cases. Reasons for this increase include HIV, rising immigration, greater transmission in congregate settings, emergence of multidrug-resistant organisms, and deterioration of local TB public health programs (4,5). However, improved TB control programs and better diagnosis and treatment of individuals with TB have helped to decrease the incidence of this disease. With respect to the year 2000, the number of cases of active TB declined by approximately 39% from 1992 and

Table 23.1   High-Risk Populations for Contracting Tuberculosis Infection and/or Disease

Persons who have had close contact with a person known or suspected to have infectious TB disease (household or enclosed areas)

Persons with *Mycobacterium tuberculosis* infection in the past 2 years or a history of uncompleted treatment for TB

Foreign-born persons who have arrived in the United States within the past 5 years or persons residing in areas with a high prevalence of TB

Residents and employees of long-term institutional settings (nursing homes, correctional facilities, mental institutions, substance abuse centers, homeless shelters)

Medically underserved low-income populations (homeless, poor, and injection and illicit drug users)

High-risk racial and ethnic minorities

Health-care workers who serve high-risk clients

Elderly persons

Persons who have human immunodeficiency virus infections

Persons with other chronic medical diseases associated with an increased risk of developing TB (chest radiograph suggestive of previous TB with partial or no treatment; diabetes mellitus; end-stage renal disease; organ transplantation, silicosis, intestinal bypass or gastrectomy; prolonged corticosteroid therapy at ≥ 15 mg prednisone per day for 1 month or other immunosuppressive therapy, cancer of the head, neck, or lung; hematologic and reticuloendothelial disease; chronic malabsorption; low body weight [<10% ideal body weight]).

Adapted from *Core Curriculum on Tuberculosis, 3rd Ed.* Atlanta, GA: Centers for Disease Control and Prevention, 1994, 1–50; *Core Curriculum on Tuberculosis, 4th Ed.* Atlanta, GA: Centers for Disease Control and Prevention, 2000, 1–75; Jerant, et al. Identification and management of tuberculosis. *Am Fam Phys* 2000;2668; American Thoracic Society. Targeted tuberculin testing and treatment of latent TB infection. *Am J Respir Crit Care Med* 2000;161:S221–S247.

by 7% from 1999 (2,6). In 2000, a total of 16,377 TB cases were reported in the United States, a rate of 5.8/100,000 persons compared with 53/100,000 persons in 1953 and 10.5/100,000 persons in 1992 (6–9). However, the current figure remains shy of the goal for TB elimination for the United States, and is projected to be less than 1 case/100,000 by 2010 (2).

Populations known to be at higher risk for developing TB can be seen in Table 23.1 (10). In 1998 to 2000, approximately 60% of all reported TB cases were from California, Florida, Illinois, New Jersey, Georgia, New York, and Texas (6–8). Between 1992 and 2000, the number of cases among United States-born persons decreased by 55%, whereas the number of cases among foreign-born persons increased by 5%. However, current TB case rates are 3.5/100,000 for United States-born and 25.8/100,000 for foreign-born persons (6). The proportion of TB cases among foreign-born persons compared with United-States-born persons has increased from 27% to 46% (6,9). Minority groups, such as African–Americans, Hispanics, and Asian Americans, comprise more than 70% of all active TB cases in the United States when compared to Caucasians (8,11). In 2000, 8% of all TB cases were resistant to isoniazid (INH), and 1% were resistant to more than one of the standard antimycobacterial agents. In 2000, half of the multidrug-resistant tuberculosis (MDR-TB) cases in the United States were reported in New York and California. Although multidrug resistance decreased from 2.7% to 0.7% in United States-born and 3.0 to 1.6% in foreign-born individuals, the death rate for persons with MDR-TB is still 40% to 60% (6,7,11).

Transmission and Pathogenesis

TB is caused by *Mycobacterium tuberculosis*, which is spread from person to person via droplet nuclei suspended in the air. A single cough can produce 3000 infective droplet nuclei, each containing from one to three microorganisms. The infecting dose is estimated to be from five to 200 microorganisms. Droplet nuclei containing the mycobacteria are inhaled into the respiratory bronchioles or alveoli. The majority bacteria are destroyed by macrophages or lie dormant in the infected tissue, but some may multiply within the macrophages and be released. The bacteria spread locally or by hematogenous and lymphatic routes to regional lymph nodes and distant organs such as the kidneys, central nervous system, and bone. Infected individuals are usually asymptomatic and noninfectious unless they develop active primary or reactivated TB disease. When a close contact is exposed to a person with active (infectious, contagious) TB disease, there is up to a 23% chance that he or she will develop a TB infection (4,10,12). After the initial exposure and subsequent infection, TB can progress to clinically active disease, remain dormant with the risk of reactivation in the future, or remain clinically silent forever. In 90% of infected individuals, TB disease will never develop. However, approximately 5% of all infected persons cannot control the multiplication of *M. tuberculosis* following the initial infection, and primary disease begins to develop within 1 to 2 years. The remaining 5% of infected patients develop latent (reactivated) disease. Fifteen to 20% of all TB cases are extrapulmonary. Extrapulmonary TB is not transmissible unless there is aerosolization of infected tissue or body fluids, such as in laryngeal TB (4,10–12).

Clinical Manifestations

Assessment for tuberculosis can be challenging, but it is necessary to treat persons with TB adequately in order to prevent the spread of the disease. When an individual is infected with *M. tuberculosis*, a variety of nonspecific signs and symptoms may be seen with the acute infection or active disease. An individual may be asymptomatic with a pulmonary TB infection. Fever, nonproductive cough, and pleuritic chest pain may be seen in primary disease. Classic symptoms, such as hemoptysis, persistent productive cough (≥ 3 weeks), weight loss, fatigue, anorexia, night sweats, and low-grade fever for more than 3 days can be seen in active or reactivated disease (10,13). Extrapulmonary TB symptoms depend on the site involved. Examples of such symptoms are back pain (Pott's disease), altered mental status (TB meningitis), and hematuria (genitourinary TB). The most common locations of extrapulmonary TB are pleural, lymphatic, skeletal, genitourinary, gastrointestinal, and the central nervous system. Further information regarding extrapulmonary TB can be reviewed in articles published by the American Thoracic Society (12,14,15). Physical findings and laboratory values tend to be nonspecific. For example, a person with pulmonary TB may have no abnormal lung sounds or may have rales or bronchial breath sounds on physical examination. Laboratory values may reveal leukocytosis, elevated monocyte or eosinophil counts, anemia, pancytopenia, or hyponatremia.

Diagnosis

The Mantoux test, or tuberculin skin test (TST), using a purified protein derivative (PPD) of the tuberculin antigen, is used to see if a person is or has been infected with *M. tuberculosis*. From 2 to 10 weeks after a patient is infected with the tubercle bacillus, a hypersensitivity reaction to the tuberculin antigen develops. One-tenth of a milliliter of five tuberculin units (TU) of PPD is placed intradermally, usually into the volar surface of the forearm. This produces a discrete, pale elevation, 6- to 10-mm in diameter. The size of the induration, not the size of the erythema, must be read within 48 to 72 hours after the injection. Table 23.2 shows the recommended definition of the reaction size to the PPD considered positive according to specific risk factors (4,10,12–14,16). Approximately 20% of patients with active TB may have a negative TST. This may be due to anergy or to factors listed in Table 23.3 (5,12,16). To prove anergy, a Mantoux test using tetanus toxoid, mumps, and *Candida* antigen should be administered. If there is more than a 3-mm reaction to any antigen or PPD, the person is not anergic. In order to look for the booster phenomenon, two-step testing is performed by doing two TSTs from 1 to 3 weeks apart. If both tests are negative, the person is probably not infected. However, if the size of the induration in the second TST is greater than 10 mm in persons less than 35 years old or greater than 15 mm in persons older than 35 years, it is held that the individual was infected with TB in the past but is not considered a new converter. The size of the induration in the second TST can be considered the person's baseline value (17).

A reactor is a person who develops a positive TST after having a negative TST more than 2 years earlier, or a person who develops a positive TST after never having been administered a TST previously. A converter is a person

Table 23.2 Positive Tuberculin Skin Test Reactions

≥ 5 mm	≥ 10 mm	≥ 15 mm
Recent close contacts of a person with active TB	Children < 4 years old. Infants, children, or adolescents who are exposed to persons in high-risk categories	Any person who does not have risk factors for TB
HIV-infected person or risk factors for HIV with unknown status	Some medically underserved, low-income populations or high-risk racial and ethnic minority groups[1]	
Chest radiograph suggestive of previously healed TB	HIV-negative injectable drug users	
Injectable or illicit drug user with unknown HIV status, HIV-positive, or BCG-vaccinated person	Recent immigrants (within 5 years) from countries with a high prevalence of TB	
Organ transplant recipients or immunosuppressed patients	Mycobacteriology laboratory personnel	
	Persons with certain medical conditions[2]	
	Residents and employees of high-risk congregate settings[3]	
	Person with recent seroconversion for TB: consider age and risk of developing or spreading TB, and whether or not to treat BCG-vaccinated person[4] who is HIV negative	

[1]Asian and Pacific Islanders, African–Americans, and Native Americans.
[2]Medical conditions include diabetes mellitus, silicosis, prolonged corticosteroid use (> 15 mg/day), or other immunosuppressive therapy; cancer of the head, neck, and lung; hematologic and reticuloendothelial disease (i.e., lymphoma, leukemia); end-stage renal disease; intestinal bypass or gastrectomy; chronic malabsorption syndrome; or low body weight (10% or more below ideal body weight)
[3]Nursing homes and other long-term facilities for elderly persons; hospitals and other health-care facilities; AIDS residential facilities; correctional facilities; homeless shelters
[4]A BCG-vaccinated person is considered PPD positive at an induration ≥ 10 mm if the person 1) has had close contact to patients with infectious TB, 2) was born or resided in a country in which TB prevalence is high, 3) is exposed continually to populations in which the prevalence of TB is high (some health-care workers, employees, and volunteers at homeless shelters or drug treatment centers)
Adapted from ATS. *Am Rev Respir Dis* 1990;142:725–35; ATS. *AJRCCM* 1994;149:359–74; CDC. Core Curr on TB 3rd ed. 1994; 1–50; CDC. *Am Rev Respir Dis* 1992;146:1623–33; ATS. *AJRCCM* 2000;161:S221–S247; CDC. Core Curr on TB 4th ed. 2000; 1–75; ATS. *AJRCCM* 2000;161:1376-95.
BCG = Bacillus-Calmette-Guerin; HIV = human immunodeficiency virus; PPD = purified protein derivative; TB = tuberculosis.

who has had a negative TST within the past 2 years who then becomes positive according to his or her risk factors. These factors are noted in Table 23.2 (4,10,12–14,16,17).

Table 23. 3   Factors That May Cause Altered Response to Tuberculin Skin Test

False-Negative
  Factors related to the person who is given the Mantoux test:
    Infections
      Viral: measles, mumps, chicken pox, and HIV
      Bacterial: typhoid fever, brucellosis, typhus, leprosy, pertussis, overwhelming TB, TB
        pleurisy
      Fungal: blastomycosis
    Live virus vaccinations: measles, mumps, polio
    Nutrition: severe malnutrition, zinc deficiency
    Lymphoproliferative diseases: chronic lymphocytic leukemia, Hodgkin's disease,
      lymphoma, sarcoidosis
    Drugs: corticosteroids, immunosuppressants
    Age: newborns, elderly
    Other: recent < 2–10 weeks since exposed to or contracted severe infection with TB,
      stress (mental illness, burns, surgery, graft vs host rejection), chronic renal failure, HIV
  Factors related to the tuberculin used: contamination, improper storage, dilution, or
    denaturation, contamination
  Factors related to the method of administration: injecting too deep or too little antigen,
    delayed administration, subcutaneous injection, injection too close to other skin tests
  Factors related to interpretation of the test and recording of the results: interpreter bias,
    error in recording, conscious or unconscious bias

False-Positive
  Factors related to the method of administration
  Factors related to cross-reactivity: reaction with nontuberculous mycobacterial antigens,
    prior BCG vaccination
  Factors related to delayed antigen recall: booster phenomenon

Adapted from American Thoracic Society. Diagnostic standards and classification of TB in adults and children. *Am J Resp Crit Care Med* 2000;161:1376–95; American Thoracic Society. Targeted tuberculin testing and treatment of latent TB infection. *Am J Respir Crit Care Med* 2000;161:S221–S247; CDC. Essential components of a TB prevention and control program. *MMWR Morbid Mortal Weekly Rep* 1995;44:19–34; CDC. *Core Curriculum on Tuberculosis*, 3rd ed. 1994, 1–50; CDC. *Core Curriculum on Tuberculosis*, 4th ed. 2000, 1–75; Jerant, et al. Identification and management of tuberculosis. *Am Fam Phys* 2000;2668.

If the TST is positive, evaluation for active disease must be done. If the workup is negative, then the person should be considered to have a nontransmissible latent tuberculosis infection (LTBI) and should be treated accordingly. Follow-up recommendations are proposed by the World Health Organization (WHO) and the Johns Hopkins Center for TB research. These suggestions are currently available on these institutions' internet websites (18,19).

Any person exposed to TB may fit into one of six different classes, depending on his or her type of exposure and evidence of infection or disease. See Table 23.4 for a description of each of these six classes. This classification system helps to place individuals into specific categories for which workup and treatment recommendations are suggested (4,12,15,18).

Further evaluation involves collecting three daily (preferably morning) sputum samples for preparing an acid-fast bacillus (AFB) smear (20) using a Ziehl–Neelsen carbofuchsin or fluorochrome stain and culture. Sputum containing 10^4 microorganisms per millimeter is needed to produce a positive smear (21). The sensitivity of a smear is about 70% (22) and that of culture is 80% to 85% with a specificity of 98.5% in active disease (4,5,17). A positive culture with supportive clinical manifestations is currently the only definitive proof of TB disease. Several culture media used include a solid-based, Lowenstein–Jensen medium, a liquid-based medium, and a Mycobacterial Growth Indicator Tube. Growth rates vary for as long as 6 weeks before identification is available (17). Approximately 35% of culture-positive specimens are associated with negative smears. Gastric aspiration, fiberoptic bronchoscopy with bronchial washings, transbronchial biopsy, urine evaluation, and body fluid examinations, depending on the suspected source of infection, should also be

Table 23.4   Classification of Tuberculosis

Class	Description
0	No *Mycobacterium tuberculosis* exposure. No history of exposure. Negative TST. No active or latent LTBI.
1	*M. tuberculosis* exposure but no evidence of infection. Negative reaction to TST. If close exposure within 3 months, follow-up testing is required and consider treatment for LTBI.
2	Tuberculosis infection but no active disease. Positive reaction to TST. Negative bacteriologic studies and no clinical or radiographic evidence of TB. Treatment for LTBI is indicated.
3	TB: active disease. Person with clinically active TB whose diagnostic procedures are complete. Clinical and/or radiographic evidence of current TB must be documented. This is most definitively established by isolation of *M. tuberculosis*, but in the absence of a positive culture the person must have a positive TST. Person remains in class 3 until treatment for current episode of TB disease is completed.
4	TB: not clinically active disease. History of previous episode(s) of TB or abnormal stable radiographic findings in a person with a positive TST reaction, negative bacteriologic studies, and no clinical and/or radiographic evidence of active, current disease. A person in this class may never have, may currently be undergoing, or may have completed a course of chemotherapy.
5	TB: suspect, diagnosis pending. A person is in this class when a diagnosis of TB is being considered, whether or not treatment has been started, until diagnostic procedures have been completed. Persons should not remain in this class for more than 3 months.

Adapted from American Thoracic Society. Diagnostic standards and classification of tuberculosis. *Am Rev Respir Dis* 1990;142:725–35; ATS. Diagnostic standards and classification of TB in adults and children. *Am J Resp Crit Care Med* 2000;161:1376-95; American Thoracic Society. Treatment of tuberculosis and tuberculosis infection in adults and children. *Am J Respir Crit Care Med* 1994;149:1359–74; CDC. *MMWR* 1995;44:19–34; CDC. *Core Curriculum on Tuberculosis, 4th Ed.* Atlanta, GA: Centers for Disease Control and Prevention, 2000:1–75; Maher D, Chaulet P, Spinaci S, Harries A. *Treatment of Tuberculosis: Guidelines for National Programmes, 2nd Ed.* Geneva, Switzerland: World Health Organization, 1997:1–78.

considered. Use of bronchoscopy or biopsy may be necessary if the individual is unable to expectorate sputum (10).

Other laboratory studies include nucleic acid probes to identify mycobacterial RNA or DNA (2,23,24), high-performance liquid chromatography (HPLC) to identify the species of mycobacterium (10), or the polymerase chain reaction (PCR). Nucleic acid amplification (NAA) on AFB smear-positive sputum has a sensitivity of 95% and a specificity 98%, but if the AFB smear is negative, the sensitivity drops to 48–53% even when the culture is positive (4,15). An enhanced NAA probe has a sensitivity of 75% to 88%, but does not replace an AFB smear and culture as the diagnostic test of choice for TB. PCRs are currently being tested to diagnose active TB (2). Possible future tests include serodiagnostic evaluation for LTBI, through the detection of interferon-α, or a combination of purified mycobacterial agents (10,12). Genetic sequencing for *M. tuberculosis* has also been completed and may be used to help develop tests to check for drug resistance and potential new vaccines (25).

Chest radiographs may help confirm either recent or prior pulmonary TB disease. Primary pulmonary TB is usually seen as a lobar infiltrate with ipsilateral hilar adenopathy with or without atelectasis. Other signs include parenchymal consolidation (especially in the lower lobes), segmental or lobar atelectasis in the anterior segment of the upper lobe or medical segment of the middle lobe, hilar or mediastinal lymphadenopathy, unilateral pleural effusion, or miliary disease (found in 1% to 7% of all TB cases) (26). With the resolution of pulmonary TB infection, nodules known as Ghon foci can develop and become calcified. If these are associated with calcified hilar lymph nodes, the radiographic finding is known as a Ranke's complex (17). Reactivated pulmonary TB usually involves the posterior segment of the right upper lobe, apicoposterior segment of the left upper lobe, and apical segments of the lower lobes. The clinician may see any of the chest radiographic findings made in primary disease, but can also see cavitation, parenchymal consolidation in the apical and posterior upper lobes, pleural thickening at the apex (apical capping), bronchiectasis with possible bronchial stenosis, or a reticulonodular infiltrate pattern. With HIV-infected persons, the radiographs can be atypical and correlate with a worsening CD4 count. Healed TB may show fibrotic scars or Ghon foci (12,26).

Treatment

Treatment of active TB depends on the location of the disease (pulmonary versus extrapulmonary), the patient's HIV status, and drug resistance or medication intolerance. Treatment is divided into the three main categories of: 1) HIV-negative persons, 2) HIV-positive persons, and 3) persons with drug-resistant TB. Treatment can be given once daily, twice weekly, or thrice weekly, and can be optimized with directly observed therapy, short course (DOTS), witnessed by health-care workers.

Treatment of Active Tuberculosis in HIV-Negative Persons

Regimens for HIV-negative individuals are based on location of disease (pulmonary versus extrapulmonary) and by whether or not the AFB smear or culture is positive or negative. The recommended regimen for smear- or culture-positive pulmonary TB begins with 2 months of rifampin (RIF), isoniazid (INH), pyrazinamide (PZA), and either ethambutol (EMB) or streptomycin (SM) followed by rifampin (RIF) and isoniazid (INH) for 4 months thereafter if the mycobacterium is sensitive to INH and RIF. This therapy can be used if the primary drug resistance to INH is less than 4%, if there is no prior treatment for TB or known exposure to a person with drug-resistant TB, and if the patient is not from a country with a high prevalence of drug resistance (4,13,14). A 9-month regimen of INH, RIF, and either SM or ethambutol (EMB) is an alternative course of treatment. The SM or EMB may be discontinued if the TB is sensitive to both INH and RIF. With pulmonary TB that is smear- and culture-negative (i.e., clinically diagnosed TB), use of RIF, INH, and pyrazinamide (PZA) for the first 2 months and then 2 more months of RIF and INH alone is suggested. Extrapulmonary TB can be treated in the same way as pulmonary TB except that in infants and children with bone and joint TB, miliary TB, or TB meningitis, 12 months of therapy should be given (4). EMB is not recommended for children younger than 8 years of age because it is difficult to monitor them for visual or color perception changes caused by the drug (14). With pregnant or lactating females, PZA should not be used because of the unknown teratogenic effects that it may have on the fetus. Streptomycin also has teratogenic effects. Therefore, the preferred regimen for pregnant patients is RIF and INH for 9 months, with EMB for the first 1 to 2 months, depending on drug sensitivities of the organism. With renal disease and hemodialysis, any of the five first-line agents should be given after hemodialysis three times a week. Again, treatment is dependent upon the location and AFB smear and culture results. See Table 23.5 for dosages and other treatment options that can be used in HIV-negative individuals (4,10,19,27). Other regimens can be reviewed in handbooks recently published by the WHO (18,28).

Treatment of Active Tuberculosis in HIV-Positive Persons

Regimens for HIV-infected individuals are based on the types of rifamycin and antiretroviral drugs used to treat the HIV infection. Initially, the use of RIF to treat TB was not recommended for patients who were starting or concurrently using a protease inhibitor (PI) or nonnucleoside reverse transcriptase inhibitor (NNRTI), because RIF decreases the efficacy of certain anti-retroviral agents, thus increasing the risk of HIV resistance and elevating the viral load (29). The PIs (ritonavir, indinavir, saquinavir, efavirenz, nelfinavir) and NNRTIs (nevirapine and delvirdine) interact with rifamycin derivatives, RIF more than rifabutin (RFB), but the nucleoside reverse transcriptase inhibitors (NRTIs) (zidovudine, didanosine, zalcitabine, stavudine, lamivudine, and abacavir) have not been found to interact with them (10). Newer guidelines indicate the probable safety of RIF for the treatment of active TB if the patient is receiving one of the following therapies: 1) the NNRTI efavirenz and two NRTIs, 2) the PI ritonavir and one or more NRTIs, or 3) a combination of two PIs (ritonavir and saquinavir) (4,30). RFB can be used with indinavir, nelfinavir, amprenavir, ritonavir, and efavirenz, but not with delavirdine or hard-gel saquinavir unless the hard-gel saquinavir is used in combination with ritonavir (Table 23.6) (30,31).

Currently, the use of INH, RFB, PZA, and EMB for the first 2 months and then INH and RFB for 4 more months (if the TB is susceptible to INH and RFB) is one of the suggested treatment options (4,32). With a delayed response to treatment, the duration of therapy needs to be extended to 9 months. An alternative SM-based regimen consisting of INH, EMB, PZA, and SM for 2 months followed by INH, PZA, and SM for 7 months may be used. EMB is used instead of SM if there is intolerance to the SM and the duration of therapy is lengthened to a total of 12 months. Table 23.7 provides more details of these regimens (4,10,14,33). Treatment for extrapulmonary TB in HIV-positive adults and children is the same as for pulmonary TB except that the duration of therapy is lengthened to 9 months. With HIV-positive pregnant women, a rifamycin-based regimen including INH, EMB, and PZA is suggested. For HIV-positive children, a course of INH, rifamycin, PZA, and EMB for 2 months and INH and rifamycin for 4 more months is recommended despite the risk of ocular complications with EMB (4).

Treatment of Active Multidrug-Resistant Tuberculosis in HIV-Positive and HIV-Negative Persons

Regimens for individuals with drug-resistant TB depend on the specific drug(s) to which the mycobacteria may be resistant, as well as on the patient's HIV status. Some recommendations for drug-resistant TB are summarized in Table 23.8 (4,10,34,35).

For HIV-negative patients with TB resistant to INH, treatment includes RIF, PZA, and EMB or SM for 6 months or RIF and EMB for 12 months. If the bacteria are resistant only to RIF, treatment is based on 2 months of INH, SM, PZA, and EMB, and then INH, SM, and PZA for 7 months. Mycobacteria resistant to INH and RIF (an example of multidrug-resistant TB) is treated with three or more drugs to which that organism is susceptible for 12

Table 23.5   Regimen Options for Treatment of Tuberculosis in HIV-Negative Persons

Indication (Total Duration)	Initial Phase		Continuation Phase		Comments
	Drugs	Time	Drugs	Time	
Pulmonary and extrapulmonary TB in adults and children (24 weeks)	INH, RIF, PZA[4], EMB (or SM)[4]	Daily x 8 weeks	INH, RIF	Daily for 2-3x/week[1] for 16 weeks[2]	EMB or SM should be continued until susceptibility to INH and RIF is seen In areas where INH resistance < 4%,
Pulmonary and extrapulmonary TB in adults and children (24 weeks)	INH, RIF, PZA[4], EMB (or SM)[4]	Daily x 2 weeks then 2x/week[1] for 6 weeks	INH, RIF	2x/week[1] for 16 weeks	EMB or SM may not be necessary with no risk factors for resistance Intermittent (2–3 times/wk)
Pulmonary and extrapulmonary TB in adults and children (24 weeks)	INH, RIF, PZA[4], EMB (or SM)[4]	Three times per week[1] for 24 weeks	Continue all four drugs for 6 months[3]		regimens should be DOT After the 8 weeks of induction phase, continue EMB or SM until susceptibility to INH and RIF is demonstrated
Smear- and culture-negative pulmonary TB in adults (16 weeks)	INH, RIF, PZA[4], EMB (or SM)[4]	Follow one of the above options for 8 weeks	INH, RIF, PZA[4], EMB, (or SM)[4]	Daily or 2-3x/week[1] for 8 weeks	Regimen should be directly observed If drug resistance is unlikely, EMB or SM may not be necessary and PZA may be d/c after 2 months
Pulmonary and extrapulmonary TB in adults and children when PZA is contraindicated (36 weeks)	INH, RIF, EMB (or SM)[4]	Daily for 4–8 weeks	INH, RIF	Daily or 2x/week[1] for 28–32 weeks[2]	EMB or SM should be continued until INH and RIF susceptibility is demonstrated In areas where primary INH resistance < 4%, EMB or SM may not be necessary for patients with no risk factors for resistance

INH = isoniazid; RIF = rifampin; PZA = pyrazinamide; EMB = ethambutol; SM = streptomycin; d/c = discontinued; TB = tuberculosis.

Note: For all patients, if susceptibility test results show resistance to any of the first-line drugs or if the patient remains symptomatic or smear or culture positive after 3 months, consult a TB medical expert.

[1] All intermittent dosing should be used with directly observed therapy (DOT).

[2] For infants and children with miliary, bone and joint, or meningeal TB, treatment should last for at least 12 months. For adults with these forms of extrapulmonary TB, response to therapy should be monitored closely. If response is slow or suboptimal, treatment may be prolonged as judged on a case-by-case basis.

[3] There is some evidence that SM may be discontinued after 4 months if the isolate is susceptible to all drugs.

[4] Avoid SM and PZA for pregnant women because of the risk of adverse effects to the fetus.

Adapted from Centers for Disease Control and Prevention. *Core Curriculum on Tuberculosis: What the Clinician Should Know.* Atlanta, GA: 2000, 1–139.

to 24 months after the AFB culture becomes negative (34). Other regimens for drug-resistant TB can be reviewed in Iseman's report on MDR-TB or in the WHO Guidelines for the treatment of MDR-TB (35,36).

If the mycobacteria in an HIV-infected patient are resistant only to INH, use of rifamycin, PZA, and EMB for at least 9 months is one of the treatment options. If the organism is resistant to RIF, use of INH, SM, PZA, and EMB for the first 2 months and then 7 months of INH, SM, and PZA is recommended. For MDR-TB, one option is an aminoglycoside and a fluoroquinolone along with other agents to which the pathogen is sensitive. The duration of therapy is at least 24 months after the AFB culture becomes negative (4).

In some cases, regardless of a patient's HIV status, surgical resection or drainage of a tuberculous empyema may be necessary (34). Surgery should be considered for persons with highly resistant TB, those intolerant of most first- and second-line drugs, or those with a large cavitary lesion. This can be done after 2 to 3 weeks of drug therapy. Postoperatively, the same regimen should be continued for at least 18 months (36).

Follow-Up

The patient with TB needs careful follow-up in order to monitor for compliance with therapy, development of drug side effects, successful completion of treatment, and cure. The goals of therapy are resolution of symptoms and progression toward negative AFB smears and cultures. During treatment, monthly or bimonthly sputum cultures should be obtained until the cultures convert to negative. To verify cure, an additional sample needs to be proven negative upon the completion of therapy. About 85% of patients taking INH and RIF become culture-negative within 2 months. If the cultures do not become negative or symptoms persist after 2 to 3 months of therapy, reassessment for drug resistance or noncompliance must be done (4,13,20). As discussed earlier, the original drug regimen can be continued or augmented by at least two drugs to which the pathogen is susceptible, or by at least three drugs if second-line agents are given when drug resistance is strongly suspected. Consider consulting a TB expert if there is resistance to any of the first-line drugs or if the patient remains smear- or culture-positive after 3 months (20). While treating MDR-TB, sputum cultures need to be obtained monthly, and a chest radiograph should be performed upon the completion of therapy (14). Other scenarios for monitoring patients with smear-positive or -negative TB can be reviewed in two manuals published by the WHO (18,28).

If the sputum culture was negative before treatment, chest radiographs and clinical evaluation can be used to monitor the efficacy of therapy. One sputum smear and culture should be obtained at the end of the second month (18).

Table 23.6   Recommendations for Coadministering Different Antiretroviral Drugs with the Antimycobacterial Drugs Rifabutin (RFB) and Rifampin (RIF)— United States, 2000

Antiretroviral Agent	Use with RFB	Use with RIF	Comments
Hard-gel capsule saquinavir (HGC)[1]	Possibly if regimen includes ritonavir[2]	Possibly, if antiretroviral regimen includes ritonavir	Coadministration of saquinavir SGC with usual dose RFB (300 mg/day or 2–3 times per week) is possible. However, the pharmacokinetic data and clinical experience are limited.
Soft-gel capsule saquinavir (SGC)[1]	Probably[3]	Same as above	The combination of saquinavir SGC or HGC and ritonavir, coadministered with 1) usual-dose RIF (600 mg/day) or 2–3 times per week), or 2) reduced-dose RFB (150 mg 2–3 times per week) is a possibility. However, the pharmacokinetic data and clinical experience for these combinations are limited. Coadministration of saquinavir HGC or SGC with RIF (in the absence of ritonavir) is not recommended because RIF markedly decreases concentrations of saquinavir.
Ritonavir	Probably	Probably	If the combination of ritonavir and RFB is used, then a substantially reduced-dose regimen of RFB (150 mg 2–3 times per week) is recommended. Coadministration of ritonavir with usual-dose RIF (600 mg/day or 2–3 times per week) is a possibility, though pharmacokinetic data and clinical experience are limited.
Indinavir	Yes	No. Because it markedly deceases ($\downarrow$) concentration of indinavir	There is limited but favorable clinical experience with coadministration of indinavir[4] with a reduced daily dose of RFB (150 mg) or with the usual dose of RFB (300 mg) 2–3 times/week.
Nelfinavir	Yes	No. Because it markedly $\downarrow$ concentrations of nelfinavir	There is limited but favorable clinical experience with coadministration nelfinavir[5] with a reduced daily dose of RFB (150 mg) or with the usual dose of RFB (300 mg 2–3 times/week).
Amprenavir	Yes	No. Because it markedly $\downarrow$ concentrations of amprenavir	Coadministration of amprenavir with a reduced daily dose of RFB (150 mg) or with the usual dose of RFB (300 mg 2–3 times per week) is a possibility, but there is no published clinical experience.
Nevirapine	Yes	Possibly	Coadministration of nevirapine with usual-dose RFB (300 mg 2–3 times per week) is a possibility based on pharmacokinetic studies. But there is no published clinical experience for the combination. Data are insufficient to assess whether dose adjustments are necessary when RIF is coadministered with nevirapine. Therefore, RIF and nevirapine should be used only in combination if clearly indicated and with careful monitoring.
Delaviridine	No	No	Contraindicated because of the marked decrease in concentration of delavirdine when administered with either RFB or RIF.
Efavirenz	Probably	Probably	Coadministration of efavirenz with an increased ($\uparrow$) dose of RFB (450 mg/day or 600 mg/day, or 600 mg 2–3 times per week) is a possibility, though there is no published clinical experience. Coadministration of efavirenz[6] with usual-dose RIF (600 mg/day or 2–3 times per week) is a possibility, though there is no published clinical experience.

[1]Usual recommended doses are 400 mg BID for each of these protease inhibitors and 400 mg of ritonavir.

[2]Despite limited data and clinical experience, the use of this combination is potentially successful; but if not used with HGC saquinavir and ritonavir, the use of either rifamycin is not recommended (Core Curriculum on TB, 2000).

[3]Based on available data and clinical experience, the successful use of this combination is likely.

[4]Usual recommended dose is 800 mg every eight hours. Some experts recommend $\uparrow$ the indinavir dose to 1000 mg every 8 hours if used with RFB.

[5] Usual recommended dose is 750 mg TID or 1250 mg BID. Some experts recommend $\uparrow$ the nelfinavir dose to 1000 if TID dosing is used and nelfinavir is used in combination with RFB.

[6]Usual recommended dose is 600 mg qd. Some experts recommend $\uparrow$ the efavirenz dose to 800 mg qd if efavirenz is used with RIF.

Adapted from Centers for Disease Control and Prevention. Updated guidelines for the use of RFB or RIF for the treatment and prevention of TB among HIV-infected patients taking PIs or NNRTIs. *MMWR Morbid Mortal Weekly Rep* 2000;49:185–9.

Table 23.7   Regimens for Treatment of Tuberculosis in HIV-Positive Persons

Initial Phase		Continuation Phase		Considerations	Comments
Drugs	**Time**	**Drugs**	**Time**		
INH RFB PZA[2] EMB[2]	Daily for 2 months or daily for 2 weeks and then 2 times a week for 6 weeks	INH RFB	Daily or 2 times per week for 4 months (18 weeks)	Monitor for RFB drug toxicity if used with PIs or NNRTIs. Can use NNRTIs with RFB May need to increase dose of PI or NNRTIs	Doses of antiretrovirals may need to be adjusted
INH SM PZA EMB	Daily for 2 months or daily for 2 weeks and then 2 times per week for 6 weeks	INH SM PZA	Two or three times per week for 7 months	Can be used with antiretroviral regimens that include PIs, NNRTIs, and NRTIs	SM is contraindicated in pregnant women If patient can't take SM for 9 months, add EMB and prolong therapy to 12 months
INH RIF PZA[2] EMB[2] (or SM)	Daily for 2 months or daily for 2 weeks and then 2–3 times per week for 6 weeks	INH RIF	Three times per week for 18 weeks	RIF can be used for treatment of active TB disease if on 1) NNRTI efavirenz and 2 NRTIs 2) PI ritonavir and one or more NRTIs or 3) combination of 2 PI ritonavir and saquinavir	SM is contraindicated in pregnant women
Same as above	Three times per week for 2 months	INH RIF PZA EMB (or SM)	Three times per week for 4 months	NRTIs can be used with RIF May need washout period between last dose of RIF and first dose of PI, NNRTI	

EMB = ethambutol; INH = isoniazid; NNRTI = non-nucleotide reverse transcriptase inhibitor; NRTI = nucleoside reverse transcriptase inhibitor; PI = protease inhibitor; PZA = pyrazinamide; RFB = rifabutin; RIF = rifampin; SM = streptomycin.
[1]Duration of therapy should be prolonged for patients with delayed response to therapy. This is checked at the 2-month induction phase by 1) lack of conversion of *Mycobacterium tuberuclosis* culture to negative or 2) lack of resolution or progression of signs or symptoms of TB.
[2]Continue PZA and EMB for the total duration of the initial phase (8 weeks). EMB can be stopped after susceptibility test results indicate *M. tuberculosis* susceptibility to INH and RIF.
Adapted from Centers for Disease Control and Prevention. *Core Curriculum on Tuberculosis*, 4th ed. Atlanta, GA: Centers for Disease Control and Prevention. 2000, 1–75; Centers for Disease Control and Prevention. Prevention and treatment of tuberculosis among patients infected with human immunodeficiency virus: principles of therapy and revised recommendations. *MMWR Morbid Mortal Weekly Rep* 1998;47(RR-20):1–53.

Table 23.8   Treatment Regimens for Drug-Resistant Tuberculosis

Drug Resistance	HIV-Negative Person	HIV-Positive Person
INH	RIF, PZA, EMB for 6 months, or RIF and EMB for 12 months, or RIF, PZA, EMB, AG for 2–3 months then RIF and EMB for 6 months. (Can use SM instead of AG if organism is sensitive)	RFB, PZA, and EMB for at least 9 months for 4 months after culture conversion. May use RIF instead of RFB in certain cases
RIF	INH, PZA, EMB for 18–24 months OR INH, SM, PZA, and EMB for 2 months then INH, SM, and PZA for 7 months	INH, PZA, and EMB for 18–24 months, or INH, PZA, SM, EMB for 2 months and then INH, PZA, SM for 7–10 months
INH, RIF	Three drugs that the organism is susceptible to for 12–24 months after culture conversion, or EMB, PZA, and FQ for 18 months after culture conversion	Aminoglycoside and FQ in addition to other agents to which the TB pathogen is sensitive for 24 months after culture conversion to negative
INH, RIF EMB	PZA, FQ + two other drugs (SM, AG) for 24 months after culture conversion	
INH, RIF, SM	AG, ethionamide, PZA, FQ, and EMB for 3 months, and then ethionamide, FQ, and EMB for 18 months	
INH, EMB (SM)	RIF, PAZ, and FQ for 9–12 months, or RIF, PZA, AG, and ethionamide for 3 months, and then RIF and ethionamide for 6 months	
INH, RIF, EMB, PZA	FQ + three other drugs (i.e., ethionamide, cycloserine, or PAS) for 24 months after conversion	

AG = aminoglycosde; EMB = ethambutol; FQ = fluoroquinolone; INH = isoniazid; PZA = pyrazinamide; RFB = rifabutin; RIF = rifampin; SM = streptomycin.
Adapted from Bradford WZM, Daley CL. Multiple drug-resistant tuberculosis. *Infect Dis Clin North Am* 1998;12:157–72.
CDC. Core Curr on TB 4th ed. 2000;1–75.
Centers for Disease Control and Prevention. Prevention and treatment of tuberculosis among patients infected with human immunodeficiency virus: principles of therapy and revised recommendations. *MMWR Morbid Mortal Weekly Rep* 1998;47(RR-20):1–53.
Crofton, Sir John. *Guidelines for the Management of Drug-Resistant Tuberculosis*. Geneva, Switzerland: World Health Organization, 1997:1–47.
Iseman MD. Treatment of multidrug-resistant tuberculosis. *N Engl J Med* 1993;329:784–91.

Chest radiographs can be made within 2 to 3 months of initiation and upon the completion of treatment. If the chest radiograph shows no improvement after 3 months of therapy, the abnormality may be the result of either previous (not current) TB or another process. Some experts suggest that routine follow-up after therapy is not needed if the treatment has been completed appropriately (13,14). Documentation of treatment outcomes should be noted. These outcomes include cure, completion of treatment, treatment failure, death, treatment interruption (for more than 2 months), or transfer out of the treatment program (18).

Antimycobacterial Agents

First-Line Antimycobacterial Agents

The first-line antimycobacterial agents that are used to treat LTBI and active TB include INH, RIF, RFB, PZA, EMB and SM. Each of these drugs has both benefits and side effects that need to be monitored when they are being used as treatment for LTBI or active disease. See Table 23.9 for a summary of dosages and adverse effects of these first-line antimycobacterial agents (4,10,18,31,35).

INH

Although INH is highly active against *M. tuberculosis* and is bactericidal, it may be contraindicated in certain groups, such as those with hypersensitivity reactions or intolerance to INH, persons with drug-resistant TB, or individuals at high risk of not completing a course of therapy (10,31). INH can cause hepatitis, peripheral neuropathy, drug-induced lupus syndrome, drowsiness, and mood changes. Signs and symptoms of hepatotoxicity include malaise, nausea, anorexia, vomiting, dark urine, icterus, jaundice, unexplained fever lasting more than 3 days, and right upper quadrant tenderness or epigastric discomfort. Some groups, such as persons with a poor nutritional status, diabetes, renal dysfunction, HIV, or seizure disorder, and expectant mothers and alcoholic individuals are at increased risk for developing INH-induced neuropathy. Therefore, pyridoxine (vitamin B6) at a dose of 10 to 50 µg/day is recommended to help prevent the neuropathy. An important drug interaction occurs with the combination of INH and phenytoin, which can cause increased serum concentrations of both drugs (4,10,31,35).

RIF

RIF, a rifamycin derivative, is a bactericidal antimycobacterial agent. It has some gastrointestinal and dermatologic side effects. It can cause gastrointestinal upset, hepatitis, rashes, and thrombocytopenic purpura, and can turn body fluids reddish-orange. RIF can increase the metabolism of certain drugs, causing decreased drug efficacy. These drugs include oral contraceptives, oral hypoglycemic agents, anticonvulsants, antidysrhythmic drugs, cardiac glycosides, clofibrate, antifungal drugs, calcium channel blockers, chloramphenicol, haldol, tricyclic antidepressants, dapsone, cyclosporine, beta-blockers, theophylline, corticosteroids, coumadin, quinidine, methadone, and clarithromycin. As noted

Table 23.9. First-Line Anti-Tuberculosis Medications

Drug (Route)	Dose in mg/kg (Maximum Dose in mg)	Adverse Reactions	Monitoring	Contraindications
INH (PO, IM)	Children Daily: 10–20 (300); Two or three times per week[1]: 20–40 (900) Adults Daily: 5 (300); Two or three times per week[1]: 15 (900)	Rash, Hepatitis Hepatic enzymes inc. Peripheral neuropathy Mild effects Drug interactions: ↑ phenytoin level ↑ disulfiram level	Baseline measurements of hepatic enzymes in adults Repeat measurements if abnormal baseline values or having symptoms of adverse reactions	Hepatitis risk increases with age and alcohol use Pyridoxine (vitamin B6) may prevent peripheral neuropathy; CNS effect
RIF[2] (PO, IV)	Children Daily: 10–20 (600); Two or three times per week[1]: 10–20 (600) Adults Daily: 10 (600); Two or three times per week[1]: 10 (600)	GI upset, Hepatitis Drug interactions Bleeding problems Flu-like sx, Rash, Fever Renal Failure Body fluids are orange Can discolor contacts	Baseline measurements of CBC, platelets, and hepatic enzymes Repeat measurements if abnormal baseline values or having symptoms of adverse reactions	Significant interactions with methadone, birth control pills, PIs, NNRTIs, other drugs Caution when used with certain PIs, NNRTIs
RFB[2] (PO, IV)	Children Daily: 10–20 (300)[3]: Two times per week[1]: 10–20 (300); Three times per week[1]: unknown Adults Daily: 5 (300)[3]: Two times per week[1]: 5 (300); Three times per week[1]: unknown	Rash, hepatitis, fever, thrombocytopenia Body fluids are orange Can discolor contact lenses With elevated RFB: Severe arthralgias, uveitis, leukopenia	Same as RIF Use adjusted daily dose of RFB[3] and monitor antiretroviral activity if on certain PIs, NNRTIs	RFB contraindicated in delavirdine Reduces levels of many drugs (methadone, dapsone, contraceptives, ketoconazole, etc.)
PZA (PO)	Children Daily: 15–20 (2 g); Two times per week[1]: 50–70 (4 g); Three times per week[1]: 50–70 (3 g) Adults Daily: 15–30 (2 g); Two times per week[1]: 50–70 (4 g); Three times per week[1]: 50–70 (3 g)	Hepatitis, rash, gastrointestinal upset, joint aches, hyperuricemia, gout (rare)	Baseline measurements of uric acid and hepatic enzymes Repeat measurements if abnormal baseline or symptoms are present	Treat hyperuricemia only if patient has symptoms May make glucose control more difficult in diabetes patients
EMB[4] (PO)	Children and Adults Daily: 15–25; Two times per week[1]: 50; Three times per week[1]: 25–30	Optic neuritis (can be unilateral). Red-green color blindness, scotoma, rash	Baseline and monthly tests of visual acuity and color vision	Not recommended in young children because inability to monitor visual or color changes
SM[5] (IM, IV)	Children Daily: 20–40 (1 g); Two to three times per week[1]: 25–30 (1.5 g) Adults Daily: 15 (1 g); Two to three times per week[1]: 25–30 (1.5 g)	Ototoxicity (hearing loss or vestibular dysfunction). Renal toxicity	Baseline and repeat hearing and renal function tests as needed	Ultrasound and warm compresses on injection site may decrease pain

CBC = complete blood count; CNS = central nervous system; EMB = ethambutol; INH = isoniazid; IM = intramuscular; IV = intravenous; PO = per os (by mouth); NNRTI = non-nucleotide reverse transcriptase inhibitor; PI = protease inhibitor; PZA = pyrazinamide; RFB = rifabutin; RIF = rifampin.

Notes: Adjust weight-based dosages as weight changes. Children defined as ≤ 12 years old. Consult product insert for detailed information.
[1] All intermittent dosing should be done by directly observed therapy; [2] RFB is contraindicated with delavirdine. See endnotes on Table 23.7 and chapter for more details regarding use of rifamycins with PIs and NNRTIs; [3] If nelfinavir, indinavir, amprenavir, or ritonavir is given with RFB, the PI concentration decreases; therefore, the daily dose of RFB is reduced from 300 mg to 150 mg when used with nelfinavir, indinavir, or amprenavir, and to 150 mg two to three times weekly when used with ritonavir. If efavirenz is given with RIF, blood concentrations of RFB decreases; therefore, the daily dose of RFB should be increased from 300 mg to 450 or 600 mg; [4] There is no maximum dosage for EMB, but in obese patients' dosages should be calculated on the basis of lean body weight; [5] Avoid or reduce dosage of SM in adults ≥ 50 years old.
Adapted from Centers for Disease Control and Prevention. Core Curriculum on Tuberculosis, 4th Ed. Atlanta, GA: Centers for Disease Control and Prevention, 2000, 1–75.

earlier, the combination of RIF and certain PIs or NNRTIs may increase RIF levels and may decrease the efficacy of certain antiretroviral agents. At higher intermittent doses, RIF can, although rarely, cause thrombocytopenia, hemolytic anemia, influenza-like syndrome, and acute renal failure (4,31).

RFB

RFB, another rifamycin derivative, is similar to RIF in its mechanism of action. It is also bactericidal. Side effects of RFB include rashes, gastrointestinal upset, myalgias, neutropenia, thrombocytopenia, dysgeusia, and orange-colored body fluids. It can decrease certain drug concentrations, as can RIF, but is recommended as an alternative to RIF if the patient is on certain PIs or NNRTIs (*see* Table 23.6) (4).

PZA and EMB

PZA and EMB are used in combination with other first-line drugs in order to produce additive bactericidal and bacteriostatic effects, respectively. PZA can cause arthralgias, hyperuricemia, and liver injury. Use of salicylates helps to relieve PZA-induced arthralgias. Gastrointestinal disturbances and hepatotoxicity may also occur with PZA. Visual acuity and color perception need to be monitored in patients taking EMB because they may develop optic neuritis at high doses. Symptoms include central scotoma, blurred vision, and red–green color blindness (4,10,18,31).

SM

SM was the first antimycobacterial agent discovered. Although it is bactericidal, it is now used in combination therapy, owing to the discovery of more effective, less toxic agents such as INH and rifamycin. SM can cause auditory and vestibular disturbances and renal toxicity. Audiometry should be performed while patients receive the drug. SM should be discontinued if vertigo, dizziness, or ataxia develops (10,14,18,34,37).

Bacillus-Calmette-Guerin Vaccine

The Bacillus-Calmette-Guerin (BCG) vaccine is used to help prevent the development of active TB. It is not recommended for the United States population as a whole because of the low risk of LTBI and disease (10). However, infants and children and high-risk health care workers may benefit from the vaccine (10,13). Infants and children may be considered for the vaccine if they are continually exposed to a person with MDR-TB, if they have more than a 10% risk per year of developing TB, or if they cannot take INH for LTBI and will be constantly exposed to a person infected with TB. Health care workers may be considered for the vaccine if they are exposed repeatedly to patients with MDR-TB or are at very high risk of being infected with MDR-TB (10).

In the United States, the Tice strain of BCG is administered percutaneously, usually in the deltoid. Three-tenths of a milliliter of the reconstituted *Mycobacterium bovis* is used in adults, and half that amount should be given to infants. The effectiveness of the vaccine ranges from 0% to 80% (38). Complications of the BCG vaccine include disseminated BCG infection, osteitis, local subcutaneous abscess, and lymphadenitis (10,14,38). In the absence of exposure to *M. tuberculosis* and infection, tuberculin reactivity caused by the vaccination wanes over time and is unlikely to persist for more than 10 years after vaccination. A diagnosis of TB should be considered for any BCG-vaccinated person who has a TST induration exceeding 10 mm if that person 1) is in contact with another person who has active TB, 2) was born or resided in a country where the prevalence of TB is high, or 3) is exposed continuously to populations in which the prevalence of TB is high, such as health-care workers, employees and volunteers at homeless shelters, and workers at drug treatment centers (38). The BCG vaccine is contraindicated in persons with an impaired immune response or immune suppression. These groups include HIV-infected patients, persons receiving immunosuppressant drugs, and persons with leukemia, lymphoma, and congenital immunodeficiency (4).

Second-Line Antimycobacterial Agents

Second-line drugs for TB are used when a patient is unable to take certain first-line agents, was exposed to drug-resistant TB, or failed treatment for TB because of noncompliance or documented new resistance. Capreomycin, kanamycin, ethionamide, para-aminosalicyclic acid (PAS), cycloserine, ciprofloxacin, ofloxacin, amikacin, and clofazimine are examples of these second-line drugs. Detailed information on dosages and side effects are provided in Table 23.10 (10,14,36). Additional information about the medications used against drug-resistant TB is provided in review articles by Iseman and the CDC (10,35,36).

Treatment for Latent Tuberculosis Infection

The Mantoux test should be done at least once on persons in a high-risk category (Table 23.11) (16,31). Specifically, a two-step Mantoux test is indicated if the person is elderly, immunocompromised, likely to be exposed to persons with TB, or newly employed by a health-care facility, or if the test is their initial TST (16,39). The frequency of tuberculin skin testing thereafter should be determined by the likelihood of exposure to active TB. For example, staff and patients of health-care facilities, nursing homes, substance abuse treatment centers, and mental or correctional facilities should be tested once a year.

Persons in a category in which the TST is considered positive (*see* Table 23.2), are considered to have LTBI, and active TB needs to be ruled out by performing a thorough history and physical examination, as well as sputum and radiographic evaluations (14). Once active TB is ruled out in an individual with a positive TST, treatment for LTBI should be considered. Currently four regimens are recommended for treating LTBI (14,20,31). INH has an increased risk of causing hepatotoxicity in TST-positive persons over the age of 35, but may still be considered for individuals at higher risk of developing active TB or spreading TB to others (4,10,20,37).

The preferred recommendation, no matter what the patient's HIV status, is 9 months of INH at a dose of 5 mg/kg/day (maximum 300 mg) in adults and 10 to 15 mg/kg/day (maximum of 300 mg) for 9 months in children (4,15,31). Treatment with INH for 6 months decreases the risk of developing active TB in 70% of infected individuals and in 90% if used for 12 months (10). Since minimal additional benefit is seen between 9 and 12 months of therapy, 9 months is the preferred duration of therapy. Direct observed therapy (DOT) is suggested if there is a high risk for active TB, if noncompliance is an issue, or both. A dose of 15 mg/kg (900 mg maximum) of INH should be used for adults and 20 to 40 mg/kg (900 mg maximum) of INH for children, two times a week and administered by health-care workers. This may reduce treatment failure and improve compliance. Another regimen involves 6 months of INH in HIV-negative persons. Four months of daily RIF is the third regimen alternative, especially for persons unable to take RIF and PZA (4,15,20,30–32,40). A fourth regimen, using RIF and PZA for 2 months, has been found to be as effective as 12 months of INH in HIV-positive persons (19). However, RIF is not recommended for the treatment of LTBI in pregnant women (20). RFB should be substituted for RIF in the case of HIV-positive persons taking most PIs or certain NNRTIs. Tables 23.6 and 23.12 provide further details regarding treatment of LTBI and recommendations for the coadministration of different antiretroviral agents with RIF or RFB (10,14,15,30,31). Although RIF-PZA for 2 months can be used in both HIV-positive and HIV-negative persons with LTBI, recent case studies have raised concerns regarding its safety. Two studies of fatal and severe hepatitis associated with RIF-PZA were reported in 2000 (43). Due to increasing numbers of severe liver injury and fatalities, revised LTBI treatment recommendations have been issued by the CDC and American Thoracic Society regarding the use of RIF-PZA: 1) RIF-PZA treatment for 2 months should be used with caution, especially in persons taking other potential hepatotoxic agents or alcohol; RIF-PZA is not recommended for patients with underlying liver disease. 2) For HIV-negative persons, 9 months of INH is the preferred treatment; 4 months of RIF is an alternative regimen. RIF-PZA for 2 months can be used when treatment completion is uncertain and the patient can be followed closely. 3) Data do not show excessive risk for severe hepatitis among HIV-infected persons. 4) No more than a 2-week supply of RIF-PZA (with a PZA dose <20 mg/kg/d) should be dispensed at one time, with re-

Table 23.10   Second-Line Anti-Tuberculosis Medications

Drug Daily Dose[1] (Maximum Dose)	Adverse Reactions	Monitoring	Comments
Capreomycin 15–30 mg/kg (1 g)	Auditory, vestibular, and renal toxicity	Evaluate vestibular and hearing function; Check BUN/creatinine	After bacteriologic conversion, dosage may be reduced to 2–3 times per week
Kanamycin 15–30 mg/kg (1 g)	Same as for capreomycin	Same as for capreomycin	Same as for capreomycin
Ethionamide 15–20 mg/kg (1 g)	GI upset, bloating, hepatotoxicity, hypersensitivity, metallic taste	Check hepatic enzymes	Start with low doses and increase as tolerated; may cause hypothyroidism if used with PAS
Para-amino-salicyclic acid 150 mg/kg (16 g)	GI upset, hepatotoxic-ity hypersensitivity, ↑ sodium load	Check hepatic enzymes; assess volume status	Start with low doses and increase as tolerated; monitor cardiac patients for volume overload
Cycloserine 15–20 mg/kg (1 g)	Psychosis, headache, rash, convulsions, depression drug interaction	Check mental status; measure serum drug levels	Start with low doses and increase as toler-ated; pyridoxine may decrease CNS effects
Ciprofloxacin 750–1500 mg/day	GI upset, restlessness dizziness, headache; hypersensitivity	Drug interactions; avoid antacids, iron, zinc, and sucralfate within 2 hours	Not approved by FDA for treatment of TB; not used in children
Ofloxacin 600–800 mg/day	Same as for ciprofloxacin	Same as for ciprofloxacin	Same as for ciprofloxacin
Levofloxacin 500 mg/day	Same as for ciprofloxacin	Same as for ciprofloxacin	Same as for ciprofloxacin
Amikacin 15–30 mg/kg (1 g)	Vestibular, auditory, and renal toxicity; dizziness, hearing loss	Evaluate hearing; measure BUN/creati-nine, serum drug levels	Not approved by FDA for treatment of TB
Clofazimine 100–300 mg/day	GI upset, abdominal pain, skin discolor-ation, urine crystal deposition	Drug interactions	Not approved by FDA for tx of TB; avoid sunlight, consider dose with meals

BUN = blood urea nitrogen; CNS = central nervous system; FDA = U.S. Food and Drug Administration; GI = gastrointestinal; TB = tuberculosis.
Notes: Doses for children are the same as for adults. Use the drugs shown in table only in consultation with a clinician experienced in the management of drug-resistant TB.
[1] Adjust weight-based dosages as patient's weight changes.
Adapted from Centers for Disease Control and Prevention. *Core Curriculum on Tuberculosis, 3rd Ed.* Atlanta, GA: Centers for Disease Control and Prevention, 1994, 1–50.
Centers for Disease Control and Prevention. *Core Curriculum on Tuberculosis, 4th Ed.* Atlanta, GA: Centers for Disease Control and Prevention, 2000, 1–75.
Bradford, WZ. Multiple drug-resistant tuberculosis. *Infect Dis Clin North Am* 1998;12:157–72.
Crofton, Sir John. Guidelines for the management of MDR-TB. Geneva, Switz: WHO. 1997;1–47.

Table 23.11   Categories of High-Risk Persons Who Should Be Considered for Mantoux Testing

Persons with signs/symptoms (cough, hemoptysis, weight loss, anorexia), laboratory, or radiograph abnormalities suggestive of clinically active TB

Recent contacts of person known to have or suspected of having clinically active TB

Persons with or at risk for HIV infection

Persons with abnormal chest radiographs compatible with previous TB

Persons with other medical conditions that increase the risk of TB (silicosis, diabetes mellitus, prolonged corticosteroid therapy, immunosuppressive therapy, some hematologic and reticuloendothelial diseases [leukemia or lymphoma], end-stage renal disease, weight loss > 10% of idea body weight, jejunoileal bypass)

Persons with organ transplants

Groups at high risk of recent infection with *Mycobacterium tuberculosis*, such as immigrants from Asia, Africa, Oceania, and Latin America

Personnel and long-term residents in some hospitals, nursing homes, correctional and mental institutions, homeless shelters

Injectable or illicit drug users, alcoholic individuals

Medically underserved, low-income populations, including some high-risk racial or ethnic minority populations (African-Americans, Hispanics, Native Americans, migrant farm workers)

Infants, children, and adolescents exposed to adults in high–TB-risk categories

Foreign-born persons recently arrived (within 5 years) in the United States or persons who have resided in areas where TB prevalence is high

Health-care workers who serve high-risk clients

American Thoracic Society. Targeted tuberculin testing and treatment of LTBI. *Am J Resp Crit Care Med* 2000;161:S221–S247; Centers for Disease Control and Prevention. *Core Curriculum on Tuberculosis, 4th Ed.* 2000:1–75.

assessment at 2, 4, and 6 weeks of treatment. 5) Serum aminotransferases and bilirubin should be measured at baseline and at 2, 4, and 6 weeks of treatment. Aminotransferases greater than five times the upper limit of normal in an asymptomatic person, levels greater than normal in a symptomatic person, or elevated bilirubin should warrant cessation of therapy (44).

Special considerations should be given to certain populations, such as persons with fibrotic lesions, HIV-infected individuals, persons with drug-resistant TB, pregnant women, and children and adolescents. If a person has a positive TST with a history of silicosis, or a chest radiograph consistent with a fibrotic lesion and no evidence of current disease, INH for 9 months, 2 months of RIF and PZA, and 4 months of RIF with or without INH can be used (10,31). Nine instead of 12 months of INH is currently used in HIV-infected individuals. Pregnant women, children, and adolescents are all treated with 9 months of INH. If there is a risk for resistance or intolerance to INH, then RIF with PZA for 2 months or RIF alone for 4 months (especially if the person is unable to take PZA) may be used (4,37). For MDR-TB (e.g., resistance to INH or RIF), one should consider observation or therapy with EMB

Table 23.12   Treatment of Latent Tuberculosis Infection*

Drug	Dose	Comments	Indications	Contraindications
INH	5 mg/kg/day in adults (300 mg) for 9 months 10–20 mg/kg/d in children (300 mg is max dose)	Can be given 2 twice weekly at 15 mg/kg (maximum 900 mg dose) 20–40 mg/kg twice weekly (maximum 900 mg dose) in children	High-risk category with positive PPD (Table 2) Use in pregnant women, children, and adolescents Use for 9 months if fibrotic lesion is seen on radiography or in children	Use with caution in active hepatitis or end-stage liver disease History of INH-induced reaction or risk for INH resistance
RIF[1] + PZA[2]	RIF 600 mg/day for 2–3 months PZA 15–30 mg/kg/day x 2–3 mo Can substitute RFB for RIF	Some PIs or NNRTIs shouldn't be given w/ RIF[3] If RFB is given, monitor for drug toxicity and adjust dosages of RFB, PIs, NNRTIs[3]	Risk of INH resistance HIV-infected persons HIV-infected person who has INH resistance but susceptible to TB	May be used in INH-intolerant patient Avoid PZA in pregnant women History of rifamycin-induced reaction Not recommended in children
EMB + PZA	EMB 15–25 mg/kg/day x 6 months PZA 15–30 mg/kg/day x 6 months	In immunocompetent patients, treat for at least 6 months Treat HIV+ patients and children for 12 months	For MDR-TB (resistance to INH and RIF) and high risk of developing TB	PZA not recommended in pregnant women Chronic severe hyperuricemia or liver disease
PZA + FQ	PZA 15–30 mg/day x 6 months Ciprofloxacin or ofloxacin x 6 months			

*Refer to text on page 474 for current recommendations on use of RIF-PZA in LTBI.
EMB = ethambutol; FQ = fluoroquinolone; HIV = human immunodeficiency virus; INH = isoniazid; IM = intramuscular; IV = intravenous; MDR-TB = multidrug-resistant tuberculosis; PO = per os (by mouth); NNRTI = non-nucleoside-reverse transcriptase inhibitor; PI = protease inhibitor; PPD = purified protein derviative; PZA = pyrazinamide; RFB = rifabutin; RIF = rifampin; TB = tuberculosis.
[1]RIF is contraindicated with hard-gel saquinavir (alone) and delavirdine. Can use RFB with indinavir, nelfinavir, amprenavir, ritonavir, efavirenz, and possibly soft-gel saquinavir and nevirapine.
[2]If PZA intolerant, use of a rifamycin (RIF or RFB) alone for LTBI for 4–6 months may be used.
[3]Refer to Table 23.7 for current recommendations in the use of rifamycins and antiretrovirals.
Adapted from American Thoracic Society. Targeted tuberculin testing and treatment of latent tuberculosis infection. *Am J Respir Crit Care Med* 2000;161:S221–S247; Centers for Disease Control and Prevention. *Core curriculum on tuberculosis: what the clinician should know, 3rd Ed.* Core curriculum on tuberculosis. Atlanta, GA: Centers for Disease Control and Prevention, 1994:1–54; Centers for Disease Control and Prevention. *Core Curriculum on Tuberculosis: What the Clinician Should Know.* 4th Ed. Atlanta, GA: Centers for Disease Control and Prevention, 2000:1–75; Centers for Disease Control and Prevention. Essential components of a tuberculosis prevention and control program; and Screening for tuberculosis and tuberculosis infection in high-risk populations: Recommendations of the advisory council for the elimination of tuberculosis. *MMWR Morbid Mortal Weekly Rep* 1995;44(RR-11):1–35; Centers for Disease Control and Prevention. Prevention and treatment of tuberculosis among patients infected with human immunodeficiency virus: principles of therapy and revised recommendations. *MMWR Morbid Mortal Weekly Rep* 1998;47(RR-20):1–53; Maher D, Chaulet P, Spinaci S, Harries A. *Treatment of Tuberculosis: Guidelines for National Programmes,* 2nd Ed. Geneva, Switzerland: World Health Organization, 1997:1–78.

and PZA or PZA and a fluoroquinolone for at least 6 months in the treatment of immunocompetent persons, or for at least 12 months in the treatment of immunocompromised patients. In children with MDR-TB, the use of EMB at 15 mg/kg/day and PZA for 9 to 12 months is recommended. Persons treated with alternative regimens should be followed for 2 years (10,31). The current recommendations for LTBI in HIV-negative and HIV-positive persons are listed in Table 23.12 (4,10,12–15,18,20,31).

Once LTBI treatment is begun, the patient needs to be evaluated on a monthly basis by the physician or other health-care personnel for signs of adverse drug effects, medication compliance, alcohol or illicit drug use, intolerance to the medication(s), and drug–drug interactions (31). If noncompliance is an issue, a pill count and urine INH metabolite studies may be needed. When INH is used, serial liver profiles should be performed at baseline and every 2 to 3 months while the patient is receiving therapy if there is suspicion of liver disorder, HIV-infection, pregnancy, or alcohol use. Baseline liver profiles may be considered in the elderly, especially if they are taking multiple medications. Active hepatitis and end-stage liver disease are relative contraindications to the use of INH or PZA. When hepatic enzyme levels exceed three to five times the upper limit of normal, or the patient reports symptoms of adverse reactions, a different antimycobacterial agent may be needed (10,31,41). Side effects of the other antimycobacterial agents are listed in Tables 23.9 and 23.10 (10).

New and Future Developments

Recent advances in the prevention and treatment of TB hold promise for improvements in the medical management of this infectious disease. The U.S. Food and Drug Administration (FDA) approved rifapentine, a member of the rifamycin class of anti-TB drugs, in June 1998. This drug eliminates both intracellular and extracellular *M. tuberculosis* by preventing gene expression. As with other drugs in its class, it can cause hepatic damage and discolor body secretions. This drug must be used with another first-line agent. Other potential therapies include a combination of INH and rifapentine (based on animal studies); an investigational new class of nitroimidazole compounds that may work against dormant mycobacteria by inhibiting glycolipid cell wall synthesis; and rifalazil, a possible newer rifamycin derivative (24,31). However, according to the Institute of Medicine, rifalazil may not go further into development because of cross-resistance. Investigations of oxazolidinone compounds and of a drug that inhibits the shikemic acid pathway are also in the preliminary testing phases (24). Other medications and better drug regimens are also being investigated. For example, rifater, a combination of INH, RIF, and PZA, was approved by the FDA in 1994. This drug was developed to treat active pulmonary TB and improve compliance. Additionally, the genome for *M. tuberculosis* has been mapped. This may lead to the development of possible vaccines, and faster and more specific tests to verify TB infection, disease, and drug resistance. Two experimental vaccines, a DNA vaccine and a vaccine using a combination of protective protein antigens in one recombinant protein, are being investigated (24).

Furthermore, DOTS has been implemented to a greater extent on an international basis. DOTS is performed by health care workers observing individuals swallowing each dose of medication while monitoring their progress toward cure. The medication is given two or three times weekly with frequent evaluation for the efficacy of the treatment protocol. The benefits of DOTS include its lower cost than traditional therapy, its 85% cure rate, and its help in preventing drug resistance and noncompliance (42). Nevertheless, only an estimated 10% of all TB patients are treated with DOTS (3).

In 1993, the WHO declared TB a global epidemic. It is estimated that one billion people will be infected and that 70 million will die from TB between 2000 and 2020. These statistics indicate that TB continues to be a threat worldwide (1). The clinician needs to be aware of the severity of TB and the potential hazards it may have for society in the United States and abroad. New tests, possible new vaccines, and more effective and cheaper drug therapies for LTBI and TB disease may help in the battle against TB. Hopefully, with better local and international efforts, such as improvements in TB programs, better innovations in the diagnosis and treatment of TB, and widespread use of DOT to help improve compliance and completion of treatment, the global threat posed by TB can be eliminated.

Summary

Although the incidence of TB has been declining nationally in the United States, it remains a deadly disease worldwide. The diagnosis and treatment of TB have undergone new developments. The preceding discussion is intended to provide a review and update on active TB and LTBI while increasing awareness of the severity of this insidious but potentially lethal disease.

REFERENCES

1. **World Health Organization.** *Tuberculosis Fact Sheet.* 2000. www.who.int/health-topics/tb.htm.
2. **Centers for Disease Control and Prevention.** Tuberculosis elimination revisited: obstacles, opportunities, and a renewed commitment. Advisory council for the elimination of tuberculosis (ACET). *MMWR Morbid Mortal Weekly Rep* 1999;48(RR-9):1–13.
3. *Stop Tuberculosis.* www.stoptb.org. 1999.

4. **Centers for Disease Control and Prevention.** *Core Curriculum on Tuberculosis: What the Clinician Should Know, 4th Ed.* Atlanta, GA: Centers for Disease Control and Prevention, 2000:1–75.

5. **Jerant AF, Bannon M, Rittenhouse S.** Identification and management of tuberculosis. *Am Fam Phys* 2000;61:2667–78.

6. **Centers for Disease Control and Prevention.** *Reported Tuberculosis in the United States,* 2000. Atlanta, GA: Centers for Disease Control and Prevention, 2001:1–78.

7. **Centers for Disease Control and Prevention.** Progress toward the elimination of tuberculosis–United States. *MMWR Morbid Mortal Weekly Rep* 1999;48:732–6.

8. **Centers for Disease Control and Prevention.** *Reported Tuberculosis in the United States,* 1999. Atlanta, GA: Centers for Disease Control and Prevention, 2000:1–80.

9. **Centers for Disease Control and Prevention.** *Status of the Tuberculosis Epidemic in the United States.* Centers for Disease Control and Prevention, 1999. cdc.gov/nchstp/tb/pubs/tbstatus/tbstatus.htm.

10. **Centers for Disease Control and Prevention.** *Core Curriculum on Tuberculosis: What the Clinician Should Know, 3rd Ed.* Core curriculum on tuberculosis. Atlanta, GA: Centers for Disease Control and Prevention, 1994:1–54.

11. **National Institute of Allergy and Infectious Diseases**–National Institutes of Health (NIAID-NIH), *Fact Sheet: Tuberculosis.* 1999. www.niaid.nih.gov/factsheets/tb.htm.

12. **American Thoracic Society.** Diagnostic standards and classification of tuberculosis. *Am Rev Respir Dis* 1990;142:725–35.

13. **American Thoracic Society.** Control of tuberculosis in the United States. *Am Rev Respir Dis* 1992;146:1623–33.

14. **American Thoracic Society.** Treatment of tuberculosis and tuberculosis infection in adults and children. *Am J Respir Crit Care Med* 1994;149:1359–74.

15. **American Thoracic Society.** Diagnostic standards and classification of tuberculosis in adults and children. *Am J Respir Crit Care Med* 2000;161:1376–95.

16. **Centers for Disease Control and Prevention.** Essential components of a tuberculosis prevention and control program; and screening for tuberculosis and tuberculosis infection in high-risk populations: Recommendations of the advisory council for the elimination of tuberculosis. *MMWR Morbid Mortal Weekly Rep* 1995;44(RR-11):1–35.

17. **Martin CG, Lazarus A.** Epidemiology and diagnosis of tuberculosis. *Postgrad Med* 2000;108:42–54.

18. **Maher D, Chaulet P, Spinaci S, Harries A.** *Treatment of Tuberculosis: Guidelines for National Programmes,* 2nd Ed. Geneva, Switzerland: World Health Organization, 1997: 1–78.

19. *Tuberculosis.* 1999, Johns Hopkins Center for Tuberculosis Research.

20. **Horsburgh C Jr., Feldman S, Ridzon R.** Practice guidelines for the treatment of tuberculosis. *Clin Infect Dis* 2000;31:633–39.

21. **Hocking T, Choi C.** Tuberculosis: a strategy to detect and treat new and reactivated infections. *Geriatrics* 1997;52:52–62.

22. **LoBue P.** Tuberculosis part II. *Disease-a-Month* 1997;43:184–274.

23. **American Thoracic Society.** Rapid diagnostic tests for tuberculosis: what is the appropriate use? *Am J Respir Crit Care Med* 1997;155:1804–14.

24. **Institute of Medicine.** *Ending Neglect: The Elimination of Tuberculosis in the United States.* Washington DC: National Academy Press, 2000:1–90.

25. **Zumla A, Grange J.** Tuberculosis. *BMJ* 1998;316:1962–64.

26. **McAdams HP, et al.** Radiologic manifestations of pulmonary tuberculosis. *Radiol Clin North Am* 1995;33:655–78.

27. **Lazarus CA, Sanders J.** Management of tuberculosis. *Postgrad Med* 2000;108:71–84.

28. **World Health Organization.** *Tuberculosis Handbook. 1st Ed.* WHO/TB/98.253. Geneva, Switzerland: World Health Organization, 1998:1–212.

29. **Centers for Disease Control and Prevention.** Prevention and treatment of tuberculosis among patients infected with human immunodeficiency virus: principles of therapy and revised recommendations. *MMWR Morbid Mortal Weekly Rep* 1998;47(RR-20): 1–53.

30. **Centers for Disease Control and Prevention.** Updated guidelines for the use of rifabutin or rifampin for the treatment and prevention of tuberculosis among HIV-infected patients taking protease inhibitors or nonnucleoside reverse transcriptase inhibitors. *MMWR Morbid Mortal Weekly Rep* 2000;49:185–9.

31. **American Thoracic Society.** Targeted tuberculin testing and treatment of latent tuberculosis infection. *Am J Respir Crit Care Med* 2000;161:S221–S247.

32. **Havlir DV, Barnes PF.** Tuberculosis in patients with human immunodeficiency virus infection. *N Engl J Med* 1999;340:367–73.

33. **Decker CF, Lazarus A.** Tuberculosis and HIV infection. *Postgrad Med* 2000;108: 57–68.

34. **Bradford WZM, Daley CL.** Multiple drug-resistant tuberculosis. *Infect Dis Clin North Am* 1998;12:157–72.

35. **Iseman MD.** Treatment of multidrug-resistant tuberculosis. *N Engl J Med* 1993; 329:784–91.

36. **Crofton SJ, Chaulet P, Maher D.** *Guidelines for the Management of Drug-Resistant Tuberculosis.* Geneva, Switzerland: World Health Organization, 1997:1–47.

37. Drugs for tuberculosis. *Med Lett Drugs Ther* 1995;37:67–70.

38. **Centers for Disease Control and Prevention.** The role of BCG vaccine in the prevention and control of tuberculosis in the United States. A joint standard by the advisory committee for the elimination of tuberculosis (ACET) and the advisory committee on immunization practices (ACIP). *MMWR Morbid Mortal Weekly Rep* 1996;45(RR-4):1–18.

39. **Menzies D, Fanning A, Yuan L, Fitzgerald M.** Tuberculosis among health care workers. *N Engl J Med* 1995;332:92–8.

40. **Markwell LMM, O'Neil KM.** Prevention of tuberculosis. *Postgrad Med* 2000;108: 87–96.

41. **Godfrey-Faussett P.** *Policy Statement Against Tuberculosis in People Living with HIV.* Geneva, Switzerland: World Health Organziation, 1997:1–20.

42. **Chaulk C, Kazandjian VA.** Directly observed therapy for treatment completion of pulmonary tuberculosis: Consensus statement of the public health tuberculosis guideline panel. *JAMA* 1998;279:943–8.

43. **Centers for Disease Control and Prevention.** Fatal and severe hepatitis associated with rifampin and pyrazinamide for the treatment of latent tuberculosis infection–New York and Georgia, 2000. *MMWR Morbid Mortal Weekly Rep* 2000;50:289-91.

44. **Centers for Disease Control and Prevention.** Update: Fatal and severe liver injuries associated with rifampin and pyrazinamide for latent tuberculosis infection, and Revisions in American Thoracic Society/CDC Recommendations–United States, 2001. *MMWR Morbid Mortal Weekly Rep* 2001;50:733-5.

24

Histoplasmosis

L. Joseph Wheat, MD

Definition

Histoplasmosis is a systemic fungal infection caused by inhalation of micro-conidia of the mold phase of *Histoplasma capsulatum* variety capsulatum. The infection begins as a focal, patchy, or diffuse pneumonitis and disseminates hematogenously to involve organs of the reticuloendothelial system before the development of specific cellular immunity to the organism. Histoplasmosis is the most prevalent endemic mycosis in the United States. Although it usually causes asymptomatic or self-limited acute pulmonary infections, severe and progressive infections do occur in some individuals.

History

The first case of histoplasmosis was described in 1905 in a patient from the Panama Canal Zone, but the organism was misidentified as *Leishmania*. Histoplasmosis was suspected to be the cause of pulmonary calcifications seen in children with negative tuberculin skin tests in 1945, thus expanding the spectrum of the disease to include benign pulmonary infections (1). Palmer (2) reported the geographic distribution of histoplasmosis in the United States in 1946 in a histoplasmin skin-test survey among student nurses and, with Edwards and coworkers (3), confirmed these findings in the mid-1950s in a skin-test survey of military recruits. Emmons (4) was the first to isolate the organism from soil, and Zeidberg and coworkers (5) noted the importance of bird droppings in the growth of *H. capsulatum* in soil.

Epidemiology

Histoplasmosis is endemic in certain areas of North America and Latin America (3), but cases also have been reported in Europe and Asia. Most cases in the United States have occurred within the Ohio and Mississippi River valleys, but exposure also may occur outside the endemic area (Fig. 24.1). Precise reasons for this endemic distribution pattern are unknown but are thought to include moderate climate, humidity, and soil characteristics including a high porosity and organic-matter content. Bird and bat excrements enhance the growth of the organism in soil by accelerating its sporulation. Birds are not susceptible to histoplasmosis and do not carry the organism, but bats actually may be infected with *H. capsulatum*, as may many other animal species. The unique growth requirements of *H. capsulatum* explain in part the localization of histoplasmosis to so-called "microfoci" (Table 24.1). Activities that disturb such sites are associated with exposure to *H. capsulatum* (*see* Table 24.1). Air currents carry the spores of the organism for miles, exposing individuals who are unaware of having had contact with a contaminated site (6). Furthermore, environmental sites that are not visibly contaminated with droppings may harbor the organism, making it difficult to suspect histoplasmosis in these areas.

Immunology, Pathogenesis, and Natural History

Infection by *H. capsulatum* is acquired by inhaling the microconidia of the organism. In the lungs, the microconidia germinate into yeasts, which attract neutrophils, macrophages, lymphocytes, and natural killer cells, all of which act to inhibit progression of the infection. Before the development of cell-mediated immunity, macrophages assist in spreading the organism to the mediastinal lymph nodes via lymphatics and throughout the reticuloendothelial system via the bloodstream.

The severity of histoplasmosis illness and attack rates correlates with the intensity of exposure and immune status of the host. Exposure in enclosed areas causes more severe illness than does outdoor exposure (7). Attack rates are higher among children than among adults because children are less likely to be immune as the result of a previous infection (8).

Cellular immunity provides the key defense against *H. capsulatum* (9). Interleukin-12 and interferon-γ arm the macrophages to kill the fungus and to halt

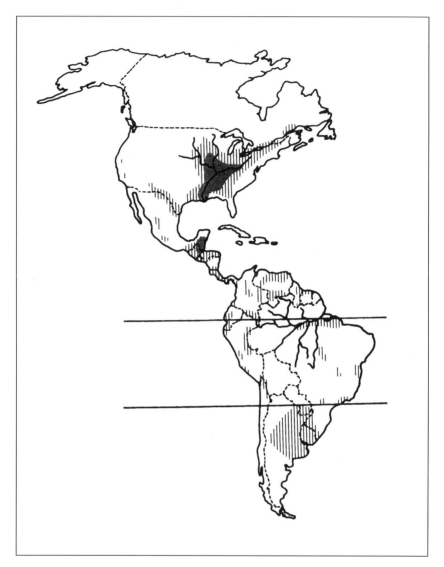

Figure 24.1 Endemic distribution of histoplasmosis in the Americas. (Republished from Rippon JW. Histoplasmosis. In Wonsiewicz M (ed). *Medical Mycology*, 3rd ed. Philadelphia: WB Saunders; 1988:424–32.)

progression of the disease (10,11). Host-defense mechanisms control the infection in immunocompetent individuals, which explains the subclinical or self-limited course characteristic of acute histoplasmosis. Individuals with underlying conditions (e.g., AIDS) that impair these defenses develop more

Table 24.1   Sources of Exposure to *Histoplasma capsulatum*

Microfocus	Activities
Caves	Spelunking
Chicken coops	Cleaning, demolition, use of bird droppings in garden
Bird roosts	Excavation, camping
Bamboo canebrakes	Cutting cane, recreation
School yards	Routine activities, cleaning
Prison grounds	Routine activities, cleaning
Decayed wood piles	Transporting or burning wood
Dead trees	Recreation, cutting wood
Contaminated chimneys	Cleaning, demolition
Old buildings	Demolition, remodeling, cleaning
Laboratories	Conducting research with *Histoplasma capsulatum*

severe and often fatal progressive disseminated manifestations of infection. Extremes of age (<1 year or >55 years (12–14) are other risk factors for progressive disseminated infection.

Reinfection with histoplasmosis occurs in patients who live in endemic areas and thus have been exposed to the fungus repeatedly. An accelerated and enhanced immune response has been postulated to follow reinfection, shortening the clinical course of the disease but increasing the inflammatory response (15,16). Illnesses of this sort are less severe and of shorter duration, and mediastinal lymphadenopathy is less common with reinfection (15). The increased inflammatory response with reinfection may play a role in the pathogenesis of the caseating tissue necrosis seen in some patients with histoplasmosis, including those with chronic pulmonary manifestations (17,18).

Reactivation of latent histoplasmosis is believed to occur in immunocompromised patients (19,20). DNA fingerprinting that shows a pattern characteristic of that found in Panamanian strains of *H. capsulatum* in five Puerto Rican immigrants to New York City supports this notion (21). However, reactivation has not been recognized as a prominent cause of histoplasmosis in patients with AIDS or among those who have undergone renal transplantation in Indianapolis (20,22,23). Cases have occurred in clusters during outbreaks involving nonimmunocompromised individuals as well, and attack rates have been low during periods free of outbreaks. This indicates that these immunocompromised individuals acquired their infections by exogenous exposure during the outbreak, not by reactivation (23). These observations and the low incidence rates in other cities within areas endemic for histoplasmosis refute the hypothesis that reactivation is a common cause of the disease in immunosuppressed individuals.

Certain manifestations of histoplasmosis are believed to result from the inflammatory response rather than the infection per se. Key examples are fibrosing mediastinitis (24,25) and a sarcoidosis-like syndrome (26); however, the pathogenesis of these forms of histoplasmosis has not been established.

Clinical Manifestations

Symptomatic infection is uncommon (<5%) following low-level exposure to *H. capsulatum* (27). In contrast, most patients exposed to a heavily contaminated site develop symptomatic infection. A significant percentage of patients (60%) with acute histoplasmosis manifest flu-like illnesses with pulmonary complaints and abnormalities on chest radiography. Less frequent manifestations include pericarditis, a rheumatologic syndrome with erythema nodosum, chronic pulmonary infection, and progressive disseminated disease (27). The more common manifestations of histoplasmosis are reviewed in Figure 24.2 and in the following sections.

Asymptomatic Histoplasmosis

Infection with *H. capsulatum* is usually asymptomatic in the healthy host, presumably because the inoculum is small and the host defense is able to restrict proliferation of the organism (16). Skin-test surveys in endemic areas indicate that over one half of individuals have had a previous infection with *H. capsulatum*, although few were believed to have had symptomatic disease. In outbreaks in Indianapolis and elsewhere, between 90% and 99% of infections were asymptomatic (6,29). Further supporting the belief that asymptomatic histoplasmosis has a high prevalence is the observation that individuals with recent evidence of the disease (based on histoplasmin skin-test conversion), rarely recall clinical illnesses consistent with acute histoplasmosis (30). Chest radiographs in patients who show skin-test conversion are abnormal in less than 10% of cases, indicating that mild exposure may be insufficient to cause pulmonary lesions. Asymptomatic infections usually are identified during epidemiologic surveys or when evaluating patients with compatible radiographic abnormalities.

Symptomatic Acute Pulmonary Histoplasmosis

Symptoms of histoplasmosis usually appear within 1 month of exposure but may occur earlier in patients with extensive pulmonary involvement after inhaling a heavy inoculum or later in patients with limited infection after exposure to a low inoculum (16). Fever, chills, headache, myalgia, anorexia, cough,

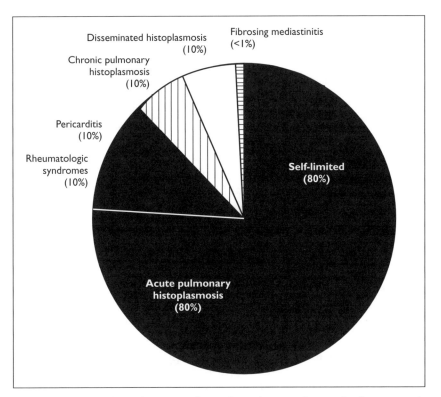

Figure 24.2 Clinical manifestations of acute histoplasmosis. In a study of symptomatic patients with acute histoplasmosis, self-limited illnesses were found to occur in 80% (28). Most of these individuals exhibited acute pulmonary illnesses characterized by flu-like symptoms accompanied by pulmonary complaints. Less commonly (in 5%–10% of cases), patients experienced rheumatologic syndromes with arthritis or arthralgia (associated with erythema nodosum or erythema multiforme) or acute pericarditis.

and sharp substernal chest pain characterize these illnesses (8,16); however, coryza and sore throat are not symptoms of histoplasmosis. Pleurisy with pleural friction rubs may occur if the lesions of pulmonary histoplasmosis abut the pleura (16). Most symptoms clear within 1 month (8), but fatigue and asthenia may persist for several months (16,29). Enlarged hilar or mediastinal lymph nodes with focal infiltrates usually are seen on radiographs, but lymph-node lesions may not be apparent (29). Infiltrates may be patchy or nodular, measuring from less than 1 cm to more than 4 cm in diameter, and they are often multiple. Infiltrates clear within 2 to 4 months in most cases (16), whereas adenopathy may persist for years (Wheat J, Unpublished data). Calcification of nodes or parenchymal granulomas occur slowly over several years in adults (Wheat J, unpublished data) but occur more rapidly in children. Rarely, nodules may cavitate in acute histoplasmosis (31). Pleural involvement is also rare (16,32,33).

Diffuse Reticulonodular or Miliary Pulmonary Histoplasmosis

Patients who have had heavy exposure to *H. capsulatum* may present with respiratory insufficiency caused by diffuse pulmonary involvement. Chest radiographs of such cases show reticulonodular or miliary infiltrates (34,35). Although patients usually recover from exposure to heavy inoculum without treatment (34), they may be severely ill or may manifest disseminated disease (35,36) and frequently remain dyspneic and fatigued for months. Although rare, restrictive ventilatory impairment caused by diffuse fibrosis may ensue (16).

Granulomatous Mediastinitis

Enlarged lymph nodes may obstruct important mediastinal structures during acute histoplasmosis (16,37). Pathologic examinations in cases of granulomatous mediastinitis show active inflammation and tissue necrosis of the mediastinal lymph nodes, rather than the fibrotic reaction characteristic of fibrosing mediastinitis. The temporal relationship of the obstructive syndrome to the acute infection is variable; obstructive symptoms may appear soon after the acute infection or months later. Symptoms are caused by compression of the airways, superior vena cava, or pulmonary vessels (16,38–40). As a result of caseous necrosis, lesions may appear lucent on computed tomography (CT) scans. These necrotic lesions may rupture into the tracheobronchial tree, producing air-filled cystic masses (16). Compression of the airways can cause respiratory difficulty (especially in young children), and prolonged obstruction can cause bronchiectasis or bronchial stenosis (16). Compression of the esophagus may cause dysphagia (16,39–41). Esophagobronchial or tracheal fistulas and traction diverticuli may develop (37,42). The esophagus also may be involved in disseminated histoplasmosis (43,44).

Enlarged and occasionally cystic mediastinal lymph nodes may be seen radiographically or on CT scans of the chest (40,45–47). These cystic lymph nodes may measure up to 10 cm in diameter and consist of a necrotic central core surrounded by granulomatous tissue, with the whole node encased in a fibrous capsule (45). Older lesions show calcification (16).

Pericarditis

Between 5% and 10% of patients with symptomatic histoplasmosis present with pericarditis. The pericarditis is caused by an immunologic reaction to the mediastinal adenitis, rather than by actual infection of the pericardium (48,49). Although rare, pericarditis may complicate disseminated histoplasmosis (49). Patients with pericarditis complain of chest pain and, on examination, may demonstrate pericardial friction rubs. Other evidence of pericarditis include enlargement of the cardiac silhouette on chest radiographs, ST-segment changes on electrocardiography, pericardial thickening or effusion on echocardiography (48,49). Hemodynamic compromise occurs in 40% of patients.

Rheumatologic Syndrome

Arthritis or arthralgia occurs in 5% to 10% of symptomatic patients with histoplasmosis, mainly in women. These patients also usually have erythema nodosum and/or erythema multiforme (50,51). Rheumatologic manifestations represent systemic inflammatory reactions to the acute infection, rather than dissemination to the joints or soft tissues. Radiography of the joints is normal, cultures of synovial fluid are negative, and patients improve without antifungal therapy. Septic arthritis is diagnosed rarely in patients with disseminated histoplasmosis.

Chronic Pulmonary Histoplasmosis

Chronic pulmonary infection follows exposure to *H. capsulatum* in patients with emphysema (17,18). Cough, dyspnea, chest pain, fatigue, fever, and sweating are typical clinical manifestations of such infection, and radiography shows apical infiltrates with cavitation that mimic findings in tuberculosis. The infection is progressive, as indicated by cavity enlargement, new cavity formation, and spread to other areas of the lungs (17,18,35). Histopathologic characteristics include emphysema, granulomas, vascular compromise, tissue necrosis, and fibrosis (17). The severity of inflammation is disproportionate to the number of organisms identified by fungal stains, suggesting that hypersensitivity to fungal antigens may be important in its pathogenesis (17).

Neoplastic or other infectious processes may complicate the course of chronic pulmonary histoplasmosis, causing confusion in the clinical management (e.g., prolonged exposure to tobacco is a risk factor for lung cancer). Tuberculosis also may coexist with chronic pulmonary histoplasmosis (17,18), and it must be excluded by tuberculin skin testing and culture. Recurrent bacterial pneumonia or bronchitis is common and should be considered in patients who seem to exhibit reactivation or progression of chronic pulmonary histoplasmosis. Aspergilloma, chronic invasive aspergillosis, atypical mycobacterial infections, and chronic pneumonia caused by a variety of other pathogens may develop in areas in which the lungs are damaged.

Broncholithiasis

Extensive calcification develops in areas of necrotic lymph nodes and pulmonary granulomas in histoplasmosis (16). The calcification may encroach on or erode into bronchi, causing hemoptysis or obstruction (40,52). Patients expectorate small stones, gravel, or gritty material and may experience life-threatening hemoptysis (52). Organisms can be demonstrated by fungal stains in the calcified nodes in some patients, but cultures are negative. Surgical therapy is often required in patients with significant hemoptysis or recurrent pneumonia and for the repair of bronchoesophageal fistulae (40).

Fibrosing Mediastinitis

Mediastinal Fibrosis
Mediastinal fibrosis represents an excessive scarring response to past infection with *H. Capsulatum* and usually (80%) occurs in individuals between the ages of 20 and 40 years (as often in women as in men) (24,25). Symptoms are more common in fibrosing mediastinitis (~80%) than in granulomatous mediastinitis (~25%) (38). Patients complain of cough, dyspnea, hemoptysis, pleurisy, and sweating, each symptom occurring in 20% to 40% of cases (25). Common sites of involvement are the superior vena cava, the airway, pulmonary arteries and veins, and the esophagus (24,25,38). Pulmonary venous occlusion, if extensive, leads to findings of pulmonary congestion that resemble those seen with mitral stenosis. Involvement of the thoracic duct, recurrent laryngeal nerve, or atrium is rare (24,38). Progressive right heart failure and respiratory insufficiency occur in nearly one third of cases (24,25). Recurrent and even fatal hemoptysis may result from 1) parenchymal damage caused by airway obstruction, vascular compromise, and tissue necrosis; or 2) dilated bronchial artery collateral vessels in patients with pulmonary artery obstruction (25). Recurrent pneumonia is common in patients with airway obstruction or bronchiectasis.

Chest radiographs may be normal or may show only subcarinal or superior mediastinal widening, whereas CT scans or pulmonary vascular imaging studies may reveal compression of mediastinal structures (24,25). The fibrosis extends from the hilar or paratracheal nodes (each in 15% to 20% of cases) and from the subcarinal nodes in approximately 30% (25). In patients with pulmonary artery obstruction, ventilation–perfusion lung scans show reduced blood flow but normal ventilation. However, pulmonary arteriography may be required to define the extent of obstruction and the status of the pulmonary veins in patients with severe manifestations of mediastinal fibrosis who are under evaluation for surgery.

Histologic and mycologic studies are often not diagnostic of histoplasmosis. Histologic findings may include only fibrosis and inflammation without granulomas. In addition to these nondiagnostic results, cultures are also usually negative. Fungal stains are positive in only approximately half of cases (24,25). These findings support the hypothesis that fibrosing mediastinitis is an excessive scarring reaction to a past infection (24,38). Biopsy of mediastinal nodes, bronchoscopy, or other invasive procedures may cause serious bleeding and should be avoided. Serologic tests are positive in two thirds of cases (25), and skin-test reactivity to histoplasmin, as evidence of previous histoplasmosis, can be demonstrated in most cases (24).

Progressive Disseminated Histoplasmosis

Although dissemination occurs during the initial infection with *H. capsulatum* in most individuals, it usually is not clinically apparent and clears spontaneously once specific cell-mediated immunity is established. Blood cultures in such cases may grow *H. capsulatum* (35). Support for this observation is derived from the demonstration of granulomas containing *H. capsulatum* in the splenic tissue of a large proportion of patients who reside in areas endemic for histoplasmosis (53).

Progressive disseminated histoplasmosis is defined as a progressive clinical illness with extrapulmonary spread of infection (12,13). Such progressive disease occurs in approximately one in 2000 cases of acute infection (13) and usually in individuals with underlying immunosuppressive conditions or at the extremes of age (14). AIDS has emerged as a major risk factor for this infection (20). Idiopathic CD4 lymphocytopenia also should be excluded in patients with disseminated histoplasmosis (54). However, between one third and two thirds of cases lack obvious risk factors for dissemination (12–14), and such patients may have unidentified defects in cellular immunity (12).

The time course of the infection is variable. Patients may present shortly after the exposure or years later and may experience asymptomatic periods interrupted by symptomatic recrudescences (12). Illnesses are more severe in immunocompromised individuals. Fever and weight loss are the most common symptoms of disseminated histoplasmosis, and hepatomegaly or splenomegaly often are present on examination (Fig. 24.3). Other common sites of involvement include the skin and oropharyngeal or gastrointestinal mucosa. Gastrointestinal involvement may be manifested in the form of ulcerations or polypoid masses, leading to misdiagnoses of colitis or malignancy (55–59). The ileocecal region is commonly involved, but lesions may occur anywhere along the gastrointestinal tract. Skin lesions may be erythematous, maculopapular, pustulonecrotic, hyperpigmented, or crateriform (60–62). Shock, respiratory distress, hepatic and renal failure, and coagulopathy may complicate severe cases (20). Involvement of the central nervous system occurs in 5% to 20% of cases, usually presenting as chronic meningitis or less

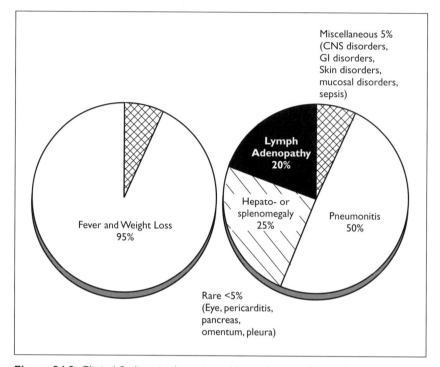

Figure 24.3 Clinical findings in disseminated histoplasmosis. These findings are based on the experience during the large outbreak in Indianapolis (13,20,23). Fever is less common in patients with localized manifestations of disseminated disease (12). Central nervous system complaints (e.g., headache, depressed mentation) were relatively common, but evidence for CNS involvement, including meningitis, was seen in only 6% of patients.

commonly as single or multiple brain lesions or diffuse encephalitis (63). Histoplasmomas also may involve the spinal cord (64,65).

At autopsy, adrenal involvement is found as a complication in 80% to 90% of cases of progressive disseminated histoplasmosis, but adrenal insufficiency is rare (<10% of cases) (12). Extensive bilateral necrosis is required to cause adrenal insufficiency. Histoplasmosis should be excluded in patients with adrenal masses or Addison's disease. Adrenal insufficiency should be suspected in patients with disseminated histoplasmosis who exhibit hypotension, hypoglycemia, hyponatremia, or hyperkalemia.

Anemia, leukopenia, or thrombocytopenia suggest bone-marrow involvement, and increased hepatic enzyme activity or bilirubin may be a clue to the presence of hepatic involvement. A marked increase in the concentration of lactic acid dehydrogenase has been an especially useful clue to the diagnosis of disseminated histoplasmosis in patients with AIDS (66). Chest radiographs are abnormal in 70% of patients, typically showing miliary, diffuse interstitial, or reticulonodular infiltrates; mediastinal adenopathy occurs in 20% of cases, whereas cavitation is rare (13,20,67).

Hypercalcemia, caused by increased sensitivity to vitamin D, has been described in progressive disseminated histoplasmosis (68,69). Other rare manifestations include chorioretinitis (70), pleuritis (71), pericarditis (72), endocarditis (73,74), peritonitis (75), pancreatitis (13), cholecystitis (76), prostatitis (77), panniculitis (78), mastitis (79), epididymitis (80), and involvement of the penis (81,82) and vagina (81). Endocarditis is manifested by systemic emboli in a person with other findings of disseminated disease but may present as isolated culture-negative endocarditis (73,83).

Presumed Ocular Histoplasmosis

The relationship between this syndrome and histoplasmosis is controversial. A choroiditis, often involving the macula and causing visual loss, has been attributed to histoplasmosis (84,85), but the scientific basis establishing *H. capsulatum* as its cause is weak. *H. capsulatum* has been demonstrated in the eye tissues of patients with this syndrome in only two cases, and culture confirmation was not included in these reports. Instead, the association has been based on histoplasmin skin-test reactivity in patients with ocular lesions, even though careful epidemiologic studies (with controls selected from the same geographic area as the cases) have not yet been performed (86). However, involvement of the eye during disseminated histoplasmosis should be distinguished from this syndrome (87).

Similarity of Clinical Findings in Histoplasmosis and Sarcoidosis

Sarcoidosis, a syndrome of unknown etiology, produces clinical findings similar to those of histoplasmosis (26). Pulmonary infiltrates with mediastinal lymphadenopathy, erythema nodosum, increased hepatic enzyme activity, and splenomegaly are seen in both conditions. Increased angiotensin-converting enzyme activity and noncaseating granulomas are shared laboratory findings in the two conditions (26,88). In some cases, histoplasmosis may trigger an inflammatory reaction typical of sarcoidosis, whereas in others sarcoidosis may be diagnosed incorrectly in patients with histoplasmosis (26). Histoplasmosis should be excluded before corticosteroid treatment for sarcoidosis is initiated. Positive fungal stains or cultures and the detection of antigen in urine or serum support a diagnosis of active histoplasmosis, not sarcoidosis. Increased titers of antibodies to *H. capsulatum*, although not excluding a diagnosis of sarcoidosis, support careful follow-up for evidence of disseminated histoplasmosis in patients who are treated with immunosuppressive medications.

Diagnosis

Although excellent laboratory methods are available, the diagnosis of histoplasmosis is in many cases missed or delayed because histoplasmosis is not considered as the differential diagnosis. Physicians must be aware of the clinical syndromes produced by histoplasmosis and must take advantage of the epidemiologic clues discussed above. Furthermore, clinicians must be familiar with the uses and limitations of a battery of serologic and mycologic tests. Diagnostic modalities for histoplasmosis include culture, special fungal stains of tissue, serologic tests for antibodies, and tests for antigens (Table 24.2). The role of each test varies with the severity of the infection (89–91). The sensitivity of these tests varies in the different clinical presentations of histoplasmosis. All are reasonably specific and can serve as the basis for diagnosis in patients with compatible clinical findings. Each test has limitations that must be recognized if the test is to be used correctly. An informational brochure describing the use of the diagnostic tests for histoplasmosis is available at the Histoplasmosis Reference Laboratory (1-800-HISTO-DGN *or* www.iupui.edu/~histodgn).

Fungal Cultures

Cultures for *H. capsulatum* are most often positive in patients with disseminated or chronic pulmonary histoplasmosis (*see* Table 24.2). In disseminated disease, the highest yield is from bone marrow or blood, which is positive in more than 75% of cases (13,20). DuPont ISOLATORS or Mycolytic blood culture bottles should be used for fungal blood cultures. The sensitivity and time to isolation in patients with positive blood cultures are inferior with other culture systems. Organisms can be found in sputum or bronchoscopy specimens from most (60%–85%) patients with chronic pulmonary histoplasmosis,

Table 24.2   Summary of Diagnostic Test Results in Histoplasmosis

	Acute Pulmonary (% Positive)	Cavitary (% Positive)	Disseminated (% Positive)
Antibody			
Immunodiffused	75	100	63
Complement fixation	89	93	63
Either immunodiffused or complement fixation	99	100	71
Antigen detection	40–75*	21	92
Culture	15	85	85

* 75% with diffuse pulmonary infiltrates (Wheat, unpublished 1995)
Modified from Williams B, Fojtasek M, Connolly-Stringfield P, Wheat J. Diagnosis of histoplasmosis by antigen detection during an outbreak in Indianapolis, Indiana. *Arch Pathol Lab Med.* 1994;118:1205–8.

but multiple specimens must be submitted (18). The sensitivity of culture is low (l0%–15%) in patients with other varieties of histoplasmosis (89). Slow growth (2–4 weeks) may delay the diagnosis in patients with positive cultures and is a significant drawback in patients with severe clinical manifestations, indicating the need for more rapid approaches (89).

Histopathology

Biopsy specimens may show granulomas in three quarters of cases, lymphohistiocytic aggregates, or diffuse mononuclear cell infiltrates (13,92). Fungal staining of lung or mediastinal lymph node tissue permits rapid diagnosis but with a lower sensitivity (<50% of culture and/or antigen positive cases) than detection by culture or antigen testing (13). Pathologists must be experienced in recognizing *H. capsulatum* to achieve this rate of success in the diagnosis of histoplasmosis. Yeast-phase organisms of *H. capsulatum* are ovoid, measure 3 to 5 µm in diameter, and exhibit narrow-based budding. *Candida glabrata, Cryptococcus neoformans, Blastomyces dermatitidis, Toxoplasma gondii, Leishmania, Pneumocystis carinii,* and staining artifacts may be misidentified as *H. capsulatum.*

Antigen Detection

Histoplasma antigen can be detected in body fluids and offers a valuable approach to the diagnosis of diffuse pulmonary or disseminated histoplasmosis (89,91), providing results within 24 to 48 hours. Antigen is found in the blood, urine, and bronchoalveolar lavage fluid of most individuals with disseminated histoplasmosis and in up to 75% of those with diffuse lung involvement during acute pulmonary histoplasmosis. Antigen is detected in the cerebrospinal fluid (CSF) of 25% to 50% of patients with *Histoplasma* meningitis (93). Cross-reactions occur in patients with paracoccidioidomycosis, blastomycosis, *Penicillium marneffi* infection, and African histoplasmosis (caused by infection with *H. capsulatum* variety duboisii) (94).

Antigen testing of serum and urine should be performed in cases of suspected disseminated or extensive pulmonary histoplasmosis. CSF should be tested in cases of histoplasmosis with evidence of meningitis and for the workup of chronic meningitis. Test results are usually negative in patients with localized acute or chronic pulmonary involvement. Antigen testing is available at the aforementioned Histoplasmosis Reference Laboratory.

Antigen concentrations decline with therapy and should become nondetectable in patients who are cured of histoplasmosis. However, antigen often fails to disappear completely in patients with AIDS (Fig. 24.4) (96–99). Patients in whom antigen levels fail to decline should be assessed carefully for response to therapy (e.g., measurement of blood concentrations of the anti-

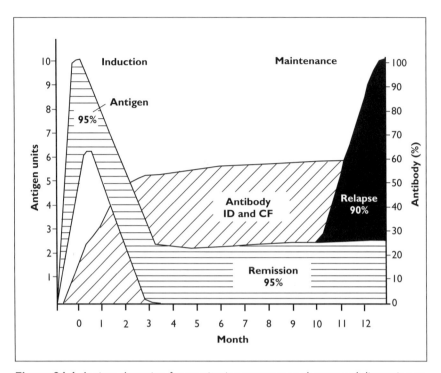

Figure 24.4 Antigen detection for monitoring response to therapy and diagnosing relapse of histoplasmosis in patients with AIDS. Antigen is detectable in the urine and serum of over 90% of patients with disseminated histoplasmosis at the time of diagnosis, and its concentration decreases in response to therapy. Antigen concentrations remain low or undetectable in 95% of patients who remain in remission and increase by at least 2 units in approximately 90% of those who relapse (95).

fungal agent being used for treatment and culture of blood). Because antigen levels rise with relapse (95), antigen detection also has been used to monitor patients receiving maintenance therapy to prevent recurrence of histoplasmosis (97–99,100). For this purpose, serum and urine specimens should be submitted for antigen testing every 4 to 6 months and at the time of suspected relapse.

Serologic Tests

Tests for antibodies to *H. capsulatum* are highly useful for the diagnosis of histoplasmosis. Antibodies appear within 4 to 12 weeks in most symptomatic infections and peak over the next few months. Standard tests include the immunodiffusion test for H and M precipitin bands and the complement fixation test with yeast and mycelial-phase antigens. Although the complement fixation test is more sensitive than the immunodiffusion test, both tests should be performed to achieve the highest sensitivity. Serologic tests are positive in approximately 90% of patients with symptomatic histoplasmosis but in a lower percentage of those with asymptomatic infection (101) and of those who are immunosuppressed (20,89). Antibody levels decline slowly over a 1- to 4-year period after recovery from histoplasmosis and may increase with relapse, but serologic tests rarely provide useful information for monitoring treatment. False-positive tests may be caused by cross-reactions to shared antigens in patients with other fungal infections, especially blastomycosis, coccidioidomycosis, and paracoccidioidomycosis. Serologic tests should be done in all cases of suspected histoplasmosis.

Histoplasmin Skin Test

High background positivity (50%–80%) in areas endemic for histoplasmosis, false-positive results in patients with other fungal diseases, and false-negative results in patients with disseminated disease limit the usefulness of the histoplasmin skin test in the diagnosis of histoplasmosis (3,102). Furthermore, skin tests boost antibody levels, compromising the interpretation of serologic tests for histoplasmosis (103).

Treatment

Infections with *H. capsulatum* are asymptomatic or self-limited in most patients, justifying observation without antifungal therapy. The likelihood that patients will require therapy depends on the size of the inoculum and on host factors that affect the course of the infection. Patients who inhale a large inoculum during exposure to a heavily contaminated site are at risk for extensive pulmonary infection and usually should be treated. Those with emphysema usually develop chronic pulmonary infection, and immunocompromised hosts experience progressive disseminated disease. Guidelines for assessing the indications for therapy are presented in Table 24.3. Specific indications and recommendations are reviewed below and summarized in Table 24.4.

Acute Pulmonary Histoplasmosis

Antifungal therapy is unnecessary in most patients with acute pulmonary histoplasmosis, because the course of disease after low-level exposure is benign in nonimmunocompromised patients. Symptoms improve within a few weeks in nearly all patients (8). Therapy may be helpful in patients who have not improved within a month and in those with more severe symptoms.

Table 24.3   Indications for Antifungal Therapy

Indicated	Not Indicated
Acute pulmonary histoplasmosis with respiratory failure or prolonged systems	Acute, self-limited pulmonary histoplasmosis
	Rheumatologic histoplasmosis
Mediastinal granuloma with symptomatic obstruction	Pericarditis
	Fibrosing mediastinitis*
Disseminated histoplasmosis	Sarcoid-like histoplasmosis
Chronic pulmonary histoplasmosis	Presumed ocular histoplasmosis

*Therapy is unlikely to be helpful in patients with fibrosing mediastinitis, but a trial can be considered (especially in patients with elevated sedimentation rates).

Acute Diffuse or Miliary Histoplasmosis

Following heavy exposure to *H. capsulatum*, patients develop diffuse pulmonary histoplasmosis, which is often complicated by respiratory compromise. Treatment is indicated in symptomatic patients with diffuse radiographic involvement, especially if they are dyspneic or hypoxic. Recovery is slow (35), and the outcome may be fatal without treatment (104). The inflammatory response seems to contribute to the pathogenesis of the respiratory compromise; patients who are hypoxic seem to benefit from a prednisone dosage of 60 mg/d for a few weeks (34,105). Corticosteroids should not be given without concurrent antifungal therapy; however, itraconazole alone could be used in patients not sufficiently ill to require hospitalization. Eight to 12 weeks of treatment with itraconazole should be adequate.

Pericarditis or Rheumatologic Syndromes

Patients with pericarditis or rheumatologic manifestations of histoplasmosis usually respond to anti-inflammatory therapy without antifungal therapy (48,49,106,107). Corticosteroids may be helpful in patients with pericardial tamponade or hemodynamic compromise (49) and might be tried before resorting to pericardial drainage or surgery. Corticosteroids should not be given for more than 2 weeks and possibly should be accompanied by itraconazole to reduce the likelihood of promoting the progressive dissemination of infection.

The joint symptoms in patients with rheumatologic manifestations may resolve spontaneously but usually require treatment with nonsteroidal anti-inflammatory drugs (107). In one reported series, patients were treated with corticosteroids (106). Antifungal therapy is not indicated unless there is evidence that the bone or joint involvement is a manifestation of disseminated disease (108).

Table 24.4   Treatment Recommendations for Histoplasmosis

Histoplasmosis Type	Severe Manifestation	Mild to Moderate Manifestation
Acute, diffuse pulmonary histoplasmosis after heavy exposure	Amphotericin B with corticosteroids followed by itraconazole for 12 weeks*	Itraconazole for 12 weeks*†
Subacute, focal pulmonary histoplasmosis	N/A	Usually resolves spontaneously; itraconazole for 6–12 weeks in those with persistent symptoms (>4 weeks)
Chronic pulmonary histoplasmosis	Amphotericin B followed by itraconazole for 12–24 months	Itraconazole for 12–24 months
Disseminated non–AIDS-related histoplasmosis	Amphotericin B followed by itraconazole for 6–18 months*	Itraconazole for 6–18 months*
Disseminated AIDS-related histoplasmosis	Amphotericin B‡ followed by itraconazole for life	Itraconazole for life§
Meningitis	Amphotericin B for 3 months followed by itraconazole or fluconazole for 12 months	Same as with a severe manifestation because of usually poor outcome
Granulomatous mediastinitis	Amphotericin B followed by itraconazole for 3–6 months	Itraconazole for 3–6 months
Fibrosing mediastinitis	Itraconazole for 3 months¶	Same as with severe manifestation
Pericarditis	Corticosteroid 1 mg/kg/d** or pericardial drainage procedure	NSAIDs for 2–12 weeks
Rheumatologic histoplasmosis	NSAIDs for 2–12 weeks	Same as with a severe manifestation

N/A = not applicable; NSAIDs = nonsteroidal anti-inflammatory drugs.

*Amphotericin B should be administered at a dosage of 0.7 mg/kg/d (50 mg/d) and itraconazole at 5 mg/kg/d (400 mg/d).

† Itraconazole blood concentrations should be measured during the second week of therapy to ensure that detectable concentrations have been achieved. If the concentration is less than 1 µg/mL, then the dose may be insufficient or drug interaction may be hindering the absorption or accelerating the metabolism of the itraconazole, requiring a dose change. If the concentrations are greater than 10 µg/mL, then the dose may be reduced.

‡ Liposomal amphotericin B (AmBisome) may be more appropriate for disseminated disease, because it was more effective than the deoxycholate formulation in a study in AIDS patients. Therapy should continue until concentrations of Histoplasma antigen are less than 4 units in urine and serum.

§ A study is currently being performed to determine whether this treatment can be stopped after 1 year if the patient's CD4 count is less than 150 cells/mL.

¶ This therapy is controversial and probably ineffective except in cases of granulomatous mediastinitis that are misdiagnosed as fibrosing mediastinitis.

** If corticosteroids are administered, concurrent antifungal therapy is recommended.

Granulomatous Mediastinitis

Enlarged lymph nodes in histoplasmosis may encroach on adjacent mediastinal structures, causing protracted symptoms. Antifungal therapy should be considered for patients with moderately severe complaints or functional limitations and for those who remain symptomatic for more than a month. Corticosteroids may be helpful in patients with airway obstruction (109). Resection of enlarged nodes has been performed in some cases (40,46,110,111) and may be helpful in patients with moderately severe complaints that are unresponsive to a 3-month trial of itraconazole. However, the resection of enlarged mediastinal lymph nodes to prevent progression to fibrosing mediastinitis (42,112) is not advised (25).

Chronic Pulmonary Histoplasmosis

Without treatment, chronic pulmonary histoplasmosis is progressive, causing loss of pulmonary function in most patients and death in up to half (35,113–115). Although some patients improve spontaneously (17,18), they remain at risk for recrudescence. Early studies showed amphotericin B to be effective in 59% to 100% of cases (113–117), both for halting progression of the illness and for reducing mortality (Table 24.5) (115). Ketoconazole and itraconazole are effective in 75% to 85% of cases (117–119). Fluconazole at 200 to 400 mg/d is less effective (64% response) than ketoconazole or itraconazole (120); however, all treatments may be complicated by recurrence after therapy is stopped. Courses of treatment of 1 to 2 years are recommended to reduce the risk of relapse.

Table 24.5   Outcome of Treatment of Chronic Pulmonary Histoplasmosis

Treatment (Reference No.)	No. of Patients	Response (%)	Deaths (%)	Relapse (%)
Amphotericin B (115)	89	59	16	10
Amphotericin B (116)	32	100		
Amphotericin B (114)	16	81	6	12
Amphotericin B (134)	56	96		9
Amphotericin B (113)	238	99		15
Itraconazole (117)	20	80	5	15
Ketoconazole (118)	23	74		4
Ketoconazole (119)	7	86		
Fluconazole (120)	11	64		29

Broncholithiasis

Antifungal therapy is not indicated for broncholithiasis resulting from histoplasmosis, because it does not represent an active infection but rather a result of mechanical trauma caused by calcified lymph nodes or parenchymal granulomas. Surgical therapy often is required in patients with significant hemoptysis or recurrent pneumonia and for repair of bronchoesophageal fistulae (40).

Fibrosing Mediastinitis

Fibrosing mediastinitis resulting from histoplasmosis is often progressive and unresponsive to antifungal therapy (24,25). Such therapy would not be expected to reverse obstruction caused by dense fibrosis, but whether it might prevent progression caused by ongoing inflammation is unknown. In one study, however, ketoconazole was thought to have been helpful (121). A short trial (3 months) of antifungal treatment is reasonable, especially if complement fixation titers and the sedimentation rate are elevated (120) or if cultures or tests for antigen are positive. Radiographic demonstration of improvement would support continuation of therapy for at least 1 year. Corticosteroid therapy has not been helpful (25,112,122), and is discouraged.

Surgery may be helpful in patients with more severe manifestations of fibrosing mediastinitis, but the risk of surgery is substantial and the benefit unpredictable. The largest review of fibrosing mediastinitis found that fewer than 40% of patients benefited and 20% died as a complication of surgery (25). Operative mortality in another report was 25% (122). In many cases, the severity of illness is insufficient to justify the risk of surgery, and the course of the untreated disease may be nonprogressive, discouraging this approach except in patients with bilateral disease or with severe clinical manifestations. Stenting has been helpful in some patients with vena cava, airway, pulmonary artery, or pulmonary vein obstruction. Creating venous bypass channels also has been tried, but with limited success, in patients with superior vena cava obstruction; however, collateral vessels usually prevent major morbidity from this complication.

Progressive Disseminated Histoplasmosis

In 80% of cases, disseminated histoplasmosis is fatal without treatment (Table 24.6) (35,115). Amphotericin B reduced the mortality from 83% in historical controls to 23% in cases surveyed by the Communicable Disease Center Cooperative Mycoses Study Group (115). Other studies have also confirmed amphotericin B's role in disseminated histoplasmosis (12,20,23, 123,124). Azole antifungal agents are also effective but usually are reserved for less severely ill patients. Itraconazole was successful in 85% to 100% of patients (100,117) compared with 56% to 70% for ketoconazole (118,119). Among patients with AIDS, itraconazole was effective in 85% (100), whereas ketoconazole, in a retrospective survey, was effective in only 10% (20). The results of these studies suggest that itraconazole is more effective than ketoconazole for the treatment of histoplasmosis. Among patients with disseminated histoplasmosis, fluconazole was effective in 86% of those without AIDS and in 74% of those with AIDS (99,120). Among AIDS patients who responded to fluconazole 800 mg/d, one third relapsed while receiving 400 mg/d for maintenance therapy (99).

Itraconazole is the treatment of choice for progressive disseminated histoplasmosis, both as the initial treatment for patients with mild or moderately severe symptoms who do not require hospitalization and for continuation of therapy in those who have improved in response to amphotericin B. Itraconazole capsules should be administered with food or a cola beverage in a loading dosage of 200 mg three times daily for 3 days to achieve steady-state blood concentrations more rapidly and thereafter should be given in a dosage of 200 mg once or twice daily, depending on the severity of the infection and the concentrations of drug achieved in the blood. A liquid formulation of itraconazole produces 50% higher blood concentrations, permitting reduction of the dosage given to some patients. The solution should be given on an empty stomach to achieve the highest concentrations in blood. A 1-year course of treatment is recommended in patients who show resolution of clinical findings

Table 24.6   Outcome of Antifungal Therapy for Disseminated Histoplasmosis

Treatment (Reference No.)	No. of Patients	Response (%)	Deaths (%)	Relapse (%)
Amphotericin B (115)	22	68	23	9
Amphotericin B (13)	43	74	16	7
Amphotericin B (135)	17	76	23	
Amphotericin B (136)	24	91	8	20
Amphotericin B (20,23)	73*	88	12	19
Itraconazole (117)	10	100		
Itraconazole (97,98,100)	59*	85		5
Ketoconazole (118)	31	56		10
Ketoconazole (119)	10	70		40
Ketoconazole (20)	11*	9		50
Fluconazole (99)	49*	74	2	31
Fluconazole (120)	14	86	7	14

*These studies were performed with AIDS patients. Relapses occurred in those who responded to induction treatment and in those who were advised to continue the medication chronically for lifelong maintenance therapy.

and clearance of antigen from urine and blood; however, a shorter course has been effective in some studies (117). Lifelong therapy is recommended in patients with AIDS (*see* section on Maintenance Therapy below).

Amphotericin B (or one of its newer lipid formulations in patients at risk for or who have significant renal impairment) is the recommended antifungal agent for patients who are sufficiently ill to require hospitalization. Amphotericin B should be administered at a dosage of 0.7–1.0 mg/kg/d, whereas the lipid formulations (Amphotec, Abelcet, and AmBisome) require higher dosages of 3 mg/kg/d. In a recent study, outcome was better in patients with AIDS and progressive disseminated histoplasmosis who were given liposomal amphotericin B (AmBisone) than in those given the deoxycholate formulations (124a). Most patients respond within 1 week and then can be treated with itraconazole. If amphotericin B is to be used for the full course of treatment, the total dose should be 35 mg/kg (100–120 mg/kg for the lipid preparations).

The outcome of treatment for endocarditis is unsatisfactory (73,74,83, 123,124). Aggressive antifungal therapy combined with resection of the infected valve provides the best outcome (in one series, 5 of 7 patients survived [83]). Amphotericin B in a dose of 35 mg/kg given over 2 to 3 months is recommended, and resection of the infected valve should be strongly considered. An additional year of treatment with itraconazole at 200 mg once or twice daily may reduce the likelihood of relapse.

Histoplasmosis of the Central Nervous System

The outcome of treatment in patients with *Histoplasma* meningitis is often is poor, justifying an aggressive approach to achieve the highest possible success. Although 60% to 80% of patients with meningitis responded to amphotericin B in one study, up to half relapsed during the next few years (63). Amphotericin B in a dose of 35 mg/kg over a period of 2 to 4 months is the regimen most commonly recommended. AmBisome achieves higher concentrations in the blood and brain than do amphotericin B and its other lipid formulations (125), providing a theoretical rationale for its use in *Histoplasma* meningitis. Furthermore, AmBisome sterilized the CSF more rapidly than did amphotericin B in patients with cryptococcal meningitis (126). Nevertheless, none of these preparations reach detectable concentrations in CSF (125–127).

To prevent relapse, administering fluconazole 800 mg/d or itraconazole 200 mg twice daily for another year should be considered. Fluconazole achieves excellent concentrations in CSF (128). Resistance to fluconazole can develop during therapy (99,129), necessitating careful follow-up of CSF findings (including culture and antigen detection). Although it is more active than fluconazole against *H. capsulatum*, itraconazole does not enter the CSF (130). Nevertheless, itraconazole has been useful for the treatment of meningitis caused by other fungi and for *Histoplasma* meningitis, using an intracranial model of experimental histoplasmosis (Wheat, unpublished data). Blood concentrations of drug and hepatic enzymes and bilirubin should be monitored in patients receiving such high doses of fluconazole. Lifelong maintenance therapy with fluconazole or itraconazole may be needed in patients who relapse after completing appropriate treatment. Relapse despite chronic maintenance therapy or failure to respond to therapy may mandate administration of amphotericin B directly into the ventricles, cisterna magnum, or lumbar arachnoid space. However, experience with intrathecal or intraventricular therapy is not encouraging (63).

Cerebritis or cerebral histoplasmomas in the absence of meningitis may be more responsive to antifungal therapy (63). Parenchymal lesions rarely require surgical excision (63). AmBisome and amphotericin B are reasonable choices for the initial treatment of such disease. Penetration of the CSF may not be required for successful therapy of parenchymal lesions; therefore, itraconazole 200 mg two or three times daily may be appropriate after patients have improved in response to amphotericin B. However, because experience with itraconazole for this indication is lacking, such cases should be monitored closely and treatment should be changed if there is clinical or radiographic evidence of disease progression.

Maintenance Treatment

Relapse of histoplasmosis is a serious problem in patients with AIDS and may occur in patients with other immunosuppressive conditions (13) or even in those without clinically apparent immune defects (131), thus necessitating chronic antifungal maintenance therapy (20). Amphotericin B given in a dosage of 50 mg weekly or biweekly is highly effective (response rate 81%–97%) but inconvenient and poorly tolerated (20,132). Itraconazole 200 mg once or twice daily is effective in at least 90% of cases (95,96) but may not be possible because of drug interaction or the inability to achieve therapeutic serum levels. Fluconazole also has been used for maintenance therapy but with less success; in one study, relapse occurred in nearly one third of patients who received fluconazole 400 mg/d (99). Thus, fluconazole should be reserved for patients who cannot take itraconazole. In patients with AIDS who have achieved a good virologic and immunologic response (CD4 count >150 cells/µL) to potent antiretroviral therapy, lifelong maintenance therapy may not be essential—a hypothesis that is to be tested in a prospective trial in development.

Prophylaxis Against Histoplasmosis in AIDS

Prophylaxis warrants consideration in patients with CD4 counts below 100 cells/µL in areas with rates of histoplasmosis above 5 cases per 100 patient-years. In a study of persons with CD4 counts below 150 cells/µL, itraconazole at 200 mg/d reduced the incidence of histoplasmosis from 6.8% (placebo group) to 2.7% (133).

Acknowledgements

Thanks to Mr. Kian Karimi for his critical review of the manuscript for this chapter. This work was supported by the Department of Veterans' Affairs and the AIDS Clinical Trials Group (A125859).

REFERENCES

1. **Christie A, Peterson JC.** Pulmonary calcification in negative reactors to tuberculin. *Am J Public Health.* 1945;35:1131–47.

2. **Palmer CE.** Nontuberculous pulmonary calcification and sensitivity to histoplasmin. *Public Health Rep.* 1945;60:513–20.

3. **Edwards LB, Acquaviva FA, Livesay VT, et al.** An atlas of sensitivity to tuberculin, PPD-B, and histoplasmin in the United States. *Am Rev Respir Dis.* 1969;99:1–18.

4. **Emmons CW.** Isolation of *Histoplasma capsulatum* from soil. *Am J Public Health.* 1949; 64:892–6.

5. **Zeidberg LD, Ajello L, Dillon A, Runyon LC.** Isolation of *Histoplasma capsulatum* from soil. *Am J Public Health.* 1952;42:930–5.

6. **Tosh FE, Doto IL, D'Alessio DJ, Medeiros AA, et al.** The second of two epidemics of histoplasmosis resulting from work on the same starling roost. *Am Rev Respir Dis.* 1966;406–13.

7. **Waldman RJ, England AC, Tauxe R, et al.** A winter outbreak of acute histoplasmosis in northern Michigan. *Am J Epidemiol.* 1983;117:68–75.

8. **Brodsky AL, Gregg MB, Kaufman L, Mallison GF.** Outbreak of histoplasmosis associated with the 1970 Earth Day activities. *Am J Med.* 1973;54:333–42.

9. **Deepe GS Jr, Bullock WE.** Histoplasmosis: a granulomatous inflammatory response. In Gallin JI, Goldstein IM, Snyderman R (eds). *Inflammation: Basic Principles and Clinical Correlates.* New York: Raven; 1988:733–49.

10. **Zhou P, Sieve MC, Tewari RP, Seder RA.** Interleukin-12 modulates the protective immune response in SCID mice infected with *Histoplasma capsulatum. Infect Immun.* 1997;65:936–42.

11. **Wu-Hsieh BA, Lee GS, Franco M, Hofman FM.** Early activation of splenic macrophages by tumor necrosis factor–alpha is important in determining the outcome of experimental histoplasmosis in mice. *Infect Immun.* 1992;60:4230–8.

12. **Goodwin RA Jr, Shapiro JL, Thurman GH, et al.** Disseminated histoplasmosis: clinical and pathologic correlations. *Medicine.* 1980;59:1–33.

13. **Sathapatayavongs B, Batteiger BE, Wheat LJ, et al.** Clinical and laboratory features of disseminated histoplasmosis during two large urban outbreaks. *Medicine.* 1983;62:263–70.

14. **Wheat LJ, Slama TG, Norton JA, et al.** Risk factors for disseminated or fatal histoplasmosis. *Ann Intern Med.* 1982;96:159–63.

15. **Goodwin RA Jr, des Prez RM.** Histoplasmosis. *Am Rev Respir Dis.* 1978;117:929–56.

16. **Goodwin RA, Loyd JE, des Prez RM.** Histoplasmosis in normal hosts. *Medicine.* 1981;60:231–66.

17. **Goodwin RA Jr, Owens FT, Snell JD, et al.** Chronic pulmonary histoplasmosis. *Medicine.* 1976;55:413–52.

18. **Wheat LJ, Wass J, Norton J, et al.** Cavitary histoplasmosis occurring during two large urban outbreaks: analysis of clinical, epidemiologic, roentgenographic, and laboratory features. *Medicine.* 1984;63:201–9.

19. **Davies SF, Khan M, Sarosi GA.** Disseminated histoplasmosis in immunologically suppressed patients. *Am J Med.* 1978;64:94–100.

20. **Wheat LJ, Connolly-Stringfield PA, Baker RL, et al.** Disseminated histoplasmosis in the acquired immune deficiency syndrome: clinical findings, diagnosis and treatment, and review of the literature. *Medicine.* 1990;69:361–374.

21. **Keath EJ, Kobayashi GS, Medoff G.** Typing of *Histoplasma capsulatum* by restriction fragment length polymorphisms in a nuclear gene. *J Clin Microbiol.* 1992;30:2104–7.

22. **Wheat LJ, Smith EJ, Sathapatayavongs B, et al.** Histoplasmosis in renal allograft recipients: two large urban outbreaks. *Arch Intern Med.* 1983;143:703–7.

23. **Wheat L.** Histoplasmosis in the acquired immunodeficiency syndrome. *Curr Top Med Mycol.* 1996;7:7–18.

24. **Goodwin RA, Nickell JA, des Prez RM.** Mediastinal fibrosis complicating healed primary histoplasmosis and tuberculosis. *Medicine.* 1972;51:227–46.

25. **Loyd JE, Tillman BF, Atkinson JB, des Prez RM.** Mediastinal fibrosis complicating histoplasmosis. *Medicine.* 1988;67:295–310.

26. **Wheat LJ, French MLV, Wass JL.** Sarcoidlike manifestations of histoplasmosis. *Arch Intern Med.* 1989;149:2421–26.

27. **Wheat LJ.** Diagnosis and management of histoplasmosis. *Eur J Clin Microbiol Infect Dis.* 1989;8:480–90.

28. **Wheat J.** Histoplasmosis: experience during outbreaks in Indianapolis and review of the literature. *Medicine.* 1997;76:339–54.

29. **Wheat LJ, Slama TG, Eitzen HE, et al.** A large urban outbreak of histoplasmosis: clinical features. *Ann Intern Med.* 1981;94:331–7.

30. **Anderson NW, Doto IL, Furcolow ML.** Clinical, X-ray, and serologic changes with *Histoplasma* infection. *Public Health Rep.* 1958;73:73–82.

31. **Chick EW, Bauman DS.** Acute cavitary histoplasmosis: fact or fiction? *Chest.* 1974; 65:479–80.

32. **Connell JV Jr, Muhn JR.** Radiographic manifestations of pulmonary histoplasmosis: a 10-year review. *Radiology.* 1975;121:281–5.

33. **Quasney MW, Leggiadro RJ.** Pleural effusion associated with histoplasmosis. *Pediatr Infect Dis J.* 1993;12:416–8.

34. **Kataria YP, Campbell PB, Burlingham BT.** Acute pulmonary histoplasmosis presenting as adult respiratory distress syndrome: effect of therapy on clinical and laboratory features. *South Med J.* 1981;74:534–7.

35. **Rubin H, Furcolow ML, Yates JL, Brasher CA.** The course and prognosis of histoplasmosis. *Am J Med.* 1959;27:278–88.

36. **Paya CV, Roberts GD, Cockerill FRI.** Transient fungemia in acute pulmonary histo-plasmosis: detection by new blood-culturing techniques. *J Infect Dis.* 1987;156:313–5.

37. **Coss KC, Wheat LJ, Conces DJ Jr, et al.** Esophageal fistula complicating mediastinal histoplasmosis: response to amphotericin B. *Am J Med.* 1987;83:343–6.

38. **Schowengerdt CG, Suyemoto R, Beachley F.** Granulomatous and fibrous medias-tinitis. *J Thorac Cardiovasc Surg.* 1969;57:365–79.

39. **Rabinowitz JG, Prater W, Silver J, et al.** Mediastinal histoplasmosis. *Mt Sinai J Med.* 1980;47:356–63.

40. **Garrett HE Jr, Roper CL.** Surgical intervention in histoplasmosis. *Ann Thorac Surg.* 1986;42:711–722.

41. **Savides TJ, Gress FG, Wheat LJ, et al.** Dysphagia due to mediastinal granulomas: diagnosis with endoscopic ultrasonography. *Gastroenterology.* 1995;109:366–73.

42. **Sakulsky SB, Harrison EG, Dines DE, Payne WS.** Mediastinal granuloma. *J Thorac Cardiovasc Surg.* 1967;54:280–90.

43. **Lee JH, Neumann DA, Welsh JD.** Disseminated histoplasmosis presenting with esophageal symptomatology. *Dig Dis.* 1977;22:831–4.

44. **Forsmark CE, Wilcox CM, Darragh TM, Cello JP.** Disseminated histoplasmosis in AIDS: an unusual case of esophageal involvement and gastrointestinal bleeding. *Gastrointest Endosc.* 1990;36:604–5.

45. **Kunkel WM Jr, Clagett OT, McDonald JR.** Mediastinal granulomas. *J Thorac Surg.* 1954;27:565–74.

46. **Landay MJ, Rollins NK.** Mediastinal histoplasmosis granuloma: evaluation with CT. *Radiology.* 1989;172:657–9.

47. **Lerner MH, Deluca SA.** Mediastinal granuloma secondary to histoplasmosis. *Am Fam Physician.* 1991;43:1649–51.

48. **Picardi JL, Kauffman CA, Schwarz J, et al.** Pericarditis caused by *Histoplasma capsu-latum. Am J Cardiol.* 1976;37:82–8.

49. **Wheat LJ, Stein L, Corya BC, et al.** Pericarditis as a manifestation of histoplasmosis during two large urban outbreaks. *Medicine.* 1983;62:110–19.

50. **Ozols II, Wheat LJ.** Erythema nodosum in an epidemic of histoplasmosis in Indi-anapolis. *Arch Dermatol.* 1981;117:709–12.

51. **Sellers TF Jr, Price WN Jr, Newberry WM Jr.** An epidemic of erythema multiforme and erythema nodosum caused by histoplasmosis. *Ann Intern Med.* 1965;62:1244–62.

52. **Arrigoni MG, Bernatz PE, Donoghue FE.** Broncholithiasis. *J Thorac Cardiovasc Surg.* 1971;62:231–7.

53. **Schwarz J, Silverman FN, Adriano SM, et al.** The relationship of splenic calcifica-tion to histoplasmosis. *N Engl J Med.* 1955;252:887–91.

54. **Smith DK, Neal JJ, Holmberg SD, The Centers for Disease Control Idiopathic CD4+ T-Lymphocytopenia Task Force.** Unexplained opportunistic infections and CD4+ T lymphocytopenia without HIV infection. *N Engl J Med.* 1993;328:374–9.

55. **Schneider RP, Edwards W.** Histoplasmosis presenting as an esophageal tumor. *Gastrointest Endosc.* 1977;23:158–9.

56. **Cimponeriu D, LoPresti P, Lavelanet M, et al.** Gastrointestinal histoplasmosis in HIV infection: two cases of colonic pseudocancer and review of the literature. *Am J Gastroenterol.* 1994;89:129–31.

57. **Lee KR, Lin F.** The radiology corner: gastrointestinal histoplasmosis, roentgenographic, clinical, and pathological correlation. *Am J Gastroenterol.* 1975;63:255–65.

58. **Lee SH, Barnes WG, Hodges GR, Dixon A.** Perforated granulomatous colitis caused by *Histoplasma capsulatum. Dis Colon Rect.* 1985;28:171–6.

59. **Morrison YY, Rathbun RC, Huycke MM.** Disseminated histoplasmosis mimicking Crohn's disease in a patient with the acquired immunodeficiency syndrome. *Am J Gastroenterol.* 1994;89:1255–7.

60. **Hazelhurst JA, Vismer HF.** Histoplasmosis presenting with unusual skin lesions in acquired immunodeficiency syndrome (AIDS). *BMJ.* 1985;II3:345–8.

61. **Barton EN, Roberts L, Ince WE, et al.** Cutaneous histoplasmosis in the acquired immune deficiency syndrome: a report of three cases from Trinidad. *Trop Geogr Med.* 1988;40:153–7.

62. **Cott GR, Smith TW, Hinthorn DR, Liu C.** Primary cutaneous histoplasmosis in immunosuppressed patients. *JAMA.* 1979;242:456–7.

63. **Wheat LJ, Batteiger BE, Sathapatayavongs B.** *Histoplasma capsulatum* infections of the central nervous system: a clinical review. *Medicine.* 1990;69:244–60.

64. **Bazan CI, New PZ.** Intramedullary spinal histoplasmosis efficacy of gadolinium enhancement. *Neuroradiology.* 1991;33:190.

65. **Livas IC, Nechay PS, Nauseef WM.** Clinical evidence of spinal and cerebral histoplasmosis 20 years after renal transplantation. *Clin Infect Dis.* 1995;20:692–5.

66. **Corcoran GR, Al-Abdely H, Flanders CD, et al.** Markedly elevated serum lactate dehydrogenase levels are a clue to the diagnosis of disseminated histoplasmosis in patients with AIDS. *Clin Infect Dis.* 1997;24:942–4.

67. **Conces DJ Jr, Stockberger SM, Tarver RD, Wheat LJ.** Disseminated histoplasmosis in AIDS: findings on chest radiographs. *Am J Roentgenol.* 1993;160:15–9.

68. **Walker JV, Baran D, Yakub N, Freeman RB.** Histoplasmosis with hypercalcemia, renal failure, and papillary necrosis: confusion with sarcoidosis. *JAMA.* 1977;237: 1350–2.

69. **Murray JJ, Heim CR.** Hypercalcemia in disseminated histoplasmosis: aggravative by vitamin D. *Am J Med.* 1985;78:881–4.

70. **Macher A, Rodrigues MM, Kaplan W, et al.** Disseminated bilateral chorioretinitis due to *Histoplasma capsulatum* in a patient with the acquired immunodeficiency syndrome. *Ophthalmology.* 1985;92:1159–64.

71. **Kilburn CD, McKinsey DS.** Recurrent massive pleural effusion due to pleural, pericardial, and epicardial fibrosis in histoplasmosis. *Chest.* 1991;100:1715–7.

72. **Young EJ, Vainrub B, Musher DM.** Pericarditis due to histoplasmosis. *JAMA.* 1978;240:1750–1.

73. **Gaynes RP, Gardner P, Causey W.** Prosthetic valve endocarditis caused by *Histoplasma capsulatum. Arch Intern Med.* 1981;141:1533–7.

74. **Rogers EW, Weyman AE, Noble RJ, Bruins SC.** Left atrial myxoma infected with *Histoplasma capsulatum. Am J Med.* 1978;64:683–90.

75. **Reddy PA, Brasher CA, Christianson C, Gorelick DF.** Peritonitis due to histoplasmosis. *Ann Intern Med.* 1969;72:79–81.

76. **Patrick CC, Flynn PM, Henwick S, Pui CH.** Disseminated histoplasmosis presenting as a cystic duct obstruction. *Pediatr Infect Dis J.* 1992;11:593–4.

77. **Zighelboim J, Goldfarb RA, Mody D, et al.** Prostatic abscess due to *Histoplasma capsulatum* in a patient with the acquired immunodeficiency syndrome. *J Urol.* 1992; 147:167–8.

78. **Pottage JC Jr, Trenholme GM, Aronson IK, Harris AA.** Panniculitis associated with histoplasmosis and alpha-1-antitrypsin deficiency. *Am J Med.* 1983;75:150–3.

79. **Osborne BM.** Granulomatous mastitis caused by *Histoplasma* and mimicking inflammatory breast carcinoma. *Hum Pathol.* 1989;20:47–52.

80. **Kauffman CA, Slama TG, Wheat LJ.** *Histoplasma capsulatum* epididymitis. *J Urol.* 1980;125:434–5.

81. **Sills M, Schwartz A, Weg JG.** Conjugal histoplasmosis: a consequence of progressive dissemination in the index case after steroid therapy. *Ann Intern Med.* 1973;79:221–4.

82. **Jayalakshmi P, Goh KL, Soo-Hoo TS, Daud A.** Disseminated histoplasmosis presenting as penile ulcer. *Aust NZ J Med.* 1990;20:175–6.

83. **Kanawaty DS, Stalker MJB, Munt PW.** Nonsurgical treatment of *Histoplasma* endocarditis involving a bioprosthetic valve. *Chest.* 1991;99:253–6.

84. **Woods AC, Wahlen HE.** The probable role of benign histoplasmosis in the etiology of granulomatous uveitis. *Am Heart J.* 1960;49:205–20.

85. **Schwarz J.** Histoplasmosis of the Eye. In *Histoplasmosis.* New York: Praeger; 1981: 317–50.

86. **Spaeth GL.** Presumed *Histoplasma* uveitis: continuing doubts as to its actual cause. In Ajello AP, Chick EM, Furcolow MMS (eds). *Histoplasmosis.* Springfield, IL: Charles C. Thomas; 1971:221–30.

87. **Specht CS, Mitchell KT, Bauman AE, Gupta M.** Ocular histoplasmosis with retinitis in a patient with acquired immune deficiency syndrome. *Ophthalmology.* 1991;98: 1356–9.

88. **Ryder KW, Jay SJ, Kiblawi SO, Hull MT.** Serum angiotensin converting enzyme activity in patients with histoplasmosis. *JAMA.* 1983;249:1888–9.

89. **Williams B, Fojtasek M, Connolly-Stringfield P, Wheat J.** Diagnosis of histoplasmosis by antigen detection during an outbreak in Indianapolis, Indiana. *Arch Pathol Lab Med.* 1994;118:1205–8.

90. **Wheat LJ, French MLV, Kohler RB, et al.** The diagnostic laboratory tests for histoplasmosis: analysis of experience in a large urban outbreak. *Ann Intern Med.* 1982; 97:680–5.

91. **Wheat LJ, Kohler RB, Tewari RP.** Diagnosis of disseminated histoplasmosis by detection of *Histoplasma capsulatum* antigen in serum and urine specimens. *N Engl J Med.* 1986;314:83–8.

92. **Kurtin PJ, McKinsey DS, Gupta MR, Driks M.** Histoplasmosis in patients with acquired immunodeficiency syndrome: hematologic and bone marrow manifestations. *Am J Clin Pathol.* 1990;93:367–72.

93. **Wheat LJ, Kohler RB, Tewari RP, et al.** Significance of *Histoplasma* antigen in the cerebrospinal fluid of patients with meningitis. *Arch Intern Med.* 1989;149:302–4.

94. **Wheat J, Wheat H, Connolly P, et al.** Cross-reactivity in *Histoplasma capsulatum* variety capsulatum antigen assays of urine samples from patients with endemic mycoses. *Clin Infect Dis.* 1997;24:1169–71.

95. **Wheat LJ, Connolly-Stringfield P, Blair R, et al.** Histoplasmosis relapse in patients with AIDS: detection using *Histoplasma capsulatum* variety capsulatum antigen levels. *Ann Intern Med.* 1991;115:936–41.

96. **Wheat LJ, Connolly-Stringfield P, Blair R, et al.** Effect of successful treatment with amphotericin B on *Histoplasma capsulatum* variety capsulatum polysaccharide antigen levels in patients with AIDS and histoplasmosis. *Am J Med.* 1992;92:153–60.

97. **Wheat J, Hafner R, Wulfson M, et al., and the NIAID Clinical Trials & Mycoses Study Group Collaborators.** Prevention of relapse of histoplasmosis with itraconazole in patients with the acquired immunodeficiency syndrome. *Ann Intern Med.* 1993;118:610–6.

98. **Hecht FM, Wheat J, Korzun AH, et al.** Itraconazole maintenance treatment for histoplasmosis in AIDS: a prospective, multicenter trial. *J Acquir Immune Defic Syndr Hum Retrovirol.* 1997;16:100–7.

99. **Wheat J, MaWhinney S, Hafner R, et al.** Treatment of histoplasmosis with fluconazole in patients with acquired immunodeficiency syndrome. *Am J Med.* 1997;103: 223–32.

100. **Wheat J, Hafner R, Korzun AH, et al., and the AIDS Clinical Trial Group.** Itraconazole treatment of disseminated histoplasmosis in patients with the acquired immunodeficiency syndrome. *Am J Med.* 1995;98:336–42.

101. **Wheat LJ.** Histoplasmosis. *Infect Dis Clin North Am.* 1988;2:841–59.

102. **Zeidberg LD, Dillon A, Gass RS.** Some factors in the epidemiology of histoplasmin sensitivity in Williamson County, Tennessee. *Am J Public Health.* 1951;41:80–9.

103. **Kaufman L, Terry RT, Schubert JH, McLaughlin D.** Effects of a single histoplasmin skin test on the serological diagnosis of histoplasmosis. *J Bacteriol.* 1967;94: 798–803.

104. **Prior JA, Saslaw S, Cole CR.** Experiences with histoplasmosis. *Ann Intern Med.* 1954;40:221–44.

105. **Wynne JW, Olsen GN.** Acute histoplasmosis presenting as the adult respiratory distress syndrome. *Chest.* 1974;66:158–61.

106. **Medeiros AA, Marty SD, Tosh FE, Chin TDY.** Erythema nodosum and erythema multiforme as clinical manifestations of histoplasmosis in a community outbreak. *N Engl J Med.* 1966;274:415–20.

107. **Rosenthal J, Brandt KD, Wheat LJ, Slama TG.** Rheumatologic manifestations of histoplasmosis in the recent Indianapolis epidemic. *Arthritis Rheum.* 1983;26:1065–70.

108. **Jones PG, Rolston K, Hopfer RL.** Septic arthritis due to *Histoplasma capsulatum* in a leukemic patient. *Ann Rheum Dis.* 1985;44:128–9.

109. **Greenwood MF, Holland P.** Tracheal obstruction secondary to *Histoplasma* mediastinal granuloma. *Chest.* 1972;62:642–5.

110. **Gilliland MD, Scott LD, Walker WE.** Esophageal obstruction caused by mediastinal histoplasmosis: beneficial results of operation. *Surgery.* 1984;95:59–62.

111. **Woods LP.** Mediastinal *Histoplasma* granuloma causing tracheal compression in a 4-year-old child. *Surgery.* 1965;58:448–52.

112. **Dines DE, Payne WS, Bernatz PE, Pairolero PC.** Mediastinal granuloma and fibrosing mediastinitis. *Chest.* 1979;75:320–4.

113. **Parker JD, Sarosi GA, Doto IL, et al.** Treatment of chronic pulmonary histoplasmosis. *N Engl J Med.* 1970;283:225–9.

114. **Sutliff WD, Andrews CE, Jones E, Terry RT.** Histoplasmosis cooperative study: Veterans Administration–Armed Forces Cooperative study on histoplasmosis. *Am Rev Respir Dis.* 1964;89:641–50.

115. **Furcolow ML.** Comparison of treated and untreated severe histoplasmosis. *JAMA.* 1963;183:121–7.

116. **Putnam LR, Sutliff WD, Larkin JC, et al.** Histoplasmosis cooperative study: chronic pulmonary histoplasmosis treated with amphotericin B alone and with amphotericin B and triple sulfonamide. *Am Rev Respir Dis.* 1968;97:96–102.

117. **Dismukes WE, Bradsher RW Jr, Cloud GC, et al. and the NIAID Mycoses Study Group.** Itraconazole therapy for blastomycosis and histoplasmosis. *Am J Med.* 1992;93:489–97.

118. **Dismukes WE, Cloud G, Bowles C, et al.** Treatment of blastomycosis and histoplasmosis with ketoconazole: results of a prospective randomized clinical trial. *Ann Intern Med.* 1985;103:861–72.

119. **Slama TG.** Treatment of disseminated and progressive cavitary histoplasmosis with ketoconazole. *Am J Med.* 1983;70–3.

120. **McKinsey DS, Kauffman CA, Pappas PG, et al.** Fluconazole therapy for histoplasmosis. *Clin Infect Dis.* 1996;23:996–1001.

121. **Urschel HC Jr, Razzuk MA, Netto GJ, et al.** Sclerosing mediastinitis: improved management with histoplasmosis titer and ketoconazole. *Ann Thorac Surg.* 1990;50:215–21.

122. **Mathisen DJ, Grillo HC.** Clinical manifestations of mediastinal fibrosis and histoplasmosis. *Ann Thorac Surg.* 1992;54:1053–8.

123. **Blair TP, Waugh RA, Pollack M, et al.** *Histoplasma capsulatum* endocarditis. *Am Heart J.* 1980;99:783–8.

124. **Berman SS, Kazlow GA, Fields BT Jr, Weinberg S.** Disseminated histoplasmosis with embolic endovascular complications: a case report. *J Vasc Surg.* 1990;12:577–80.

124a. **Wheat LJ, et al.** *Antimicrob Agents Chemother.* 2001;45:2354–7.

125. **Groll A, Giri N, Gonzalez C, et al.** *Penetration of lipid formulations of amphotericin B into cerebrospinal fluid and brain tissue.* Paper Presented at the 97th International Conference on Antimicrobial Agents and Chemotherapy, Toronto, Ontario,1997;A-90:19.

126. **Leenders A, Reiss P, Portegies P, et al.** Liposomal amphotericin B (AmBisome) compared with amphotericin B both followed by oral fluconazole in the treatment of AIDS-associated cryptococcal meningitis. *AIDS.* 1997;11:1463–71.

127. **Dugoni B, Guglielmo BJ, Hollander H.** Amphotericin B concentration in cerebrospinal fluid of patients with AIDS and cryptococcal meningitis. *Clin Pharm.* 1989;8:220–1.

128. **Tucker RM, Williams PL, Arathoon EG, et al.** Pharmacokinetics of fluconazole in cerebrospinal fluid and serum in human coccidioidal meningitis. *Antimicrob Agents Chemother.* 1988;32:369–73.

129. **Wheat J, Marichal P, Vanden Bossche H, et al.** Hypothesis on the mechanism of resistance to fluconazole in *Histoplasma capsulatum. Antimicrob Agents Chemother.* 1997;41:410–4.

130. **de Gans J, Portegies P, Tiessens G, et al.** Itraconazole compared with amphotericin B plus flucytosine in AIDS patients with cryptococcal meningitis. *AIDS.* 1992;6:185–190.

131. **Paya CV, Hermans PE, van Scoy RE, et al.** Repeatedly relapsing disseminated histoplasmosis: clinical observations during long-term follow-up. *J Infect Dis.* 1987;156:308–12.

132. **McKinsey DS, Gupta MR, Riddler SA, et al.** Long-term amphotericin B therapy for disseminated histoplasmosis in patients with the acquired immune deficiency syndrome. *Ann Intern Med.* 1989;111:655–9.

133. **McKinsey D, Wheat J, Cloud G, et al.** *Itraconazole is effective primary prophylaxis against systemic fungal infections in patients with advanced HIV infection.* Paper presented at the 36th International Conference on Antimicrobial Agents and Chemotherapy, New Orleans, Louisiana, 1996;LB9:9.

25

Blastomycosis

Burton C. West, MD

Epidemiology and Etiology

Blastomycosis is a sporadic deep fungal infection in humans that is caused by
the organism *Blastomyces dermatitidis*. It is diagnosed principally in the United
States, occurring infrequently in Latin America, southern Canada, and Africa
and rarely elsewhere. Some cases outside of North America and Africa involve individuals who have visited an area endemic for the disease; however,
there are some cases in which the subject has never traveled.

In the United States, blastomycosis is distributed mainly in the Midwest
and South often in association with river valleys, especially the Mississippi
and the Ohio rivers and their tributaries. Generally, it is seen in residents
from the shores of the Great Lakes to the Gulf of Mexico. Although most
cases occur to the east of the central areas of Oklahoma and Texas and west
of the Appalachian mountains, U.S. citizens have become infected from
prairie dogs as far west as Colorado and from unknown sources in California.
Furthermore, endemic acquisition of blastomycosis has occurred as far east as
Virginia, the Carolinas, and Florida. Interestingly, virtually all cases of the disease in Arkansas occur south of a diagonal line drawn in a northeasterly direction from Texarkana to the Missouri "boot." The terrain south of this line
is a coastal plain with pinewoods and farms, whereas the land north of the
line consists of the hardwood-forested Ozark mountains where there have
been almost no cases (1) (Abernathy RS, personal communication).

Infectious disease specialists in the areas endemic for blastomycosis accumulate experience through many cases, although rarely more than 30 in a lifetime of practice (2). When a case occurs outside of an endemic area, its notoriety often gains it a place in the major medical literature; thus, a case of pulmonary blastomycosis that was diagnosed at a Boston hospital was reported in the *New England Journal of Medicine* (3).

Although not a zoonosis, blastomycosis is a well-known canine infection and is occasionally found in other domestic and wild mammals, yet dog owners do not seem to acquire the disease from their animals.

Occupation is a risk factor. There is limited evidence that *B. dermatitidis* comes from trees or tree products or perhaps soil, which would explain the association between the infection and people employed in the timber or lumber industries, farming, and other outdoor occupations. Loggers, timber men, sawmill workers, farmers, and laborers are at increased risk. Small clusters of cases of blastomycosis from a circumscribed geographic area suggest a common point source for human inhalation and subsequent infection with the yeast (4,5); however, despite many efforts to identify the organism in nature, only a few researchers have recovered it (6). Even then, culturing the relevant soil or wood at a later date usually fails to yield positive results. Thus, a reservoir of *B. dermatitidis* remains unproven but strongly inferred. A vector, if any, is unknown and unsuspected. Inhalation of yeast leads to infection but, as in primary tuberculosis, probably not in everyone. The yeast has not been recovered from the air or consistently from any environmental source, yet it is known to be present in the air and environment, at least periodically.

Natural History and Clinical Manifestations

Parallels between tuberculosis and deep fungal infections are numerous, and blastomycosis is no exception. *B. dermatitidis* is normally inhaled, causing a pulmonary infection that may not be symptomatic and that may not progress. A classic presentation of blastomycosis (and other deep fungal infections) is a somewhat indolent pneumonia that neither responds to antibacterial therapy nor proves to be tuberculosis (i.e., a nonresolving, nontuberculous pulmonary infiltrate). From a primary pulmonary infection, the yeast may disseminate to the rest of the body and cause a progressive primary or even miliary blastomycosis. As with primary pulmonary tuberculosis, the more typical clinical manifestation of blastomycosis is a mildly symptomatic fungemia that occurs with seeding of tissues that only later, under the influence of unknown stimuli, become active as sites of infection. Although a long dormancy period for such disseminated fungi is not well established in blastomycosis, it does offer a reasonable explanation for the range of presentations encountered clinically.

In addition to pulmonary infections, which themselves may be gradually progressive, without evidence of disease elsewhere, dissemination may occur without evidence of a primary pulmonary infection or may be combined with an active pneumonia.

Cavitation can occur, and blastomycosis can coexist with tuberculosis or cryptococcosis, making the second major infectious diagnosis difficult. Other sites in the respiratory tract that have been infected include the pharynx, larynx, and pleura. The larynx is a particularly noteworthy site for chronic granulomatous inflammation. *B. dermatitidis* can cause a lesion that appears grossly identical to carcinoma of the larynx. In at least one tragic case, a well-intentioned otolaryngologist performed a radical laryngectomy without waiting for a histology report. When the biopsy specimen was examined, it exhibited an infection with *B. dermatitidis*.

Another infection site in some patients is the throat. However, it is unclear if *B. dermatitidis* can be primarily inoculated into the throat by becoming directly embedded there during inhalation or if such infections actually follow lymphohematogenous dissemination from a primary infection of the lower respiratory tract. In any case, chronic pharyngeal lesions may appear with bleeding and irritation that suggest malignancy. It is not unusual for ear, nose, and throat surgeons who find such a suspicious lesion to make the diagnosis with a surgical biopsy and only then conclude that blastomycosis is the cause of chronic pharyngitis or a chronic pharyngeal lesion. The organism also has been known to involve the ears, sinuses, and mouth; however, this is distinctly rare (7).

During the dissemination of *B. dermatitidis* from the lung, the sites most often infected clinically are the skin and the bones, particularly the long bones. Skin lesions seem to be of two types, but the distinction is difficult. The first type consists of deep, nodular skin lesions that range from a few millimeters to 2 cm across, are tan or brown, and are asymptomatic until they break down. These lesions are often multiple and are in different stages at the time of clinical presentation but generally reflect a crop of hematogenously disseminated lesions. The second kind of lesion is clearly related to a deep-seated infection, most often proven to have its origin in the underlying bones that harbor osteomyelitis caused by *B. dermatitidis*. The infection drains very gradually to the surface, causing ulcerated, indolent, "angry-looking" lesions that may cover from 10 to 300 cm^2 of skin and drain pus at a slow rate but that are not highly symptomatic. This latter feature often markedly delays the decision to seek medical care.

Blastomycotic osteomyelitis occurs in different bones, generally in proportion to the size of each. Consequently, the long bones are infected most frequently but probably not preferentially. The vertebrae, wrist, and ribs are occasionally infected as well. Osteomyelitis of the cranium actually may lyse many of the cranial bones and is usually associated with an indolent, slow drainage of pus into the scalp. One such case illustrates the perils of outpatient treatment of pneumonia. A young deliveryman was treated on an outpatient basis with oral penicillin for a mildly symptomatic but densely consolidated pneumonia. He did not return for adequate follow-up, but a radiograph taken 6 months later showed scarring and some resolution. Two and a half years later, the young man presented with a bulging, 3- by 5-cm abscess over the zygomatic arch. The aspirate of the abscess contained gross pus that teemed with *B. dermatitidis*. On further careful history, the patient was found to have multiple sinuses that drained indolently into his scalp that were hidden by an "afro" haircut. Although many of the flat cranial bones had been lysed by the infection, there was quite remarkably no evidence of meningitis. Treated with amphotericin B, the patient improved dramatically. In retrospect, he was determined to have had the inoculating blastomycotic pneumonia for 3 years before this devastating osteomyelitis.

Osteomyelitis caused by *B. dermatitidis* may be more common than the frequency with which it is diagnosed. A seemingly superficial, chronic, slowly draining, inflammatory, macular, irregular skin lesion actually indicates an underlying osteomyelitis. The fistulous connection to deeper structures is not obvious. Radiography of the underlying bone and identification of the organism in the drainage fluid should establish blastomycotic osteomyelitis rather easily. However, in cases without skin lesions, there may be swelling or tenderness over an infected bone. Such an example was the patient with the pharyngeal lesion discussed previously. That patient had a sore wrist that was tender and swollen. Radiography showed a lytic lesion in the head of the radius. Chest radiographs, originally determined to be normal, showed some minimal perihilar infiltrates. All of these findings were due to blastomycosis and resolved with a course of amphotericin B. The infiltrates and the lytic lesion provided a baseline against which to determine the success of therapy and for long-term follow-up. Resolution of such abnormalities may be needed to determine the duration of therapy.

In autopsy series of blastomycosis, the prostate was sometimes infected; clinically, this can be important. For example, a patient who presented with a lower urinary tract obstruction and in whom a Foley catheter was placed was given a diagnosis of a low-grade urinary tract infection, for which he received antimicrobial therapy. Although there was no diagnosis of prostatitis, the patient continued to have fever during a month of catheter drainage. As part of a reassessment, he underwent a rectal examination, at which time his prostate was found to be enlarged and slightly tender. No further evaluation was conducted, but within 24 hours the patient developed an acute fever and began having pulmonary symptoms. Within 1 week, he had a miliary pattern on his chest radiograph, was producing sputum, and had a high fever. Direct microscopic examination of the sputum revealed budding yeasts consistent with the size and morphology of *B. dermatitidis*. The yeasts were easy to find without any special stains, and the organism grew in quantity from the sputum. What clearly happened was that chronic blastomycosis was present in the prostate, accounting for the low-grade fever and some of the urinary tract abnormalities. It was not recognized, and yet turned out to be the source of a hematogenous or miliary dissemination of the organism from the prostate at the time the prostate was massaged during an examination. This was a dramatic and partly iatrogenic clinical event.

Joints, intra-abdominal organs, and the heart are rarely infected by *B. dermatitidis*. Nonetheless, the organism may cause septic arthritis, granulomatous hepatitis, infiltrative bowel disease, and clinical renal disease.

Infection of the central nervous system with *B. dermatitidis* consists of two forms: chronic meningitis and abscess. Blastomycotic meningitis is more difficult to diagnose than is tuberculous or coccidioidal meningitis, because the organism is not seen in the cerebrospinal fluid, and cultures are nearly always negative. Waiting to take the aggressive diagnostic step of performing a biopsy on the brain and meninges results in clinical disaster or death (8). Brain abscess should be diagnosed with neurosurgical biopsy or excision, and this approach is usually undertaken, because the indolent abscess acts like a slow-growing brain tumor. Once the abscess is imaged, the decision to operate is usually made easily. Treatment for blastomycosis of the central nervous system is with amphotericin B in both immunocompetent and immunocompromised patients.

Host Factors and Pathogenesis

As in other deep fungal infections in patients who are not known specifically to be immunocompromised, there is the clinical suspicion that a defect may exist in the host defenses of patients who develop blastomycosis. If such a defect exists, it is still undefined. Immunocompromised patients (e.g., those with transplants, myelosuppression, or AIDS) tend to have rapidly progressive blastomycosis that may manifest itself as a miliary infection or as adult respiratory distress syndrome and that may be rapidly fatal. Blastomycosis can be an index infection that converts HIV infection to AIDS, but this is an infrequent event. Other deep fungal infections have served this function far more often.

Little is known about fungal virulence factors, but an adhesin from *B. Dermatitidis* was recently shown to be responsible for the adherence of the organism to lung tissue, for its binding and entry into macrophages, and for its virulence (9).

Diagnosis

Because of the virtual worthlessness of skin and serologic tests for blastomycosis, these tools are useful neither for epidemiologic study nor for diagnosis of the disease. Microscopic visualization or culture of *B. dermatitidis* from human pus or tissues is needed for diagnosis. Blastomycosis is diagnosed infrequently and is probably underdiagnosed. Nevertheless, direct microscopic diagnosis and isolation of the yeast by culture are standard methods that are remarkably accurate, sensitive, and easy to perform. It is far more difficult to consider the diagnosis than it is to prove it once seriously considered. Therefore, understanding the range of its manifestations and having a high index of suspicion for blastomycosis when these manifestations are present is the first step in diagnosing the disease.

Except in its advanced stages, blastomycosis has an indolent or even quiescent appearance and is of relatively little concern to physicians occupied with acutely ill patients. Because the presentation is rarely the same in any two people, the diagnosis is not contemplated easily on the basis of a particular complaint or physical finding. Cases of extrapulmonary blastomycosis without skin lesions are difficult to diagnose, because sputum or tissue is normally required to find the organism or to obtain an adequate specimen for fungal culture.

Clinical Microbiology

Microscopic visualization or culture of *B. dermatitidis* establishes the diagnosis of blastomycosis by the direct examination of purulent material, sputum, or another body fluid that contains the organism. *B. dermatitidis* in pus can be observed directly without any staining; a saline wet mount with the right light can reveal the organisms almost as easily as stained purulence. However, virtually any stain that enhances the contrast of a fungal organism is useful. Among these are wet pus treated with potassium hydroxide or lactophenol blue and dried smears stained with Gram's stain, methylene blue, Wright's stain, or any other handy stain. Pap stains are quite effective in demonstrating the organism in sputum. Similarly, tissues may be stained with nearly any of these aforementioned stains. The classic fungal stains are the best, including Gomori's methenamine silver or periodic acid-Schiff stains.

Recognizing the morphology of the organism is more important than ordering the correct stain. The organism is 8 to 16 mm in diameter, generally round, and not encapsulated in the true sense (as are most *Cryptococcus neoformans*). The mother–daughter budding is broad based, in contrast with *C. neoformans*, which has narrow-based budding. With *B. dermatitidis*, the connection between the daughter and the mother cells encompasses almost the entire diameter of the daughter cell until separation occurs. Inoculation of specimens onto ordinary and fungal media usually results in growth in less than 1 week; but some strains take longer to grow. Currently, molecular nucleic acid probes are used to confirm culture isolates of *B. dermatitidis* rather than for the direct diagnosis of blastomycosis from body fluids or tissues.

Treatment

Amphotericin B remains the "gold standard" in the treatment of deep fungal infections, including blastomycosis. No prospective trials are available to support a recommendation for any of the newer formulations of amphotericin B; however, at great additional expense, the results obtained with these formulations are expected to be similar to that of amphotericin B. Of the organisms that cause deep fungal infections, *B. dermatitidis* is the most susceptible to amphotericin B; therefore, blastomycosis treatment usually does not require a dosage greater than 20–30 mg/d of amphotericin B. Amphotericin B should be diluted in ample 5% glucose-in-water, because mixing the colloidal suspension in a salt solution causes the colloidal particles to coalesce, essentially precipitating them. The usual 20–30-mg/d dosage of amphotericin B for blastomycosis is routinely diluted in 1 L of 5% dextrose in water and infused through a peripheral or central vein over a period of 4 hours. Two hours should be the minimum duration of an infusion, but most experienced clinicians prefer a 4-hour infusion. Amphotericin B is the treatment of choice for patients with *B. dermatitidis* meningitis, those with disseminated or extensive disease, and individuals who are immunocompromised (e.g., AIDS patients) (Table 25.1 and Fig. 25.1).

The dosing of amphotericin B may be based on one of three methods, each of which has an empirical rationale. The first is a regimen of 20–30 mg/d for most adult patients with blastomycosis, which is usually effective but results in conceptually less rigorous dosing, particularly for large or small patients.

The second dosing method is the total-dose regimen, which for many deep fungal infections is 2.5 g; however, it is generally lower for blastomycosis. with 1.5 g total dose usually being sufficient. Both methods may be combined to avoid excess daily dosing and its accompanying adverse effects and to avoid too short a course of treatment, which might result in treatment failure or relapse. A combined course of this type consists of amphotericin B 20–25 mg/d for 10 weeks.

The third method is applicable to all of the usual deep fungal infections, including blastomycosis, which are treated with approximately 0.5 mg/kg/d. Later in the course of therapy, usually after 1 to 3 weeks, a switch may be made to alternate-day therapy at twice the daily dose (i.e., up to 1 mg/kg),

Table 25.1   Guidelines for the Treatment of Various Forms of Blastomycosis*

Disease	Preferred Treatment	Alternative Treatment
Pulmonary		
Life threatening	Initiate amphotericin B at 20–30 mg per dose up to a total dose of 1.5 g	Initiate with amphotericin B and switch to itraconazole after the patient's condition has stabilized
Mild to moderate	Itraconazole 200–400 mg/d	Ketoconazole 400–800 mg/d or fluconazole 800 mg/d
Disseminated		
CNS	Initiate amphotericin B at 0.7–1.0 mg/kg/d up to a total dose of 2 g	For patients unable to tolerate a full course of amphotericin B, consider fluconazole 800 mg/d
Non-CNS		
Life threatening	As with disseminated CNS disease, but up to a total dose of 1.5–2.5 g	Initiate with amphotericin B and switch to itraconazole after patient has stabilized
Non–life threatening		Ketoconazole 400–800 mg/d or fluconazole 400–800 mg/d
Immunocompromised host*	Initiate amphotericin B at 0.7–1.0 mg/kg/d up to a total dose of 1.5–2.5 g; AIDS patients may need lifetime suppression with itraconazole 100–200 mg/d	After a primary course of amphotericin B, suppressive therapy should be continued with itraconazole 200–400 mg/kg/d; for patients with CNS disease or those who cannot tolerate itraconazole, consider fluconazole 800 mg/d
Special circumstance		
Pregnancy	≤50 mg/d of amphotericin B, up to total dose of 1.5–2.5 g	—
Pediatrics	≤30 mg/kg total dose of amphotericin B	Itraconazole 5–7 mg/kg/d

Modified from Chapman SW, Bradsher RW, Campbell GD Jr, et al. Practice guidelines for the management of patients with blastomycosis. *Clin Infect Dis.* 2000;30:679–683.
* Including AIDS patients.

which saves infusions, visits, and money (10). Many patients can be treated outside the hospital after being stabilized either with daily or alternate-day therapy. Alternate-day therapy works well, but its main drawback is that the higher dose on alternate days may take a greater toll from a higher likelihood

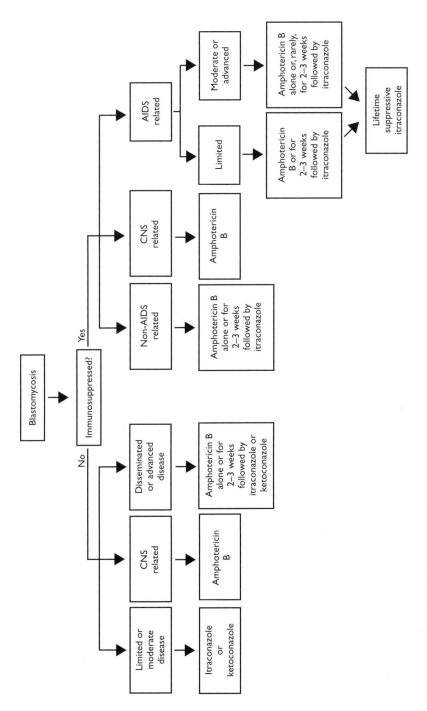

Figure 25.1 Algorithm for the treatment of blastomycosis.

of adverse effects than with the smaller daily dose and, consequently, from a loss of a sense of well-being. The advantage of using either 0.5 or 1.0 mg/kg/d for treatment of blastomycosis is that the course of treatment is usually shorter than with the 2.5 g total-dose formula used in other deep fungal infections or even with a 10-week formula, with a cure being likely at a total dose of approximately 1.5 g in the immunocompetent patient.

Immunosuppressed patients and those with severe disease, and especially central nervous system infection, should receive the more aggressive daily dosing, with amphotericin B being given as a 0.5-mg/kg/d infusion and a total dose that rationally may be 2.5 g, instead of the treatment outlined for mild to moderate disease. Usually, no more than 50 mg/d should be infused, because side effects are more likely above this dose (*see* section on Adverse Reactions).

Treatment with itraconazole or ketoconazole has been used with good success in selected cases of blastomycosis. If the patient is not seriously ill or toxic, one of these two agents may be selected for treatment. Immunocompromised patients are not usually treated with an azole, at least not initially. If such a patient is moderately ill and requires hospitalization for more than just diagnosis, an initial course of amphotericin B followed either by itraconazole or ketoconazole is reasonable treatment. For AIDS patients, treatment may be switched to itraconazole in a therapeutic dosage (e.g., 200–400 mg/d) after 2 to 3 weeks of amphotericin B if they are doing well with this regimen. However, this is easier said than done because so many of the pharmaceuticals used to treat AIDS interact in adverse ways with itraconazole. Treating blastomycosis with ketoconazole was popular for a while, but it is used less frequently today. Ketoconazole may be used effectively in immunocompetent patients who have minimal to moderate blastomycosis, but it should not be used in patients who are toxic or have extensive clinical disease. Such patients should be treated, at least initially, with amphotericin B. Ketoconazole is administered orally, initially at a dosage of 400 mg/d. Disease progression or failure to improve should prompt the clinician to increase the dosage to 800 mg/d. Treatment with ketoconazole alone should be given for 6 months.

Currently, itraconazole is recommended for the treatment of mild to moderate blastomycosis. Because it does not interfere with androgen or corticosteroid metabolism (as ketoconazole does), itraconazole is preferred to ketoconazole and has become popular because of its oral route of administration and its effectiveness. In the immunocompetent host, a dosage of 200 mg/d for 6 months is usually, but not always, curative; some patients require 400 mg/d. Itraconazole also is recommended as the second phase of treatment to complete a course of antifungal therapy after an initial 1- to 3-week course of intravenous amphotericin B in cases of moderate and, in selected cases, advanced disease.

Generally, blastomycosis treatment must be continued for a prolonged period. Amphotericin B may be administered for a 10-week period in a modest (not maximal) dosage, usually daily. In blastomycosis, it is the duration of amphotericin B therapy as much as its daily dose or the total dose that governs success in this relatively easily treated deep fungal infection. However, the cost of this classic treatment renders its use to be infrequent. An azole, especially itraconazole, can be used from the outset in mild to moderate disease or after an initial (1–3 week) course of amphotericin B. Azole therapy, even if it follows a 1- to 3-week first-phase course of treatment with amphotericin B, should be given daily for 6 months.

Immunocompromised patients should receive therapy with amphotericin B, either for the full therapeutic course or for a minimum of 2 to 3 weeks followed by oral itraconazole therapy for 6 months. The follow-up of immunocompromised patients must be done carefully; however, only in AIDS patients is blastomycosis usually considered incurable, requiring life-long suppression. A test for cure should be considered for every immunocompromised patient with a periodic follow-up at 3, 6, and 12 months after completion of the patient's antifungal regimen. AIDS patients are followed routinely at 3- to 4-month intervals, at which consideration must be given to the patient's previously treated blastomycosis.

Complications of blastomycosis treatment with ketoconazole or itraconazole are understood and limit the use of these drugs. Prolongation of the electrocardiographic QT interval, including ventricular arrhythmias, when ketoconazole or itraconazole is used with astemizole, terfenadine, or cisapride has made such combinations contraindicated. Multiple additional drug interactions are caused by these antifungal agents' inhibition of the cytochrome P450 pathway, making individualization of treatment with either drug a requirement when prescribing it. During treatment with ketoconazole or itraconazole, any other drug metabolized by the cytochrome P450 3A enzyme system reaches higher-than-expected levels, with predictable toxicity.

Conversely, drugs that induce the cytochrome P450 enzyme system (e.g., rifampin), reduce the blood levels of ketoconazole or itraconazole, resulting in subtherapeutic levels of these drugs and possible drug failure in the treatment of blastomycosis.

Ketoconazole inhibits androgen synthesis, reducing testosterone levels in some men. High-dose therapy (800 mg/d), which is sometimes required in the treatment of blastomycosis, may result in male gynecomastia and impotence and in alterations in the adrenal–pituitary axis in both sexes. Hypersensitivity, hepatic toxicity, fever, nausea, and psychiatric abnormalities are known to occur with the use of this drug.

Additionally, itraconazole has caused changes in ideation in some patients. Nausea, hepatic toxicity (usually reflected by increased hepatic enzyme levels), and rash are the common adverse reactions to itraconazole.

Amphotericin B is a wonderful, life-saving drug; nonetheless, patients treated with it routinely and unpredictably experience fever, chills, nausea, and vomiting. Prophylaxis for these possible events can be achieved in part by routine orders for antipyretics and antinausea drugs. A standard order is for an aspirin suppository (325 mg) and trimethobenzamide hydrochloride (Tigan) administered in tablet form (100 or 250 mg), as an injection (100 mg), or as a suppository (200 mg) just before and subsequent to the first daily infusion(s) of amphotericin B and every 3 hours thereafter for two additional doses. This schedule prevents the reactions that can occur hours after the infusion has ended. After a week or 10 days of therapy have been completed, one may try to reduce or eliminate these prophylactic measures, thus individualizing therapy. Severe chills in patients who have been given amphotericin B can be managed by the use of meperidine, if given early enough in the chill; however, routine use of this drug is not indicated. Alternatives to the routine use of aspirin is acetaminophen given as a suppository or, in patients who do not experience nausea and vomiting, in tablet form. Small quantities of hydrocortisone (20–40 mg) added to the amphotericin B infusion may reduce fever and chills if the usual antipyretic agents do not work. Experienced clinicians use a 1-mg test dose of amphotericin B diluted in 100 to 500 ml of 5% dextrose in water and infused over 1 hour to check the reactions of the patient empirically. If the infusion is tolerated, then the first therapeutic dose of amphotericin B may be given 1 or 2 hours later. Because patients occasionally have a profound reaction (including hypotension) to the test dose of amphotericin B, this approach is appropriately conservative. Most patients, however, do not require a treatment delay of more than a few hours by this test procedure. The next dose should be therapeutic; a 20-mg dose is effective for this purpose.

Impaired renal function also routinely occurs in patients who receive amphotericin B; however, the kidneys do not excrete the drug. The overall dosing of amphotericin B need not be changed in renal insufficiency, but the doses administered should be reduced temporarily if the serum creatinine concentration rises quickly over a period of a few days. Significant renal insufficiency caused by amphotericin B is not usually an adverse effect that is associated with the daily and total doses of the drug required for the treatment of blastomycosis.

Summary

Blastomycosis is uncommon; however, because it is normally an indolent, slowly progressive infection, time is on the side of the thoughtful clinician. The wide range of manifestations does not make blastomycosis an easy diagnosis. However, if the patient returns upon failure to improve or gets no better with nonspecific therapy and if the physician considers blastomycosis in the differential diagnosis, the disease may be discovered quickly. Although effective drug treatments for blastomycosis are readily available, their adverse side effects, long duration, and multiple drug interactions require patience on the part of both the physician and patient.

Acknowledgements

Support for this work was given from Huron Hospital's Department of Medicine. The author also thanks Cindy Storm for her contributions.

REFERENCES

1. **Editorial.** *JAMA*. 1969;208:1695–6.
2. **Vasquez JE, Mehta JB, Agrawal R, Sarubbi FA.** Blastomycosis in northeastern Tennessee. *Chest*. 1998;114:436–43.
3. **Palmer PE, McFadden SW.** Blastomycosis: report of an unusual case. *N Engl J Med*. 1968;279:979–83.
4. **Lowry PW, Kelso KY, McFarland LM.** Blastomycosis in Washington Parish, Louisiana, 1976–1985. *Am J Epidemiol*. 1989 130:151–9.
5. **Frye MD, Seifer FD.** An outbreak of blastomycosis in eastern Tennessee. *Mycopathologia*. 1991;116:15–21.
6. **Baumgardner DJ, Paretsky DP.** The *in vitro* isolation of *Blastomyces dermatitidis* from a woodpile in north-central Wisconsin, US. *Med Mycol*. 1999;37:163–8.
7. **Farr RC, Gardner G, Acker JD, et al.** Blastomycotic cranial osteomyelitis. *Am J Otol*. 1992;13:582–6.
8. **Benzel EC, King JW, Mirfakhraee M, et al.** Blastomycotic meningitis. *Surg Neurol*. 1986;26:192–6.
9. **Brandhorst TT, Wuthrich M, Warner T, Klein B.** Targeted gene disruption reveals an adhesin indispensable for pathogenicity of *Blastomyces dermatitidis*. *J Exp Med*. 1999; 189:1207–16.
10. **Bennett JE.** Antifungal agents. In Mandell GL, Bennett JE, Dolin R (eds). *Principles and Practice of Infectious Diseases*, 4th ed. New York: Churchill Livingstone; 1995:401–10.
11. **Chapman SW, Bradsher RW, Campbell GD Jr, et al.** Practice guidelines for the management of patients with blastomycosis. *Clin Infect Dis*. 2000;30:679–83.

26

Coccidioidomycosis

Francisco L. Sapico, MD

History

The migration of population in increasing numbers to the southwestern part of the United States and the climatic changes that have occurred in the past decade have made coccidioidomycosis an increasingly significant health problem, resulting in an increase in the number of cases of this disease.

The very first case of human coccidioidomycosis reported in the literature involved an Argentinean cavalryman in the Chaco region of that country who, in 1892, developed a nonhealing lesion on his right cheek (1). A medical intern named Alejandro Posadas first reported this case as one of mycosis fungoides. Shortly thereafter, the first cases of coccidioidomycosis in the United States were reported by Rixford and Gilchrist (2). These cases, from the San Joaquin Valley in California, were described as being caused by a protozoon, and the term *Coccidioides immitis* was coined for the cause of the disease manifested in these cases. The true fungal nature of the microorganism that causes the disease was later demonstrated by Ophüls and Moffitt (3), fulfilling Robert Koch's postulates in guinea pigs. Much of the more recent knowledge of this disease's epidemiology was reported by Dickson (4) and later by Smith (5) in their classic works on "valley fever."

Epidemiology

The geographic areas endemic for coccidioidomycosis are confined to the western hemisphere. Specifically, these areas conform to the so-called *lower Sonoran life zone* (8), which is defined as areas of low elevation, arid climate, yearly rainfall ranging from 5 to 20 inches, hot summers, few episodes of winter freezing, and having an alkaline soil. California, Arizona, New Mexico, Texas, and localized areas in Nevada and Utah are places in the United States where coccidioidomycosis is endemic. Other endemic areas are the northern part of Mexico, including Baja California and the Sonora desert. In Central America, small microfoci of coccidioidomycosis have been described in Guatemala, Honduras, and El Salvador. In South America, the countries of Venezuela, Argentina, Colombia, Bolivia, and Paraguay have known endemic areas.

Acquisition of the disease outside the confines of its known endemic areas is rare. However, fomite-associated cases (e.g., those from farm products, including cotton grown in endemic areas) have been described in such distant areas as in the state of Georgia (U.S.) and Naples, Italy (9,10). Laboratory-acquired cases also have been known to occur (11).

It has been shown that the number of new cases of coccidioidomycosis increases during summers that follow periods of relatively heavy rainfall (12). Severe climatic changes, consisting specifically of severe droughts for several years in succession, followed by heavy rainfalls, also have been reported to result in increased numbers of cases. Thus, for example, a five- to 10-fold increase in the number of cases was observed in California from 1991 to 1993, following relatively heavy rainfall after a drought of 6-years' duration (13). Increases after earth movement (e.g., earthquakes) also have been described. This happened in 1994 after the Northridge earthquake in Southern California (14). Additionally, severe dust storms have been associated with outbreaks of coccidioidomycosis in areas with low or no known endemicity (15).

Much has been written about a predilection for more severe coccidioidomycosis in certain individuals and racial groups. Men, pregnant women, immunocompromised individuals, and darker-skinned peoples (e.g., blacks, Hispanics of Native American descent, Filipinos, other Asians) have been reported to be at increased risk (16,17). The risk of extrapulmonary dissemination in immunocompetent white individuals is less than 1%. Increased numbers of cases and more severe disease have been seen in organ-transplant recipients and in HIV-infected individuals (18–20).

Etiology

The fungus *C. immitis* propagates in the soil in the form of barrel-shaped, end-to-end arthroconidia. These arthroconidia are very small (2–5 µm in length), easily carried by the wind, and readily inhaled by a potential host. Almost all cases of coccidioidomycosis are acquired via the respiratory route, although rare cases of primary cutaneous disease have been reported (6).

Once inhaled by a susceptible host, the arthroconidia of *C. immitis* are transformed into round cells that multiply by endosporulation. These round cells are called *spherules*, and each spherule is capable of forming hundreds to thousands of endospores within a few days. Each endospore, after rupture, is in turn capable of forming new batch of spherules. Although the presence of *C. immitis* in lung tissue elicits a variety of inflammatory cell responses, it is clear that T-cell–mediated immunity plays the most important role in the containment of coccidioidomycosis (7). Animal-to-human or human-to-human transmission of the disease has not been demonstrated definitively.

Clinical Manifestations

Most patients (~66%) who develop acute infection with *C. immitis* either have no symptoms or have a mild cough that is not sufficiently severe to cause them to seek medical attention.

Primary pulmonary infection is the most common form of coccidioidomycosis. The most common symptoms are nonspecific and include fatigue, cough, chest pain, dyspnea, and hemoptysis (21). Fever may be seen in close to one half of patients, and arthralgia and/or myalgia also may be present. A diffuse, evanescent, maculopapular rash is uncommon, but erythema nodosum (usually associated with a good prognosis) may be seen in approximately 25% of women but in only 3% of men. Erythema multiforme is seen less commonly but seems to be more common in children. Chest radiography may reveal pneumonitis, nodules, or cavitation and may not distinguish pulmonary coccidioidomycosis readily from other pathologies. Early pleural effusion and hilar adenopathy may be part of the primary disease. The acute infection almost always resolves even without therapy, although the illness may sometimes last for several weeks. Approximately 5% of patients may be left with asymptomatic residua in their lungs, either in the form of nodules or thin-walled cavities. In a few individuals, the acute pulmonary infection may evolve into a progressive pneumonia or a chronic lung infection (22).

Symptomatic extrapulmonary (disseminated) coccidioidomycosis may become manifest in the meninges, bones, joints, skin, soft tissues, genitourinary tract, and virtually every organ system of the body. Skin lesions on the face are relatively common, and those found in the nasolabial fold sometimes are associated with intracranial spread of infection. Bone lesions often involve the skull, vertebrae, hands, feet, ankle, and knee joints and are often found in areas of bony prominence or next to tendon or ligament attachments. In the spine, "skip" lesions (with normal intervening vertebrae between pathologic ones) are not uncommon (23). In general, extrapulmonary infection becomes manifest within a year after primary infection. However, dissemination may become manifest much later if immunity becomes impaired (e.g., with immunosuppressive therapy or HIV disease).

Diagnosis

Isolation of *C. immitis* from clinical specimens is a definitive way of making the diagnosis of coccidioidomycosis. The organism is a fairly rapidly growing organism, with colonies being detectable within a few days. DNA probes can confirm the identity of the mycelial forms isolated (24). Spherules seen in tissue specimens usually are not easily confused with other pathogens.

The classic serologic tests used in the past for identifying *C. immitis* have been the tube precipitin (TP) test and the tube complement-fixation (CF) test. The TP test is positive in early disease (before the CF test becomes positive) and becomes negative after several months. The CF test becomes positive after a few months and stays positive much longer than the TP test. CF titers of 1:32 or higher are significantly associated with extrapulmonary dissemination of coccidioidomycosis, and the titers can be used for follow-up while the patient receives chemotherapy (25). The immunodiffusion tube precipitin (IDTP) test is fairly equivalent to the classic TP test, but occasional false-positive results have been reported. The immunodiffusion complement-fixation (IDCF) test mimics the CF test, but it is a qualitative rather than quantitative and may not be as useful for follow-up as is the CF test while the patient receives chemotherapy. The IDCF test may be able to determine whether the antibody present in a patient's serum is IgM or IgG (26). Enzyme immunoassay tests also have been devised for *C. immitis*.

Cerebrospinal fluid (CSF) cultures are not very sensitive in the diagnosis of coccidioidal meningitis (27). A CF test performed with overnight binding, however, has been reported to have a 95% sensitivity (28). Patients with coccidioidal meningitis usually show lymphocytic pleocytosis, decreased glucose levels (although not as low as in pyogenic disease), and a moderate increase in CSF protein. An increased spinal opening pressure may be seen in most cases.

Mild to moderate eosinophilia (5%–10%) may be seen during the second or third week of acute illness. Clinical improvement is associated with the decline of this eosinophil count. Persistent, high-grade eosinophilia (>20%) has been associated with disseminated disease (29). Eosinophilic pleocytosis also has been seen in coccidioidal meningitis (30); however, the prognostic significance of this finding is unclear.

Fungemia is seen occasionally in disseminated coccidioidomycosis. It occurs primarily in immunocompromised patients (including in those with AIDS) and is associated with a poor prognosis (31).

Treatment

Most patients with primary pulmonary coccidioidomycosis recover without therapy. However, patients with more severe primary infection may require therapy (Table 26.1). Other factors often considered that weigh in favor of therapy include CF titer, negative coccidioidal skin test (signifying anergy), patient's race being one that is predisposed to dissemination, exposure to large inocula (e.g., laboratory exposure), and immunosuppressed states. The duration of fluconazole therapy indicated for these patients is unclear and has varied from 1 month to 1 year, depending on the physician involved.

Prolonged therapy is indicated for patients with disseminated disease. Because of its rapidity of action, amphotericin B is often the preferred initial therapy. Often, a minimum total dose of 1 g is given until the patient has improved clinically, followed by long-term treatment with fluconazole. A test dose of 1 mg of amphotericin B has been recommended by the manufacturer; however, some authorities give the full dosage of 0.6 to 1.0 mg/kg/d after the patient shows tolerance to the first few drops of the infusion. Slow escalation of the dosage is no longer commonly practiced. The total daily dose of fluconazole has varied from 400 mg to as high as 1600 mg (the higher doses are used for meningitis). Liver enzymes and a complete blood count should be monitored regularly during azole therapy. Most authorities feel that disseminated coccidioidomycosis often requires a treatment of indefinite duration, because relapses are common after treatment is stopped. One study found that a negative serial coccidioidin skin test and a peak CF titer of 1:256 are good predictors for future relapse (32).

Meningitis is a particularly difficult form of coccidioidomycosis to treat. Amphotericin B, the standard of therapy for many years, has to be given intrathecally as well as intravenously for this form of the disease. Intrathecal administration usually necessitates cisternal injection or administration through a cisternal Ommaya reservoir (33). The average tolerated dose of intrathecal amphotericin B is 0.5 mg; however, lower doses are given initially and then slowly increased. Intrathecal amphotericin B is given daily at the start of treatment and is then decreased in frequency from every other day to once every 6 weeks as clinical improvement occurs and CF titers and leukocyte counts progressively decrease. The minimum duration of therapy usually has been 1 year, but close clinical and CSF follow-up are necessary after the cessation of therapy because relapse is common. Side effects of intrathecal therapy with amphotericin B may include pain, headaches, paresthesia, nerve palsies, arachnoiditis, and direct neurotoxic effects. Ommaya reservoirs can become blocked or superinfected.

The availability of oral azoles has simplified the treatment of coccidioidal meningitis. Fluconazole is well absorbed, diffuses well into the CSF, and is as-

Table 26.1   Treatment Recommendations for Coccidioidomycosis

Primary Pulmonary Disease
Patients without Dissemination Risk
  Observe or treat with either of the following for 3–6 months or for 3 months after
    resolution of clinical infection:
      Fluconazole 400 mg/d
      Itraconazole 200 mg bid

Patients with Dissemination Risk or Progressive Pulmonary Disease
  Treat with either of the following for 3–6 months or for 3 months after resolution of
    clinical infection:
      Fluconazole at least 400 mg/d
      Itraconazole at least 200 mg bid

Pulmonary Cavity (Uncomplicated) or Fibronodular Disease
      Fluconazole 400 mg/d for 6–12 months

Progressive Pulmonary or Disseminated (Nonmeningeal) Disease*
Patients with Immediately Life-Threatening Disease
  Treat with one of the following:
      Amphotericin B 0.6–1.0 mg/kg to ~2000 mg/d total[†]
      Fluconazole at least 400 mg/d
      Itraconazole at least 200 mg bid

Patients with Slowly Progressive or Stable Disease
  Treat with either of the following:
      Fluconazole at least 400 mg/d
      Itraconazole at least 200 mg bid

Meningitis*
  Treat with one of the following:
      Fluconazole at least 400 mg/d
      Itraconazole at least 200 mg bid
      Amphotericin B injected directly into cerebrospinal fluid in combination with systemic
      therapy, followed by oral fluconazole

HIV-Infected Patients
      Lifelong suppressive therapy with fluconazole or itraconazole[‡]

Pregnant Patients
      Amphotericin B 0.6–1.0 mg/kg/d

---

* Duration of therapy should be at least 1 year if not lifelong
[†] Switch to fluconazole or itraconazole when disease is under control.
[‡] After control of the infection with amphotericin B or, in the case of mild disease in low-risk patients,
fluconazole or itraconazole.
Adapted from Derensinski SC. Coccidioidomycosis. In David Schlossberg (ed). *Current Therapy of Infec-
tious Diseases.* St. Louis: Mosby; 2001:717–9.

sociated with fewer side effects than is ketoconazole. Doses have ranged from 800 to 1600 mg. Suppressive therapy, guided by CSF formula improvement and CF titers, has to be given for prolonged periods (years). There is growing evidence that maintenance therapy for coccidioidal meningitis may have to be lifelong (34).

There is some evidence that itraconazole therapy may be effective for coccidioidal meningitis, despite the finding of negligible CSF levels of the drug at the usual dosages of 300 to 400 mg/d (35). More clinical experience is needed with this antifungal agent for this disease.

Newer preparations of amphotericin B (lipid-associated or liposomal) may be used for patients who develop toxicity (particularly renal) with the regular formulation of amphotericin B.

Future Directions for Research

An effective vaccine is desperately needed for coccidioidomycosis, especially to protect populations living in endemic areas, immunocompromised patients, highly susceptible racial groups, and population groups likely to be exposed to high inocula of *C. immitis* (e.g., microbiology laboratory personnel, military recruits in training maneuvers in endemic areas).

Newer, more effectively fungicidal drugs need to be developed. The antifungal drugs available now are primarily fungistatic against *C. immitis*. Drugs that will cure and not merely suppress coccidioidomycosis need to be discovered.

REFERENCES

1. **Deresinsky SM.** History of coccidioidomycosis: "Dust to dust." In Stevens DA (ed). *Coccidioidomycosis.* New York: Plenum Publishing Corporation; 1980:1–20.
2. **Rixford E, Gilchrist TC.** Two cases of protozoan (coccidioidal) infection of the skin and other organs. *Johns Hopkins Hosp Rep.* 1896;1:209–68.
3. **Ophüls W, Moffitt HC.** A new pathogenic mould (formerly described as a protozoan: *Coccidioides immitis* pyogenes): preliminary report. *Philadelphia Med J.* 1900;5: 1471–2.
4. **Dickson EC.** "Valley fever" of the San Joaquin Valley and the fungus *Coccidioides. Calif West Med.* 1937;47:151–5.
5. **Smith CE.** Reminiscences of the flying chlamydospore and its allies. In Ajello L (ed). *Coccidioidomycosis.* Tucson, AZ: University of Arizona Press; 1967:xiii–xxii.
6. **Winn WA.** Primary cutaneous coccidioidomycosis: reevaluation of its potentiality based on study of three new cases. *Arch Dermatol.* 1965;92:221–8.
7. **Galgiani JN.** Coccidioidomycosis. *West J Med.* 1993;159:153–71.
8. **Maddy KT.** The geographic distribution of *Coccidioides immitis* and possible ecologic implications. *Ariz Med.* 1958;15:178–88.

9. **Rothman PE, Graves RG Jr, Harris JC Jr, Anslow JM.** Coccidioidomycosis: possible fomite transmission. *Am J Dis Child.* 1969;118:792–801.

10. **Albert BL, Sellers TF.** Coccidioidomycosis from fomites. *Arch Intern Med.* 1963; 112:253–61.

11. **Johnson JE, Perry JER, Fekety FR, et al.** Laboratory acquired coccidioidomycosis. *Ann Intern Med.* 1964;60:941–56.

12. **Smith CE, Beard RR, Rosenberger HG, Whiting EG.** Effect of season and dust control on coccidioidomycosis. *JAMA.* 1946;132:833–8.

13. **Pappagianis D.** Marked increase in cases of coccidioidomycosis in California: 1991, 1992, and 1993. *Clin Infect Dis.* 1994;19(Suppl 1):S14–8.

14. **Schneider E, Hajjeh RA, Spiegel RA, et al.** A coccidioidomycosis outbreak following the Northridge, California, earthquake. *JAMA.* 1997;277:904–8.

15. **Flynn NM, Hoeprich PD, Kawachi MM, et al.** An unusual outbreak of windborne coccidioidomycosis. *N Engl J Med.* 1979;301:358–62.

16. **Pappagianis D.** Epidemiology of coccidioidomycosis. *Curr Top Med Mycol.* 1988;2: 199–238.

17. **Stevens DA.** Coccidioidomycosis. In Warnock DW, Richardson MD (eds). *Fungal Infection in the Compromised Patient,* 2nd ed. Chichester, UK: John Wiley; 1991:207–14.

18. **Holt CD, Winston DJ, Kuback B, et al.** Coccidioidomycosis in liver transplant patients. *Clin Infect Dis.* 1997;24:216–21.

19. **Galgiani JN, Ampel NM.** Coccidioidomycosis in HIV-infected patients. *J Infect Dis.* 1990;162:1165–9.

20. **Singh VR, Smith DK, Lawrence J, et al.** Coccidioidomycosis in patients infected with HIV: review of 91 cases at a single institution. *Clin Infect Dis.* 1996;23:563–8.

21. **Galgiani JW.** Coccidioidomycosis. *West J Med.* 1993;159:153–71.

22. **Stevens DA.** Coccidioidomycosis. *N Engl J Med.* 1995;332:1077–82.

23. **Herron LD, Kessel P, Smilovitz D.** Treatment of coccidioidal spinal infection: experience in 16 cases. *J Spinal Disord.* 1997;10:215–22.

24. **Stockton L, Clark KA, Hunt JM, Roberts GD.** Evaluation of commercially available acridinium ester-labeled chemiluminiscent DNA probes for culture identification of *Blastomyces dermatitidis, Coccidioides immitis, Cryptococcus neoformans,* and *Histoplasma capsulatum. J Clin Microbiol.* 1993;31:845–50.

25. **Pappagianis D, Zimmer BL.** Serology of coccidioidomycosis. *Clin Microbiol Rev.* 1990;3:247–68.

26. **Galgiani JN, Grace GM, Lundergan LL.** New serologic tests for early detection of coccidioidomycosis. *J Infect Dis.* 1991;163:671–4.

27. **Bouza E., Dreyer JS, Hewitt WL, Meyer RD.** Coccidioidal meningitis: an analysis of thirty-one cases and review of literature. *Medicine.* 1981;60:139–72.

28. **Caudill RG, Smith CE, Reinarz JA.** Coccidioidal meningitis: a diagnostic challenge. *Am J Med.* 1970;49:360–5.

29. **Harley WB, Blaser MJ.** Disseminated coccidioidomycosis associated with extreme eosinophilia. *Clin Infect Dis.* 1994;18:627–9.

30. **Ragland AS, Arsura E, Ismail Y, Johnson R.** Eosinophilic pleocytosis in coccidioidal meningitis: frequency and significance. *Am J Med.* 1993;95:254–7.

31. **Ampel NM, Ryan KJ, Carry PJ, et al.** Fungemia due to *Coccidioides immitis*: an analysis of 16 episodes in 15 patients and a review of literature. *Medicine.* 1986;65:312–21.

32. **Oldfield EC III, Bone WD, Martin CR, et al.** Prediction of relapse after treatment of coccidioidomycosis. *Clin Infect Dis.* 1997;25:1205–10.

33. **Einstein HE, Johnson RH.** Coccidioidomycosis: new aspects of epidemiology and therapy. *Clin Infect Dis.* 1993;16:349–56.

34. **Demsnup DH, Galgiani JN, Graybill JR, et al.** Is it ever safe to stop azole therapy for *Coccidioides immitis* meningitis? *Ann Intern Med.* 1996;124:305–10.

35. **Tucker RM, Denning DW, Dupont B, Stevens DA.** Itraconazole therapy for chronic coccidioidal meningitis. *Ann Intern Med.* 1990;112:108–12.

27

Viral Respiratory Infections Including Influenza

Jason W. Chien, MD

John L. Johnson, MD

Two percent to 15% of community-acquired pneumonia in children and adults is caused by viruses. Although influenza and respiratory syncytial viruses (RSVs) are the most common causes of respiratory illness, parainfluenza viruses, adenoviruses, and other agents are also significant viral pathogens (Table 27.1) (1). The true proportion of community-acquired viral pneumonia in adults is probably closer to the lower end of the aforementioned 2%-to-15% range. In a meta-analysis of 122 studies performed from 1966 to 1995, a viral cause was confirmed in 3% of 7113 cases (2). The frequency of reported viral pneumonia has increased during the past decade, most likely as the result of a combination of better diagnostic techniques and increasing risk for viral pneumonia among the growing immunocompromised population. This chapter focuses on modern diagnostic techniques and treatment for viral respiratory infections and on the most frequent viral pathogens that cause severe lower respiratory disease in adults.

Clinical Manifestations

Diagnosing viral infections of the lower respiratory tract can be challenging. The clinical presentation of viral pneumonia varies, is often nonspecific, and can be mimicked by other processes (e.g., severe community-acquired or atypical pneumonia; acute lung injury from a systemic inflammatory syndrome; noninfectious, diffuse lung processes such as hypersensitivity pneumonitis).

Table 27.1   Common Causes of Viral Pneumonia in Adults and Children

Children	Adults
Respiratory syncytial virus	Influenza A and B
Parainfluenza virus types 1–3	Herpes simplex virus type I
Adenovirus	Varicella-zoster virus
Influenza A and B	Adenovirus
Varicella-zoster virus	Cytomegalovirus
Herpes simplex virus type I	Hantavirus

Clinical suspicion should be based on the combination of epidemiologic characteristics and constitutional symptoms such as fever, chills, nonproductive cough, rhinitis, myalgias, headaches, and fatigue. Although findings such as wheezing, rales, increased fremitus, and signs of widespread bronchial inflammation are often found on physical examination to accompany viral processes, they are also seen in pyogenic pneumonia. Unfortunately, the radiologic features of viral pneumonia are also nonspecific. Findings may mimic those of bacterial pneumonia and can range from patchy bronchopneumonia to fleeting infiltrates or more characteristic diffuse interstitial infiltrates (Figs. 27.1 and 27.2). Cavitation and pleural effusions, although possible, are rare (*see* Fig. 27.1). Because severe leukocytosis is uncommon in viral pneumonia, a total white blood cell count of less than 15,000 cells/mm^3 in the setting of severe pneumonia should also suggest a viral cause.

Laboratory Diagnosis of Viral Pneumonia

Viral Culture and Antigen Detection

An etiologic diagnosis of viral pneumonia can be made by isolating and identifying the viral pathogen through viral culture or by isolating its DNA or antigens in lung tissue or the secretions of the lower respiratory tract (3). Most respiratory viruses can be isolated by cell culture of specimens from the upper and lower respiratory tract, which include specimens obtained from nasopharyngeal swab, sputum, and bronchoalveolar lavage (BAL), or biopsy. Nasopharyngeal swabs or washings are useful for culture of RSV, influenza viruses, parainfluenza viruses, and adenoviruses. For best results, viral cultures should be obtained early during the course of illness. Specimens should be placed in viral transport media, kept on ice or refrigerated, and transported

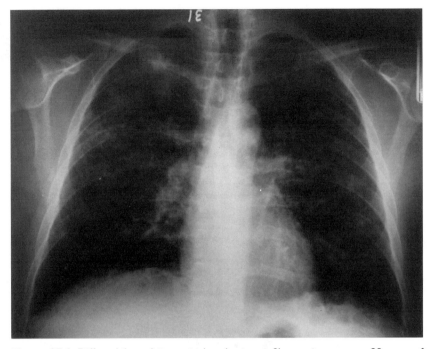

Figure 27.1 Diffuse, bilateral, interstitial, and acinar infiltrates in a woman 23 years of age who has varicella pneumonia.

quickly to the laboratory where they are first centrifuged and filtered to remove mucus and other debris. Cell cultures are incubated at 35°C and examined microscopically to detect the cytologic changes known as the viral cytopathic effect (CPE) as evidence of viral growth. CPE is manifested either in the form of degenerative changes or through the formation of syncytial collections of multinucleated giant cells. Viral growth also can be detected via hemadsorption testing by adding guinea pig erythrocytes to cultured cell monolayers and noting the adherence of red blood cells to the monolayer. When CPE is observed or hemadsorption tests are positive, the responsible virus is identified by further testing. Immunofluorescence-type enzyme-linked immunosorbent assays (ELISA) and nucleic-acid probes can be used to identify influenza A and B viruses, parainfluenza viruses, adenoviruses, RSV, herpes simplex virus (HSV), and cytomegalovirus (CMV) in cell cultures.

Because CMV grows very slowly in conventional fibroblast cell culture, it often requires 14 to 18 days to produce a CPE. Shell vial culture systems are now used widely to speed the detection of CMV, RSV, HSV, adenovirus, influenza virus, parainfluenza virus, and other viral pathogens. In the shell-vial culture method, prepared clinical specimens are inoculated onto adherent cell

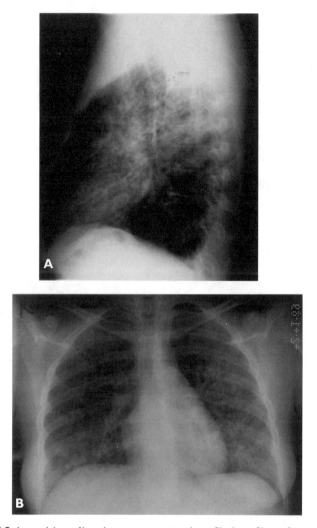

Figure 27.2 Lateral (*part A*) and posteroanterior (*part B*) chest films of a man 47 years of age who has varicella pneumonia. Note the multiple small, bilateral, discrete nodules that can be seen most optimally in the upper lobes of the lateral film. There are also small, bibasilar, pleural effusions.

monolayers grown on round cover slips in small vials. The vials are centrifuged at low speed for 1 hour, after which fresh culture medium is added, and then the vials are examined serially to detect viral antigen or DNA expression.

Rapid antigen-detection assay tests on ELISA methods are available for identifying HSV, RSV, influenza A and B viruses, parainfluenza virus types 1 through 4, CMV, and other respiratory viruses (3). Antigen-detection tests can be used alone or in conjunction with viral culture. These tests can be performed directly on properly collected specimens and can be completed within 1 to 3 hours. Unlike viral culture, antigen-detection tests are specific for each virus. Many laboratories use panels of antibodies to common respiratory viruses for screening clinical specimens. For example, the respiratory antigen panel routinely includes influenza virus, parainfluenza virus, adenovirus, and RSV. Antigen detection tests continue to give positive results for several days to weeks after viable virus can no longer be detected in culture, and they may be useful in the evaluation of patients who present late after the onset of symptoms or of patients who received previous treatment with antiviral agents. Overall, the sensitivity of antigen-detection tests is lower than that of viral culture, and the principal advantage of these tests is their speed. A recently developed molecular diagnostic technique—the multiplex reverse transcription-polymerase chain reaction (RT-PCR) assay—overcomes the low sensitivity of antigen detection, the delay inherent in viral culture, and the limitation of assaying for only one type of virus per specimen with traditional polymerase chain reaction (PCR) assay (4). This assay permits rapid detection of RSV, parainfluenza virus types 1, 2, and 3, and adenovirus in a single-step multiplex RT-PCR with high sensitivity and specificity.

Test results should be interpreted with caution. Although the recovery of influenza virus, parainfluenza virus, and RSV confirms the diagnosis of viral pneumonia caused by these pathogens, the significance of respiratory secretions and tissue cultures that are positive for herpesviruses such as CMV and HSV must be established by correlation with clinical and histologic findings. This is because herpesviruses can establish latency and are often shed intermittently in the absence of invasive disease. A culture that is positive for herpesviruses alone is not diagnostic of active disease.

Cytology and Histology

Respiratory secretions, BAL samples, and tissue specimens can be examined with cytologic and histologic methods (3). Although intranuclear inclusions are often seen in cells infected with DNA viruses, cytoplasmic inclusions usually are present in cells infected by RNA viruses. For instance, infection with CMV (a DNA virus) is associated with the presence of characteristic "owl's eye" cells, which appear as large cells with basophilic intranuclear inclusions and a surrounding clear zone (Fig. 27.3). Although the presence of viral inclusions is diagnostic of a viral infection, cytologic methods have low sensitivity, and the absence of inclusions does not exclude infection or active disease reliably.

The laboratory studies used in the diagnosis of viral respiratory infections are summarized in Table 27.2.

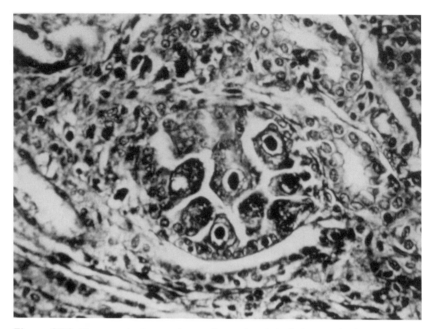

Figure 27.3 Cytomegalovirus nuclear and cytoplasmic inclusions in the lung.

Treatment

A decision to treat for viral pneumonia empirically should be made only after considering pyogenic causes of pulmonary infection. Empirical therapy for community-acquired pneumonia (especially atypical pneumonia) should be instituted until its absence is confirmed. An aggressive diagnostic approach, with the aid of fiberoptic bronchoscopy, is useful for ruling out pyogenic as well as noninfectious causes of diffuse pulmonary disease. As is discussed below, there are only a few options of proven efficacy available for treating viral pulmonary infections. However, because acyclovir and ganciclovir have relatively benign side-effect profiles, these antiviral agents should be considered for empirical therapy whenever herpes viruses such as varicella zoster virus (VZV), HSV, and CMV are possible causes of pulmonary infection. If a noninfectious cause (e.g., hypersensitivity pneumonitis) is a serious consideration and if corticosteroids are indicated, one should make every effort to rule out an infectious process before initiating corticosteroid therapy.

Table 27.2 Diagnostic Techniques for Viral Infections

Virus	Method of Diagnosis
Herpesviruses	
HSV	Tracheal aspirate or BAL for viral cultures and antigen testing by ELISA
VZV	Samples from lesions for Tzanck smears, viral culture, and immunofluorescent assays; serum for immunofluorescent assays, complement fixation, neutralizing antibody test, and enzyme immunoassay
CMV	BAL specimens for cytology, viral culture, and DNA PCR; serum for DNA PCR and antigen testing
Paramyxoviruses	
RSV	Tracheal aspirate or BAL for viral culture and antigen testing by ELISA and fluorescein conjugate monoclonal or polyclonal antibody
Parainfluenza virus	Nasal and bronchial secretions for viral culture and immunofluorescent assays (serotypes 1, 2, and 3); serum for complement fixation and hemagglutination
Measles virus	BAL specimens for cytology; tracheal, respiratory secretions, or BAL samples for viral culture and immunofluorescent assays
Influenza virus	Respiratory secretions for viral cultures and immunofluorescent and ELISA assays
Adenovirus	Respiratory secretions for viral culture, complement fixation, hemagglutination inhibition, and neutralization
Hantavirus	Serum for hantavirus IgM antibodies or acute and convalescent IgG antibody; tissue for immunohistochemistry and RT-PCR

BAL = bronchoalveolar lavage; CMV = cytomegalovirus; ELISA = enzyme-linked immunosorbent assay; HSV = herpes simplex virus; IgG = immunoglobulin G; IgM = immunoglobulin M; PCR = polymerase chain reaction; RSV = respiratory syncytial virus; RT-PCR = reverse transcription-polymerase chain reaction; VZV = varicella-zoster virus.

Herpesviruses

The family Herpesviridae consists of large, double-stranded, DNA-containing, enveloped viruses that vary widely in their ability to infect different types of cells and that share the common ability to induce lifelong latent infection. This latter aspect of the herpesviruses is of particular concern for seropositive individuals with immunosuppression whose immune systems may be unable to contain the virus in its latent form. The members of the Herpesviridae that more commonly cause respiratory infection are HSV, VZV, and CMV.

Herpes Simplex Virus

Despite the ability of HSV to cause a wide spectrum of diseases in the human host, it rarely causes lower respiratory tract infections (LRI). This is most likely due to the virus' predilection for infecting squamous epithelium. Unfortunately, a number of factors (e.g., traumatic endotracheal intubation, burns, radiation therapy, cytotoxic chemotherapy, acute respiratory distress syndrome [ARDS], smoking) promote squamous metaplasia of the tracheobronchial tree and predispose the host to LRI with HSV (5). Immunocompromised patients (e.g., those who receive cancer chemotherapy, are neutropenic, are HIV positive, have congenital cell-mediated immunodeficiency, are burn victims, are severely debilitated or malnourished as a result of prolonged hospitalization) are at particular risk for HSV pneumonia (6). Although the lung is often involved in disseminated HSV infection, disseminated disease is not commonly associated with mucocutaneous HSV infections. Less than 10% of HSV-seropositive transplant recipients with mucocutaneous herpes infection develop visceral dissemination (7).

Pathogenesis
Pneumonia caused by HSV develops via two principal mechanisms. First, focal or multifocal infiltrates correlate with antecedent upper airway infection with HSV. This pattern is most likely due to direct extension of infection from the upper to the lower respiratory tract, to aspiration of infectious secretions, or to reactivation of dormant HSV in vagal ganglia (5). These patients often have tracheitis or esophagitis, and usually have oral mucocutaneous lesions before they develop pulmonary disease. Second, diffuse interstitial infiltrates may follow viremia caused by dissemination of HSV from genital or oral lesions or transfusion of HSV-infected blood (5). Early dissemination also may be reflected by other organ dysfunction, such as increased liver enzyme activities.

Clinical Manifestations
The spectrum of respiratory diseases caused by HSV infection ranges from oropharyngitis to membranous tracheobronchitis and diffuse or localized pneumonia but usually localizes to the trachea and large bronchi, producing a thick, inflammatory membrane that can ultimately create significant resistance to ventilation. HSV pneumonia is an uncommon type of community-acquired pneumonia and usually develops after a prolonged and complicated hospital stay. Dyspnea and cough are the most common clinical complaints. Fever, tachypnea, intractable wheezing, chest pain, or hemoptysis also occur. Cutaneous, genital, or oral mucocutaneous lesions often herald pulmonary or disseminated disease.

Diagnosis
The diagnosis of HSV pneumonia should be based on clinical suspicion, radiographic findings, isolation of HSV from the lungs, and histologic findings of a necrotizing or hemorrhagic pneumonia in appropriate specimens.

Focal lesions on chest radiographs begin as small nodules best seen in the periphery, away from normal vascular markings. As the disease progresses, the nodules may coalesce to form extensive infiltrates. It should be noted that HSV pneumonia may present initially as a focal or segmental pneumonia due to the spread of infection from upper airway lesions but ultimately can extend to other areas of the lung, producing diffuse infiltrates similar to the pattern seen with viremic HSV infection (7).

Because HSV can be isolated from oropharyngeal secretions in from 2% to 25% of normal hosts, positive sputum cultures for HSV are often difficult to interpret (6). The diagnostic use of tracheal aspirates allows one to bypass the upper respiratory tract, which significantly improves diagnostic specificity; however, upper airway secretions can still contaminate such aspirates. Bronchoscopy is especially useful for direct sampling of mucosal ulcers and for obtaining bronchial brushings, washings, and biopsy specimens for histologic and cytologic examination. The presence of Cowdry type A intranuclear inclusion bodies in lower respiratory secretions significantly increases the specificity of an HSV pneumonia diagnosis. Mucocutaneous lesions also should be investigated for the presence of HSV. Scrapings from the base of ulcerated lesions can be examined with Wright or Giemsa stains for multinucleated giant cells and intranuclear inclusions (Fig. 27.4). Specimens also can be examined by immunofluorescence staining with specific polyclonal or monoclonal antibodies, electron microscopy, or ELISA. Appropriate viral cultures of mucosal

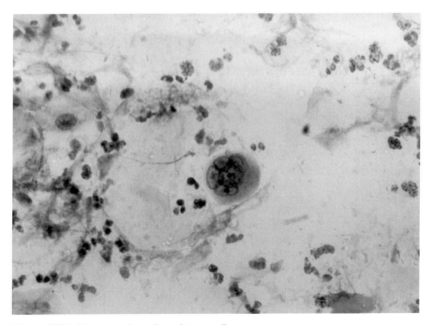

Figure 27.4 Herpes multinucleated giant cell.

lesions, blood, and respiratory secretions should always be obtained in cases of suspected herpetic pneumonia. Serologic assays have little diagnostic use.

Treatment

Because oral acyclovir is poorly absorbed, acyclovir given intravenously at a dose of 5–10 mg/kg or 250 mg/m^2 every 8 hours is currently the treatment of choice for HSV pneumonia (Table 27.3). Over half of all cases of HSV pneumonia are complicated by other infections (5); therefore, empirical broad-spectrum antibiotic therapy, including an antistaphylococcal drug (either nafcillin or vancomycin, depending on the local prevalence of methicillin-resistant *Staphylococcus aureus*), should be instituted in patients with progressive HSV pneumonia that does not respond appropriately to antiviral therapy. If deterioration continues despite the addition of antibiotics, a definitive diagnostic procedure such as bronchoscopy or open-lung biopsy should be performed to seek other opportunistic organisms such as *Aspergillus*, *Candida*, and *Pneumocystis carinii*. The role of adjunctive corticosteroids is still controversial, and their use should not be considered standard care, especially in already immunocompromised hosts. Ventilation support often is needed because of severe hypoxemia. Fluid management is of special concern because fulminant pneumonia is frequently associated with pulmonary edema and alveolar hemorrhage. Efforts to prevent HSV pneumonia should focus on chemoprophylaxis of high-risk, seropositive patients during induction of immunosuppression for transplantation. Passive or active immunization has not been proven helpful.

Table 27.3   Treatment of Severe Respiratory Tract Infections

Virus	Therapy
Herpesviruses	
HSV	Acyclovir
VZV	Acyclovir, VZIG
CMV	Ganciclovir, foscarnet, IVIG
Paramyxoviruses	
RSV	Ribavirin*, RSVIG
Parainfluenza	Supportive care, ribavirin*
Measles virus	Supportive care, IVIG, ribavirin*
Influenza virus	Amantidine, rimantadine, neuraminidase inhibitors (e.g., zanamivir, oseltamivir)
Adenovirus	Ribavirin*
Hantavirus	Supportive care, ribavirin*

IVIG = intravenous immunoglobulin; RSVIG = respiratory syncytial virus immunoglobulin; VZIG = varicella-zoster immunoglobulin.
* Presently not considered standard care or still under investigation.

Varicella-Zoster Virus

A highly contagious herpesvirus infection, VZV is transmitted among humans by direct contact with skin lesions or aerosolization of respiratory tract secretions. The incubation period ranges from 10 to 21 days. Primary infection with VZV causes chicken pox, a febrile illness with malaise and a characteristic, generalized "dewdrop-on-rose-petal" vesicular rash that lasts 4 to 5 days. VZV also causes herpes zoster, a dermatologic manifestation of reactivated latent virus from nerve ganglia. Respiratory tract involvement is an uncommon complication of herpes zoster in otherwise healthy individuals. Adults, pregnant and postpartum women, immunocompromised patients (e.g., those with hematologic malignancies), and HIV-infected children may have more severe disease and are at increased risk for complications such as pneumonia, secondary bacterial infections of skin lesions, encephalitis, hepatitis, and Reye's syndrome. Approximately 10% of adults with varicella have lower respiratory tract symptoms, and approximately 1 in 400 develops overt pneumonia. Five percent of women of childbearing age in the United States have no antibodies against varicella and are at risk for varicella pneumonia. Pneumonia is a more frequent complication of varicella infection in pregnant women than it is in other adults and is more common in the third trimester. Mortality rates of up to 45% have been reported in pregnant women with varicella pneumonia.

Pulmonary manifestations of varicella pneumonia correlate with the severity of the rash. Mild cases of varicella pneumonia usually improve as the rash begins to subside. Long-term respiratory sequelae are infrequent, although small, scattered, punctate lung calcifications may persist on chest radiographs. The mortality rate in severe cases of varicella pneumonia with overt respiratory failure is approximately 50%.

Diagnosis
Varicella pneumonia characteristically presents with patchy diffuse infiltrates that sometimes have the appearance of small nodules or miliary lesions (see Fig. 27.2). Lesions may be more prominent in the lower lung fields or perihilar regions. The hilar lymph nodes may be enlarged. Pleural effusions occur infrequently and are small when present. Varicella pneumonia often can be diagnosed clinically in the setting of the typical rash. However, the rash may be atypical or absent in immunosuppressed patients, and further laboratory testing is warranted. The virus can be isolated from the fluid of the skin vesicles, blood, respiratory tract secretions, and cerebrospinal fluid. Tzanck smears on cutaneous lesions coupled with rapid immunofluorescence tests for antigen can speed the diagnosis. Serologic assays include immunofluorescence assays, complement fixation (CF) tests, neutralizing antibody tests, and enzyme immunoassay.

Treatment

Management of varicella pneumonia includes respiratory isolation of the patient until skin lesions heal (varicella is highly contagious), supportive care, antiviral therapy, and active and passive immunization. For patients at high risk for complications of varicella, the use of varicella-zoster immunoglobulin (VZIG) can decrease the risk of infection or severity of illness substantially if administered within 96 hours of exposure. Acyclovir given intravenously at 10 mg/kg every 8 hours for 7 to 10 days has been shown to be effective in immunocompromised patients. No teratogenic effects have been seen in pregnant women (8). The clearance of acyclovir is primarily renal, and the dose should be adjusted for renal insufficiency.

Immunization

In March 1995, a live attenuated varicella vaccine was licensed in the United States for use in healthy individuals aged over 12 months. The vaccine is nearly 100% protective against severe varicella disease and is recommended for routine vaccination of all healthy children at 12 to 18 months of age (9). Vaccination of susceptible individuals (i.e., those without a reliable history of varicella infection or without detectable serum antibodies) aged over 13 years is recommended for health care workers and family contacts of immunocompromised patients, teachers, daycare workers, staff and residents in institutional settings, and nonpregnant women of childbearing age. The vaccine should not be given to pregnant women. Adults should receive two 0.5-mL subcutaneous doses of the vaccine administered 4 to 8 weeks apart. Intramuscular VZIG at 12.5 U per 10 kg (maximum 625 U) is indicated for passive immunization of immunosuppressed children exposed to varicella or zoster, neonates whose mothers became infected with VZV shortly before delivery, and neonates with postnatal exposure to zoster (9). VZIG is also indicated in immunocompromised adults (i.e., those with primary or acquired immunodeficiency or neoplastic diseases or who receive immunosuppressive agents), pregnant women, and susceptible hospital personnel with substantial exposure to cases of zoster.

Cytomegalovirus

Infection with CMV is frequent among the general population and is almost always asymptomatic. Seropositivity to CMV varies between 50% and 80% in healthy adults in the United States. Acute CMV infection causes a mononucleosis-like syndrome in the immunocompetent host, which is associated with pneumonia in 6% of cases (10). However, because of its ability to reactivate from a latent state, CMV has become a serious cause of morbidity and mortality with the advent of immunosuppression in organ and bone marrow transplantation and in HIV infection. Although CMV disease in these patient groups can involve nearly any organ system, CMV pneumonia results in the highest mortality.

Pathogenesis

CMV infection in the immunocompromised host occurs through one of two mechanisms. In CMV-seropositive transplant patients, reactivation of latent endogenous virus during profound immunosuppression accounts for approximately 70% of the cases of CMV disease. In a retrospective analysis, acquisition of the virus from CMV-seropositive bone marrow, blood products, or donor organs was found to have led to disease in approximately 36% of CMV-seronegative organ recipients (11). CMV pneumonia typically occurs 6 to 12 weeks after transplantation in 10% to 40% of bone-marrow recipients (12). However, late occurrences (3–9 months after transplantation) are now more frequent because of the use of posttransplant antiviral prophylaxis. Risk factors for developing CMV disease include CMV seropositivity, donor seropositivity, older age, total-body irradiation, and acute graft-versus-host disease (11–13). A CMV-positive serologic status of the bone-marrow donor and the use of granulocyte transfusions from seropositive donors also increase the rate of CMV disease (~2.5-fold) (11).

Clinical Manifestations

Clinical symptoms of CMV pneumonia are subacute and nonspecific. In the normal adult, a dry cough, tachypnea, and low-grade temperatures are the usual complaints. Immunocompromised patients tend to have a more subacute presentation with similar symptoms. Severe hypoxemia and the development of respiratory failure that requires mechanical ventilation are poor prognostic indicators. Patterns seen on chest radiography are nonspecific but typically include interstitial infiltrates, alveolar consolidation, or a reticulonodular pattern (13,14). A miliary pattern also has been described with acute viremia in patients with primary CMV infection (15).

Diagnosis

The diagnosis of CMV pneumonia is challenging and should be based on the evaluation of clinical features, quantitative cultures of BAL specimens (16), transbronchial or open-lung biopsy, and serologic studies (e.g., viral culture, PCR for the DNA of CMV). Important cytopathologic findings in respiratory secretions and tissues include typical large "owl's eye" cells that contain basophilic intranuclear inclusions with a surrounding clear zone (*see* Fig. 27.3). Unfortunately, much controversy surrounds the use of BAL specimens for the diagnosis of CMV pneumonia (17). CMV is often found in the presence of other pulmonary pathogens, such as *Pneumocystis carinii*, making it difficult to determine whether the CMV in such cases is a true pathogen. PCR for the DNA of CMV performed on BAL specimens has a high negative predictive value but a low positive predictive value. Studies of patients with bone marrow and lung transplants have suggested that the use of quantitative BAL cultures is also useful in predicting the development of CMV pneumonia (16,18,19). The definitive diagnosis of CMV pneumonia must be based on histologic demonstration of invasive disease in affected tissues.

Treatment

Because CMV infection and pneumonia usually are self-limited in the immunocompetent host, there are currently no data about treating CMV pneumonia in this setting. Treatment of CMV pneumonia in immunocompromised patients has focused on prevention, acute therapy, and passive immunization with immunoglobulins (20). The high incidence and severe morbidity of CMV pneumonia among posttransplant patients (especially CMV-seropositive individuals) has led to the widespread use of prophylactic acyclovir and ganciclovir before and after transplantation (12,19,21). Preemptive therapy based on the detection of CMV in BAL specimens, CMV antigenemia, or CMV seropositivity by PCR after transplantation also has been shown to reduce the incidence of posttransplant CMV pneumonia significantly (13). The recommended treatment for acute CMV pneumonia is intravenous ganciclovir 2.5 mg/kg every 8 hours for 20 days followed by 2 weeks of oral therapy three to five times per week at 5 mg/kg/d for a total of 20 doses. Ganciclovir prevents the replication of CMV DNA by inhibiting the virus' DNA polymerase.

High-dose intravenous immunoglobulin in conjunction with ganciclovir also has been used successfully for the treatment of CMV pneumonia. This combination therapy is based on the premise that lung injury is not due to direct damage by the virus but instead is probably the result of a T-cell response to a virally induced antigen on cells of the lung. Immunoglobulins act by blocking host T-cell recognition of CMV antigens on infected cells. Unfortunately, the use of combined therapy involving high-dose intravenous immunoglobulin with ganciclovir has never been evaluated in a randomized trial. Foscarnet, a competitive inhibitor of CMV replication, is an alternative drug used in cases of ganciclovir-resistant CMV infection—a situation more frequently encountered in HIV-infected patients who receive chronic suppressive ganciclovir therapy for their disease. Despite major advances in the prevention, diagnosis, and treatment of CMV pneumonia, the mortality rate for this disease remains high, ranging from 40% to as high as 90% in some series.

Paramyxoviruses

The paramyxovirus family consists of enveloped, single-stranded RNA viruses that were first recognized to be causes of respiratory tract infections among children. Three members of this family—RSV, parainfluenza virus, and measles virus—are important causes of respiratory tract infections in both children and adults.

Respiratory Syncytial Virus

Among infants and children, RSV is the most common cause of LRI; it is also the responsible pathogen in 40% to 50% of children hospitalized for bronchiolitis and in 25% of children hospitalized for pneumonia (22). Premature infants and children with bronchopulmonary dysplasia, congenital heart disease, or immunodeficiency are at the highest risk for severe disease. Unfortunately, immunity is incomplete and reinfection can occur later in life, presenting as mild URI or tracheobronchitis. Since 1986, RSV has been recognized as a cause of LRI in the elderly and in immunocompromised adults (22–24). It ranks second to influenza as the most prevalent viral pathogen in the elderly. RSV infections in elderly and immunocompromised patients may originate both in the community and in health care facilities (25,26). Infection may present as a seasonal URI during the winter months or as an outbreak in a hospital, nursing home, or long-term care facility. When pneumonia is present, the infection has a mortality rate that ranges from 11% to 78%, depending on the degree of underlying immunocompromise (27).

Clinical Manifestations

Unlike herpesvirus infections, asymptomatic RSV infections are rare, even in cases of reinfection. RSV infection may manifest as a mild URI or as LRI in the form of tracheobronchitis, bronchiolitis, pneumonia, or, rarely, croup. In children, RSV causes nasal congestion, sinusitis, otitis media, coryza, and pharyngitis. In general, the manifestations of RSV infection are similar to that of immunocompromised and elderly patients, except that the lower respiratory tract is involved in up to 80% of childhood cases. RSV infection typically presents with fever, nonproductive cough, anorexia, and dyspnea. On physical examination, wheezing and rales are commonly seen. Bronchial wall thickening and hyperinflation are distinctive radiographic features of LRI caused by RSV in hospitalized children (24). However, among adults, chest radiography generally demonstrates bilateral interstitial or patchy infiltrates, sometimes with lobar consolidation (25%) or pleural effusions (5%) (27).

Diagnosis

The diagnosis of RSV infection can be made by examining the respiratory tract secretions. Nasopharyngeal sampling is easily performed, but BAL is twice as sensitive a diagnostic technique (albeit more invasive). The "gold standard" for diagnosing RSV infection is viral culture but may require several days for results. The more rapid and recommended test is identification of the RSV antigen with a fluorescein-conjugated monoclonal or polyclonal antibody or ELISA, both of which have a sensitivity and specificity of 80% to 95% (22). A rise of more than fourfold in RSV-specific IgG demonstrates infection with RSV (28). However, serologic measurement of convalescent antibody titers (as is done with these methods) is useful only for retrospective diagnosis.

Treatment

Ribavirin, a nucleoside analogue of guanosine, is the only effective antiviral agent currently available for treating RSV pneumonia. Because of its high toxicity profile when administered intravenously, ribavirin is delivered as a small-particle aerosol. Although early pediatric investigations demonstrated some positive therapeutic results with its use, several more recent studies have found evidence to the contrary (29). Ribavirin therapy among immunocompromised adults generally has been unsuccessful; however, in one case series, mortality decreased by as much as 30% (26). Prophylactic use of ribavirin among high-risk patients has not been shown to diminish the frequency of severe RSV infections. Given these findings and the high cost of ribavirin therapy, current recommendations are that ribavirin therapy be considered only in severe illness.

RSV immunoglobulin is a pooled product containing IgG antibodies against RSV. When given to high-risk patients (e.g., premature neonates, patients with bronchopulmonary dysplasia or congenital heart disease), monthly treatment with RSV immunoglobulin was found to reduce the numbers of both hospitalizations and hospital days significantly, with fewer admissions to and shorter stays in the intensive care unit. Overall, these patients also had fewer mild LRIs of any cause (30). Unfortunately, the safety and efficacy RSV immunoglobulin have not been established (31). A new alternative is palivizumab, which is an intramuscularly administered, humanized, monoclonal antibody preparation that recently has been approved by the U.S. Food and Drug Administration for use in children infected with RSV (32). The decision to approve this antibody preparation was based on the IMpact-RSV clinical trials, which showed a 55% reduction in the risk of hospitalization attributable to RSV infection in high-risk pediatric patients (33). Among children at high risk for RSV infection, palivizumab is preferred over RSV immunoglobulin because of its ease of administration, a lack of interference with the measles-mumps-rubella vaccine and the varicella vaccine, and the absence of complications associated with the intravenous administration of human immunoglobulin products. There are currently no data about the use of palivizumab in adults.

Attempts to develop a vaccine for RSV infection have not been successful. To date, only two studies of candidate RSV vaccines have been completed in the elderly (28). Although the vaccines in both trials were well tolerated without significant side effects, the rise in serum IgG was not found to be statistically significant.

Parainfluenza Virus

All of the four serotypes of parainfluenza virus can produce respiratory disease in humans. Parainfluenza virus is a common virus that infects most individuals during childhood; from 90% to 100% of children have antibodies to parainfluenza type 3 by 5 years of age (27). Unfortunately, immunity is transient, and reinfection (manifesting as mild URI) can occur in older children and adults. Depending on the serotype of the infecting virus, infection in children can cause croup, bronchitis, pharyngitis, or pneumonia. Because previous episodes of infection confer partial immunity, URIs caused by parainfluenza virus in adults are usually mild and self-limited and rarely cause pneumonia. Since 1979, however, parainfluenza virus has been noted to cause severe pneumonia in immunocompromised hosts during the winter months, and outbreaks have been reported in extended-care facilities in the United States.

The serotypes of parainfluenza virus differ in their epidemic patterns. Infection with serotypes 1 and 2 typically occurs during fall and usually causes croup or laryngotracheobronchitis in late childhood. URI is associated with serotype 4. Serotype 3 is a common cause of bronchiolitis and pneumonia in infants and of croup and tracheobronchitis in older children. It also has been associated with pneumonia in bone marrow and renal transplant patients (24). Depending on whether the infection is primary or secondary, symptoms can range from a very mild illness to life-threatening croup or bronchiolitis. Immunocompetent adults typically develop mild URI symptoms; however, in immunosuppressed individuals, parainfluenza virus infection can result in life-threatening pneumonia. Signs and symptom of parainfluenza virus pneumonia include fever, cough, coryza, and dyspnea with rales or wheezing. Radiographic findings range from normal to focal or diffuse interstitial infiltrates or diffuse alveolar interstitial infiltrates consistent with acute lung injury.

Diagnosis and Treatment

Diagnosis of parainfluenza virus infection is made on the basis of clinical characteristics and demonstration of the virus in specimens from the respiratory tract. The virus can be cultured from the nasopharynx, but this requires 5 to 14 days for identification. Therefore, rapid immunofluorescence-type antigen-detection tests performed on nasal and bronchial secretions for serotypes 1, 2, and 3 are preferred. No rapid test is currently available for serotype 4. Serologic assays based on neutralization, hemagglutination inhibition, and CF assays are also available. Test results should be interpreted with the realization that parainfluenza virus has such a predilection for the upper respiratory tract that a positive result may be found in the presence of minimal respiratory tract symptoms or even in the absence of such symptoms. Treatment is supportive. Ribavirin has been used to treat LRIs with some benefit in uncontrolled studies, but no effect of this drug has been demonstrated in the transplant population. No available vaccines are effective against parainfluenza virus infection.

Measles Virus

Measles virus typically causes a febrile illness, with a typical erythematous maculopapular rash in children and mild pneumonia in healthy adults. Severe respiratory involvement is more frequent in children than in adults, and pneumonia is the leading cause of death from measles in children. Although measles is rarely a cause of severe LRI in immunocompetent adults, it may result in more severe pneumonia in immunocompromised and malnourished hosts (34).

Measles is highly contagious and is transmitted from person to person by aerosolized droplet nuclei by infected individuals with a cough. The peak incidence of cases in the United States occurs in the late winter and early spring. The incubation period is 10 to 14 days. A 2- to 3-day prodrome with fever, cough, headache, conjunctivitis, and coryza usually precedes the onset of the rash.

Clinical Manifestations and Diagnosis

Respiratory complications of measles include primary viral pneumonia, secondary bacterial pneumonia, and atypical measles pneumonia. Primary measles pneumonia typically occurs in immunosuppressed adults, such as patients with hematologic malignancies or those with primary or secondary immunodeficiency. Primary measles virus pneumonia is characterized histologically by diffuse bronchiolar and alveolar inflammation with characteristic multinucleated giant cells that contain eosinophilic nuclear and cytoplasmic inclusions. Atypical pneumonia tends to occur in the immunocompromised host and in healthy individuals who received killed measles vaccine from 1964 to 1967. In these cases, the patient may not present with classic clinical findings. For instance, the rash may be atypical (i.e., beginning on the hands and feet and then spreading to the trunk) or absent. A severe and often fatal pneumonia, called Hecht's giant cell pneumonia, is more frequent in patients with atypical measles (24).

The diagnosis of measles virus pneumonia often can be made on clinical grounds in the presence of the characteristic erythematous maculopapular rash of measles, which usually begins on the face and then spreads to the trunk and finally to the extremities. Laboratory studies may be helpful if the rash is atypical or absent. The virus can be cultured from throat washings and respiratory secretions with a visible CPE in culture after 6 to 10 days of incubation. Newer rapid immunofluorescence assays also can be used to detect measles virus antigens in respiratory secretions.

The oropharynx should be inspected for the Koplik's spots that are pathognomonic of measles virus infection. These are small, raised, white spots that are most prominent on the buccal mucosa opposite the molar teeth during the early stages of measles. In primary measles pneumonia, chest radiography usually reveals diffuse, fine reticular and alveolar infiltrates. As in varicella, the course of primary measles pneumonia parallels that of the rash. The presence of patchy alveolar infiltrates and atelectasis is more suggestive of secondary bacterial pneumonia. The virus can be cultured from throat washings and respiratory secretions and produces a visible CPE in culture after 6-to-10-days' incubation. Newer rapid immunofluorescence assays also can be used to detect measles virus antigens in respiratory secretions.

Treatment
Treatment of measles is primarily supportive. Postexposure prophylaxis of immunocompromised individuals with intravenous immunoglobulin is effective if given within 72 hours after exposure to infectious cases of measles. Vaccination of healthy susceptible individuals is accomplished in a two-dose schedule. The measles vaccine is a live, attenuated virus vaccine and should not be given to pregnant women or severely immunocompromised individuals (35,36). HIV-infected children and immunosuppressed adults with measles virus pneumonia have been treated successfully with intravenous and aerosolized ribavirin in doses similar to those used in severe RSV infection (37).

Influenza Viruses

Influenza viruses are enveloped, single-stranded RNA viruses of the family Orthomyxoviridae. Influenza viruses are classified as type A, B, or C on the basis of antigenic differences in their internal matrix and nuclear proteins and are subtyped on the basis of differences in surface hemagglutinin (H) and neuraminidase (N) glycoproteins (38). Influenza A virus, the leading cause of influenza in adults in the United States, is responsible for up to 90% of cases of epidemic influenza. Influenza epidemics occur almost annually during the winter months and are associated with 10,000 to 40,000 excess deaths in the United States during severe outbreaks. Eighty percent of these deaths occur in individuals over 65 years of age. Those with emphysema, congestive heart failure, hemoglobinopathies, and immunosuppression are at increased risk for severe disease (38a).

Influenza is transmitted by respiratory secretions from individuals who are actively shedding the virus. The incubation period in humans is short, ranging from 1 to 5 days. The virus infects and kills ciliated respiratory epithelial cells, causing diffuse inflammation throughout the tracheobronchial tree. Therefore, transient increases in airway reactivity are frequent, and wheezing may be present.

Influenza manifests as an acute febrile respiratory illness that is associated with cough, sore throat, headache, myalgia, and malaise. The illness is usually self-limited, with major symptoms typically easing within 3 to 5 days. However, influenza may be complicated either by direct involvement of the lung parenchyma, or more seriously by superimposed bacterial infection with *Streptococcus pneumoniae*, *S. aureus*, *Haemophilus influenzae*, or gram-negative pathogens. In the case of infection with gram-negative pathogens, there is often a history of initial easing of influenza symptoms followed by clinical deterioration, return of fever, and pneumonia several days later. Patients suspected of having bacterial pneumonia as a consequence of influenza require culture of blood and respiratory secretions and appropriate antibiotic coverage for bacterial pathogens.

Diagnosis

During community outbreaks of influenza in the winter months, the diagnosis can be made confidently on the basis of typical clinical symptoms. At other times, laboratory confirmation is required. Influenza virus can be isolated from respiratory secretions by tissue culture. Immunofluorescence- and ELISA-based antigen-detection methods for respiratory and nasopharyngeal secretions have a sensitivity exceeding 80%. A fourfold increase in acute and convalescent serum hemagglutination inhibition, enzyme immunoassay, CF, or neutralization antibody titers is diagnostic but requires several weeks for completion and is mainly of epidemiologic importance.

Several office-based and point-of-care tests (e.g., Flu OIA, Quickvue, ZymeTx, Directogen Flu A) are now available for rapidly diagnosing influenza. These are either immunoassays for detecting viral nucleoproteins or enzyme assays for detecting viral neuraminidase, and both types require 10 to 20 minutes to perform on nasal or throat swabs, aspirates, or sputum. Their specificity for influenza is high, but their sensitivity is intermediate (60%–75%), and a negative rapid test result does not rule out influenza (39).

Vaccination

Annual vaccination of high-risk individuals before each year's influenza season is the most effective measure for decreasing morbidity and mortality from influenza. Humoral and, to a lesser degree, mucosal immunity are required for protection against influenza. Antibodies against the hemagglutinin antigen and, to a lesser degree, against neuraminadase are the major determinants of host immunity. The surface antigens of influenza A viruses, especially the hemagglutinin antigens, undergo periodic changes. Minor changes caused by point mutations are known as *antigenic drifts*, whereas major changes or *antigenic shifts* are due to genetic rearrangement between strains. Antigenic shifts result in the expression of new hemagglutinin and neuraminidase proteins to which few or no members of the human population have immunity and are therefore associated with pandemic disease that has severe morbidity and mortality. The rapid loss of mucosal immunity and these antigenic drifts and shifts are the factors that necessitate annual vaccination against influenza.

The influenza vaccine given in a particular year contains the three virus strains (usually two type A and one type B strain) expected to be the strains most likely to be transmitted in the United States during that year on the basis of epidemiologic surveillance. Inactivated trivalent whole-virus, split-virus, and purified surface-antigen vaccines are available. Whole-virus vaccines are prepared by culturing the virus in chicken eggs and then inactivating it with formalin. Split-virus products are made by chemical disruption of the viral envelope. Split-virus and whole-virus vaccines have similar efficacy; however, split-virus vaccines may cause fewer side effects in children.

The effectiveness of a particular influenza vaccine depends on the age and general health status of the individual receiving the vaccine and on the antigenic similarity of the influenza strains in the vaccine to those being transmitted in the community. In years when the vaccine is well matched to circulating strains of influenza virus, vaccine efficacy in healthy adults ranges between 70% and 90% (40). Immunocompromised individuals and adults over 65 years of age receive less vaccine but still benefit substantially; vaccination is highly beneficial in preventing severe influenza and death in these high-risk groups. Annual influenza vaccination is recommended for all individuals in high-risk groups aged 6 months or older (Table 27.4) and for healthy individuals wishing to decrease their risk of contracting influenza. Health care workers and other staff in chronic care facilities and household contacts of high-risk individuals also should be vaccinated. The optimal time for influenza vaccination in the United States is from October through mid-November, because the influenza season usually occurs from late December through early March. Individuals who are vaccinated after an outbreak of influenza in the community require at least 2 weeks for effective antibody titers to develop.

Chemoprophylaxis with amantadine or rimantidine, which does not interfere with the development of protective antibodies, should be considered when outbreaks of influenza A occur in institutions such as nursing homes that house high-risk individuals. Both amantadine and rimantidine are oral

Table 27.4   High-Risk Groups for Complicated Influenza

Age >65 years
Nursing home residents
Adults and children with chronic cardiopulmonary disease
Immunocompromised adults with diabetes mellitus, renal failure, HIV infection, or other
   immunosuppressive disease
Patients receiving chronic corticosteroids or other immunosuppressive medications
Pregnant women who will be in the second and third trimester of pregnancy during
   influenza season

tricyclic amines that target the influenza A M2 protein, a membrane protein
that is essential for viral replication. Both drugs prevent viral uncoating after
cell entry, are highly active against the influenza A virus, and are approved in
the United States for preventing and treating influenza A infection. All individuals in these institutions should be treated for at least 2 weeks or for 1
week after the end of the outbreak regardless of previous influenza vaccination (40). Chemoprophylaxis also should be given to unvaccinated health care
workers and other staff members who care for high-risk individuals in the institution. The new neuraminidase inhibitors have been used as prophylactic
agents for influenza (40a). These agents have been shown to be effective for
preventing influenza and are well tolerated.

Treatment

Treatment of uncomplicated influenza is supportive, consisting of rest and the
administration of antipyretic and analgesic agents as needed. In adults with
uncomplicated influenza, treatment with amantadine or rimantidine within 48
hours after the onset of symptoms decreases the duration of fever and symptoms by several days (40). However, amantadine and rimantidine are active
only against the influenza A virus, and their efficacy in patients with influenza
pneumonia or severe influenza is unknown. The usual adult dosage for both
amantidine and rimantidine is 100 mg twice daily. Because amantadine and rimantidine are excreted unchanged in the urine and are approximately 75%
metabolized in the liver, individuals with severe hepatic and renal dysfunction
should receive no more than 100 mg/d. Amantadine and rimantidine should
not be used in pregnant women and are also teratogenic in animals. Side effects of amantadine include edema, anorexia, nausea, nervousness, insomnia,
and lightheadedness. Rimantidine is less likely than amantadine to cause side
effects that involve the central nervous system. Confusion, hallucinations, and
seizures also have been reported with these drugs and are more frequent in
the elderly.

Influenza virus neuraminidase, which is critical for viral attachment to surface epithelial cells, for the agglutination of the virus to red blood cells, and for the release of mature virions, has been the target for developing a new class of antiviral agents called neuraminidase inhibitors (41). These inhibitors block the release of virions from infected cells and decrease viral spread in the respiratory tract. Zanamivir, the first agent of this class, is poorly bioavailable by mouth and is administered by intranasal inhalation as a dry powder. It has been shown to be effective for the prevention and early treatment of influenza infection if started within the first 48 hours of symptoms and given at 10 mg twice daily for 5 days (42,43). In rare instances, Zanamivir may cause bronchospasm in patients with asthma or chronic obstructive lung disease. Oseltamivir, a recently licensed oral neuraminidase inhibitor, can be used for preventing influenza when given at a dosage of 75 mg/d for 6 weeks during periods of local disease activity and for treating influenza when given at 75 or 150 mg twice daily for 5 days if started within 36 hours of symptom onset (44–46). Early treatment with zanamivir and oseltamivir reduces the severity and duration of such symptoms as cough and fever by 1 to 2 days and decreases severe influenza-related complications. The main side effects of oseltamivir are minor self-limited nausea and vomiting during the first 1 to 2 days of administration. The drug is better tolerated when taken with food. Zanamivir and oseltamivir have no recognized, clinically significant interactions with other drugs.

Adenoviruses

Adenoviruses are nonenveloped, icosahedral DNA viruses that cause many types of URI, including pharyngitis, bronchiolitis, and pneumonia. Aside from infecting the respiratory tract, adenoviruses can infect the conjunctiva and the gastrointestinal and genitourinary tracts. Most cases of respiratory adenovirus infection are mild. However, severe pneumonia has been reported in outbreaks in adults in communal living settings, such as long-term psychiatric hospitals and military-recruit training centers. Adenovirus pneumonia also has been reported in immunocompromised patients such as transplant, oncology, and HIV- infected patients.

There are 41 human serotypes of adenoviruses. Most cases of severe disease are caused by types 3 and 7. Type 4 is associated with outbreaks in military recruits. LRI caused by adenoviruses results in necrotizing bronchitis and bronchiolitis. Individuals with adenovirus pneumonia present with fever, cough, malaise, hoarseness, and sore throat and less frequently with cervical lymphadenopathy and conjunctivitis. Radiologic manifestations of adenovirus pneumonia range from patchy lower-lobe infiltrates to diffuse interstitial infiltrates and cannot be differentiated from the radiographic manifestations of other community-acquired pneumonia. The diagnosis can be established by viral culture of respiratory secretions and serologic CF, hemagglutination inhibition, and neutralization testing. A CPE of viral growth is visible in cultures of kidney, HEP-2, or HeLa cells after 2 to 20 days of incubation. Rapid antigen-detection assays also are available for identifying adenoviruses. Treatment is primarily supportive. Ribavirin has *in vitro* activity against adenoviruses and has been used anecdotally with success for treating severe adenovirus pneumonia in adults (47,48). However, there are currently no formal recommendations about its use. Although vaccines against adenovirus serotypes 5 and 7 have been developed, they are not recommended for general use; however, they have been used in military-recruit populations (49).

Hantaviruses

Members of the family Bunyaviridae, the hantaviruses are spherical, lipid-enveloped, single-strand RNA viruses that parasitize small rodents and can be transmitted to humans. Different strains of hantavirus have different rodent species as their predominant hosts. The most frequently recovered hantavirus in the United States is the Sin Nombre virus, which is transmitted by the deer mouse (*Permyscus maniculatus*) and several rodent species. Rodent species that harbor the four different hantavirus strains that are associated with hantavirus pulmonary syndrome (HPS) in the United States are distributed throughout the lower 48 states. Infected rodents chronically excrete virus in their urine, feces, and saliva. Aerosolization of their excreta is believed to be the major mode of transmission of hantaviruses from rodents to humans. Hantavirus infection also can be transmitted by direct contact or via bites from infected rodents. Human interpersonal transmission of hantaviruses is not known to occur.

Clinical Manifestations and Natural History

An influenza-like prodrome with rapid progression to ARDS and respiratory failure characterizes HPS. Initial symptoms include fever, myalgia of large muscle groups, dyspnea, cough, headache, nausea, and diarrhea. The prodromal phase is followed within several days by hypotension, tachycardia, and tachypnea that frequently and rapidly progress to shock and ARDS. Common laboratory abnormalities include severe leukocytosis with a left shift, atypical lymphocytosis, thrombocytopenia, hemoconcentration, prolongation of the activated partial thromboplastin and prothrombin times, hypoproteinemia, increased serum lactate dehydrogenase levels, and proteinuria. The initial chest radiograph usually shows rapidly progressive, bilateral pulmonary infiltrates in 65% of cases.

The high mortality of HPS is due to ARDS with diffuse pulmonary capillary leakage and multiple organ system failure (50). Autopsy may reveal large, serous, pleural effusions and severe pulmonary edema. Microscopic changes present in the lungs of fatal cases include intra-alveolar pulmonary edema with scant to moderate numbers of hyaline membranes and interstitial lymphoid infiltrates and little evidence of a viral CPE or viral inclusion bodies.

Diagnosis and Treatment

The diagnosis of HPS is made by serologic testing for hantavirus IgM antibodies or from a fourfold increase in acute and convalescent IgG antibody titers. Hantavirus antigens also can be detected in tissue by immunohistochemistry and RT-PCR. Current therapy for HPS is primarily supportive. Admission to the intensive care unit and inotropic and vasopressor support are frequently required. Fluid administration should be monitored carefully. In a controlled trial conducted in China, intravenous ribavirin (when given early after presentation) reduced mortality in patients with hemorrhagic fever and renal failure syndrome from hantavirus infection (51). Intravenous ribavirin is presently available in the United States as an investigational drug for treating HPS (52). A double-blind, placebo-controlled trial of ribavirin in HPS is currently in progress in the United States.

Prevention

Because hantavirus is transmitted through contact with rodents, environmental factors play a large role in sporadic cases of HPS throughout the United States and Canada (53). Worsening socioeconomic problems, such as poor housing conditions, also lead to increased contact with rodents. Minimizing human exposure to rodents and their excreta can prevent HPS. The most effective measure for minimizing exposure is rodent control, such as proper food storage, eliminating rodent nesting sites, adequate ventilation of infested areas before human entry, use of 10% bleach solution to disinfect infested areas, and use of gloves when handling dead rodents.

Summary

Most of the common respiratory viruses cause mild, self-limited illnesses in adults. Elderly and immunocompromised individuals are at increased risk for severe pneumonia. Clinical and radiographic features of viral pneumonia are often nonspecific. Newer and faster methods for viral culture and viral antigen detection have improved the definitive diagnosis of viral pneumonia in recent years. Preventive measures focus on the following:

- Limiting the exposure of sick patients to active cases of chicken pox and influenza
- Annual influenza vaccination
- Broad use of varicella vaccine in children and susceptible adults
- The use of hyperimmunoglobulin such as VZIG in high-risk patients
- Chemoprophylaxis against influenza with amantadine, rimantidine, or a neuraminidase inhibitor and against CMV with acyclovir or ganciclovir in high-risk groups.

Treatment of viral pneumonia is primarily supportive. Neuraminidase inhibitors are beneficial for influenza pneumonia when given early, as are acyclovir for herpes and varicella pneumonia, ganciclovir and immune globulin in CMV pneumonia, and possibly ribavirin for severe RSV, adenovirus, and hantavirus pneumonia.

REFERENCES

1. **Bartlett JG, Mundy LM.** Community-acquired pneumonia. *N Engl J Med.* 1995; 333:1618–24.

2. **Fine MJ, Smith MA, Carson CA, et al.** Prognosis and outcomes of patients with community-acquired pneumonia: a meta-analysis. *JAMA.* 1996;275:134–41.

3. **Leland DS, Emanuel D.** Laboratory diagnosis of viral infections of the lung. *Semin Respir Infect.* 1995;10:189–98.

4. **Osiowy C.** Direct detection of respiratory syncytial virus, parainfluenza virus, and adenovirus in clinical respiratory specimens by a multiplex reverse transcription-PCR assay. *J Clin Microbiol.* 1998;36:3149–54.

5. **Ramsey PG, Fife KH, Hackman RC, Meyers JD, Corey L.** Herpes simplex virus pneumonia: clinical, virologic, and pathologic features in 20 patients. *Ann Intern Med.* 1982;97:813–20.

6. **Graham BS, Snell JD Jr.** Herpes simplex virus infection of the adult lower respiratory tract. *Medicine.* 1983;62:384–93.

7. **Feldman S, Stokes DC.** Varicella zoster and herpes simplex virus pneumonias. *Semin Respir Infect.* 1987;2:84–94.

8. **Mahmood W, Sacks SL.** Anti-infective therapy for viral pneumonia. *Semin Respir Infect.* 1995;10:270–81.

9. **Advisory Committee on Immunization Practices (ACIP).** Prevention of varicella: recommendations of the ACIP. *MMWR Morbid Mortal Wkly Rep.* 1996;45:1–36.

10. **Klemola E, Von Essen R, Henle G, et al.** Infectious mononucleosis–like disease with negative heterophil agglutination test: clinical features in relation to Epstein–Barr virus and cytomegalovirus antibodies. *J Infect Dis.* 1970;121:608–14.

11. **Meyers JD, Flournoy N, Thomas ED.** Risk factors for cytomegalovirus infection after human marrow transplantation. *J Infect Dis.* 1986;153:478–88.

12. **Soubani AO, Miller KB, Hassoun PM.** Pulmonary complications of bone marrow transplantation. *Chest.* 1996;109:1066–77.

13. **Ljungman P.** Cytomegalovirus pneumonia: presentation, diagnosis, and treatment. *Semin Respir Infect.* 1995;10:209–15.

14. **Mera JR, Whimbey E, Elting L, et al.** Cytomegalovirus pneumonia in adult non-transplantation patients with cancer: review of 20 cases occurring from 1964 through 1990. *Clin Infect Dis.* 1996;22:1046–50.

15. **Smith C.** Cytomegalovirus pneumonia: state of the art. *Chest* 1989:182–7S.

16. **Storch GA, Ettinger NA, Ockner D, et al.** Quantitative cultures of the cell fraction and supernatant of bronchoalveolar lavage fluid for the diagnosis of cytomegalovirus pneumonitis in lung transplant recipients. *J Infect Dis.* 1993;168:1502–6.

17. **Ruutu P, Ruutu T, Volin L, et al.** Cytomegalovirus is frequently isolated in bronchoalveolar lavage fluid of bone-marrow transplant recipients without pneumonia. *Ann Intern Med.* 1990;112:913–6.

18. **Slavin MA, Gleaves CA, Schoch HG, et al.** Quantification of cytomegalovirus in bronchoalveolar lavage fluid after allogeneic marrow transplantation by centrifugation culture. *J Clin Microbiol.* 1992;30:2776–9.

19. **Schmidt GM, Horak DA, Niland JC, et al.** A randomized controlled trial of prophylactic ganciclovir for cytomegalovirus pulmonary infection in recipients of allogeneic bone marrow transplants: the City of Hope–Stanford–Syntex CMV Study Group. *N Engl J Med.* 1991;324:1005–11.

20. **Meyers JD, Reed EC, Shepp DH, et al.** Acyclovir for prevention of cytomegalovirus infection and disease after allogeneic marrow transplantation. *N Engl J Med.* 1988; 318:70–5.

21. **Crumpacker C, Marlowe S, Zhang JL, et al.** Treatment of cytomegalovirus pneumonia. *Rev Infect Dis.* 1988;10(Suppl 3):S538–46.

22. **Heilman CA.** From the National Institute of Allergy and Infectious Diseases and the World Health Organization: Respiratory syncytial and parainfluenza viruses. *J Infect Dis.* 1990;161:402–6.

23. **Mlinaric-Galinovic G, Falsey AR, Walsh EE.** Respiratory syncytial virus infection in the elderly. *Eur J Clin Microbiol Infect Dis.* 1996;15:777–81.

24. **Yang E, Rubin BK.** "Childhood" viruses as a cause of pneumonia in adults. *Semin Respir Infect.* 1995;10:232–43.

25. **Dowell SF, Anderson LJ, Gary HE Jr, et al.** Respiratory syncytial virus is an important cause of community-acquired lower respiratory infection among hospitalized adults. *J Infect Dis.* 1996;174:456–62.

26. **Harrington RD, Hooton TM, Hackman RC, et al.** An outbreak of respiratory syncytial virus in a bone marrow transplant center. *J Infect Dis.* 1992;165:987–93.

27. **Wendt CH, Hertz MI.** Respiratory syncytial virus and parainfluenza virus infections in the immunocompromised host. *Semin Respir Infect.* 1995;10:224–31.

28. **Falsey AR, McCann RM, Hall WJ, et al.** Evaluation of four methods for the diagnosis of respiratory syncytial virus infection in older adults. *J Am Geriatr Soc.* 1996; 44:71–3.

29. **American Academy of Pediatrics Committee on Infectious Diseases.** Reassessment of the indications for ribavirin therapy in respiratory syncytial virus infections. *Pediatrics.* 1996;97:137–40.

30. **Wandstrat TL.** Respiratory syncytial virus immune globulin intravenous. *Ann Pharmacother.* 1997;31:83–8.

31. **Rodriguez WJ, Gruber WC, Groothuis JR, et al.** Respiratory syncytial virus immune globulin treatment of RSV lower respiratory tract infection in previously healthy children. *Pediatrics.* 1997;100:937–42.

32. **AUTHORS?** Prevention of respiratory syncytial virus infections: indications for the use of palivizumab and update on the use of RSV-IGIV. *Pediatrics.* 1998;102:1211–6.

33. **The IMpact-RSV Study Group.** Palivizumab, a humanized respiratory syncytial virus monoclonal antibody, reduces hospitalization from respiratory syncytial virus infection in high-risk infants. *Pediatrics.* 1998;102:531–7.

34. **Kaplan LJ, Daum RS, Smaron M, et al.** Severe measles in immunocompromised patients. *JAMA.* 1992;267:1237–41.

35. **Angel JB, Walpita P, Lerch RA, et al.** Vaccine-associated measles pneumonitis in an adult with AIDS. *Ann Intern Med.* 1998;129:104–6.

36. Measles pneumonitis following measles-mumps-rubella vaccination of a patient with HIV infection, 1993. *MMWR Morbid Mortal Wkly Rep.* 1996;45:603–6.

37. **Forni AL, Schluger NW, Roberts RB.** Severe measles pneumonitis in adults: evaluation of clinical characteristics and therapy with intravenous ribavirin. *Clin Infect Dis.* 1994;19:454–62.

38. **Cox NJ, Subbarao K.** Influenza. *Lancet.* 1999;354:1277–82.

38a. **Piedra PA.** Influenza virus pneumonia: pathogenesis, treatment, and prevention. *Semin Respir Infect.* 1995;10:216–23.

39. **Advisory Committee on Immunization Practices (ACIP).** Rapid diagnostic tests for influenza. *Med Lett Drugs Ther.* 2000;121–2.

40. Prevention and control of influenza: recommendations of the Centers for Disease Control and Prevention. *MMWR Morbid Mortal Wkly Rep.* 1998;47:1–26.

40a. **Welliver R, Monte AS, Carewicz O, et al.** Effectiveness of oseltamivir in preventing influenza in household contacts: a randomized controlled trial. *JAMA.* 2001; 285:748–54.

41. **Gubareva LV, Kaiser L, Hayden FG.** Influenza virus neuraminidase inhibitors. *Lancet.* 2000;355:827–35.

42. **Hayden FG, Osterhaus AD, Treanor JJ, et al.** Efficacy and safety of the neuraminidase inhibitor zanamivir in the treatment of influenzavirus infections: GG167 Influenza Study Group. *N Engl J Med.* 1997;337:874–80.

43. **Hayden FG, Treanor JJ, Betts RF, et al.** Safety and efficacy of the neuraminidase inhibitor GG167 in experimental human influenza. *JAMA.* 1996;275:295–9.

44. **Hayden FG, Atmar RL, Schilling M, et al.** Use of the selective oral neuraminidase inhibitor oseltamivir to prevent influenza (See comments). *N Engl J Med.* 1999;341: 1336–43.

45. **Nicholson KG, Aoki FY, Osterhaus AD, et al.** Efficacy and safety of oseltamivir in treatment of acute influenza: a randomised controlled trial: Neuraminidase Inhibitor Flu Treatment Investigator Group. *Lancet.* 2000;355:1845–50.

46. **Treanor JJ, Hayden FG, Vrooman PS, et al.** Efficacy and safety of the oral neuraminidase inhibitor oseltamivir in treating acute influenza: a randomized controlled trial: U.S. Oral Neuraminidase Study Group (See comments). *JAMA.* 2000;283: 1016–24.

47. **Wulffraat NM, Geelen SP, van Dijken PJ, et al.** Recovery from adenovirus pneumonia in a severe combined immunodeficiency patient treated with intravenous ribavirin. *Transplantation.* 1995;59:927.

48. **Maslo C, Girard PM, Urban T, et al.** Ribavirin therapy for adenovirus pneumonia in an AIDS patient. *Am J Respir Crit Care Med.* 1997;156:1263–4.

49. **Gurwith MJ, Horwith GS, Impellizzeri CA, et al.** Current use and future directions of adenovirus vaccine. *Semin Respir Infect.* 1989;4:299–303.

50. **Duchin JS, Koster FT, Peters CJ, et al.** Hantavirus pulmonary syndrome: a clinical description of 17 patients with a newly recognized disease: Hantavirus Study Group. *N Engl J Med.* 1994;330:949–55.

51. **Huggins JW, Hsiang CM, Cosgriff TM, et al.** Prospective, double-blind, concurrent, placebo-controlled clinical trial of intravenous ribavirin therapy of hemorrhagic fever with renal syndrome. *J Infect Dis.* 1991;164:1119–27.

52. **Chapman LE, Mertz GJ, Peters CJ, et al.** Intravenous ribavirin for hantavirus pulmonary syndrome: safety and tolerance during 1 year of open-label experience: Ribavirin Study Group. *Antivir Ther.* 1999;4:211–9.

53. Hantavirus pulmonary syndrome: Colorado and New Mexico, 1998. *MMWR Morbid Mortal Wkly Rep.* 1998;47:449–52.

28

Joint Infections

William G. Gardner, MD

The acutely swollen joint presents the physician with a diagnostic and therapeutic challenge. The differential diagnosis is extensive, including noninfectious causes of joint inflammation, reactive arthritis caused by infection at a site remote from the joint, and infections within the joint space (1,2). Septic arthritis, which is caused by direct invasion of the joint space by a pyogenic microorganism, can be difficult to differentiate from joint swelling of reactive or noninfectious origin. However, it is extremely important to establish a correct diagnosis and institute the proper therapy to ensure a satisfactory outcome. Unrecognized and untreated bacterial infection of a joint can lead to permanent injury and even death (3,4). Because it is often difficult to establish a specific diagnosis at an early point, empirical antimicrobial therapy may be necessary if the clinical setting suggests an infectious cause.

Pathogenesis

Joint infection most often results from the hematogenous spread of microorganisms to the joint from a primary site of infection elsewhere in the body. Several factors contribute to seeding of the joint, including the vascular nature of the synovial membrane and the absence of a limiting basement membrane (2). When bacteria reach the joint space, they prompt an intense inflammatory response with release of proteolytic enzymes from synovial lining cells and neutrophils. The inflammatory response is further enhanced by the production of cytokines, such as interleukin-1 and tumor necrosis factor (TNF). Additionally, the infecting bacteria release proteolytic enzymes and collagenases that, along with the host inflammatory response, damage the articular cartilage if not properly treated (5).

Inoculum size and other virulence factors of specific bacteria are important in the pathogenesis of joint infection. For example, *Staphylococcus aureus*, the most common pathogen in septic arthritis, has a predilection for infecting joints that is partly the result of its specific binding properties for collagen and articular cartilage. Recent studies also have suggested that strains of *S. aureus* that produce certain types of capsular polysaccharides may cause septic arthritis more often than other strains (6). The capsular polysaccharide may protect the microorganism from phagocytosis and intracellular killing by macrophages.

Microorganisms also may reach the joint space by inoculation at surgery, during joint aspiration or injection, and after trauma (7,8). The incidence of septic arthritis after intra-articular injections is low. Such arthritis may occur in patients with rheumatoid arthritis who receive intra-articular injections of corticosteroids for acute flare-ups of their arthritis (9). Septic arthritis also has been reported after arthroscopy, occurring in 0.12% of cases in one large series (10). Coagulase-negative staphylococci and *S. aureus* are the most common pathogens in septic arthritis, but gram-negative bacilli and anaerobic organisms are sometimes found. In children, septic arthritis may result from extension of a contiguous focus of osteomyelitis into the joint. This is uncommon in adults, but septic arthritis may result from a contiguous cellulitis, abscess, or septic bursitis.

Joint inflammation also may result from an infectious process at a site remote from the joint or may be a postinfectious complication, such as occurs with acute rheumatic fever. This is not septic arthritis, because no infectious agent can be cultured from the joint space. Examples of reactive arthritides include Reiter's syndrome, the arthropathies associated with enteric infections, and the chronic arthritis of Lyme disease. The list of infectious agents associated with reactive arthritis is steadily growing. The pathogenesis of the joint inflammation associated with these agents is unclear but probably involves more than one mechanism. In some cases, intra-articular persistence of viable (but nonculturable) bacteria such as *Chlamydia trachomatis* may be responsible for ongoing inflammation. In others, only bacterial antigens are found in synovial tissue, causing an immune-mediated arthritis. Recent studies suggest that the distinction between infectious and reactive arthritis is less clear than previously thought (11,12).

Several factors have been recognized as predisposing to the pathogenesis of septic arthritis, and these are listed in Table 28.1. Infections at extra-articular sites, such as urogenital or rectal *Neisseria gonorrhoeae* infection, may lead to bacteremia with subsequent infection of one or more joints. Preexisting joint disease, especially advanced rheumatoid arthritis, creates an excellent environment for bacterial growth if the bacteria are seeded during an intra-articu-

Table 28.1   Predisposing Factors for Infectious Arthritis

Chronic Serious Illness
Cancer
Hepatic cirrhosis
Diabetes mellitus

Impaired Host Defense Mechanisms
Immunosuppressive drugs
Hypogammaglobulinemia
Complement deficiencies
Disorders of chemotaxis or intracellular killing

Previous Arthritis or Joint Damage
Rheumatoid arthritis
Crystal-induced arthritis
Severe osteoarthritis

Extra-articular Infection

Systemic Lupus Erythematosus

Intravenous Drug Abuse

Joint Trauma

Intra-articular Injections

lar injection or through bacteremia (9,13). Often there is a history of blunt trauma preceding the joint infection. This trauma may injure the vascular supply, allowing bacteria to enter the joint and establish an infection. Immunologic abnormalities (e.g., immunoglobulin deficiency, complement deficiency, phagocytic defect) are also important factors that predispose to septic arthritis, especially when the latter is caused by *Neisseria* (2).

Etiology of Septic Arthritis

Infectious arthritis may be caused by a wide variety of microorganisms, including pyogenic bacteria, mycobacteria, fungi, and viruses. Additionally, noninfectious joint inflammation of various causes may mimic infectious arthritis and must be considered in the differential diagnosis. Several factors are important in determining the microbial etiology of a case of septic arthritis, including the clinical setting, predisposing factors or conditions, and the age of the patient. Table 28.2 lists the relative frequency of several common bacterial causes of infectious arthritis in various age groups (14).

In neonates and infants under 1 year of age, the most common bacterial sources of septic arthritis are *S. aureus*, group B streptococcus, and gram-negative bacilli (e.g., *Escherichia coli*). *Haemophilus influenzae* was a previously common agent of septic arthritis in children between the ages of 1 and 5 years, but the widespread use of *H. influenzae* vaccine has decreased its frequency markedly. In children 5 to 15 years of age, *S. aureus* accounts for almost 50% of cases (15).

N. gonorrhoeae should be considered a possible pathogen in sexually active adolescents and adults with septic arthritis. Certain strains of *N. gonorrhoeae* are more likely than others to cause disseminated disease and arthritis; however, urogenital infection has occurred with decreasing frequency over the past two decades, with a subsequent decrease in the incidence of gonococcal joint infection (16). In contrast, the frequency of joint infection caused by *N. meningitidis* has increased over the same period for reasons that remain unclear.

In the adult population, *S. aureus* is the most common bacterial agent of septic arthritis; however, in certain clinical settings or in persons with predisposing conditions (Table 28.3), other microorganisms must be considered (14). This becomes important when selecting initial empirical antimicrobial therapy for septic arthritis, because routine antistaphylococcal drugs do not inhibit some of these pathogens.

In recent years, an increasing proportion of cases of septic arthritis have been caused by gram-negative bacilli. A particular factor or condition usually predisposes to the gram-negative infection. In individuals who abuse intravenous drugs, *Pseudomonas aeruginosa* and *Serratia* species may be involved and may infect the sternoclavicular or sacroiliac joints (17,18). *Aeromonas hydrophila*

Table 28.2   Etiology of Septic Arthritis by Age*

Microorganism	Age (years)				
	<1	1–5	5–15	15–50	>50
Staphylococcus aureus	+++	+++	+++	++	++++
Streptococcus species[†]	++	++	++	+	++
Streptococcus pneumoniae	++	++	+	—	+
Haemophilus influenzae	+	+	+	—	—
Neisseria gonorrhoeae	—	—	+	++++	+
Neisseria meningitidis	—	—	+	+	+
Gram-negative bacilli[‡]	++	++	++	+	++

* Plus signs indicate the frequency of each pathogen, with "+" signifying an uncommon occurrence and "++++" signifying a very common occurrence.

[†] Includes *Streptococcus* groups A and B, *viridans* streptococci, and micro-aerophilic *Streptococcus* species

[‡] Includes Enterobacteriaceae and *Pseudomonas aeruginosa*.

Table 28.3   Pathogens Associated with Specific Clinical Settings or Predisposing Conditions

Clinical Setting or Predisposing Condition	Pathogen
Neonatal arthritis	Group B *Streptococcus, Staphylococcus aureus*
Adolescent or sexually active adult	*Neisseria gonorrhoeae*
Elderly with urinary infection	*Escherichia coli, Proteus mirabilis*
Immunocompromised adult	*S. aureus, Pseudomonas aeruginosa*
	Other gram-negative bacilli
Adult with alcoholism, rheumatoid arthritis, or immunoglobulin deficiency	*Streptococcus pneumoniae*
Intravenous drug user	*P. aeruginosa, Serratia* species
Animal bite wound	*Pasteurella multocida, S. aureus*
Human bite wound	*Eikenella corrodens, S. aureus*
	Anaerobic bacteria
History of tick bite	*Borrelia burgdorferi*
Systemic lupus erythematosus	*Salmonella* species
Erythematous papulopustular skin lesions	*Neisseria gonorrhoeae, N. meningitidis*
Arthritis following bacterial enteritis	*Sterile reactive arthritis*

may cause arthritis in those with acute leukemia (19). *E. coli* and *Proteus mirabilis* may be associated with septic arthritis in elderly people who have urinary infections (20). *Salmonella* arthritis is associated with systemic lupus erythematosus, especially in those who are chronic carriers of *Salmonella* (21). Septic arthritis occurring after bite wounds from dogs or cats is often caused by *Pasteurella multocida*, whereas arthritis associated with human bites may be caused by *Eikenella corrodens* (22,23).

Anaerobic bacteria are an uncommon cause of septic arthritis. When an anaerobic joint infection occurs, it is usually in a setting of chronic debilitating disease, posttraumatic infection, or total joint arthroplasty (24). Nearly half of all anaerobic joint infections are polymicrobial. *Peptococcus* species are the most common anaerobic bacteria associated with posttraumatic and postoperative anaerobic septic arthritis, whereas *Bacteroides* species are responsible for most cases of septic arthritis associated with chronic debilitating disease. A recent review of septic arthritis caused by *Clostridium* species indicated that prompt diagnosis and proper management with open arthrotomy promise a good outcome (25).

Inflammatory arthritis also may be associated with viral infections. Such arthritis is usually polyarticular, which is in contrast with bacterial arthritis. For example, rubella in young women commonly causes a polyarthritis, usually beginning within 7 days after onset of the characteristic rash in this disease and persisting for several weeks. The arthritis in rubella usually involves the small joints of the hands and, less commonly, the wrists and knees. A similar arthritis may occur in women who have received a rubella vaccine (26).

Other viral arthritides in adults include the arthritis associated with hepatitis B infection, which is related to antigen–antibody complexes. Joint inflammation usually occurs in the pre-icteric phase and resolves with the onset of jaundice (27). Men infected with the mumps virus may develop a polyarthritis similar to that of rubella infection in young women (28). Additionally, parvovirus B19 may cause a self-limiting polyarthritis that 1) is acute and symmetrical; 2) involves the hands, wrists, and knees; and 3) lasts from 2 to 4 weeks (29). Several other viral infections have been associated with arthritis, including infection with HIV, hepatitis A and C viruses, and lymphocytic choriomeningitis virus (30).

Clinical Features of Septic Arthritis

Generally, septic arthritis is divided into gonococcal and nongonococcal arthritis. In nongonococcal septic arthritis, it is extremely important to recognize the infection early and to begin treatment promptly to achieve a good outcome. Gonococcal arthritis usually runs a less virulent course (2).

Nongonococcal arthritis is monoarticular in 80% to 90% of cases. Although the knee is the most commonly affected joint, any joint may be involved. The onset is usually abrupt, with fever and joint pain; however, fever may be absent in the elderly, in patients with severe underlying disease, and in those who take corticosteroids. On examination, the affected joint is erythematous, warm, and swollen, with a significant effusion present in most cases. A key point in the diagnosis of nongonococcal arthritis is the severe pain that occurs with attempted movement of the joint or with weight bearing (2,31).

Gonococcal arthritis usually has a much different clinical presentation than does nongonococcal arthritis, commonly taking the form of a polyarthritis that is often migratory with associated painful tenosynovitis. The knees, wrists, hands, and ankles are normally affected. Fever and chills are common. Joint effusions, when present, are usually small and difficult to tap. The synovial fluid leukocyte count may be less than 50,000 cells/mm^3, and synovial fluid cultures are usually negative. However, blood cultures and cultures of primary sites (e.g., urethra, cervix, rectum) are often positive for *N. gonorrhoeae*. Skin manifestations of disseminated gonococcal disease, which are present in two thirds of cases, are a key to the diagnosis of gonococcal arthritis. The skin lesions, often noted on the extremities, begin as painful maculopapular lesions that become pustular with a central area of necrosis (16,32). The lesions are not specific for gonococcal infection and occasionally may be seen in cases of infection caused by other microorganisms, including *S. aureus*, *N. meningitidis*, group A streptococci, and *H. influenzae*. However, in the right clinical setting, they are helpful in supporting the diagnosis of gonococcal arthritis. The primary genitourinary infection in cases of gonococcal arthritis is often not clinically apparent, and patients may be completely asymptomatic. Disseminated gonococcal infection with arthritis occurs more often in women than in men and is commonly seen during menstruation or pregnancy (2).

Untreated gonococcal polyarthritis may either resolve spontaneously or settle into a single large joint, mimicking nongonococcal arthritis. On rare occasions, monoarticular arthritis caused by *N. gonorrhoeae* may develop in the absence of preceding skin lesions and polyarthritis (33). In both of the aforementioned situations, the synovial fluid findings are similar to those in nongonococcal arthritis, with leukocyte counts in excess of 50,000 cells/mm^3. Joint-fluid cultures for *N. gonorrhoeae* are more likely to be positive, and blood cultures are usually negative. Generally, the higher the synovial fluid leukocyte count is, the more likely the culture is positive. Gonococcal monoarthritis usually responds well to appropriate antimicrobial therapy and percutaneous needle drainage. Open surgical drainage of the joint is rarely needed.

Diagnosis

Septic arthritis must be considered in any patient who presents with one or more acutely swollen joints. As shown in Table 28.4, the differential diagnosis is broad and includes both infectious and noninfectious conditions. Several factors should be considered in making the diagnosis, including the age of the patient, the duration of symptoms, the presence of recent or remote trauma, the status of the patient's immune system, and the possibility of infection at another site (2).

Laboratory features that may help in establishing a diagnosis include the peripheral blood leukocyte count, which is usually mildly increased in septic arthritis but also may be increased in noninfectious inflammatory arthritis (8,31). However, the count in either of these conditions also may be normal. The erythrocyte sedimentation rate and C-reactive protein concentration usually are elevated, reflecting acute inflammation; however, these measurements are not specific for septic arthritis. Peripheral blood cultures are positive for the etiologic organism in 40% to 50% of cases of nongonococcal arthritis but in less than 10% of cases of gonococcal arthritis (2,8). Cultures of the urethra, cervix, rectum, and pharynx should be obtained in cases in which gonococcal arthritis is being considered. If performed correctly with selective culture media for *N. gonorrhoeae*, cultures of the primary site of infection are more likely to be positive than are cultures of blood or synovial fluid (33).

Table 28.4   Differential Diagnosis of the Inflamed Joint

Infectious Arthritis
Nongonococcal arthritis
Infective endocarditis
Gonococcal arthritis
Whipple's disease
Viral arthritis
Lyme disease

Postinfectious Arthritis
Rheumatic fever
Poststreptococcal arthritis

Reactive Arthritis
Reiter's syndrome
Postdysenteric reactive arthritis

Crystal-Induced Arthropathy
Gout
Calcium pyrophosphate deposition disease
Hydroxyapetite crystalline arthritis

Endocrine Diseases
Diabetic neuropathic arthropathy
Hyperparathyroidism
Hyperthyroidism
Hypothyroidism
Acromegaly

Gastrointestinal Diseases
Inflammatory bowel disease
Primary biliary cirrhosis

Metabolic Disorders
Hyperlipoproteinemia
Hemochromatosis
Alkaptonuria (ochronosis)
Wilson's disease

Hematologic Diseases
Sickle cell disease
Hemophilia
Leukemia

Immunologic Diseases
Rheumatoid arthritis
Hypogammaglobulinemia
Systemic lupus erythematosus
Serum sickness

Miscellaneous Disorders
Psoriatic arthritis
Behçet's disease
Osteoarthritis
Amyloidosis
Traumatic arthritis
Familial Mediterranean fever
Sarcoidosis
Sweet's syndrome
Neuropathic joint disease
Hemarthrosis

The most important and helpful diagnostic study in cases of suspected infectious arthritis is the examination of the synovial fluid; therefore, arthrocentesis should be performed on any acutely swollen joint with a clinically apparent effusion. Features of the synovial fluid examination in infectious arthritis compared with those in several noninfectious causes of joint swelling are listed in Table 28.5. The fluid should be analyzed for volume, turbidity, color, and viscosity. Cell analysis should include a total leukocyte count and differential. The normal, noninfected joint has a scant amount of synovial fluid that is nonturbid, viscous, and contains fewer than 200 leukocytes/mm^3. Joint effusions seen in osteoarthritis may have leukocyte counts of up to 2000

Table 28.5 Synovial Fluid Findings in Acute Arthritis

Disorder	Appearance	Viscosity	WBC* (cells/mm^3)	PMNs in WBC	Gram Stain	Culture	Crystals
Osteoarthritis	Clear to mildly turbid	High	200–2000	<30%	Negative	Negative	Negative
Nongonococcal septic arthritis	Turbid, purulent	Low	>50,000	>90%	Positive 75%	Positive 85%–95%	Negative
Gonococcal polyarthritis	Turbid	Low	10,000–50,000	>90%	Positive <25%	Positive 25%	Negative
Gout and pseudogout	Turbid	Low	3000–50,000	—	Negative	Negative	Positive
Rheumatoid arthritis	Turbid	Low	3000–50,000	>70%	Negative	Negative	Negative
Reactive arthritis	Turbid	Low	3000–50,000	>70%	Negative	Negative	Negative

* Cell counts may vary widely

leukocytes/mm^3 and are considered noninflammatory. The joint fluid in non-gonococcal septic arthritis usually has a total count that exceeds 50,000 leukocytes/mm^3, with a predominance of neutrophils. However, the range is broad and the cell count may be low early in the disease (34,35). The cell count in gonococcal polyarthritis and noninfectious arthritis is usually less than 50,000 leukocytes/mm^3.

The joint fluid also should be analyzed for crystals, because crystalline deposition disease may mimic septic arthritis. Polarized light microscopy can be helpful in differentiating gout (characterized by fine, tapered crystals with weakly negative birefringence) and calcium pyrophosphate deposition (broad rhomboid-shaped crystals with strongly positive birefringence) from septic arthritis. It is important to remember that the presence of crystals does not exclude infection, because septic and crystal-induced arthritis may occur simultaneously (36). Synovial fluid glucose, lactic dehydrogenase, and protein levels are abnormal in both infectious and noninfectious arthritis and are of little value in making a specific diagnosis (8). A recent study examined levels of TNF in synovial fluid in infectious and noninfectious arthritis. The results showed that nearly all patients with infectious arthritis had increased TNF levels, and that these levels were significantly higher than those of patients with noninfectious inflammatory arthritis. A similar difference was not seen with other inflammatory cytokines (37). This may become useful as assays for TNF become more readily available.

Gram stain of the synovial fluid is positive in more than 65% of cases of nongonococcal septic arthritis (2). The Gram stain can be quite helpful in the presumptive identification of the etiologic microorganism and in the selection of the initial antimicrobial therapy in patients with suspected septic arthritis. Although the exact identification of the etiologic pathogen is not possible with Gram stain alone, general categorization into gram-positive and -negative organisms narrows the choice of antimicrobial agents considerably. Gram stain is especially helpful in cases in which antimicrobial therapy has been given before joint-fluid analysis, yielding negative cultures. Gram stain should be interpreted by an experienced laboratory technician to avoid false-positive results from artifact or precipitated stain.

The definitive laboratory examination for the diagnosis of infection and the determination of appropriate antimicrobial therapy in suspected septic arthritis is synovial fluid culture. Cultures are positive in nearly all cases of nongonococcal septic arthritis unless the patient has been given an antimicrobial agent (2,8). The specimen should be cultured with both aerobic and anaerobic techniques and on chocolate agar in 5% to 10% carbon dioxide to support the growth of *N. gonorrhoeae* and *N. meningitidis*. In contrast to the situation in nongonococcal arthritis, synovial fluid cultures are positive in less than 25% of cases of gonococcal arthritis (38).

Some investigators have used polymerase chain reaction (PCR) technology to diagnose infectious arthritis caused by fastidious microorganisms or microorganisms that are difficult to culture, such as *Kingella kingae* and *Borrelia burgdorferi* (39). However, this technology is not readily available in the clinical setting and has several limitations, including a high incidence of false-positive results. One study that used PCR to seek viral DNA in joint effusions found DNA sequences of one or more viruses in several patients with early arthritis of a noninfectious cause. The investigators postulated that the viral DNA sequences were actually within the leukocytes and macrophages that had migrated into the inflamed joints and that the viruses from which the sequences had come were unlikely to be the etiologic agents of the arthritis (40). This same problem could occur with bacterial organisms that are harbored intracellularly. Nevertheless, although caution must be exercised in interpreting PCR results, this technology will undoubtedly become more important in the diagnosis of infectious arthritis.

Radiographic studies are of limited value in the diagnosis of septic arthritis. The most common radiographic feature of the disease is periarticular soft tissue swelling. Joint-space widening may be seen early in the disease as the result of effusion. As the disease progresses and the articular cartilage is destroyed, the joint space becomes narrowed (41,42). Rarely, radiographic studies show adjacent bone disease. Computed tomography may help in identifying hip-joint effusions (43). Magnetic resonance imaging is also useful in detecting joint and tendon-sheath effusions (44). However, these studies are expensive and usually unnecessary for the diagnosis of septic arthritis. Technetium-99m bone scans, gallium-67 scans, and indium-111 scans are usually positive in septic arthritis but are of limited value in distinguishing infectious from noninfectious joint disease (45).

Treatment

The treatment of septic arthritis has three facets: antimicrobial therapy, drainage of the infected joint, and restoring normal function of the joint. Because the identity of the infecting pathogen is often unknown, selecting the initial antimicrobial therapy often must be empirical. However, important clues to the identity of the infecting pathogen may be found in the clinical history and physical examination. Predisposing factors and specific clinical settings (*see* Table 28.3) also may suggest a likely pathogen. Additionally, a Gram stain of aspirated synovial fluid is often helpful in separating gram-positive from -negative infection, and the morphology of the microorganism visualized with the stain may suggest a specific bacterial species.

When a specific microorganism cannot be identified, empirical therapy must include one or more antimicrobial agents that are effective against the most likely pathogens for the patient's age group. Once culture results become available, specific therapy (preferably with a single agent) should be selected. Single-drug therapy is sufficient for most infections, including those caused by staphylococci, most streptococci, *Neisseria* species, and most Gram-negative bacilli. To achieve synergy, combination therapy is indicated for infections caused by *Enterococcus faecalis* and *P. aeruginosa*. Infections caused by *viridans* streptococci strains that are intermediately sensitive to penicillin also may respond better to combination therapy than to single-drug therapy (46).

Most antibiotics achieve therapeutic levels in synovial fluid when given systemically in the appropriate dose (47). The practice of injecting an antimicrobial agent directly into a joint is unnecessary and not recommended (48), because it may produce excessively high concentrations of antibiotic in the synovial fluid, increasing the inflammatory response. An exception to this is the use of amphotericin B in treating infectious arthritis caused by fungi, in which intra-articular injection of small doses of the drug has proven safe and effective (49).

Measuring antibacterial activity (ABA) in serum and synovial fluid has been suggested as a means of ensuring that the dose of antimicrobial agent used in a case of septic arthritis is appropriate and that there is adequate penetration of the agent into the infected joint (50). To measure ABA, a sample of the patient's synovial fluid is aspirated approximately 1 hour after administering a dose of antimicrobial agent. The fluid is serially diluted to determine the highest dilution that inhibits *in vitro* growth of the pathogen previously isolated from the fluid. A peak ABA titer of 1:8 or greater in the joint fluid is considered adequate when treating gram-negative bacilli or *S. aureus*, but a titer of 1:32 or greater is suggested for streptococci (51). However, data that support the efficacy of the ABA test in treating joint infections are limited, and this test is generally not recommended or necessary. Even so, it may be considered when using oral antimicrobial therapy to ensure adequate absorption of the orally administered agent.

The optimal duration of antimicrobial therapy for septic arthritis is not well established and varies with the causative pathogen, the adequacy of host defenses, and the clinical response (31,51). Disseminated gonococcal infection with polyarthritis usually is cured with a 7- to 10-day course of antibiotic therapy, whereas acute nongonococcal suppurative arthritis requires a longer duration of therapy. Infections caused by most streptococci and by *H. influenzae* usually respond to a 2-week course of antimicrobial therapy, whereas *S. aureus* and gram-negative bacillus infections are treated for 3 to 4 weeks. If staphylococcal bacteremia occurs, the risk of endocarditis and other metastatic infection often necessitates 4 to 6 weeks of parenteral therapy. The antimicrobial agents of choice for common pathogens that cause septic arthritis are listed in Table 28.6.

The second facet of treatment for septic arthritis is drainage of pus from the affected joint. Drainage decompresses the joint and removes inflammatory cells, degradative enzymes, and fibrinous debris. In nongonococcal suppurative arthritis, adequate drainage is essential for a satisfactory outcome (2). However, the effusions in septic arthritis caused by *N. gonorrhoeae* or *N. meningitidis* are rarely large enough to require drainage, and these conditions respond well with antimicrobial therapy alone. When effusions are present, needle aspiration is almost always adequate and surgical drainage is rarely indicated.

The efficacy of repeated needle aspiration compared with surgical arthrotomy in septic arthritis has long been a subject of debate. No prospective controlled studies have compared medical and surgical drainage. An early study by Goldenberg and coworkers (52) indicated a better result with needle aspiration than with surgical drainage, but the difference was not statistically sig-

Table 28.6   Antimicrobial Agents of Choice for Common Pathogens That Cause Septic Arthritis

Pathogen*	Drug Regimen[†]	Alternative Drugs
Staphylococcus aureus	Nafcillin 2 g IV q6h	Vancomycin, cefazolin, clindamycin
Staphylococcus epidermidis	Vancomycin 1 g IV q12h	TMP-SMX
Methicillin-resistant S. aureus	Vancomycin 1 g IV q12h	TMP-SMX, doxycycline, linezolid
Streptococcus groups A, B, C, and G	Penicillin G 2 MU IV q4h	Vancomycin, cefazolin, erythromycin
Enterococcus faecalis	Penicillin G 2 MU IV q4h (or ampicillin 2 g q6h) + gentamicin 1 mg/kg IM/IV q8h	Vancomycin with gentamicin
Neisseria gonorrhoeae	Ceftriaxone 1 g IV q24h	Spectinomycin, ciprofloxacin, or other quinolones
Neisseria meningitidis	Penicillin G 2 MU IV q4h	Ceftriaxone
Haemophilus influenzae		
beta-Lactamase negative	Ampicillin 2 g IV q6h	Cefuroxime, TMP-SMX
beta-Lactamase positive	Ceftriaxone 2 g IV q24h	TMP-SMX
Pseudomonas aeruginosa	Piperacillin 4 g IV q6h + tobramycin 5–7 mg/kg IV	Ceftazidime with aminoglycoside or ciprofloxacin

IM = intramuscularly; IV = intravenously; MU = million units; TMP-SMX = trimethoprim–sulfamethoxazole.
* Duration of drug regimen is determined by pathogen: 2 weeks for *Streptococcus*, *Haemophilus*, *Neisseria*, and *Enterococcus* species, and 3 weeks for *Staphylococcus* species and gram-negative bacilli.
[†] Dose may vary with body weight and renal function.

nificant. However, the study did clearly show the importance of early therapy to a good outcome. A subsequent retrospective analysis of several studies showed no significant difference in outcome with medical and surgical therapy but did confirm the importance to outcome of early diagnosis and treatment (53). It is very likely that the drainage method used on a joint effusion has little effect on outcome so long as the drainage procedure is effective in removing the effusion.

If needle aspiration is selected as the technique for drainage, the affected joint should be aspirated at least daily until fluid no longer accumulates. Repeat cultures and leukocyte counts on the joint fluid are useful in monitoring the response to therapy. The joint fluid should become sterile over a period of 48 to 96 hours, and the leukocyte count should steadily decline. Positive synovial fluid cultures after 7 days of therapy and high synovial fluid leukocyte counts after 5 days are associated with a poor outcome (54). Therefore, if fluid continues to reaccumulate after 2 to 3 days of needle aspiration or if there is worsening of systemic sepsis, surgical drainage should be considered.

Recent advances in arthroscopic technique have made surgical drainage of infected joints more attractive and, in most cases, the preferred approach (55). Open surgical drainage usually is reserved for severe infections with loculated debris within the infected joint and for infections involving the shoulder and hip. Hip infections require open surgical arthrotomy to relieve the pressure on intracapsular vascular structures completely and to prevent ischemic destruction of the epiphyseal plate or femoral head (56). In most other cases, arthroscopic drainage is preferable to repeated needle aspiration.

Many surgeons insert a closed suction drainage system postoperatively to irrigate an infected joint continuously and to deliver intra-articular antimicrobial agents. This practice has not proven beneficial and is probably unnecessary, because most systemically administered antimicrobial agents reach adequate levels in synovial fluid (48). Furthermore, local antimicrobial therapy does not eliminate the need for systemic therapy. Systems for irrigating the joint space function well only for a short time and serve as a potential source of superinfection in the joint (57). If used, these irrigation systems should remain in place for no longer than 48 hours. Irrigating an infected joint with an antimicrobial solution at the time of arthroscopy is sometimes done, but its efficacy has not been established.

Traditionally, intra-articular corticosteroids have been contraindicated in the treatment of acute septic arthritis. However, recent studies in a rabbit model of staphylococcal septic arthritis and anecdotal reports with human patients have suggested that, when used in conjunction with appropriate antimicrobial therapy, corticosteroids may help decrease synovitis in such disease (58,59). The rationale for using corticosteroids is to decrease cytokine production and to diminish the activation of chondrocyte proteases, which con-

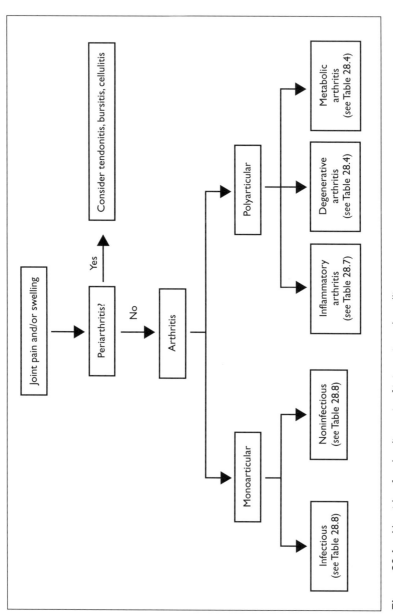

Figure 28.1   Algorithm for the diagnosis of joint pain and swelling.

tribute to the inflammatory response and to joint damage. In the rabbit model, the use of intra-articular corticosteroids produced improvement in joint histologic–histochemical parameters without adverse effects (58). There may be clinical settings in which corticosteroids are a useful adjunct in treating septic arthritis, but further studies of this are needed. For now, the use of systemic or intra-articular corticosteroids remains controversial and is not recommended.

The third facet of treatment for septic arthritis is the restoration of normal function of the affected joint. During the initial presentation and early treatment period, any movement of the joint can be very painful. Immobilization during this phase of treatment alleviates pain; however, after adequate decompression and a response to initial treatment, passive motion should be initiated to prevent fibrous adhesions and permanent joint injury (60). Whenever possible, continuous passive motion is preferred to intermittent passive or active motion. When the inflammatory process is controlled, appropriate physical therapy may be required to ensure the return of normal joint function.

Outcome

Several factors have been identified as important in influencing the outcome of septic arthritis. These include the causative microorganism, the duration of symptoms before the beginning of appropriate antimicrobial therapy, the adequacy of drainage of the infected joint, the particular joint or joints involved, and the host factors of age and underlying disease (3,7,31,54). Generally, gonococcal arthritis has a much better prognosis than does nongonococcal arthritis and rarely requires surgery (7). Arthritis caused by gram-negative or anaerobic bacteria has been associated with a poor outcome in some series but not in others (2,21,24,31); however, more important than the microbial cause is the presence of underlying disease, because most deaths of patients with septic arthritis occur in those with serious underlying or chronic disease (3,31). The overall mortality rate for nongonococcal septic arthritis is approximately 10% but varies with the aforementioned factors (3).

Delay in instituting appropriate antimicrobial therapy is associated with a poor outcome in septic arthritis. The duration of symptoms before therapy is begun is inversely related to outcome (4,34,54). The outcome also is related to the time required to sterilize the synovial fluid after therapy has begun. Patients in whom this requires more than 7 days have a poor outcome (54). The synovial fluid leukocyte response also can be used as a prognostic indicator, because patients with persistently high synovial fluid leukocyte counts on repeated aspirations have a poor outcome (3).

Table 28.7   Differential Diagnosis of Acute Polyarticular Inflammatory Arthritis

Symmetrical	Asymmetrical
Rheumatoid arthritis	Neisseria infection
Systemic lupus erythematosis	Lyme disease
Other connective tissue diseases	Sarcoidosis
Crystal deposition disease	Henoch–Schönlein purpura
Hepatitis B	Ankylosing spondylitis
Rubella	Reiter's syndrome
Subacute bacterial endocarditis	Enteropathic arthropathy
Rheumatic fever	Psoriatic arthritis
Hypersensitivity reactions	Behçet's syndrome
Psoriatic arthritis	Whipple's disease

Table 28.8   Differential Diagnosis of Acute Monoarticular Arthritis

Infection
Trauma
Crystal-induced arthropathy
Hemarthrosis
Neuropathic joint
Mechanical internal derangement
Reactive (e.g., Reiter's disease, enteric-associated diseases)

Algorithms for Acute Joint Pain

The patient who complains chiefly of joint pain presents a diagnostic challenge for the primary care physician. A systematic approach, beginning with a thorough medical history and comprehensive physical examination, is essential in establishing the correct diagnosis. Figure 28.1 is an algorithm that illustrates the approach to patients with joint pain with or without swelling. First, a clinical evaluation should be performed to determine whether the pain is more likely the result of a periarticular inflammation (e.g., tendonitis, bursitis, cellulitis) or the result of a true arthritis. Although infection must always be considered, many cases of polyarticular arthritis have a noninfectious cause (*see* Table 28.4). Additionally, polyarticular inflammatory arthritis can be divided into those conditions that present with a symmetrical arthritis and those that present with an asymmetrical arthritis (Table 28.7). The major causes of acute monoarticular arthritis are listed in Table 28.8. It is important to recognize that there is considerable overlap among the causes of polyarticular and monoarticular disease.

Figure 28.2 is an algorithm that illustrates the approach to patients with monoarticular arthritis, but it also can be applied to the patient with polyarthritis. If a joint effusion is present, arthrocentesis is indicated. In the ab-

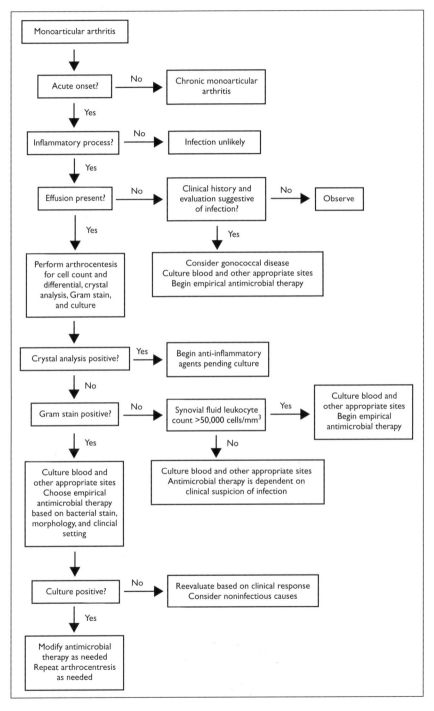

Figure 28.2 Algorithm for the management of monoarticular arthritis.

sence of an effusion, especially in the patient with polyarthritis, gonococcal disease should be considered. Synovial fluid leukocyte counts greater than 50,000 cells/mm^3 strongly support an infectious cause; however, cell counts of this magnitude may be found occasionally in crystal-induced arthritis. The decision about whether or not to begin antimicrobial therapy depends on both clinical and laboratory findings, and the initial choice of antimicrobial agent is often empirical. Once culture results are available, the clinical response should be assessed and antimicrobial therapy should be altered, if appropriate. If the culture results are negative, noninfectious causes should be reconsidered.

REFERENCES

1. **Fink CW.** Reactive arthritis. *Pediatr Infect Dis J.* 1988;7:58–65.

2. **Goldenberg DL, Reed JI.** Bacterial arthritis. *N Engl J Med.* 1985;312:764–71.

3. **Goldenberg DL, Cohen AS.** Acute infectious arthritis: a review of patients with non-gonococcal joint infections (with emphasis on therapy and prognosis). *Am J Med.* 1976;60:369–77.

4. **Kelly PJ, Martin WJ, Coventry MB.** Bacterial (suppurative) arthritis in adults. *J Bone Joint Surg.* 1970;52A:1595–1602.

5. **Daniel D, Akeson W, Amiel D, et al.** Lavage of septic joints in rabbits: effects of chondrolysis. *J Bone Joint Surg.* 1976;58-A:393–5.

6. **Nilsson M, Lee JC, Bremell T, et al.** The role of staphylococcal polysaccharide microcapsule expression in septicemia and septic arthritis. *Infect Immun.* 1997;65:4216–21.

7. **Manshady BM, Thompson GR, Weiss JJ.** Septic arthritis in a general hospital, 1966–77. *J Rheumatol.* 1980;7:523–30.

8. **Sharp JT, Lidsky MD, Duffy J, Duncan MW.** Infectious arthritis. *Arch Intern Med.* 1979;139:1125–30.

9. **Goldenberg DL.** Infectious arthritis complicating rheumatoid arthritis and other chronic rheumatic disorders. *Arthritis Rheum.* 1989;32:496–502.

10. **Sherman OH, Fox JM, Snyder SJ.** Arthroscopy: no problem surgery. *J Bone Joint Surg.* 1986;68A:256–65.

11. **Kuipers, JG, Kohler L, Zeidler H.** Reactive or infectious arthritis. *Ann Rheum Dis.* 1999;58:661–4.

12. **Keat A.** Reiter's syndrome and reactive arthritis in perspective. *N Engl J Med.* 1983;309:1606–15.

13. **Gardnerr GC, Weisman MH.** Pyarthrosis in patients with rheumatoid arthritis: a report of 13 cases and a review of the literature from the past 40 years. *Am J Med.* 1990;88:503–11.

14. **Reiman P, Gardner W.** Septic arthritis. In: Fu FH, Harner CD, Vince KG (eds). *Knee Surgery.* Baltimore: Williams and Wilkins; 1994:443–55.

15. **Cooper C, Cawley MID.** Bacterial arthritis in an English health district: a 10 year review. *Ann Rheum Dis.* 1986;45:458–63.

16. **Rompalo AM, Hook III EW, Roberts PL, et al.** The acute arthritis-dermatitis syndrome. The changing importance of *Neisseria gonorrhoeae* and *Neisseria meningitidis.* *Arch Intern Med.* 1987;147:281–3.

17. **Roca RP, Yoshikawa TT.** Primary skeletal infections in heroin users: a clinical characterization, diagnosis and therapy. *Clin Orthop Rel Res.* 1979;144:238–48.

18. **Gifford DB, Patzakis M, Ivler D, Swezey RL.** Septic arthritis due to Pseudomonas in heroin addicts. *J Bone Joint Surg.* 1975;57a:631–5.

19. **Chmel H, Armstrong D.** Acute arthritis caused by *Aeromonas hydrophila. Arthritis Rheum.* 1976;19:169.

20. **Newman ED, Davis DE, Harrington TM.** Septic arthritis due to gram negative bacilli: older patients with good outcome. *J Rheum.* 1988;15:659–62.

21. **Medina F, Fraga A, Lavalle C.** *Salmonella* septic arthritis in systemic lupus erythematous. The importance of chronic carrier state. *J Rheumatol.* 1989;16:203–8.

22. **Ewing R, Fainstein V, Musher D, et al.** Articular and skeletal infections caused by *Pasteurella multocida. South Med J.* 1980;73:1349–52.

23. **Bilos ZJ, Kucharchuk A, Metzger W.** *Eikenella corrodens* in human bites. *Clin Orthop Rel Res.* 1978;134:320–4.

24. **Fitzgerald RH, Rosenblatt JE, Tenney JH, Bourgault AM.** Anaerobic septic arthritis. *Clin Orthop Rel Res.* 1982;164:141–8.

25. **Gredlein CM, Silverman ML, Downey MS.** Polymicrobial septic arthritis due to *Clostridium* species: case report and review. *Clin Infect Dis.* 2000;30:590–4.

26. **Tingle AJ, Allen M, Petty RE.** Rubella-associated arthritis. Comparative study of joint manifestations associated with natural rubella infection and RA27/3 rubella immunization. *Ann Rheum Dis.* 1986;45:110–4.

27. **Hyer FH, Gottlieb NL.** Rheumatic syndromes associated with hepatitis B antigenemia. *IM.* 1981;2:43–9.

28. **Gordon SC, Lauter CB.** Mumps arthritis: a review of the literature. *Rev Infect Dis.* 1984;6:338–344.

29. **Woolf AD, Campion GV, Chishick A, et al.** Clinical manifestations of human parvovirus B19 in adults. *Arch Intern Med.* 1989;149:1153–6.

30. **Rynes RI, Goldenberg DL, Digiacoma R, et al.** Acquired immunodeficiency syndrome-associated arthritis. *Am J Med.* 1988;84:810–6.

31. **Rosenthal J, Bole GG, Robinson WD.** Acute nongonococcal infectious arthritis. Evaluation of risk factors, therapy, and outcome. *Arthritis Rheum.* 1980;23:889–96.

32. **Keiser H, Ruben FL, Wolinsky E, Kushner I.** Clinical forms of gonococcal arthritis. *N Engl J Med.* 1968;279:234–40.

33. **Gelfand SG, Masi AT, Garcia-Kutzbach A.** Spectrum of gonococcal arthritis: Evidence for sequential stages and clinical subgroups. *J Rheumatol.* 1975;2:83–90.

34. **Argen RJ, Wilson CH, Wood P.** Suppurative arthritis. *Arch Intern Med.* 1966; 117:661–6.

35. **McCutchan HJ, Fisher RC.** Synovial leukocytosis in infectious arthritis. *Clin Orthop Rel Res.* 1990;256:226–30.

36. **Baer PA, Tenebaum J, Fam AG.** Coexistent septic and crystal arthritis. Report of four cases and literature review. *J Rheumatol.* 1986;13:3.

37. **Jeng GW, Wang CR, Liu ST, et al.** Measurement of synovial tumor necrosis factor in diagnosing emergency patients with bacterial arthritis. *Am J Emerg Med.* 1997; 15:626–9.

38. **O'Brian JP, Goldenberg DL, Rice PA.** Disseminated gonococcal infection: a prospective analysis of 49 patients and a review of pathophysiology and immune mechanisms. *Medicine.* 1983;62:395–406.

39. **Yagupsky P.** Diagnosis of *Kingella kingae* arthritis by polymerase chain reaction analysis. *Clin Infect Dis.* 1999;29:704–5.

40. **Stahl H, Hubner B, Seidl B, Liebert UG.** Detection of multiple viral DNA species in synovial tissue and fluid of patients with early arthritis. *Ann Rheum Dis.* 2000;59:342–6.

41. **Mitchell M, Howard B, Haller J.** Septic arthritis. *Radiol Clin North Am.* 1988;26: 1295–1313.

42. **Gelman MI, Ward JR.** Septic arthritis: a complication of rheumatoid arthritis. *Radiology.* 1977;122:17–23.

43. **Hendrix RW, Fisher MR.** Imaging of septic arthritis. *Clin Rheum Dis.* 1986;12:459–77.

44. **Beltran J, Noto AM, McGhee RB.** Infections of the musculoskeletal system: High-field-strength MR imaging. *Radiology.* 1987;164:449–54.

45. **Tumeh SS.** Scintigraphy in the evaluation of arthropathy. *Radiol Clin North Am.* 1996; 34:215–31.

46. **Johnson CC, Tunkel AL.** Viridans streptococci and groups C and G streptococci. In: Mandell GL, Douglas RG, Bennett JE (eds). *Principles and Practice of Infectious Diseases,* 5th ed. New York: Churchill Livingstone; 2000:2167–83.

47. **Nelson J.** Antibiotic concentrations in septic joint effusions. *N Eng J Med.* 1971;284: 349–53.

48. **Parker RH, Schmid FR.** Antibacterial activity of synovial fluid during therapy of septic arthritis. *Arthritis Rheum.* 1971;14:96–104.

49. **Downs NJ, Hinthorn D, Mhatre VR, Liu C.** Intra-articular amphotericin B treatment of *Sporothrix schenckii* arthritis. *Arch Intern Med.* 1989;149:954–5.

50. **Sattar MA, Barrett SP, Cawley MID.** Concentrations of some antibiotics in synovial fluid after oral administration, with special reference to antistaphylococcal activity. *Ann Rheum Dis.* 1983;42:67–74.

51. **Syrogiannopoulos GA, Nelson JD.** Duration of antimicrobial therapy for acute suppurative osteoarticular infections. *Lancet.* 1988;37–40.

52. **Goldenberg DL, Brandt KD, Cohen AS, Cathcart ES.** Treatment of septic arthritis: comparison of needle aspiration and surgery as initial modes of joint drainage. *Arthritis Rheum.* 1975;18:83–90.

53. **Broy SB, Schmid FR.** A comparison of medical drainage (needle aspiration) and surgical drainage (arthrotomy or arthroscopy) in the initial treatment of infected joints. *Clin Rheum Dis.* 1986;12:501–22.

54. **Ho G, Su EY.** Therapy for septic arthritis. *JAMA.* 1986;247:797–800.

55. **Jackson RW.** The septic knee: arthroscopic treatment. *Arthroscopy.* 1985;1:194–7.

56. **Wilson N, DiPaola M.** Acute septic arthritis in infancy and childhood: 10 year experience. *J Bone Joint Surg.* 1986;68B:584–7.

57. **Sledge CB.** Surgery in infectious arthritis. *Clin Rheum Dis.* 1978;4:159–65.

58. **Wysenbeek AJ, Volchek J, Amit M, et al.** Treatment of staphylococcal septic arthritis in rabbits by systemic antibiotics and intra-articular corticosteroids. *Ann Rheum Dis.* 1998;57:687–90.

59. **Lane SE, Merry P.** Intra-articular corticosteroids in septic arthritis: beneficial or barmy? *Ann Rheum Dis.* 2000;59:240.

60. **Salter RB.** The biologic concept of continuous passive motion of synovial joints. *Clin Orthop.* 1989;242:12–25.

29

Osteomyelitis

Jon T. Mader, MD
Jue Wang, MD
Mark E. Shirtliff, PhD
Jason Calhoun, MD

Osteomyelitis is commonly characterized by infection of the cortical and/or medullary portions of bone. The term *osteo* refers to bone and the term *myelo* to the marrow cavity, both of which are involved in the disease. Osteomyelitis is progressive and results in the inflammatory destruction of bone, in bone necrosis, and in new bone formation. Although there are many etiologic microorganisms, osteomyelitis is predominantly of bacterial origin.

Etiology

For the purpose of discussing the etiology of osteomyelitis, Waldvogel's staging system (Table 29.1) is used because it is based on the etiology of the infection (1–3). His staging system describes three categories of osteomyelitis: hematogenous osteomyelitis, osteomyelitis with a contiguous focus, and osteomyelitis associated with a vascular insufficiency. Additionally, each of these categories can be either acute or chronic.

Acute Osteomyelitis

Acute Hematogenous Osteomyelitis
Hematogenous osteomyelitis occurs primarily in infants and children. In these cases, the disease most often begins in the tibial and femoral metaphyses, be-

Table 29.1 Osteomyelitis: Waldvogel's Classification

Hematogenous osteomyelitis
Osteomyelitis due to contiguous focus of infection
No generalized vascular disease
Generalized vascular disease
Chronic osteomyelitis (necrotic bone)

cause the anatomy and histology of the long-bone metaphyses make them susceptible to infection (4). In the metaphyses, the nonanastomosing capillary ends of the nutrient arteries that supply the bone make sharp loops in the area of the epiphyseal growth plates and enter a system of sinusoidal veins connected with the venous network of the medullary cavity. There are no functionally active phagocytic cells in the lining of the afferent loops of these metaphyseal capillaries, and blood flow through them slows considerably and becomes more turbulent (5). For these reasons, any obstruction of the capillary ends can lead to avascular necrosis. Because children bear the greatest amount of mechanical stress on their epiphyseal growth plates, they are at greater risk than are adults or infants for trauma in this area. When minor trauma occurs in an infant, it may cause a small hematoma or bone necrosis, which can be invaded by an infecting pathogen. The targets of infection are the large sinusoids that form from the terminal vessels of the growth plates.

At the onset of hematogenous osteomyelitis, the acute infection is regularly focal. Subsequently, many cumulative physiologic factors add to the extension of the infection by compromising the medullary circulation. These factors include leukocyte breakdown, increased bone pressure, decreased pH, and decreased oxygen tension. As it progresses, the infection swells laterally through haversian and Volkmann's canal systems, perforating the bony cortex and lifting the periosteum from the surface of the bone. At this point in the progression of the disease, the periosteal and endosteal circulations are lost, leaving large segments of dead cortical and cancellous bone. In infants, because capillaries extend across the growth plate, infection can spread into the epiphysis and the joint space. In children over 1 year of age, the capillaries no longer penetrate the growth plate, and therefore the epiphysis and joint space are protected from spreading infection. However, because the growth plate in adults has been resorbed completely, infection can pass into the joint space. A single pathogenic species is most commonly recovered from bone cultures of hematogenous osteomyelitis, with *Staphylococcus aureus* being the most commonly isolated organism (6).

Although normally described as a disease of children, hematogenous osteomyelitis has been reported in older age groups. In adults, hematogenous osteomyelitis usually occurs in the vertebrae or in the bones of the wrist and ankle. It is thought that vertebral osteomyelitis begins with an infected embolus within the vertebral body. The resulting ischemia and infarct lead to bone destruction and to the infection's spread into the contiguous disk space. The lumbar vertebral bodies are the most common sites of infection in vertebral osteomyelitis, followed by (in order of frequency of infection) the thoracic and cervical vertebrae. The infection can spread rapidly in the axial skeleton via the abundant venous networks of the spine. Commonly, patients with vertebral osteomyelitis have a history of chronic skin infections, urinary tract infections, and intravenous drug use. The osteomyelitis in such cases is typically monomicrobial, with *S. aureus* again being the most frequent pathogen (1–3).

Acute Osteomyelitis Secondary to a Contiguous Focus of Infection with Normal Vascularity

Contiguous osteomyelitis occurs when bacteria are introduced exogenously into bone by trauma or by the extension of an adjacent soft tissue infection. The most common factors that contribute to contiguous osteomyelitis are open fractures, joint infections, and soft tissue infections. Traumatic injury often deprives the bone and surrounding tissues of vascularization, providing a good matrix for the survival of bacteria. Another important source of contiguous osteomyelitis is an infection that originates from surgical contamination, including that of hardware and joint prosthetic devices. The most common site of contiguous osteomyelitis is the tibia, and the most common cause is trauma (6). This is because the mid-portion of the tibia lacks dense vascularity and has little surrounding soft tissue, which limits its degree of protection and recovery from injury. Bone necrosis, soft tissue damage, and loss of bone stability often result from this form of osteomyelitis. Unlike hematogenous osteomyelitis, multiple species of organisms are often isolated from the infected bone in contiguous osteomyelitis, with *S. aureus* and *S. epidermidis* the most prevalent pathogens. Also isolated are gram-negative bacilli and anaerobic microorganisms.

Acute Osteomyelitis Secondary to a Contiguous Focus of Infection with Generalized Vascular Insufficiency

Neuropathy, ischemia, and immunopathy are the three pathophysiologic factors responsible for infection in the diabetic foot (7,8). Neuropathy and vascular compromise make the feet of diabetic individuals more susceptible to minor trauma (e.g., skin ulceration, tissue breakdown) and, along with immunopathy, set the stage for infection (8). One third of diabetic foot infections that require hospitalization are accompanied by osteomyelitis; in such cases, the small bones of the feet are the most common sites of infection. A delayed inflammatory response, stemming from poor tissue perfusion, predisposes the bone to infection in these patients. The disease begins in a claudicated area of traumatized skin. Most often, the infection gains entry through a cutaneous portal (e.g., a diabetic foot ulcer), which leads to cellulitis. Although it is only a local infection, the cellulitis can spread contiguously to tendons, a joint capsule, or bone. However, only when the infection penetrates the medullary cavity can the resulting condition be diagnosed as osteomyelitis. Osteomyelitis is present if a diabetic foot ulcer extends to the bone. Multiple aerobic organisms are isolated from the infected bone in such cases. Additionally, because of the ischemic environment, anaerobic organisms are often isolated from the infected bone as well.

Chronic Osteomyelitis

Although the pathologies of acute and chronic osteomyelitis are similar, some characteristics that are unique to each of these two states of infection distinguish them from one another. Pathologic features of chronic osteomyelitis are the presence of necrotic bone, the formation of new bone, and the exudation of polymorphonuclear leukocytes joined by large numbers of lymphocytes, histiocytes, and occasionally plasma cells.

The hallmark of chronic osteomyelitis is infected dead bone within a compromised soft tissue envelope. The cause of the infection is variable: Pathogenic organisms can reach the bone through hematogenous seeding, open trauma, or contiguous spread. Once the infection is established, an involucrum of fibrous tissue and chronic inflammatory cells forms around the granulations and dead bone. After the infection is contained, there is a decrease in vascularization of the infection site, and the metabolic demands of an effective inflammatory response cannot be satisfied. The revascularization and resorption of the dead bone and scar tissue are similarly affected. The process of resorption eventually subsides, and the haversian canals are sealed by scar tissue. The bacteria responsible for the infection are enclosed in a glycocalyx and are metabolically inactive. The coexistence of infected, nonviable tissues and an ineffective host response leads to chronicity of the infection. The nidus of persistent contamination must be removed before the infection can regress.

New bone formation is another characteristic of chronic osteomyelitis. New bone develops from the surviving fragments of periosteum, endosteum, and cortex in the region of the infection and is produced by a vascular reaction to the infection. The newly forming bone may extend outward from the periosteum and along the intact periosteal and endosteal surfaces, thereby surrounding the dead bone and forming an involucrum. This involucrum is irregularly shaped and contains openings through which pus may permeate into the surrounding soft tissues, forming a sinus tract that allows pus to travel from the involucrum to the skin surface. The involucrum may increase in density gradually and form part or all of a new bone shaft. Depending on the size of the affected bone and the duration of the infection, the amount and density of the new bone may increase progressively for weeks or months. New endosteal bone may proliferate and obstruct the medullary canal. Once the sequestrum has been removed surgically, the remaining cavity may be filled with new bone, especially in children. In adults, however, the cavity may persist or may be filled with fibrous tissue that connects with the skin surface through a sinus tract.

Clinical Manifestations

Local findings that lead to the diagnosis of osteomyelitis are often absent in neonates (9). When present, these local findings include edema and decreased motion of a limb. A joint effusion adjacent to the site of bone infection is present in 60% to 70% of cases of osteomyelitis. In contrast with infants, children with hematogenous osteomyelitis have fever of abrupt onset, irritability, lethargy, and local signs of inflammation that are typically present for 3 weeks or less from the time that the bone infection began. Although there may be a minimal increase in temperature, systemic toxicity is absent in 50% of children with hematogenous osteomyelitis. Children with the disease have complaints referable to the involved bone, such as pain of 1- to 3-months' duration in the affected limb. Infants and children with hematogenous osteomyelitis usually have normal soft tissue that envelops the infected bone and are capable of an efficient immune response to the infection.

In hematogenous vertebral osteomyelitis in adults, the clinical signs of soft tissue extension often dominate the findings at presentation and may lead to misdiagnosis and improper treatment, unless the possibility of osteomyelitis is considered. Patients with hematogenous vertebral osteomyelitis present with vague symptoms and signs that include dull, constant back pain, spasms of the paravertebral muscles, point tenderness over the involved vertebral body, and no (or only a low-grade) fever. There is localized pain and tenderness of the involved bone segments in at least 90% of cases (10). The pain, usually of insidious onset, progresses slowly over a period from 3 weeks to 3 months. An acute clinical presentation of chills, swelling, and erythema over the involved bone is seen occasionally.

The clinical features of osteomyelitis with a contiguous focus and normal vascularity include low-grade fever, local pain, draining sinuses, tenderness, and erythema over the involved bone. The infection usually manifests within 1 month after the inoculation of organism(s) via trauma, surgery, or soft tissue infection. The patient is often afebrile and frequently has loss of bone stability, bone necrosis, and soft tissue damage. In patients who have vascular disease, the clinical features are more subtle and are usually associated with foot ulcers, which render this form of bone infection difficult to diagnose. Patients can present with an apparently localized process that includes an ingrown toenail, a perforating foot ulcer, cellulitis, or a deep-space infection. Furthermore, concurrent peripheral neuropathy often blunts the patient's perception of pain. Fever and toxicity are frequently absent.

There are no exact criteria for defining the transition from acute to chronic osteomyelitis. The hallmark of chronic osteomyelitis is the presence of dead bone (1–3). Involucrum, local bone loss, persistent drainage, and/or sinus tracts are the common features of chronic osteomyelitis. Patients with chronic osteomyelitis present with chronic pain and drainage. Fever is usually of a low grade or is absent. The erythrocyte sedimentation rate (ESR) is often increased, reflecting chronic inflammation; however, the leukocyte count is usually normal. Squamous cell carcinoma and amyloidosis are rare complications of chronic osteomyelitis.

Classification

Osteomyelitis can be classified by duration, pathogenesis, location, extent, and host status. Osteomyelitis is currently classified according to Waldvogel's (see Table 29.1) or the Cierny–Mader (Table 29.2) system (1–3,11). Although Waldvogel's system remains the most popular classification system, it is limited to the etiology of the infection and does not lend itself well to the identification of different clinical features of the disease for diagnosis and treatment. For this reason, the Cierny–Mader classification system is used in this chapter as a model for discussion of the diagnosis and treatment of osteomyelitis. It is based on the anatomy of the bone infection and the physiology of the host and allows the staging of long-bone osteomyelitis and the development of comprehensive treatment guidelines for each stage of the disease.

The Cierny–Mader classification is based on the status of the disease process, regardless of etiology, localization, or chronicity. The anatomical categories of osteomyelitis in the Cierny–Mader system are medullary, superficial, localized, and diffuse. Stage 1, or medullary osteomyelitis, denotes an infection that is confined to the intramedullary surfaces of the bone (e.g., hematogenous osteomyelitis, infection of intramedullary rods). Stage 2, or superficial osteomyelitis (a true contiguous-focus infection of bone), occurs when an exposed, infected, or necrotic surface of bone lies at the base of a soft tissue wound. Stage 3 or localized osteomyelitis is usually characterized by a full-thickness cortical sequestration that can be removed surgically without compromising bone stability. Stage 4, or diffuse osteomyelitis, is a process that involves all structural components of the bone; its arrest usually requires an

Table 29.2 Cierny and Mader Staging System

Anatomic Type

Stage 1—Medullary osteomyelitis
Stage 2—Superficial osteomyelitis
Stage 3—Localized osteomyelitis
Stage 4—Diffuse osteomyelitis

Physiologic Class

Type A host—Normal host
Type B host—Systemically compromised host (Bs)
  Local compromise (Bl)
  Systemic & local compromise (Bls)
Type C host—Treatment worse than the disease

Systemic or Local Factors That Affect Immune Surveillance, Metabolism, and Local Vascularity

Systemic (Bs)

Malnutrition
Renal, hepatic failure
Diabetes mellitus
Chronic hypoxia
Immune disease
Malignancy
Extremes of age
Immunosuppression or immune deficiency

Local (Bl)

Chronic lymphedema
Venous stasis
Major vessel compromise
Arteritis
Extensive scarring
Radiation fibrosis
Small vessel disease
Neuropathy
Tobacco abuse

intercalary resection of the bone. Diffuse osteomyelitis includes infections in which there is a loss of bone stability, either before or after debridement surgery.

According to the Cierny–Mader system, the patient is classified as an A, B, or C host (*see* Table 29.2): An A host represents a patient with normal physiologic, metabolic, and immunologic capabilities; a B host is either systemically compromised, locally compromised, or both; and a C host is a patient in whom the morbidity of treatment is worse than that of the disease itself. The terms acute and chronic osteomyelitis are not used in this staging system, because areas of macronecrosis must be removed regardless of the acuity or chronicity of an uncontrolled infection. The stages of osteomyelitis in the Cierny–Mader system are dynamic and may be altered by treatment or by changes in the host.

Diagnosis

It is important that the physician recognize the clinical signs of osteomyelitis in its earliest stages. Most presentations of osteomyelitis, such as radiographic features or draining sinus tracts, are late complications of the disease. When osteomyelitis is first discovered through radiographic manifestations, the diagnosis is already late and the treatment is more costly and difficult. Making the diagnosis at an early stage gives the patient the best opportunity for full recovery.

Culture and Microbiology

The most determinate diagnostic tool for osteomyelitis is isolation of the causative pathogen through bone, blood, or joint culture (12–14). With stage 1 hematogenous osteomyelitis, a blood or joint culture can eliminate the need for a bone biopsy when radiographs and nucleotide scans show evidence of osteomyelitis. It should be noted that only 50% of patients with hematogenous osteomyelitis have positive blood cultures; however, for all other stages of the disease, it is necessary to obtain a bone culture from debridement surgery or deep bone biopsy to make a diagnosis. Sinus tract culture should not be used as a diagnostic technique because it has proven a poor indicator of gram-negative infection (15). Antimicrobial treatment of osteomyelitis should be based on susceptibility tests of culture isolates. If possible, the cultures should be made before any antibiotic is given and after the patient has ceased receiving antibiotic therapy for 24 to 48 hours. Furthermore, both fungi and mycobacteria should be considered to be pathogens in immunocompromised patients. In osteomyelitis that occurs after a foot-puncture wound, *Pseudomonas aeruginosa* is the most commonly found organism.

Hematologic Findings

In acute osteomyelitis, there is leukergy, increased ESR, and increased C-reactive protein (CRP) level and white blood cell (WBC) count before treatment is begun (16–18). In cases of chronic disease, the WBC count rarely exceeds

15,000 cells/mm3 and is most often normal. The ESR, CRP level, and WBC count may fall with appropriate treatment, but they often increase after debridement surgery. Return of the ESR and CRP to normal during the course of therapy is a favorable prognostic sign.

Imaging Studies

Radiologic evaluation of osteomyelitis can be used to support or refute clinically suspected disease; no radiologic technique can confirm or rule out the presence of osteomyelitis absolutely. Because the radiologic approaches and techniques used for investigating osteomyelitis are numerous and diverse, there is confusion about which is most effective.

It is difficult to interpret changes on plain radiography in early stage 1 osteomyelitis, because the changes often lag behind the evolution of infection by at least 2 weeks (19). The first radiographic changes to occur are soft tissue swelling, periosteal thickening, and focal osteopenia; however, these findings are subtle and often missed. The most diagnostic changes are delayed and occur in association with an indolent infection of several months' duration. It should be remembered that at the beginning of antibiotic therapy, the patient shows clinical improvement before radiographic improvement is evident.

In stage 2 osteomyelitis, the outer cortex of the bone is involved. In these cases there is evidence of periosteal thickening and/or sclerosis. Osteomyelitis of stages 3 and 4 may be more evident than the disease in its earlier stages; soft tissue swelling, osteopenia, lytic changes, and sclerosis are all characteristic findings. Small and large sequestra also may be present. Because of the degree of sclerosis and nonspecific radiographic changes, it is often difficult to estimate the scope of the infection by visualization on films. Therefore, the physician must carefully evaluate the disease clinically and possibly surgically as well. Although it is the least sensitive diagnostic technique, plain radiography is the most informative technique when there is a clinical suspicion of osteomyelitis.

Radionucleotide scans, computed tomography (CT), and magnetic resonance imaging (MRI) are often used to diagnose osteomyelitis in cases in which it is ambiguous and to determine the extent of bone and soft tissue infection. In most cases, these diagnostic tests are not required for osteomyelitis of the long bones.

The technetium-99m methyldiphosphonate scan demonstrates increased isotope accumulation in areas of osteoblastic activity and increased vascularity (20). A second class of radiopharmaceuticals used for the evaluation of osteomyelitis includes gallium-67 citrate and indium-111 chloride; both become bound to transferrin, which leaks from the blood into areas of inflammation. These scans also show increased isotope uptake in malignant tumors and in areas in which polymorphonuclear leukocytes or macrophages are concentrated. Because they do not show bone detail well, these scans do not readily distinguish between bone and soft tissue inflammation. Three-phase technitium-99m methyldiphosphonate scans help resolve this problem.

Indium-111–labeled leukocyte scans are less useful in the evaluation of chronic osteomyelitis (21). These scans are positive in approximately 40% of patients with acute osteomyelitis and in 60% of patients with septic arthritis. Chronic osteomyelitis, bony metastases, and degenerative arthritis often yield negative scans.

Computed axial tomography (CAT) may be useful in the diagnosis of osteomyelitis by measuring the increased marrow density that occurs early in the infection (22). CAT is also useful in identifying areas of devitalized bone, and reveals the involvement of surrounding soft tissues. In a difficult infection, the CAT scan may assist in selecting the most appropriate surgical approach (23).

Magnetic resonance imaging has become the most useful diagnostic tool for identifying and determining the extent of musculoskeletal sepsis (24,25). The spatial resolution of MRI makes it useful in differentiating bone from soft tissue infections. MRI displays greater anatomic detail than does radionuclide scanning and has greater specificity for abnormalities than do either CT or radiography. Moreover, MRI does not expose patients to ionizing radiation. The main disadvantage of MRI is its poor resolution of the cortex, which could yield many false-negative results in cases of isolated cortical infection (26).

Initial MRI screening usually consists of both T1- and T2-weighted spin echo pulse sequences. In a T1-weighted study, edema and fluid are dark, whereas fat (including the fatty marrow of bone) is bright. In a T2-weighted study, the reverse is true. The typical appearance of osteomyelitis is of a localized area of abnormal marrow with a decreased signal intensity (darker appearance) on T1-weighted images and increased signal intensity on T2-weighted images. Occasionally, however, there also may be a decreased signal intensity on T2-weighted images. Cellulitis is seen as a diffuse area of intermediate signal intensity on T1-weighted images of soft tissue and as an increased signal intensity on T2-weighted images of the same tissue. Because it may be difficult to differentiate infection from neoplasm on the basis of MRI alone, further clinical and radiographic confirmation may be necessary.

Osteomyelitis with Vascular Insufficiency

For patients with vascular disease, the diagnosis of osteomyelitis can become a challenge because of coexisting clinical effects. It is essential, however, that the physician recognize osteomyelitis in its early stages to arrest the infection and prevent amputation caused by complications of peripheral vascular disease.

Clinical evaluation is the most important step in diagnosing osteomyelitis in patients with vascular disease. Any ulcer or skin laceration near a bony area of the foot that has persisted for more than 1 to 2 weeks should be considered a risk factor for underlying osteomyelitis. When the bone can be visualized, treatment for osteomyelitis can begin immediately and can be adjusted when culture results are known. In all other cases, radiographic evidence is necessary to confirm the existence of the disease.

Patients with both osteomyelitis and vascular disease often have radiographs that show patchy bone destruction, a periosteal reaction, and ill-defined bone margins. CT scans, although more sensitive, are less useful than radiographs for identifying infections of the foot bones because of the small amount of bone and adjacent soft tissue in the extremities. Radionuclide scans yield positive findings in cases of both soft tissue and bone inflammation. Consequently, a positive scan may indicate only a soft tissue infection. In studies of patients with osteomyelitis with complicating soft tissue infections of the foot, MRI proved to be diagnostically better than plain radiography, bone scanning, gallium-67 scanning, and WBC scanning (27). MRI is also useful in distinguishing areas of neuropathy, which are identified by a low signal intensity on all pulse sequences within bony structures and soft tissue. This contrasts with osteomyelitis, in which marrow gives a high signal intensity on all pulse sequences except for T1-weighted sequences. Because of their high cost, MRI studies should be reserved for patients who have a questionable diagnosis of osteomyelitis.

Vertebral Osteomyelitis

The most common radiographic feature of vertebral osteomyelitis is faint lucency at the edge of the affected vertebral body, with loss of clear demarcation of the cortical margin. MRI is the simplest and most effective method for determining osteomyelitis of the spine. Involvement of the vertebral bodies, discs, and paravertebral region is detected easily. Disease-induced changes in MRI scans include increased enhancement on T1-weighted images and increased intensity on T2-weighted images. Consistently, infection has been associated with an early decreased intensity of the vertebral marrow on T1-weighted images and an enhanced intensity of the same area with gadolinium-enhanced contrast studies. Significant changes on T2-weighted images also have been shown to be early signs of infection.

Treatment

Many factors must be considered in determining the appropriate course of treatment for the patient with osteomyelitis and especially the effect that treatment will have on the patient. If curative measures will adversely effect the patient's quality of life, simple suppression of the disease with oral antibiotic therapy may be preferred. If the patient is a good surgical candidate, foreign material and sequestra must be removed. Appropriate treatment of osteomyelitis includes adequate drainage, thorough debridement, obliteration of dead space, wound protection, stabilization if necessary, and specific antimicrobial coverage. If the patient is a compromised host, an effort should be made to correct or improve the host's defect(s).

Medical Management

After cultures are obtained from a patient with osteomyelitis, a parenteral antimicrobial regimen is begun to eliminate the clinically suspected pathogens (Table 29.3). Once the causative pathogen has been identified, the specific class(es) of antimicrobial drugs for its eradication can be selected through appropriate methods of sensitivity testing (28).

Stage 1, or hematogenous osteomyelitis, in children usually can be treated with antimicrobial drugs alone (29). Antibiotic therapy without surgery is possible because children's bones are very vascular and because children have an effective immune response to infection. It is recommended that children with osteomyelitis initially receive 2 weeks of parenteral antibiotic therapy followed by an oral antibiotic regimen. Oral therapy should be given for 4 to 6 weeks. Because the quinolone class of antimicrobial drugs has been shown to cause articular damage in young animals, this class of drugs should not be used in pediatric patients.

Stage 1 osteomyelitis is more refractory to therapy in adults than in children and is usually treated with antimicrobial drugs and surgery. The patient is given 4 weeks of appropriate parenteral antimicrobial therapy, dating from the initiation of therapy or after the last major debridement surgery. For methicillin-sensitive S. aureus (MSSA) and Streptococcus species, the antimicrobial agent initially chosen should be clindamycin, nafcillin, or cefazolin. Clindamycin may the drug of first choice for sequential intravenous/oral therapy because of its excellent bone penetration and bioavailability. If the initial medical management fails and the patient is clinically compromised by a recurrent infection, medullary and/or soft tissue debridement is necessary, in conjunction with another 4-week course of antibiotic therapy.

As noted earlier, an infected intramedullary rod can cause stage 1 osteomyelitis. If the bone is stable, the rod can be removed. The patient is given a 4-week course of antibiotic therapy beginning at the time of rod removal. If the bone is unstable, the patient is given suppressive oral antibiotic therapy until bone stability is achieved. Once stability is achieved, the rod is removed and the patient is given a 4-week course of antibiotic therapy, again beginning at the time of rod removal.

Stage 2, or superficial osteomyelitis, occurs when an exposed infected, necrotic surface of bone lies at the base of a soft tissue wound. After superfi-

Table 29.3 Initial Choice of Antibiotics for Therapy of Infectious Arthritis and Osteomyelitis (Adult Doses)

Organism	Antibiotics of First Choice*	Alternative Antibiotics
Staphylococcus aureus	Nafcillin 2 g q6h or clindamycin 900 mg q8h	Vancomycin, cefazolin
Methicillin-resistant S. aureus	Vancomycin 1 g q12h	TMP-SMX + rifampin, minocycline + rifampin Linezolid
S. epidermidis	Vancomycin 1 g q12h or nafcillin 2 g q6h	Cefazolin, clindamycin
Group A Streptococcus	Penicillin G 2 MU q4h	Clindamycin, cefazolin
Group B Streptococcus	Penicillin G 2 MU q4h	Clindamycin, cefazolin
Enterococcus species	Ampicillin 2 g q6h ± Gentamicin 5 mg/kg/d q8h	Vancomycin, ampicillin–sulbactam
Vancomycin-resistant Enterococcus species	Quinupristin/dalfopristin Linezolid	Chloramphenicol + rifampin
Escherichia coli	Ampicillin 2 g q6h or cefazolin 2 g q8h	Ceftriaxone, cefotaxime
Proteus mirabilis	Ampicillin 2 g q6h or cefazolin 2 g q8h	Ceftriaxone, cefotaxime
P. vulgaris, P. rettgeri, Morganella morganii	Cefotaxime 2 g q6h ± gentamicin 5 mg/kg/d q8h	Ceftriaxone, piperacillin–tazobactam
Serratia marcescens	Cefotaxime 2 g q6h ± gentamicin 5 mg/kg/d q8h Levofloxacin 500 mg/d	Ciprofloxacin, mezlocillin + gentamicin
Pseudomonas aeruginosa	Cefepime 2 g q12h or ceftazidime 2 g q8h ± tobramycin 5 mg/kg/d q8h	Ciprofloxacin, amikacin
Bacteroides fragilis group	Clindamycin 900 mg q8h	Metronidazole, ampicillin–sulbactam
Peptostreptococcus species	Clindamycin 900 mg q8h	Penicillin, metronidazole, ampicillin–sulbactam

MU = million units; TMP-SMX = trimethoprim–sulfamethoxazole.
* Doses may need to be modified in patients with renal dysfunction.

cial bony debridement and soft tissue treatment, the patient is given a 2-week course of antibiotic therapy. The arrest rate for stage 2 osteomyelitis with such treatment is approximately 80% (10).

In stages 3 and 4 osteomyelitis, the patient is given from 4 to 6 weeks of parenteral antimicrobial therapy beginning after the last major debridement surgery. Without adequate debridement, most antibiotic regimens fail no matter what the duration of therapy. Even when all necrotic tissue has been debrided adequately, the remaining bed of tissue must be considered contaminated with the causative pathogen(s). Consequently, it is important to give the patient at least 4 weeks of antibiotic treatment. The arrest rate for stages 3 and 4 osteomyelitis with such treatment is approximately 90% (10).

Hospital lengths of stay for osteomyelitis have been decreased in recent years by the development of outpatient catheters and oral antibiotic therapy. Intravenous therapy can be given on an outpatient basis with long-term intravenous access catheters, such as Hickman or Groshong catheters (30,31).

In addition to outpatient intravenous therapy, oral therapy with quinolones for gram-negative organisms is being used for adult patients with osteomyelitis (32,33). The second-generation quinolones (e.g., ciprofloxacin, ofloxacin) have poor activity against *Streptococcus*, *Enterococcus*, and anaerobic bacteria. The third-generation quinolones (e.g., levofloxacin, gatifloxacin) have excellent activity against *Streptococcus* but provide minimal coverage of anaerobic organisms. None of the quinolones provides reliable coverage of *Enterococcus*. The currently available quinolones provide variable coverage of *S. aureus* and *S. epidermidis*, and resistance to the second-generation quinolones is increasing. MSSA should be covered with another oral antimicrobial agent, such as clindamycin or amoxicillin–clavulanate. Before being moved to an oral antimicrobial regimen, the patient should be given 2 weeks of parenteral antibiotic therapy; it is important to ascertain whether the organism(s) isolated from the patient's infection are sensitive to the oral regimen. The patient must be compliant with treatment and have close outpatient follow-up.

A combination of parenteral and oral antibiotic therapy has been used in some situations. Osteomyelitis caused by MSSA has been treated successfully with the combination of a semisynthetic penicillin and rifampin, and osteomyelitis caused by methicillin-resistant *S. aureus* (MRSA) has been treated successfully with a combination of vancomycin and rifampin.

Surgical Management

Surgical management of osteomyelitis can be very challenging. The principles of surgically treating any infection are equally applicable to the treatment of infection in bone. These include adequate drainage, extensive debridement of all necrotic tissue, obliteration of dead spaces, adequate soft tissue coverage of the treated bone, restoration of an effective blood supply, and stabilization of the patient. The goal of debridement in osteomyelitis is to leave healthy, viable bone tissue and conditions that can lead to the rapid formation of new bone. However, even when all necrotic tissue has been debrided adequately, the remaining bed of tissue must be considered to be contaminated with the etiologic pathogen.

The challenge in treating osteomyelitis compared with that of an infection of soft tissue alone is the need for bone debridement. In cases of chronic osteomyelitis, debridement is essential for cure. Adequate debridement may leave the large-bone defect known as a "dead space." To arrest the disease and maintain the integrity of the bone, appropriate management of any dead space created by debridement surgery is mandatory. The goal of dead-space management is to replace dead bone and scar tissue with durable, vascularized bone tissue.

Allowing the bone to become revascularized is the best way to ensure the arrest of the infection in osteomyelitis. Complete wound closure should be attained whenever possible. Cancellous bone grafts allow the filling of the dead space that remains after debridement surgery with tissue that allows revascularization (34). These grafts also can be placed beneath local or transferred tissues where soft tissue reconstruction is necessary. Careful preoperative planning is critical to conserving the patient's limited cancellous bone reserves. Open cancellous grafts are useful when a free tissue transfer is not a treatment option and when local tissue flaps are inadequate.

Antibiotic-impregnated acrylic beads may be used to sterilize and to maintain dead space temporarily (35,36). The beads are usually removed within 2 to 4 weeks and then replaced with a cancellous bone graft. The antibiotics most commonly used in impregnated beads are vancomycin, tobramycin, and gentamicin. Local delivery of antibiotics (e.g., amikacin, clindamycin) into dead space has been accomplished with an implantable pump.

If pathologic movement of bone is present at the site of infection, measures must be taken to achieve permanent stability of the affected skeletal unit. Stability may be achieved with plates, screws, and rods, and/or an external fixator. External is preferred to internal fixation because of the tendency of medullary rods to become secondarily infected and thereby extend the original bone infection. An Ilizarov external fixator allows bone reconstruction of segmental defects and difficult infected nonunions (37,38). This external fixation method is based on the theory of distraction histogenesis, whereby bone is fractured in the metaphyseal region and slowly lengthened. The growth of new bone in the metaphyseal region pushes a segment of healthy bone into the defect left by surgery. The Ilizarov method also may be used to compress nonunions and to correct malunions. Infected pseudarthroses with segmental osseous defects also may be treated by debridement and microvascular bone transfers. Vascularized bone transfer is a useful procedure for treating infected segmental osseous defects of long bones of more than 3 cm length. Vascularized bone transfers can be performed 1 month or more after the successful treatment of a bone infection.

Adequate soft tissue coverage of the bone is necessary to arrest osteomyelitis. Small soft tissue defects may be covered with a split-thickness skin graft. Local tissue flaps or free flaps may be used to fill dead space (39,40). Although local muscle flaps are useful because of their ease of placement, they are often of limited use because of the locality of the bone infection in osteomyelitis. For areas such as the distal tibia, microsurgical implantation of a muscle flap is necessary. In the presence of a large soft tissue defect or with an inadequate soft tissue envelope, local muscle flaps and free vascularized muscle flaps may be placed in a one- or two-stage procedure. Local and free muscle flaps, when combined with antibiotic therapy and surgical debridement of all nonviable osseous and soft tissue, have a success rate of from 66% to 100% in chronic osteomyelitis (41). Local muscle flaps and free vascularized muscle transfers improve the local biological environment by bringing in a blood supply important to host-defense mechanisms, antibiotic delivery, and osseous and soft tissue healing.

Special Treatments

Osteomyelitis with Vascular Insufficiency

Determination of the vascular status of the tissue at the infection site is crucial in the evaluation of patients in whom osteomyelitis is accompanied by vascular insufficiency. Although several methods can be used to determine the vascular status of such patients, measuring cutaneous oxygen tension and pulse pressure is the most commonly used method. Cutaneous oxygen tensions are measured with a modified Clark electrode that is applied to the skin surface. The results provide guidelines for determining the location of adequately perfused tissue. The tensions recorded in this manner are also helpful for predicting the benefit of local debridement surgery and in selecting surgical margins at which healing can be expected to occur. Revascularization, if possible, or hyperbaric oxygen therapy facilitates healing in areas where oxygen tensions are of borderline normality.

The patient who has osteomyelitis with vascular insufficiency may be managed with suppressive antibiotic therapy, local debridement surgery, or ablative surgery. The choice of treatment is based on tissue oxygen perfusion at the infection site, extent of the osteomyelitis, and patient preference. The patient can be offered long-term suppressive antibiotic therapy when a definitive surgical procedure might lead to unacceptable morbidity or disability or in cases in which the patient refuses local debridement or ablative surgery. However, even with suppressive antibiotic therapy amputation of the involved bone may ultimately be necessary.

Local debridement surgery and a 4-week course of antibiotic therapy may be used for the patient who has osteomyelitis in bone that is amenable to debridement. Unless good tissue oxygen tensions are present, the wound fails to heal and ultimately requires an ablative procedure. As noted earlier, hyperbaric oxygen therapy facilitates healing in areas of borderline-normal oxygen tension.

The patient with extensive osteomyelitis and poor tissue oxygen perfusion usually requires some type of ablative surgery. Digital and ray resections, transmetatarsal amputations, mid-foot disarticulations, and Chopart's, Lisfranc's, and Syme's amputations (amputation of the foot with retention of the heel pad) permit the patient to ambulate without a prosthesis. The level of amputation is determined by the vascularity and potential viability of the tissues proximal to the site of infection. Hyperbaric oxygen therapy facilitates healing if surgery is performed in or through areas of low oxygen tension as measured cutaneously. When infected bone is transected surgically, the patient is given 4 weeks of antibiotic therapy. Two weeks of antibiotic therapy are given when the infected bone is excised completely, but some residual soft tissue infection remains. When amputation is performed proximal to a site of bone and soft tissue infection, the patient should be given from 1 to 3 days of antibiotic therapy.

Vertebral Osteomyelitis

Biopsy and debridement cultures dictate the choice of antibiotic(s) to be used in treating vertebral osteomyelitis. Antibiotic therapy is given for 4 to 6 weeks and is dated from the initiation of therapy or from the last major debridement surgery. Open surgical treatment is usually necessary only in cases in which the patient develops an extension of an original infection (e.g., paravertebral or epidural abscess, when medical management fails, when bone instability is likely to occur). The neurological status of the patient must be monitored closely in such cases. Surgical fusion of the involved vertebrae is usually not required, because bone fusion occurs spontaneously within 1 to 12 months after appropriate antibiotic therapy. The frequency of a successful outcome for patients treated with bed rest alone is not substantially different from that for ambulatory patients stabilized with a cast, corset, or brace.

Prevention

Most cases of long-bone osteomyelitis are posttraumatic or postoperative. With the increasing number of accidents and orthopedic procedures performed, it is unlikely that the infection rate will decrease. Patients with diabetes mellitus can prevent osteomyelitis by minimizing foot trauma and by preventing foot ulcers (8). This includes education about proper foot care, including daily inspection of the feet. Daily foot washing and the use of moisturizing creams are necessary to avoid breaking of the skin. Furthermore, patients should avoid activities that might cause unnecessary trauma to vasculitic neuropathic feet. This includes walking barefoot or wearing improperly fitted shoes. The only way to reduce the frequency of contiguous-focus osteomyelitis in diabetic patients is to prevent the development of diabetic foot ulcers or aggressively prevent diabetic foot ulcers from involving bone through treatment of the infection, wound care, and the off-loading of pressure points.

Acknowledgments

The authors thank Melinda Stevens, Steve Bergquist, and Donna Milner Mader for manuscript research and preparation.

REFERENCES

1. **Waldvogel FA, Medoff G, Swartz MN.** Osteomyelitis: a review of clinical features, therapeutic considerations and unusual aspects. *N Engl J Med.* 1970;282:316–22.

2. **Waldvogel FA, Medoff G, Swartz MN.** Osteomyelitis: a review of clinical features, therapeutic considerations and unusual aspects (second of three parts). *N Engl J Med.* 1970;282:260–6.

3. **Waldvogel FA, Medoff G, Swartz MN.** Osteomyelitis: a review of clinical features, therapeutic considerations and unusual aspects. *N Engl J Med.* 1970;282:198–206.

4. **Trueta J, Morgan JD.** The vascular contribution to osteogenesis. Studies by the injection method. *J Bone Joint Surg.* 1960;42B:97–109.

5. **Hobo T.** Zur Pathogenese de akuten haematatogenen Osteomyelitis, mit Beruckishtigun der Vitalfarbungslehre. *Acta School Med Univ Imp Kioto.* 1922;4:1–29.

6. **Mader JT, Wilson KJ.** Comparative evaluation of cefamandole and cephalothin in the treatment of experimental *Staphylococcus aureus* osteomyelitis in rabbits. *J Bone Joint Surg Am.* 1983;65:507–13.

7. **Caputo GM, Cavanagh PR, Ulbrecht JS, et al.** Assessment and management of foot disease in patients with diabetes. *N Engl J Med.* 1994;331:854–60.

8. **Calhoun JH, Cantrell J, Cobos J, et al.** Treatment of diabetic foot infections: Wagner classification, therapy, and outcome. *Foot Ankle.* 1988;9:101–6.

9. **Ish-Horowicz MR, McIntyre P, Nade S.** Bone and joint infections caused by multiply resistant *Staphylococcus aureus* in a neonatal intensive care unit. *Pediatr Infect Dis J.* 1992;11:82–7.

10. **Cierny G.** Chronic osteomyelitis: results of treatment. *Instr Course Lect.* 1990;39: 495–508:495–508.

11. **Cierny GI, Mader JT, Penninck JJ.** A clinical staging system for adult osteomyelitis. *Contemp Orthop.* 1985;10: 17–37.

12. **Perry CR, Pearson RL, Miller GA.** Accuracy of cultures of material from swabbing of the superficial aspect of the wound and needle biopsy in the preoperative assessment of osteomyelitis. *J Bone Joint Surg Am.* 1991;73:745–9.

13. **Mader JT, Calhoun JH.** Osteomyelitis. In: Mandell GL, Douglas RG, Bennett JE Jr, eds. *Principles and Practice of Infectious Diseases.* New York: Churchill Livingstone; 1995:1039–51.

14. **Cierny G, Mader JT.** Approach to adult osteomyelitis. *Orthop Rev.* 1987;16:259–70.

15. **Mackowiak PA, Jones SR, Smith JW.** Diagnostic value of sinus-tract cultures in chronic osteomyelitis. *JAMA.* 1978;239:2772–5.

16. **Otremski I, Newman RJ, Kahn PJ, et al.** Leukergy–a new diagnostic test for bone infection. *J Bone Joint Surg Br.* 1993;75:734–6.

17. **Roine I, Faingezicht I, Arguedas A, et al.** Serial serum C-reactive protein to monitor recovery from acute hematogenous osteomyelitis in children. *Pediatr Infect Dis J.* 1995;14:40–4.

18. **Unkila-Kallio L, Kallio MJ, Eskola J, Peltola H.** Serum C-reactive protein, erythrocyte sedimentation rate, and white blood cell count in acute hematogenous osteomyelitis of children. *Pediatrics.* 1994;93:59–62.

19. **Butt WP.** The radiology of infection. *Clin Orthop.* 1973;96:20–30:20–30.

20. **Rosenthall L, Lisbona R, Hernandez M, Hadjipavlou A.** 99mTc-PP and 67Ga imaging following insertion of orthopedic devices. *Radiology.* 1979;133:717–21.

21. **Propst-Proctor SL, Dillingham MF, McDougall IR, Goodwin D.** The white blood cell scan in orthopedics. *Clin Orthop.* 1982;157–65.

22. **Kuhn JP, Berger PE.** Computed tomographic diagnosis of osteomyelitis. *Radiology.* 1979;130:503–6.

23. **Seltzer SE.** Value of computed tomography in planning medical and surgical treatment of chronic osteomyelitis. *J Comput Assist Tomogr.* 1984;8:482–7.

24. **Tehranzadeh J, Wang F, Mesgarzadeh M.** Magnetic resonance imaging of osteomyelitis. *Crit Rev Diagn Imaging.* 1992;33:495–534.

25. **Modic MT, Pflanze W, Feiglin DH, Belhobek G.** Magnetic resonance imaging of musculoskeletal infections. *Radiol Clin North Am.* 1986;24:247–58.

26. **Erdman WA, Tamburro F, Jayson HT, et al.** Osteomyelitis: characteristics and pitfalls of diagnosis with MR imaging. *Radiology.* 1991;180:533–9.

27. **McAndrew PT, Clark C.** MRI is best technique for imaging acute osteomyelitis [letter; comment]. *BMJ.* 1998;316:147.

28. **Ericsson HM, Sherris JC.** Antibiotic sensitivity testing. Report of an international collaborative study. *Acta Pathol Microbiol Scand B Microbiol Immunol.* 1971;217.

29. **Tetzlaff TR, McCracken GHJ, Nelson JD.** Oral antibiotic therapy for skeletal infections of children. II. Therapy of osteomyelitis and suppurative arthritis. *J Pediatr.* 1978;92:485–90.

30. **Couch L, Cierny G, Mader JT.** Inpatient and outpatient use of the Hickman catheter for adults with osteomyelitis. *Clin Orthop.* 1987;226–35.

31. **Hickman RO, Buckner CD, Clift RA, et al.** A modified right atrial catheter for access to the venous system in marrow transplant recipients. *Surg Gynecol Obstet.* 1979; 148:871–5.

32. **Mader J.T.** Fluoroquinolones in bone and joint infections. In: Sanders WE Jr, Sanders CC, eds. *Fluoroquinolones in the Treatment of Infectious Diseases.* Chicago: Physicians Scientists; 1990:71–86.

33. **Mader JT, Cantrell JS, Calhoun J.** Oral ciprofloxacin compared with standard parenteral antibiotic therapy for chronic osteomyelitis in adults. *J Bone Joint Surg Am.* 1990;72:104–10.

34. **Minami A, Kaneda K, Itoga H.** Treatment of infected segmental defect of long bone with vascularized bone transfer. *J Reconstr Microsurg.* 1992;8:75–82.

35. **Henry SL, Seligson D, Mangino P, Popham GJ.** Antibiotic-impregnated beads. Part I: Bead implantation versus systemic therapy. *Orthop Rev.* 1991;20:242–7.

36. **Calhoun JH, Mader JT.** Antibiotic beads in the management of surgical infections. *Am J Surg.* 1989;157:443–9.

37. **Calhoun JH, Anger DM, Mader J, Ledbetter BR.** The Ilizarov technique in the treatment of osteomyelitis. *Texas Med.* 1991;87:56–9.

38. **Green SA.** Osteomyelitis. The Ilizarov perspective. *Orthop Clin North Am.* 1991;22: 515–21.

39. **May JWJ, Jupiter JB, Gallico GG, et al.** Treatment of chronic traumatic bone wounds. Microvascular free tissue transfer: a 13-year experience in 96 patients. *Ann Surg.* 1991;214:241–50.

40. **Anthony JP, Mathes SJ, Alpert BS.** The muscle flap in the treatment of chronic lower extremity osteomyelitis: results in patients over 5 years after treatment. *Plast Reconstr Surg.* 1991;88:311–8.

41. **Gayle LB, Lineaweaver WC, Oliva A, et al.** Treatment of chronic osteomyelitis of the lower extremities with debridement and microvascular muscle transfer. *Clin Plast Surg.* 1992;19:895–903.

30

Skin Infections

Thomas M. File Jr., MD, MS

B acterial skin infections range from mild pyodermas to life-threatening necrotizing infections (1–4). The manifestations of bacterial skin infections result from the interaction of bacterial virulence factors with the immune status and underlying conditions of the host (Table 30.1).

The skin represents an effective physical barrier against invasion by microorganisms. The normal skin of healthy individuals is resistant to invasion by bacteria that may reside on the skin surface. Infection of the skin usually occurs when there is a defect in the integrity of the epidermis, allowing microorganisms that have colonized the skin to invade the underlying tissues and cause clinical effects. Such defects may result from surgery or trauma or may follow relatively innocuous events, such as an insect bite or abrasion. Skin lesions also may result from the hematogenesis spread of bacteria or bacterial toxins from distant sites of infections.

Pathogenesis and Risk Factors

Most bacteria decrease in number when applied to the surface of the keratinized layers of normal skin. A variety of physical characteristics of the skin act to reduce bacterial multiplication:

- The relatively low pH (~5.5) of the skin environment
- The presence of natural antibacterial substances in the secretions of the sebaceous glands
- The relative dryness of normal skin
- Bacterial interference (the suppressive effect of "normal flora" on the growth of pathogens)

Table 30.1 Microbe and Host Factors That Affect Bacterial Skin Infections

Bacterial Virulence Factors	Local Defense Factors	Host Conditions
Adherence factors (e.g., fibrils M protein of *Streptococcus pyogenes*)	Intact skin (barrier effect)	Abnormalities of epidermis (eczema, dermatitis)
Antiphagocytic factors (e.g., M protein of *S. pyogenes*)	Low pH, relative dryness	Breaks of skin (abrasions, trauma, surgical incision)
Enzymes (proteinases, hyaluronidases)	Antibacterial secretions of sebaceous glands	
Toxins (i.e., toxic shock syndrome toxin)		Ulcers (diabetic foot pressure sores)
Beta-lactamase production (reduces susceptibility to beta-lactam antibiotics)		Ischemia, immunosuppression, presence of foreign body (e.g., catheter)

Normal skin is colonized with a variety of microorganisms that are classified as resident flora, including *Propionibacterium* species, coagulase-negative staphylococci, and *Corynebacterium* species. For the most part, these organisms are not pathogenic. When a foreign body (e.g., intravenous catheter) is present, such resident organisms may cause localized infection and bacteremia. The skin may be colonized transiently by *Staphylococcus aureus* and beta-hemolytic streptococci, which are more likely to cause invasive disease. Additionally, members of the Enterobacteriaceae family, *Pseudomonas* species, *Enterococcus* species, and a variety of anaerobes from fecal sources are particularly prone to colonizing the lower extremities. Colonization of normal skin with pathogenic organisms usually precedes clinical infection. Subsequently, minimal trauma may cause an epidermal defect that allows organisms on the skin surface to cross the keratinized layers that normally protect against infection and to cause disease. Although the etiologic pathogens that are associated with many of the pyodermas are fairly predictable (usually *S. aureus* or beta-hemolytic *Streptococcus* species), other organisms (e.g., *Pseudomonas* in whirlpool-bath folliculitis, anaerobes and Enterobacteriaceae in chronic hidradenitis suppurativa) may be involved. *S. aureus* often colonizes patients both in and out of the hospital setting. Common sites for colonization include the anterior nares or perineum. Approximately 50% of patients may be found to carry *S. aureus* transiently at any given time. Individuals who are prone to colonization include health care workers, patients with diabetes, patients who undergo chronic hemodialysis, and users of illicit intravenous drugs (5). Most patients with staphylococcal folliculitis or furunculosis experience a self-limiting infection. Certain patients, however, are especially prone to recurrent infections, including those who have hypogammaglobulinemia, diabetes mellitus, cancer or organ transplants (who are also receiving immunosuppressive drugs), chronic granulomatous disease of childhood, and Job's syndrome. Additionally, poor hygiene, obesity, folliculosis, chronic dermatitis, seborrhea, psoriasis, malnutrition, and occupational trauma all may predispose the patient to recurrent *S. aureus* pyoderma.

The pathogenicity of specific microorganisms is determined in part by virulence factors (6). Local invasiveness is an important element in group A streptococcal infection (e.g., *Streptococcus pyogenes*), which depends on the antiphagocytic M protein of the bacterial cell envelope (7, 8). Several extracellular products associated with *S. pyogenes* may contribute to the manifestations of skin infection. These include hyaluronidase, proteinase, deoxyribonuclease, and streptokinase, all of which cause liquefaction of pus and enhance the spread of infection throughout tissue planes (9). Toxins and enzymes seem to play a role in the ability of *S. aureus* to produce disease (10). Alpha- and delta-toxins may contribute to disease manifestations by damaging tissue membranes. Exfoliative toxin, which is produced by certain strains of *S. aureus*, causes separation between the epidermis and the dermis, resulting in the scalded-skin syndrome. Both *S. aureus* and *S. pyogenes* may produce pyogenic toxins associated with a toxic shock syndrome. The staphylococcal toxic shock syndrome characterized by hypotension, rash, and multisystem involvement is caused by strains of *S. aureus* that produce an exotoxin, toxic shock syndrome toxin 1 (11). More recently, serious skin infections caused by *S. pyogenes* and characterized by necrotizing fasciitis have been described and called *group A streptococcal toxic shock syndrome* (*see* Chapter 31). The pathogenesis of skin infections associated with gram-negative bacilli (e.g., exotoxins produced by *Pseudomonas aeruginosa*) and anaerobes may be caused by elaboration of a variety of extracellular toxins. In the case of *Clostridium perfringens*, elaboration of collagenases, specific toxins, and proteases seems to play an important role in producing the spreading necrotizing infection that may be associated with this organism.

Several host factors contribute to the predisposition to skin infections, including a reduced vascular supply, compromised immune system, disruption of lymphatic or venous drainage, the presence of underlying conditions (e.g., dermatitis), and the presence of a foreign body (e.g., intravenous catheter, suture).

This chapter reviews the clinical aspects of superficial bacterial skin infections, which are often referred to as *primary pyodermas*.

Clinical Manifestations and Natural History

Primary superficial skin infections, or pyodermas, usually occur on relatively normal skin and are most often caused by beta-hemolytic streptococci (most

Table 30.2 Common Microbial Etiology and Treatment of Superficial Skin Infections

Infection	Microorganisms	Treatment and Comments
Impetigo	*Streptococcus pyogenes, Staphylococcus aureus**	Oral: Antistaphylococcal penicillins,[†] first-generation cephalosporins,[‡] macrolide, clindamycin Topical: Mupirocin, Bacitracin
Erysipelas	*S. pyogenes* and other beta-hemolytic streptococci; rarely *S. aureus*	Oral: Penicillin VK and penicillin G, antistaphylococcal penicillins (if there is a concern for *S. aureus* infection), first-generation cephalosporins, macrolide, clindamycin
Cellulitis	*S. aureus,** *S. pyogenes*	Oral: Antistaphylococcal penicillins, first-generation cephalosporins, clindamycin IV: Antistaphylococcal penicillins, first-generation cephalosporins, clindamycin
Folliculitis, furuncles, carbuncles	*S. aureus**	Oral: Antistaphylococcal penicillins, erythromycin (250–500 mg q6h) hours, clindamycin (150–300 mg q6h), new macrolides[§] IV: Nafcillin, first-generation cephalosporins, vancomycin
Whirlpool folliculitis	*Pseudomonas aeruginosa*	Self-limiting, treatment not necessary
Hidradenitis suppurativa	Acute: *S. aureus*[¶] Chronic: *S. aureus*, Enterobacteriaceae, *Pseudomonas* species, anaerobes	Antistaphylococcal agents Empirical: Beta-lactam/beta-lactamase inhibitor,[**] cefoxitin (1–2 g q6h), cefotetan (1–2 g q12h), imipenem (0.5–1.0 g q6–8h), meropenem (0.5–1 g q8h), clindamycin + fluoroquinolone[††]

* Duration of therapy of most superficial skin infections is 7–14 days; hidradenitis suppurativa may require longer duration.

[†] Oral antistaphylococcal penicillins include cloxacillin (250–500 mg q6h) and dicloxacillin (250–500 mg q6h); parenteral antistaphylococcal penicillins include oxacillin (0.5–2.0 g q4–6h), and nafcillin (0.5–2.0 g q6h).

[‡] Oral first-generation cephalosporins include cephalexin (250–500 mg q6h) and cefadroxyl (250–500 mg q12h); parenteral first-generation cephalosporins include cephalothin (0.5–2.0 g q4–6h), and cefazolin (0.5–1 g q8h).

[§] The new macrolides are azithromycin (500 mg on day 1, followed by 250 mg/d), clarithromycin (500 mg q12h), and clarithromycin XL (1000 mg/d).

[¶] Therapy for *S. aureus* is directed against methicillin-susceptible strains; see text for discussion.

[**] Oral beta-lactam/beta-lactamase inhibitors include amoxicillin–clavulanate (500–875 mg q12h); parenteral beta-lactam/beta-lactamase inhibitors include ampicillin–sulbactam (1.5–3.0 g q6h), ticarcillin–clavulanate (3.1 g q4–6h), and piperacillin–tazobactam (3.375–4.5 g q6h).

[††] Base definitive therapy on culture results.

commonly group A streptococci) or *S. aureus* (Table 30.2). Such infections are often mild, and most do not require parenteral antibiotic therapy or hospitalization. They often occur in patients who do not exhibit any significant underlying condition. The infections include folliculitis, furunculosis, carbunculosis, impetigo, cellulitis, erysipelas, and hidradenitis suppurativa.

Folliculitis

Folliculitis is an infection located within hair follicles and the apocrine glands. The lesions are usually from 2 to 5 mm in diameter. Folliculitis is most commonly caused by *S. aureus*; however, in immunocompromised patients the etiologic agent may be gram-negative bacilli or *Candida* species. A specific form of *Pseudomonas* folliculitis has been described in association with whirlpool bathing or use of a hot tub. Recently, an outbreak of pustular dermatitis was described among mud-wrestling college students; organisms isolated from the pustules included *Enterobacter cloacae* and *Citrobacter* species (12). The pathogenesis of this condition may resemble that of pseudomonal folliculitis, with organisms from mud possibly entering the skin through hair follicles or through breaks in the skin that occurred during the wrestling.

Folliculitis originates in the hair follicle and is defined by its anatomical features. Clinically, the lesions present as 2- to 5-mm erythematous papules that surround the hair follicle and often exhibit central pustulation. Systemic manifestations are rare. Sycosis barbae is a distinctive form of deep folliculitis that is often chronic and seen in bearded areas.

Patients with whirlpool-bath folliculitis develop generalized, fine, papular pustules from which *P. aeruginosa* may be isolated (13). The modified apocrine glands of the external canal of the ear and the areolae of the breasts are structures that are particularly susceptible to this infection. The most common sign of this syndrome is a generalized rash accompanied by otitis externa, mastitis, malaise, and fever. The average incubation period is approximately 2 days. *Pseudomonas* infection may follow immersion in swimming pools, Jacuzzis, or whirlpool baths in which the organism may reside in higher numbers if the chlorination or the pH of the system is not adjusted properly. The disease is usually self-limited. Systemic antibiotic therapy is not indicated for treating whirlpool-bath folliculitis unless cellulitis develops.

Furuncle and Carbuncle

Folliculitis that extends beyond the hair follicle and into the subcutaneous tissues may give rise to a furuncle or carbuncle. A furuncle is a deeper inflammatory nodule that often follows folliculitis. Furuncles usually measure less than 5 mm in diameter. A carbuncle is a larger, deeper lesion and often occurs as a confluent infection that comprises multiple furuncles. *S. aureus* is the organism most often associated with furunculosis and carbunculosis.

Clinically, a furuncle begins as an erythematous, firm, tender, nodular lesion that progresses to a fluctuant mass that may drain pus spontaneously.

They occur in skin areas that are subject to friction and perspiration and that contain hair follicles (e.g., the neck, face, axillae, buttocks). Predisposing factors include obesity, corticosteroid use, defects in neutrophil function, and probably diabetes mellitus.

Carbuncles are more serious lesions that often are located at the back of the neck, on the back, or in the region of the thigh. Fever and malaise are frequent accompaniments of a carbuncle, and sepsis may occur. Blood stream infection also may occur with carbuncles (less so with furuncles) and may result in metastatic foci of infection (e.g., endocarditis, osteomyelitis). Furuncles on the upper lip and nose may be associated with the spread of infection via emissary veins to the cavernous sinus.

Impetigo

Impetigo is a vesicular (initially), crusted (later), superficial, intraepithelial infection of the skin that is associated with *S. aureus* and beta-hemolytic streptococci (alone or in combination). Mixtures of group A streptococci and *S. aureus* are isolated from approximately half of patients with nonbullous impetigo. Mixed flora of anaerobic streptococci with *Prevotella* or *Fusobacterium* species can be found in infections of the head and neck, whereas enteric gram-negative bacilli (often mixed with *Bacteroides fragilis*) can be isolated from infections of the buttock (3). A relatively specific form of impetigo (bullous impetigo) has been identified as a primarily staphylococcal disease. Non–group A streptococci (i.e., groups B, C, and G) may be responsible for isolated cases of nonbullous impetigo. Because impetigo is a very superficial infection, vesiculopustules develop just beneath the stratum corneum and it is generally not associated with any systemic manifestations of infection. The disease begins with vesicular lesions that rapidly become pustular and crusted. A honey-colored crust over slightly erythematous areas of inflammation is characteristic; Nikolsky's sign and scarring do not occur. Regional lymphadenopathy without systemic symptoms is common. The early vesicular lesions of impetigo may resemble the initial lesions of varicella or herpes simplex; however, the crusts that form in these viral infections are usually harder.

Impetigo appears primarily in young children during warm, humid months. Predisposing conditions include minor trauma, insect bites, poor hygiene, and preexisting skin disease. Spread of the disease within families is common through direct contact with infectious material. Bullous impetigo is more often associated with *S. aureus* than is the nonbullous form of the disease. As in the nonbullous form, the lesions initially appear as vesicles but progress to flaccid bullous lesions filled with yellow fluid. When these lesions rupture, light brown crusts form. These crusts and the bullous lesions are characteristic of the condition. Regional lymphadenopathy is found less commonly in the bullous form of impetigo. Fever and constitutional symptoms are uncommon in both the bullous and nonbullous forms of the disease.

Cellulitis

Cellulitis is a diffuse, spreading, and nonsuppurative infection of the skin and subcutaneous tissues that presents with localized redness, warmth, swelling, and tenderness of the skin. Both *S. aureus* and beta-hemolytic streptococci are associated with cellulitis. The lesion in cellulitis is often very red, hot, and swollen, but the borders of the lesion are usually not clearly demarcated. Previous trauma (laceration, abrasion) may precede the development of cellulitis. Within days of the trauma, local tenderness, pain, and erythema develop. Fever, chills, malaise, and regional lymphadenitis commonly accompany the infection. If the condition is untreated, local abscesses may develop, and areas of overlying skin also may become necrotic. Because of this, cellulitis may be mistaken for a number of other clinical disorders, including deep venous thrombosis, erythema nodosum, allergic reactions, reactions to insect bites, and reactions to chemical irritants.

The microbiology of cellulitis and its correlation with the site of infection were recently investigated with more than 200 swab and 64 needle-aspirate specimens (14). The greatest recovery of anaerobic bacteria (predominantly *Peptostreptococcus, B. fragilis, Prevotella,* and *Clostridium*) was from the neck, trunk, groin, external genitalia, and leg area. Aerobes (predominantly *S. aureus,* group A streptococci, and *Escherichia coli*) outnumbered anaerobes in the arm and hand areas. Certain clinical findings correlated with the following pathogens: 1) swelling and tenderness with *Clostridium* species, *S. aureus,* and group A streptococci; 2) regional adenopathy with *B. fragilis;* 3) gangrene and necrosis with anaerobes and Enterobacteriaceae; and 4) a foul odor or gas in tissues containing anaerobes.

A frustrating problem for some patients is recurrent cellulitis at sites of previous surgery. This problem has been associated particularly with saphenous venectomy for coronary bypass surgery, stripping of varicose veins, and procedures that affect lymphatic drainage (e.g., neoplasia, radiation therapy, surgery) (15,16). Recurrent cellulitis also has been seen after radical mastectomy. Patients with recurrent cellulitis following surgery may experience acute pain, fever, and erythema of acute onset at the site of the surgical scar. Tinea pedis is often an associated finding; however, I and my colleagues recently reported an instance of underlying psoriasis (16). Although pathogens are often not isolated from sites of recurrent cellulitis, an underlying skin disorder (e.g., tinea pedis) may predispose to invasion of *Streptococcus* species. Cellulitis often recurs if the underlying skin disorder is not controlled.

Erysipelas

Erysipelas is a distinctive form of cellulitis that involves the superficial epidermis. It differs from cellulitis because the lesion is indurated and red, with a well-demarcated border. Additionally, it is usually painful, and the condition is often complicated by lymphangitis. Erysipelas is more common in children and in older adults. The face and lower extremities are the most frequent sites of involvement (7). Because erysipelas tends to produce lymphatic obstruction, it can recur in an originally affected area of the skin. Occasionally, the infection extends more deeply, producing cellulitis, subcutaneous abscess, and necrosis. Fever and systemic symptoms are found in most cases; bacteremia is found in approximately 5% of patients (4). Patients who have venous or lymphatic insufficiency (e.g., recurrent cellulitis after venectomy or radical mastectomy) have been reported to have a high relapse rate for cellulitis. The lesions of cellulitis should be differentiated from those of erythema nodosum, shingles, erysipeloid, and the skin lesions of Lyme disease.

Hidradenitis Suppurativa

Hidradenitis suppurativa is a suppurative disease that affects the apocrine glands in the axillary, genital, or perianal areas. The disease rarely has systemic manifestations. Acute infection usually results from obstruction to drainage of the apocrine gland. The lesion seems to result from plugging of the apocrine gland ducts, causing dilation and eventual rupture of the glands and inflammation of the surrounding tissue. Acute infection is often caused by *S. aureus*. Chronic hidradenitis suppurativa is characterized by recurrent disease. The initial step in the disease is the formation of nodules that slowly become fluctuant and drain. Eventually, with repeated crops of lesions, sinus tracts form and cause intermittent drainage and cicatricial scarring. In some patients, infection is associated with cellulitis of the scalp (acne conglobata); such patients may experience a distinctive spondyloarthropathy. The lesions in this condition are usually bilateral and vary from a few to many, with widespread involvement. Culture of aspirate from the lesions frequently yields a mixture of aerobic and anaerobic organisms.

Diagnosis

The diagnosis of pyodermas usually is made clinically on the basis of the manifestations described in the preceding sections of this chapter. Although the skin is easily accessible for culture, isolation of an infecting organism in cases of pyoderma has not been consistent, usually because of the presence of contaminated normal skin flora. Additionally, because bacterial products or toxins, rather than the bacteria themselves, are the sources of certain skin lesions, the number of bacteria at the site of the pathology may be too small to allow consistent culture of pathogens. Therefore, the etiologic diagnosis and management of bacterial skin infections, especially in the office setting, often is based on the clinical presentation and less commonly on microbiologic techniques. In patients who have skin and soft tissue infections that require hospitalization, a more aggressive approach is needed to identify the etiologic agent because outpatient therapy has failed for some reason (e.g., misdiagnosis, wrong therapy choice, noncompliance).

Culture of lesions in folliculitis, furunculosis, carbunculosis, impetigo, and hidradenitis suppurativa usually yields the etiologic agent. Although *Staphylococcus* is often found, certain special circumstances suggest the presence of other organisms. Exposure to hot tubs should alert the physician to the possible role of *P. aeruginosa*; patients who have *Candida* folliculitis may have systemic *Candida* infection. Culture in impetigo may be achieved by removing the superficial crust of a lesion with sterile saline and by culturing the surface of the lesion. Blood culture is usually not helpful in cases of pyoderma; however, patients who present with systemic manifestations of disease and who have carbuncles may have bacteremia, for which blood culture is appropriate.

The diagnosis of cellulitis is usually made clinically, because generally the condition is a closed-skin infection and is not associated with drainage that can be submitted for culture. Ascertaining a specific bacteriologic cause for cellulitis is difficult. Usually, as with cellulitis, the diagnosis of erysipelas is also made clinically. Leukocytosis is a common occurrence in both conditions. In patients who have erysipelas, culture of the pharynx frequently yields *S. pyogenes*.

Numerous studies have evaluated the use of intradermal needle aspiration in the bacteriologic diagnosis of cellulitis, but the value of the technique remains controversial (17–19). Recent studies have reported rates of isolation of pathogenic organisms that range from 5% to 36% (20–22). The most common pathogens isolated in studies of needle aspirates are staphylococci and streptococci. A similar method of needle aspiration was used in most of these studies. Briefly, it involves cleansing the site of aspiration with povidone–iodine solution and, without prior anesthesia, puncturing the skin over the area with a 22-gauge needle attached to a disposable plastic syringe. The contents of the syringe, consisting of 1 mL of sterile isotonic saline, are injected subcutaneously, and the resulting fluid is then aspirated with the needle kept in the subcutaneous tissue. The aspirated material is promptly taken to the microbiology laboratory and immediately inoculated into culture medium. Generally, needle aspiration is not recommended for the diagnosis of superficial skin infections but may be appropriate in selected circumstances (e.g., treatment failure, immunosuppression).

Treatment

When a patient presents with a skin or soft tissue infection, an initial consideration for treatment is whether the clinical illness is severe enough to warrant hospital admission. Most superficial pyodermas are without systemic symptoms and can be managed in the outpatient setting with oral antimicrobial agents. There are no well-documented criteria for choice of a site of care (i.e., outpatient vs. inpatient). Consideration of hospitalization should be based on illness severity (i.e., the extent of abnormality of vital signs and of soft tissue involvement; see Chapter 31), patient age, presence of comorbid conditions that may be affected by an acute infection (e.g., diabetes, congestive heart failure), and the need for close observation or surgical management. When the decision to hospitalize is made, the following factors should be taken into consideration: extent of infection, presence of devitalized tissues, state of the patient's vascular supply, patient's immune and nutritional status, and the etiologic agent and its antimicrobial susceptibility pattern. Additionally, timely surgical intervention should be considered for deep infections.

Antimicrobial therapy plays an important role in the management of skin and soft tissue infections. Often, the etiologic agent is unknown when therapy is begun. For uncomplicated folliculitis, local measures (e.g., warm compresses, topical antimicrobial agents such as Bactroban and bacitracin) are usually sufficient. For other pyodermas, oral agents that have a spectrum of activity against the common infecting organisms (e.g., *Staphylococcus*, *Streptococcus*) are preferred for outpatients. For hospitalized patients, empirical antimicrobial therapy is initiated to combat or prevent life-threatening infections. Therefore, the ideal agent(s) should cover the most common pathogens associated with life-threatening skin infections. Beta-lactam/beta-lactamase–inhibitor combinations, carbapenems, trovafloxacin, and combinations that have activity against staphylococci, streptococci, aerobic gram-negative rods, and anaerobic organisms have been shown to have consistent success. Table 30.2 lists our recommendations for agents that treat common superficial bacterial infections after the specific bacteriologic cause has been identified.

Of increasing concern is the emergence of antimicrobial resistance among isolates of *S. aureus* that are associated with skin infection . Previously, this was primarily limited to nosocomial infection, but recent reports of outpatient methicillin-resistant *S. aureus* (MRSA) infection in both children and adults are increasing (23,24). At present, the only parenterally administered antimicrobial agents that are universally active against MRSA are vancomycin (even though rare isolates with intermediate resistance to vancomycin have been described recently), quinupristin–dalfopristin, and linezolid. Among these drugs, only linezolid is also available for oral administration. Other oral agents that may have activity against MRSA are trimethoprim–sulfamethoxazole and minocycline, but this requires confirmation through in vitro–susceptibility testing. The newer fluoroquinolones (i.e., gatifloxacin, moxifloxacin, gemifloxacin) usually have good activity against methicillin-sensitive *S. aureus* but generally are not considered effective against MRSA. If active in vitro, oral rifampin can be added for antimicrobial efficacy but should never be used as monotherapy because of the possibility of rapid emergence of resistance.

Surgical intervention is usually not required for superficial bacterial infections; however, the role of surgery cannot be overestimated in deeper or necrotizing skin infections (*see* Chapter 31). However, surgical drainage is indicated for furuncles, carbuncles, and hidradenitis suppurativa with large and fluctuant lesions. Antibiotic treatment should be continued until evidence of acute inflammation has subsided.

Treatment of hidradenitis suppurativa is difficult, particularly when the disease process is chronic, because of deep-seated abscesses and scar tissue that are inaccessible to antimicrobial agents. Antimicrobial therapy accompanied by the local application of moist heat is often helpful in the initial phases of infection. Surgical drainage is required in the management of abscesses. Radical excision of tissue with subsequent skin grafting is often necessary for severe cases that exhibit extensive scarring.

Prevention

The management of patients with recurrent furunculosis presents a troublesome problem because most patients do not have definable underlying defects. However, a higher rate of colonization with *S. aureus* has been observed in subgroups of patients (e.g., diabetic patients, dialysis patients) with this condition. Therefore, because even small scratches or blisters may be colonized more rapidly and infected at an early stage, we recommend the use of topical antibiotics (e.g., mupirocin, bacitracin, neomycin) for the early treatment of abrasions in such patients. In one comparative study of the efficacy of topical mupirocin (2%) cream with oral cephalexin in treating secondarily infected traumatic skin lesions (e.g., lacerations), pathogen-eradication rates in the patients who could be evaluated were 100% for both treatment groups (25).

Preventive management of recurrent furunculosis involves the following measures:

- **Institute a regimen of meticulous skin care with antibacterial soaps (e.g., Phisoderm) and frequent washing:** Because infections (particularly impetigo) may be spread among family members, a separate towel and washcloth (carefully washed in hot water before use) should be reserved for each patient. Chlorhexidine solution or hexachlorophene also may be used to reduce staphylococcal skin colonization.

- **Systemic antibiotic treatment should be instituted for active infection:** However, prolonged treatment (e.g., 2 months) seems to be no more effective than a 10- to 14-day course of treatment in preventing recurrences (4).
- **Further measures aimed at preventing a carrier state can be considered if infection continues to recur:** Nasal application of 2% mupirocin ointment in a soft, white paraffin base for 5 days can eliminate colonization of *S. aureus* in otherwise healthy patients for up to 90 days. Oral antibiotics (e.g., rifampin with another antimicrobial agent to prevent resistance) can be used in an attempt to eradicate a carrier state. In one very limited study, prophylaxis of oral clindamycin (150 mg qid for 3 months), without an accompanying intranasal antimicrobial agent, reduced the frequency of recurrent staphylococcal skin infections (4).

The likelihood of recurrent cellulitis at sites of previous surgery (e.g., after coronary artery bypass surgery or mastectomy) also may be reduced by reducing skin colonization with antibacterial soaps and by controlling tinea pedis in the case of recurrent cellulitis of the lower extremities after coronary artery bypass surgery. Prolonged antimicrobial prophylaxis with erythromycin has been shown to be effective and safe for preventing subsequent recurrent episodes of soft tissue infections in such patients (26). However, it is our recommendation that, in the case of recurrent cellulitis of the lower extremities, systemic antibiotic therapy should be reserved only for patients who do not respond to antibacterial soaps and control of tinea pedis.

REFERENCES

1. **File TM Jr, Tan JS.** Treatment of bacterial skin and soft tissue infections. *Surg Gynecol Obstet.* 1991;S172:17–24.

2. **Finch R.** Skin and soft tissue infections. *Lancet.* 1988;1:164–8.

3. **Brook I.** Cellulitis and fasciitis. *Curr Treat Op Infect Dis.* 2000;2:127–46.

4. **Swartz MN.** Cellulitis and subcutaneous tissue infections. In Mandell GL, Bennett JE, Dolin R (eds). *Principles and Practice of Infectious Diseases*, 4th ed. New York: Churchill Livingstone; 2000:1037–57.

5. **Waldvogel FA.** *Staphylococcus aureus*. In Mandell GL, Douglas RG Jr, Bennett JE (eds). *Principles and Practice of Infectious Diseases*, 4th ed. New York: Churchill Livingstone; 1995:1754–76.

6. **Schluter B, Konig W.** Microbial pathogenicity and host defense mechanisms: crucial parameters of posttraumatic infections. *Thorac Cardiovasc Surg.* 1990;38:339–47.

7. **Musher D.** The gram-positive cocci. Part I: Streptococci. *Hosp Pract.* 1988;23:63–76.

8. **Bisno AL, Stevens DL.** Streptococcal infections of skin and soft tissues. *N Engl J Med* 1996;334:240–5.

9. **Bisno A.** *Streptococcus pyogenes.* In Mandell GL, Douglas RG Jr, Bennett JE (eds). *Principles and Practice of Infectious Diseases,* 4th ed. New York: Churchill Livingstone; 1995: 1786–98.

10. **Musher D.** The gram-positive cocci. Part II: Staphylococci. Hosp Pract. 1988;23: 179–93.

11. **File TM Jr, Tan JS, DiPersio J.** Group A streptococcal necrotizing fasciitis: Diagnosing and treating the "flesh-eating bacteria syndrome." *Cleve Clinic J Med.* 1998; 65(5):241–9.

12. **Alder AI, Altman J.** An outbreak of mud-wrestling–induced pustular dermatitis in college students. JAMA. 1993;269:502–4.

13. **Jacobson JA.** Pool-associated *Pseudomonas aeruginosa* dermatitis and other bathing-associated infections. *Infect Control Hosp Epidemiol.* 1985;6:398–401.

14. **Brook I, Frazier EH.** Clinical features and aerobic and anaerobic characteristics of cellulitis. *Arch Surg.* 1995;130:786–92.

15. **Baddour LM, Bisno AL.** Recurrent cellulitis after saphenous venectomy for coronary bypass. *Ann Intern Med.* 1982;97:493–6.

16. **File TM, Tan JS, Maseelall EA, et al.** Recurrent cellulitis after bypass surgery associated with psoriasis. *JAMA.* 1984;252:1681.

17. **Newell PM, Norden CW.** Value of needle aspiration in bacteriologic diagnosis of cellulitis in adults. *J Clin Microbiol.* 1988;26:401–4.

18. **Bernard P, Bedane C, Mounier M, et al.** Streptococcal cause of erysipelas and cellulitis in adults: a microbiologic study using a direct immunofluorescence technique. *Arch Dermatol.* 1989;125:779–82.

19. **Kielhofner MA, Brown B, Dall L.** Influence of underlying disease process on the utility of cellulitis needle aspirates. *Arch Intern Med.* 1988;148:2451–2.

20. **Lebre C, Girard-Pipau F, Roujeau JC, et al.** Value of fine-needle aspiration in infectious cellulitis. *Arch Dermatol.* 1996;132:842–3.

21. **Hook EW III, Hooton TM, Horton CA, et al.** Microbiologic evaluation of cutaneous cellulitis in adults. *Arch Intern Med.* 1986;146:295–7.

22. **Sachs MK.** The optimum use of needle aspiration in bacteriologic diagnosis of cellulitis in adults. *Arch Intern Med.* 1990;150:1907–12.

23. **Herold BC, Immergluck LC, Maranan MC, et al.** Community-acquired methicillin-resistant *Staphylococcus aureus* in children with no identified predisposing risk. *JAMA.* 1998;279:593–8.

24. **Moreno F, Crisp C, Jorgenson JH, et al.** Methicillin-resistant *Staphylococcus aureus* as a community organism. *Clin Infect.* 1995;21:1308–12.

25. **Henkel TJ, Bottonfield G, Drehobl M, et al.** Comparison of mupirocin calcium cream with oral cephalexin in the treatment of secondarily infected traumatic lesions. 20th International Congress of Chemotherapy. 1997, Sydney, Australia, Abstract No. 5308.

26. **Kremer M, Zuckerman R, Avraham Z, Raz R.** Long-term antimicrobial therapy in the prevention of recurrent soft-tissue infections. *J Infect.* 1991;22:37–40.

31

Necrotizing Soft Tissue Infections

Thomas M. File Jr., MD, MS

Necrotizing soft tissue infections include infections of the skin and skin structures that share a clinical picture that is characterized by necrosis of the skin and associated tissues (e.g., subcutaneous tissue, fascia, muscle) (1–5). These infections occur less frequently than do pyoderma but require an aggressive early response for optimal management. They often progress rapidly and dramatically, and they frequently require urgent, aggressive surgical excision of tissue. Additionally, these infections are often deep and devastating, because they can cause major destruction of tissue and may have a fatal outcome.

Generally, necrotizing soft tissue infections are classified into specific entities (e.g., necrotizing fasciitis, clostridial myonecrosis, synergistic necrotizing cellulitis) according to selected characteristics (Table 31.1) (3–6). However, the initial clinical manifestations of such infections may not be distinct. I agree with other clinicians that the classification of these infections into precise categories is often difficult and is not significant to the initial management of the patient (1,6a).

Etiology

Necrotizing soft tissue infections can be classified etiologically as either polymicrobial (involving mixed aerobes and anaerobes) or monomicrobial infectious processes.

Table 31.1 Characteristics of the Common Severe Necrotizing Soft Tissue Infections

Characteristic	Anaerobic Gas-Forming Cellulitis	Synergistic Necrotizing Cellulitis	Clostridial Myonecrosis (Gas Gangrene)	Streptococcal Myonecrosis	Necrotizing Fasciitis
Predisposing condition	Trauma	Diabetes, previous local and/or perirectal lesions	Trauma or surgical wound	Trauma, surgery	Diabetes, trauma, surgery, perineal infection
Incubation	>3 days	3–14 days	1–4 days	3–4 days	1–4 days
Etiology	Clostridia, others	Mixed aerobes and anaerobes	Clostridia, especially C. perfringens	Anaerobic streptococci	Type I: polymicrobial (aerobic and anaerobic) Type II: S. pyogenes
Systemic toxicity	Minimal	Moderate to severe	Severe	Minimal until late in the course	Moderate to severe
Course	Gradual	Acute	Acute	Subacute	Acute to subacute
Wound findings					
Local pain	Minimal	Moderate to severe	Severe	Late in the course	Minimal to moderate
Skin appearance	Swollen, minimal discoloration	Erythematous or gangrenous	Tense and blanched, yellow-bronze in color, and necrotic with hemorrhagic bullae	Erythematous or yellow-bronze in color	Blanched, erythematous, and necrotic with hemorrhagic bullae
Gas	Abundant	Variable	Usually present	Variable	Variable
Muscle involvement	None	Variable	Myonecrosis	Myonecrosis	None
Discharge	Thin, dark; sweet or foul odor	Dark or "dishwater" pus; putrid odor	Serosanguineous; sweet or foul odor	Seropurulent	Seropurulent or "dishwater" pus; putrid odor
Gram stain findings	PMNLs, gram-positive bacilli	PMNLs, mixed flora	Sparse PMNLs, gram-positive bacilli	PMNLs, gram-positive bacilli	PMNLs, mixed flora, gram-positive cocci
Surgical therapy	Debridement	Wide filleting incisions	Extensive incision, amputation	Excision of necrotic muscle	Wide filleting incisions

PMNLs = polymorphonuclear leukocytes.
Modified from Gorbach SL. IDCP guidelines: necrotizing skin and soft tissue infections. *Infect Dis Clin Pract.* 1996;5:406–72.

Polymicrobial Infectious Processes

Polymicrobial infections are commonly found in the perineal area and lower extremities. In such cases, the fecal flora contribute to other skin pathogens. Gram-positive organism (e.g., *Staphylococcus, Streptococcus, Enterococcus sp.*), gram-negative enteric bacilli, and anaerobes are often isolated from such infections. In combination, these bacteria may induce the formation of abscesses as well as severe necrotizing infections.

Clinical medicine has numerous examples of mixed bacterial infections. The polymicrobial nature of peritonitis and intra-abdominal abscess formation is well known to surgeons. Aspiration of oropharyngeal secretions may lead to necrotizing mixed aerobic/anaerobic pneumonitis, which is often more serious than pneumonia that is caused by a single organism. Polymicrobial causes of skin and soft issue infections may be found in surgical-site infections, bite-wound infections, pressure-ulcer infections, and diabetic foot infections. The evaluating physician must be aware of the possibility of a synergistic poly-microbial infection in such cases so that appropriate early therapy can be initiated.

The pathogenic role of mixed aerobic/anaerobic infections has been well demonstrated in a number of anatomical models of infection (6). Weinstein and coworkers first published results of a rat model of peritonitis/intra-abdominal abscess that demonstrated a biphasic process of infection (7). The first phase manifested itself by peritonitis that was caused by facultative aerobes, whereas anaerobes were predominant in the second phase. Using an animal model that more closely resembles skin and soft tissue infections, Brook (8) evaluated the effect of subcutaneously inoculating various combinations of aerobes and anaerobes into mice. The mice were then challenged with either a single organism or a mixture of *Bacteroides* species and facultative aerobic organisms. The bacterial strains tested included *Bacteroides fragilis, Escherichia coli, B. melaninogenicus, Klebsiella pneumoniae, Pseudomonas aeruginosa, Staphylococcus aureus, Streptococcus pyogenes,* and *E. fecalis,* all of which are organisms commonly found in the mixed aerobic/anaerobic skin and soft tissue infections of humans. Infection caused by individual isolates was relatively innocuous, but combinations of facultative organisms and aerobes showed a synergistic effect, as manifested by the formation of abscesses and by significant animal mortality. This synergistic effect was demonstrated for *Bacteroides* species in conjunction with all of the facultative aerobic organisms tested. The effect also was seen among most peptostreptococci, *P. aeruginosa,* and *S. aureus.*

Brook (8) electively treated inoculated animals with a variety of antibiotics that were chosen specifically to cover aerobes, anaerobes, or both of these components of mixed infections. Antimicrobial agents that were directed at one component of a mixed infection did not eliminate the infection or the untreated organisms completely; therefore, the abscesses persisted. Treatment aimed at both components was required to achieve significant reductions in the numbers of both contributing agents. Using another model of soft tissue infection, Kelly (9) demonstrated synergy between *E. coli* and *B. fragilis* when these organisms were injected subcutaneously into guinea pigs. A certain threshold count or number of organisms was required for this synergistic effect to occur. When the size of the *E. coli* or *B. fragilis* inoculum was below a critical threshold (10^4 *B. fragilis* or 10^3 *E. coli*), there was no abscess or necrosis, whereas when bacterial numbers were above the threshold, significant bacterial growth, abscess formation, and necrosis were present.

These animal studies and others tend to confirm the observation that mixed aerobic/anaerobic infections are often more virulent than monomicrobial infections caused by the same organisms. Mackowiak (10) proposed the following four principles by which microorganisms may interact to produce a synergistic infection:

1. An effect on host defenses (most commonly inhibition of phagocytosis)
2. Supplementation of vital nutrients
3. Provision of environmental conditions that are favorable for growth
4. Increased virulence of the infecting organisms

Monomicrobial Infectious Processes

Several individual pathogens may cause necrotizing soft tissue infections. The most clinically significant of these infections are caused by *Clostridium* species and *S. pyogenes*.

Clostridia may play a role in various infections of skin, subcutaneous tissue, and muscle (5) that include crepitant cellulitis, pyomyositis, and clostridial myonecrosis (gas gangrene). *Clostridium perfringens* is the major causative species of such infections and accounts for approximately 80% of cases. Other species that cause such infections include *C. septicum*, *C. novyi*, *C. sordellii*, *C. histolyticum*, and *C. bifermentans*. Clostridial species that have been implicated in necrotizing soft tissue infections produce various exotoxins that contribute to the pathophysiology of such infections. Clostridia are anaerobic and therefore require an anaerobic environment for multiplication and production of these necrotizing toxins. The clostridial organisms that cause necrotizing soft tissue infections can be of either endogenous or exogenous origin, in that they may be present in the patient's normal gastrointestinal flora or may come from soil contamination in wounds caused by, for example, motorcycle or lawn mower accidents.

The past decade has seen an increasing number of reports of necrotizing fasciitis caused by the group A streptococcus (GAS) *S. pyogenes* (11,12). Such infections may appear suddenly, sometimes in previously healthy patients with no history of a wound or injury, and can progress within hours to necrosis of an entire limb, often culminating in amputation or death. The lay media quickly named this disease the "flesh-eating bacteria syndrome." GAS produce a number of surface components and extracellular products that are believed to play important roles in the pathogenesis of necrotizing soft tissue infections. Such components include M proteins, hyaluronic acid capsules, and pyrogenic exotoxins (streptococcal pyrogenic exotoxins Spe-A, Spe-B, and Spe-C). Streptococcal pyrogenic exotoxins belong to a group of proteins called *super antigens*, which in some individuals may activate a much larger proportion of T cells than do conventional peptide antigens and may cause various cytokines to be produced. These cytokines, in turn, are thought to be responsible for the manifestations of streptococcal toxic shock syndrome and necrotizing fasciitis (13).

Other single pathogens associated with necrotizing soft tissue infections include group B streptococci, *Staphylococcus* species, *Vibrio vulnificus* (in cases of salt-water injury), *Aeromonas hydrophila* (in cases of fresh-water injury), Enterobacteriaceae, *P. aeruginosa*, and *Yersinia enterocolitica* (14–19).

Clinical Manifestations

Clinical features that suggest necrotizing soft tissue infections include the following:
- Severe, constant pain
- Bullous lesions
- Gas in soft tissues that is detected by palpation, radiography, or scanning; the gas is produced by metabolic activity of the infecting aerobic and/or anaerobic bacteria; when anaerobes are present, there is often a distinctive putrid odor
- Systemic toxicity manifested by fever and occasionally by delirium
- A tendency toward the rapid spread of infection centrally along fascial planes

The inflammatory reaction in tissues with necrotizing soft tissue infections is often much different from that seen in pyodermas caused by staphylococci, because there is often an associated serous, putrid, dish-watery discharge in the former compared with the purulent discharge associated with abscess formation in the latter. Necrotizing soft tissue infections frequently occur in association with previous trauma, surgery, or other sources of tissue damage. Diabetes mellitus is a common underlying condition (20). Infections associated with preexisting ulcers (e.g., foot ulcers, decubitus ulcers) may progress to necrotizing infections. Tissue necrosis is characteristic and can occur by any of the following means: 1) pressure necrosis in infected areas of the fascia or skin, 2) vascular thrombosis caused by anaerobic organisms via heparinase production or by direct acceleration of coagulation, and 3) extracellular toxins produced by bacteria (e.g., the necrotoxins of *C. perfringens*). The clinical characteristics of the more common necrotizing soft tissue infections are given in Table 31.1. Many of these conditions are differentiated from one another on the basis of anatomic extent of disease, which often can be determined only at the time of surgical intervention. The following sections discuss further salient clinical features of necrotizing soft tissue syndromes.

Polymicrobial Infections

Necrotizing fasciitis refers to deep tissue infections that involve the fascial cleft between the subcutaneous tissue and underlying muscle. Necrotizing fasciitis can be classified into two types: type I is associated with polymicrobial (mixed aerobic and anaerobic) infection, whereas type II is associated with *S. pyogenes* as the most prominent pathogen (21). Examples of polymicrobial infections (type I) include diabetic foot infections, decubitus ulcer infections, postoperative infections, and infections associated with trauma and bite wounds. Necrosis of the overlying cutaneous layer often results from the ischemic effects of vascular thrombosis. The most distinguishing clinical feature of such necrosis is the hard, wooden feel of the subcutaneous tissues. In cellulitis or erysipelas, the subcutaneous tissues can be palpated and are yielding, whereas, in fasciitis, the underlying tissues are firm and the fascial planes and muscle groups cannot be discerned by palpation. It is often possible to observe a broader erythematous track in the skin along the route of the fascial plane as the infection advances. If there is an open wound, probing its edges with a blunt instrument permits ready dissection of the superficial fascial planes well beyond the wound margins. Remarkably little pain may be associated with this procedure because of anesthesia from the necrosis of nerve endings. Infection of the fascial cleft may spread rapidly but is occasionally indolent. In the more indolent cases, biopsy has been useful (22).

Fournier's gangrene is a form of necrotizing fasciitis that involves the fascial planes of the scrotum and/or perineum, which may spread to involve the abdominal wall or thighs. Synergistic necrotizing cellulitis resembles type I necrotizing fasciitis because both are caused by a mixed aerobic/anaerobic infection; however, with necrotizing cellulitis, there is often extension beneath the fascia and that involves the muscle. Just as in clostridial myonecrosis, amputation is required when there is muscle involvement of an extremity. Progressive bacterial synergistic gangrene (often referred to as Meleney's gangrene) is an indolent process characterized by poor healing, often after a surgical operation. The presentation may be one of a slowly progressive (often over several weeks), expanding necrosis. Local pain and tenderness are nearly always present, but fever and systemic toxicity are not associated with this condition as often as the other syndromes discussed in this chapter.

The term *pyomyositis* describes a discrete abscess that develops within individual muscle groups and is caused primarily by *S. aureus* but occasionally by other gram-positive organisms or gram-negative enteric rods. Because of its geographic distribution, this condition is often referred to as *tropical pyomyositis*, but cases are being recognized increasingly in temperate climates, especially among patients with HIV infection or diabetes. Presenting findings are localized pain in a single muscle group, muscle spasm, and fever. The disease most often occurs in an extremity, but any muscle group may be involved. Palpation of a discrete abscess in cases of pyomyositis may not always be possible, because the infection may be localized deep within a muscle; however, the affected area has a firm, woody feel on palpation in addition to being painful and tender.

Clostridial Necrotizing Infections

The clinical picture of clostridial myonecrosis, or classic gas gangrene, is well described (2,5). Clostridial myonecrosis may occur within hours of an initiating insult or surgery and is often associated with sudden pain that increases in severity and extends beyond the wound. Systemic toxicity, indicated by tachycardia and mental contusion, is common. A thin, watery discharge is often noted early in the process, and large hemorrhagic bullae may appear in the vicinity of the wound. Microscopic examination of the discharge often reveals gram-positive rods and a paucity of polymorphonuclear leukocytes. The lack of polymorphonuclear leukocytes is attributable, in part, to clostridial toxins that cause the lysis of white blood cell membranes and subsequent cell death. The characteristic finding in clostridial myonecrosis is necrotic infected muscle. As the disease progresses, the muscle loses viability and turns black. Early diagnosis is essential so that the devitalized tissue can be resected completely.

It should be stressed that, although classic gangrene implies infection by *Clostridium* species (e.g., *C. perfringens*), the isolation of these organisms does not necessarily indicate clinical disease because they can colonize or contaminate wounds (either postsurgically or posttraumatically) without invading tissue. Additionally, *C. perfringens* may cause only cellulitis (anaerobic cellulitis) without deep tissue involvement. In such cases, there may be an abundance of gas formation but without severe pain or systemic toxicity.

Group A Streptococcal Necrotizing Fasciitis

Necrotizing fasciitis caused by GAS tends to occur sporadically. In the largest population surveillance study of GAS necrotizing fasciitis, the incidence was reported to be 0.4 cases per 100,000 population (23). Secondary cases are rare but have been reported among family members, intimate contacts, and medical personnel who care for affected patients (24). Large outbreaks of necrotizing fasciitis caused by GAS have not occurred because the vast majority of people have acquired immunity to one or more of the streptococcal variance factors. However, GAS necrotizing fasciitis can occur in any age group, including young, previously healthy individuals. Infection often occurs after a penetrating or blunt injury to the site of fasciitis but may occur without any noticeable preceding injury. Other predisposing factors include varicella, chronic skin conditions (e.g., decubitus, ischemic ulcers, psoriasis), and previous surgery.

My own experiences and that of other clinicians suggest that the use of nonsteroidal anti-inflammatory drugs (NSAIDs) has a positive association with the progression of invasive GAS infection, including necrotizing fasciitis. Stevens (25) found several cases in which pain from such infection was attributed erroneously to phlebitis, muscle pain, bursitis, or arthritis. Many of the affected patients received NSAIDs but not antibiotics, and the disease progressed even though the NSAIDs reduced the signs and symptoms of inflammation. In many cases, GAS necrotizing fasciitis was not diagnosed until signs of shock or tissue gangrene were apparent. The use of NSAIDs may enhance the production of tumor necrosis factor, probably by preventing feedback inhibitors with prostaglandin E2. NSAIDs may predispose to GAS necrotizing fasciitis by inhibiting granulocyte function, augmenting cytokine production, and attenuating the cardinal manifestations of inflammation in patients with GAS cellulitis.

The most common primary sites of GAS necrotizing fasciitis are the extremities. Among my patients, the upper extremities have been involved most commonly. However, other authors have found the lower extremities to be the most common primary sites of such disease (23). GAS necrotizing fasciitis usually follows a specific sequence, in which diffuse erythema and swelling, exquisite tenderness, and pain are the first signs and symptoms, with lymphangitis and lymphadenitis infrequently observed initially. Bullae filled with clear liquid are the next signs to occur; commonly these bullous lesions rapidly become maroon or violaceous. Frank cutaneous gangrene follows, evolving rapidly and extending along fascial planes as the last step in the sequence. In some patients, necrosis proceeds less quickly. Kaul and coworkers (23) described a subset of patients with diabetes, peripheral vascular disease, or both in whom chronic ischemia may have contributed to soft tissue necrosis and in whom the progression of necrosis was less rapid. Anesthesia of the overlying skin provides a clue to the existence of necrotizing fasciitis rather than just simple cellulitis in the subjacent tissues. As tissue necrosis progresses, pain may disappear because thrombosis in small blood vessels leads to the destruction of the superficial nerves in the underlying subcutaneous tissues. Toxic shock syndrome is linked to streptococcal necrotizing fasciitis in approximately 50% of cases. Table 31.2 lists the criteria for diagnosing these two conditions.

Table 31.2   Case Definitions of Streptococcal Toxic Shock Syndrome* and Necrotizing Fasciitis

Streptococcal Toxic Shock Syndrome: Definite Case
GAS organism isolated from a normally sterile site
  and
Hypotension
  and at least two of the following:
Renal impairment
Coagulopathy
Liver abnormalities
Acute respiratory distress syndrome
Extensive tissue necrosis (i.e., necrotizing fasciitis)
Erythematous rash

Streptococcal Toxic Shock Syndrome: Probable Case
Same as above except that GAS organism is isolated from a *non*sterile site

Necrotizing Fasciitis: Definite Case
Necrosis of soft tissues with involvement of the fascia
  and
Serious systemic disease, including one or more of the following:
  Death
  Shock (systolic blood pressure <90 mm Hg)
  Disseminated intravascular coagulopathy
  Respiratory, hepatic, or renal failure
  and
GAS organism isolated from a normally sterile site

Necrotizing Fasciitis: Probable Case
Necrosis of soft tissues with involvement of the fascia
  and
Serious systemic disease (as above)
  and either of the following:
Serologic confirmation of GAS infection by a fourfold rise against streptolysin O or
  DNAase B
  or
Histologic confirmation of gram-positive cocci in a necrotic soft tissue injection

---

GAS = group A streptococci.
*Any GAS infection associated with early onset of shock and organ failure.
Republished with permission from Working Group on Severe Streptococcal Infections. Defining the group A streptococcal toxic shock syndrome: rationale and consensus definition. *JAMA*. 1993;269:390–1.

Diagnosis

Although the diagnosis of necrotizing fasciitis and other necrotizing soft tissue infections may be clear in the later stages of these diseases (i.e., because of the extensive necrosis that occurs), these conditions are often difficult to differentiate from primary cellulitis with presentation at an early stage. However, their distinction is important because cellulitis can be treated with antimicrobial agents without surgical management, whereas deep, necrotizing soft tissue infections require timely surgical debridement and excision of tissue in addition to the use of antimicrobial agents.

Clinical characteristics that should lead to the consideration of deep, necrotizing soft tissue infections are listed in Table 31.3. In cellulitis, bullae may be observed without fasciitis and also may be associated with toxins (e.g., from a brown recluse spider bite) and with primarily dermatologic conditions (e.g., pyoderma gangrenosum). However, fever with unexplained severe musculoskeletal pain is an important clue to imminent necrotizing fasciitis. Other conditions that may mimic the early manifestations of necrotizing soft tissue infections include trauma with hematoma (although fever and leukocytosis are usually absent), phlebitis, bursitis, and arthritis. Of note is that gas in subcutaneous tissue can occur from such noninfectious processes as 1) subcutaneous emphysema secondary to local trauma or after surgical procedures, 2) the use of hydrogen peroxide, and 3) from the introduction of air during irrigation.

Leukocytosis is usually present in most deep, necrotizing soft tissue infections. Gram staining of smears made from aspirates or debrided tissue often reveals causative organisms (e.g., gram-positive cocci in GAS necrotizing fasciitis). In contrast, I have found that a Gram stain is rarely positive in cases of non–necrotizing cellulitis. An increased serum creatinine kinase level is often a clue to the presence of necrotizing fasciitis or myositis. Additionally, blood cultures are often positive in necrotizing soft tissue infections (23). Kaul and coworkers (23) found that bacteremia predicted increased mortality in necrotiz-

Table 31.3   Clues That Help Distinguish Necrotizing Fasciitis from Cellulitis

Severe pain followed by anesthesia
Rapidly spreading swelling and inflammation
Bullae
Necrosis (late appearance)
Toxic shock syndrome
Elevated creatinine kinase level
Predisposing factors (*Varicella* infection, NSAID use)

NSAID = nonsteroidal anti-inflammatory drug.

ing fasciitis; however, bacteremia is not a clinically useful marker for such disease because it can be detected only 24 to 48 hours after presentation. Similarly, the presence of GAS bacteremia does not distinguish necrotizing fasciitis from cellulitis reliably, because bacteremia also can occur in non–necrotizing cellulitis.

The most definitive diagnostic test for a necrotizing soft tissue infections is therapeutic surgical exploration to define the extent of infection of the involved tissues (e.g., subcutaneous, fascia, muscle). Whenever a necrotizing soft tissue infection is considered in a differential diagnosis, immediate surgical evaluation is imperative. Diagnostic studies performed before surgical incision and drainage may include radiography (to demonstrate soft tissue swelling or the presence of gas), computed tomography or ultrasound (to detect fluid or abscesses and to direct needle aspiration), and biopsy. Computed tomography, magnetic resonance imaging, and routine soft tissue radiography may be helpful in demonstrating the involvement of subcutaneous tissue beyond the visible cutaneous abnormality in a necrotizing soft tissue infection. However, these studies should not delay surgical evaluation if such an infection is suspected; they should serve to expedite and direct surgical intervention.

Treatment

The management of necrotizing soft tissue infections requires expeditious evaluation and early surgical intervention. Kaul and coworkers (23) reported that, without appropriate surgical intervention, the mortality rate in necrotizing fasciitis approached 100%. McHenry and coworkers (20) reported that survival in necrotizing fasciitis correlated with the timing of surgery. Thus, regardless of the microbial cause of a necrotizing soft tissue infection, the primary treatment is urgent surgery accompanied by antibiotic therapy with agents active against the most likely pathogens (i.e., streptococci, staphylococci, enterococci, clostridia, and mixed aerobic/anaerobic flora).

Surgical Therapy

Surgery for necrotizing soft tissue infections has three goals: 1) to remove all necrotic tissue by radical debridement, 2) to preserve as much viable skin as possible, and 3) to maintain hemostasis. Amputation may be necessary to remove all nonviable tissues (which is particularly important for myonecrosis). A "second-look" procedure may be and often is necessary within 12 to 24 hours to reculture and further remove any necrotic and infected materials that may have been missed in the initial procedure. Multiple debridements may be necessary: McHenry and coworkers (20) reported a case series of 65 patients with necrotizing fasciitis, each of whom needed an average of three surgical debridements and several of whom needed amputations to control the infection. General principles in the care of necrotizing fasciitis, which also apply to many other necrotizing soft tissue infections, are listed in Table 31.4.

Empirical Antimicrobial Therapy

Because it is difficult to determine the microbial cause of a necrotizing soft tissue infection on the basis of its clinical presentation, empirical antibiotic therapy should be begun as soon the condition is suspected. The antimicrobial agents chosen for use should have activity against streptococci, staphylococci, clostridia, and mixed aerobic/anaerobic organisms. The combination of a beta-lactam drug plus a beta-lactamase inhibitor (e.g., ticarcillin–clavulanate, piperacillin–tazobactam) or the use of a single carbapenem should provide adequate coverage.

Penicillin is ineffective for treating necrotizing soft tissue infections in the presence of a large inoculum of bacteria. Furthermore, Stevens and coworkers (26) demonstrated that streptococci do not express penicillin-binding proteins on their membranes during the stationary phase of their cell cycle (i.e., when they are not dividing). Clindamycin has shown a greater efficacy than penicillin in formidable, experimentally induced streptococcal infection (27). Un-

Table 31.4   General Principles in the Care of Patients with Necrotizing Fasciitis

Principles
- Patients with necrotizing fasciitis or myonecrosis who do not undergo exploration and debridement will surely die.
- Devitalized tissue, including muscle, fascia, and skin, must be removed.
- Appropriate surgical debridement in certain locations of the body (e.g., head, neck, thorax, abdomen) may be virtually impossible.
- Multiple debridements over the course of several weeks are usually necessary.
- Extensive reconstructive surgery is generally necessary.

Corollaries
- Adequate debridement can rarely be performed in one step.
- Skin overlying necrotic fascia may remain viable; if it appears viable at the time of initial debridement, it may be spared for a second look during follow-up debridement.
- Patients with established necrotizing fasciitis are frequently poor surgical risks, with high rates of surgical mortality and morbidity; however, without the operation, patients face a mortality rate of virtually 100%.
- If primary care physicians are concerned that a deeper infection might be present, surgical evaluation is warranted.

Adapted from Stevens DL. Necrotizing fasciitis: Don't wait to make a diagnosis. *Infect Med.* 1997;14:684–88.

like the beta-lactam drugs, clindamycin inhibits bacterial protein synthesis and is unaffected by inoculum size or the stage of bacterial growth in streptococcal infection (27). Additionally, clindamycin suppresses the synthesis of bacterial toxin and enhances the phagocytosis of streptococci.

We recommend initial therapy with the combination of a beta-lactam drug and beta-lactamase inhibitor plus clindamycin until the cause of a necrotizing soft tissue infection is known. Once the results of appropriate cultures are available, antimicrobial therapy should be specified for the pathogens isolated. The duration of therapy varies with the extent of infection, clinical course of the patient, and presence or absence of metastatic infection; however, a minimum of 2 weeks of therapy is usually required. Tetanus prophylaxis should be given to patients whose immunization status is not up to date (Table 31.5).

Other Therapies

Hyperbaric oxygen is debated as a therapy for necrotizing soft tissue infections (2,12). It has long been recommended for the treatment of clostridial myonecrosis and more recently has been applied to other necrotizing infections. However, the role of hyperbaric oxygen is adjunctive at best. Its benefits are far clearer in clostridial myonecrosis than in other necrotizing infections because hyperbaric oxygen is bactericidal for *C. perfringens* and may reduce the genesis of exotoxin in clostridial myonecrosis but does not neutralize toxin that is already present. The use of hyperbaric oxygen therapy should be limited to specialized centers where complications can be minimized, and this therapy should never take precedence over surgical debridement of necrotizing soft tissue infections.

Intravenous immunoglobulin (IVIG) has been shown to have some beneficial effect in treating the toxic shock syndrome associated with GAS necrotizing fasciitis (28). This effect may come from the ability of IVIG to neutralize

---

Table 31.5   Recommended Empirical Therapy for Necrotizing Fasciitis

Surgical debridement, amputation
Antimicrobial therapy
  Clindamycin 600–900 mg every 8 hours*
   plus one of the following:
  Piperacillin–tazobactam 3.375–4.5 g every 6 hours
  Ticarcillin–clavulanate 3.1 g every 4–6 hours
  Imipenem–cilastin 500–750 mg every 6–8 hours
Tetanus toxoid
Intravenous immunoglobulin[†]

---

* Use clindamycin and ciprofloxacin in beta-lactam–intolerant patients.
[†] Consider in severe cases only; see text.

superantigen. Kaul and coworkers (29) observed a beneficial effect of IVIG in 21 consecutive patients with GAS-associated toxic shock syndrome who received a single dose of 2 g/kg, with a repeated dose at 48 hours if the they remained unstable. The proportion of cases with 30-day survival was higher among patients treated with IVIG than in a control group (67% vs. 34%; $p =$ 0.02). However, the findings of this study must be considered on the basis of the control group having been an historical one. Because it is unlikely that a randomized controlled trial of IVIG therapy for GAS-associated toxic shock syndrome will be performed, it seems reasonable at this time to consider IVIG for patients with severe necrotizing fasciitis caused by GAS.

Prevention

Because necrotizing soft tissue infections often occur as complications of less serious cutaneous infections (e.g., diabetic lower-extremity ulcers), attention should be focused on preventing the pressure ulcers and wounds of patients with identifiable risk factors for necrotizing infections. Patients with conditions such as diabetes need to be educated about their predisposition to infection and alerted to the early signs of infection. Hopefully, the early treatment of superficial infections in such patients can ward off the serious complication of deep, necrotizing infection (30).

Outbreaks of necrotizing GAS infections (especially clusters of toxic shock syndrome and necrotizing fasciitis) have raised concern about the transmissibility of the invasive etiologic strains of GAS and the need for prophylaxis against such infections. Although some clinicians support this strategy, it has not been verified by clinical data. Two possible strategies for preventing GAS infection are based on observations of their transmission within families and to health care providers. The first strategy is to give preventive treatment to individuals who have come in contact with the secretions or culture specimens of patients infected with GAS. The second strategy is to treat patients whose cultures are positive for GAS (31). Recently, the Ontario Ministry of Health developed guidelines for the preventive treatment of close contacts of people with serious GAS disease (Donald A. Low, personal communication). These guidelines state that chemoprophylaxis may be considered for contacts of patients with invasive GAS infection who present with toxic shock syndrome or necrotizing fasciitis or who die within 7 days of diagnosis. Significant contacts include the following:

- Household contacts (all contacts living in the same household as the case patient within the 7 days before the case patient's having become ill).
- Individuals who share sleeping arrangements with the case patient.

- Any individuals who have had direct contact with the mucous membrane or oral or nasal secretions of a case patient within 76 days before onset of the case patient's illness.

A 10-day course of treatment with a cephalosporin (or erythromycin if the contact is allergic) is recommended for all such contacts. No controlled studies support such a recommendation, but it seems a reasonable approach based on what is known about GAS-related disease.

REFERENCES

1. **File TM Jr, Tan JS.** Treatment of necrotizing soft tissue infections. *Compl Surg.* 1993;(Suppl):43–9.
2. **Lewis RT.** Necrotizing soft tissue infections. *Infect Dis Clin North Am.* 1992;6:693–701.
3. **Gorbach SL.** IDCP Guidelines: necrotizing skin and soft tissue infections. Part I: Necrotizing fasciitis. *Infect Dis Clin Pract.* 1996;5:406–11.
4. **Gorbach SL.** IDCP Guidelines: necrotizing skin and soft tissue infections. Part II: Myositis, Meleney's gangrene, pyomyositis, necrotizing cellulitis, nonclostridial cellulitis, and Fournier's gangrene. *Infect Dis Clin Pract.* 1996;5:463–72.
5. **Swartz MN.** Cellulitis and subcutaneous tissue infections. In Mandell GL, Bennett JE, Dolin R (eds). *Principles and Practice of Infectious Diseases,* 4th ed. Philadelphia: WB Saunders; 1995:909–29.
6. **File TM Jr, Tan JS.** The triple threat of gram-positive cocci, gram-negative bacilli, and anaerobes. In CE Nord (ed). *The Role of Piperacillin/Tazobactam in the Treatment of Skin and Soft Tissue Infections.* PharmaLibri: Montreal; 1994.
6a. **Dellinger EP.** Severe necrotizing soft tissue infections: multiple disease entities requiring a common approach. *JAMA.* 1981;246:1717–21.
7. **Weinstein WM, Onderdonk AB, Bartlett JG, et al.** Experimental intra-abdominal abscesses in rats: development of an experimental model. *Infect Immunol.* 1974;10:1250.
8. **Brook I.** Synergistic aerobic and anaerobic infections. *Clin Ther.* 1987;20(Suppl A)19–35.
9. **Kelly MJ.** The quantitative and histological demonstration of pathogenic synergy between *Escherichia coli* and *Bacteroides fragilis* in guinea pig wounds. *J Med Microbiol.* 1978;11:511–22.
10. **Mackowiak PA.** Microbial synergism in human infections (second of two parts). *N Engl J Med.* 1978;298:83–7.
11. **Stevens DL.** Invasive group A streptococcus infection. *Clin Infect Dis.* 1992;14:2–13.
12. **File TM Jr, Tan JS, DiPersio JR.** Group A streptococcal necrotizing fasciitis: diagnosing and treating the "flesh-eating bacteria syndrome." *Cleve Clin J Med.* 1998;65:241–9.
13. **Stevens DL, Bryant AE, Hackett SP, et al.** Group A streptococcal bacteremia: the role of tumor necrosis factor in shock and organ failure. *J Infect Dis.* 1996;173:619–26.
14. **Gardan M, Low DE, Saginur R, Miller MA.** Group B streptococcal necrotizing fasciitis and streptococcal toxic shock–like syndrome in adults. *Arch Intern Med.* 1998;158:1704–8.

15. **Bodemer C, Panhans A, Chretien-Marquet B, et al.** Staphylococcal necrotizing fasciitis in the mammary region in childhood: a report of five cases. *J Pediatr.* 1997; 131:466–9.

16. **Halow KD, Harner RC, Fontenelle LJ.** Primary skin infections secondary to *Vibrio vulnificus*: the role of operative intervention. *J Am Coll Surg.* 1996;183:329–34.

17. **Furusu A, Yoshizuka N, Abe K, et al.** *Aeromonas hydrophila* necrotizing fasciitis and gas gangrene in a diabetic patient on haemodialysis. *Nephrol Dial Transplant.* 1997;12: 1730–4.

18. **Schreuder F, Chatoo M.** Another cause of necrotizing fasciitis? *J Infect.* 1997; 35:177–8.

19. **Zipper RP, Bustamante MA, Khatib R.** *Serratia marcescens*: a single pathogen in necrotizing fasciitis. *Clin Infect Dis.* 1996;23:648–9.

20. **McHenry CR, Piotrowski JJ, Petrinic D, Malangoni MA.** Determinants of mortality for necrotizing soft tissue infections. *Ann Surg.* 1995;221:556–63.

21. **Guilano A, Lewis F, Hadley K, Balisdell FW.** Bacteriology of necrotizing fasciitis. *Am J Surg.* 1977;134:52–7.

22. **Stamenkovic I, Lew PD.** Early recognition of potentially fatal necrotizing fasciitis. *N Engl J Med.* 1984;310:1689–93.

23. **Kaul R, McGeer A, Low D, et al.** Population-based surveillance of group A streptococcal necrotizing fasciitis: clinical features, prognostic indicators, and microbiologic analysis of seventy-seven cases. *Am J Med.* 1997;103:18–24.

24. **DiPersio JR, File TM, Stevens DL, et al.** Spread of serious disease-producing M3 clones of group A *Streptococcus* among family members and health care workers. *Clin Infect Dis.* 1996;22:490–5.

25. **Stevens DL.** Could nonsteroidal anti-inflammatory drugs (NSAIDs) enhance the progression of bacterial infections to toxic shock syndrome? *Clin Infect Dis.* 1995;21: 977–80.

26. **Stevens DL, Yan S, Bryant AE.** Penicillin-binding protein expression at different growth stages determines penicillin efficacy *in vitro* and *in vivo*: an explanation for the inoculum effect. *J Infect Dis.* 1993;167:1401–5.

27. **Stevens DL, Gibbons AE, Bergstrom R, Winn V.** The Eagle effect revisited: efficacy of clindamycin, erythromycin, and penicillin in the treatment of streptococcal myositis. *J Infect Dis.* 1988;158:23–8.

28. **Norrby-Teglund A, Kaul R, Low DE, et al.** Plasma from patients with severe group A streptococcal infections treated with normal polyspecific IgG inhibits streptococci: superantigen-induced T cell proliferation and cytokine expression. *J Immunol.* 1996; 156:3057–64.

29. **Kaul R, McGeer A, Norrby-Teglund A, et al.** Intravenous immunoglobulin therapy for streptococcal toxic shock syndrome: a comparative observational study. *Clin Infect Dis.* 1999;28:800–7.

30. **File TM Jr, Tan JS.** Diabetic foot infections: treat now or pay later. *Infect Med.* 1993;10:19–20.

31. **Gamba M-A, Martinelli M, Schaad HJ, et al.** Familial transmission of a serious disease-producing group A *Streptococcus* clone: case report and review. *Clin Infect Dis.* 1997;24:1118–21.

32

Foot Infections in Patients with Diabetes Mellitus

Francisco L. Sapico, MD

James S. Tan, MD

Foot infections in diabetic patients are responsible for 50% to 70% of all non–trauma-related amputations performed in hospitals throughout the United States. These amputations have been associated with a 3% to 7% mortality rate and an approximate 36% complication rate (1,2). The average hospital stay for the diabetic patient with foot infection has been reported to range from 22 to 36 days, and in some areas more than 40% of patients remain hospitalized for 3 months (3,4). Considering that 6% to 12% of the population of the United States has diabetes (either diagnosed or undiagnosed) (5), it is easy to recognize that the incidence of diabetic foot infections reaches massive proportions. Therefore, the prevention and optimal management of this disease is of paramount importance in decreasing the morbidity, mortality, and financial burden it incurs.

Pathophysiology

The diabetic patient's susceptibility to foot infection is caused by three metabolic abnormalities associated with the disease: neuropathy, vasculopathy, and immunopathy. These abnormalities are highly prevalent in diabetic patients.

Neuropathy is manifested by autonomic nerve dysfunction, peripheral mononeuropathy, and polyneuropathy, all of which affect the lower extremities to a greater extent than the upper extremities. Autonomic nerve dysfunction reduces sweating and impairs vasomotor responses, resulting in dryness, fissuring, and cracking of the skin and in the formation of calluses at points of increased stress on the skin. Insensitivity to pain may result in physical trauma, thermal or chemical injury, or ischemic damage from unperceived shoe tightness or chronic pressure. The patient may walk on parts of the foot that are injured or poorly adapted for weight bearing, leading to microfractures, ligament tears, and progressive articular damage (Charcot's osteoarthropathy). Neuropathy also may result in uneven weakening of the extrinsic muscles of the foot, leading to toe deformity, prominent metatarsal heads on the plantar side, loss of the plantar arch, or foot drop.

Vasculopathy may result in both macro- and microangiopathy. The vascular disease process, in conjunction with autonomic vasomotor impairment, may cause local hypoxia, atrophy, and necrosis. The combination of neuropathy and vasculopathy may accelerate the process of soft tissue breakdown. Deficient circulation may retard wound healing, and open wounds invite infection.

Immunopathy manifests in several ways. Metabolic abnormalities have been implicated in defects in polymorphonuclear leukocyte function (adherence, chemotaxis, phagocytosis, and microbial killing) (6-8). Poor wound healing, defective granuloma formation, and prolonged persistence of abscesses have been described in animals rendered experimentally diabetic (9,10).

Classification and Clinical Manifestations

Foot infections in diabetes can vary in both severity and clinical presentation (11). Most of these infections arise from some type of trauma, whether from improperly fitting footwear or from puncture or other mechanical injury of the foot. Infections of the diabetic foot can range in severity from the relatively mild (e.g., early infection of a ruptured blister, infected abrasion, corn, or callus; an early web-space infection; paronychia; infected superficial ulcer; mild cellulitis) to the more severe (e.g., crepitant anaerobic cellulitis, abscess of the plantar space, infected gangrene, osteomyelitis, necrotizing fasciitis, nonclostridial myonecrosis).

Foot infections in diabetes have been classified according to their depth of involvement, anatomical location, and severity. Patients with superficial infections of the foot may not manifest signs of systemic toxicity. Paronychia, infected ingrown toenails, infected shallow ulcers, and web-space infections are examples of such superficial infections. Web-space infections are particularly dangerous, because they frequently are missed during routine examinations and because the web spaces are in close proximity to the digital arteries. Edema around these arteries may result in digital gangrene. Additionally, bacteria may gain access to deeper structures by contiguous spread along the tendons. Superficial infections, including dermatophytic infections, may result in cellulitis and deeper tissue involvement in the diabetic foot.

Deep infections of the foot can be subdivided into the three categories: cellulitis of the dorsal foot, deep infection of the plantar space, and infection of a foot ulcer (12,13). Any of these conditions may result in osteomyelitis, sepsis, limb loss, and even death.

Cellulitis of the dorsal foot may begin as an infection at the nail base or in the web space, with subsequent spread to the rest of the foot. Systemic symptoms, such as fever and chills, are common.

Deep infections of the plantar space most often originate from infections of a web space, nail bed, or, less commonly, from direct puncture. Infections of the medial or lateral plantar space are not as dangerous as those of the central space, which may result in loss of skin creases and the longitudinal arch of the foot and may present with swelling behind the medial malleolus. Complications of deep infections of the plantar space may include gangrene of one or more toes, ischemic necrosis of intrinsic foot muscles, suppurative tendinitis, arthritis, and sepsis.

Approximately 15% of all diabetic patients develop foot ulcers during the course of their illness (14). Spread of infection from the ulcer may result in deep-space infection and may be responsible for three fourths of all foot amputations among diabetic patients (15). Neuropathic ulcers are commonly found on the soles of the feet at the sites of bony prominences, such as metatarsal heads, and are often surrounded by a halo of hyperkeratinization but generally have a good blood supply (mal perforans). Ulcers that are caused by vascular insufficiency are usually seen at the tips of the toes or on the heel.

Foot infections in diabetes also have been classified according to clinical severity as mild, moderate (potentially limb-threatening), and severe (potentially life-threatening) (16). Mild infections usually include 1) superficial infections of ulcers without a purulent discharge, and 2) infections in the absence of cellulitis or in the presence of mild cellulitis and without associated systemic toxicity. Moderate infections include those of ulcers that extend to deeper tissues and/or have associated purulence, cellulitis, systemic toxicity, or moderate necrosis. Severe infections are associated with systemic toxicity with or without septic shock, with bacteremia or with marked necrosis or gangrene of the foot.

Microbiology

Early and milder infections of the diabetic foot (e.g., localized cellulitis, infected superficial ulcers without concomitant necrosis and/or gangrene) are generally of monomicrobial origin (17,18). *Staphylococcus aureus*, aerobic strepto-cocci, enterococci, and coagulase-negative staphylococci are generally isolated from these lesions. Occasionally, gram-negative aerobic bacilli (e.g., *Klebsiella*, *Proteus mirabilis*, *Pseudomonas aeruginosa*) may be recovered; however, anaerobes are isolated infrequently from these types of lesions. Despite care in method-ology to avoid isolating skin-colonizing bacteria in cases of chronic, nonheal-ing ulcers (i.e., by debriding the base of the ulcer with a dermal curette or a scalpel to avoid such contamination before specimen collection), it may not be possible to exclude completely such contamination in these types of lesions.

In contrast to such early and milder infections, more severe infections of the diabetic foot, especially when associated with necrotic tissue and/or gan-grene, are generally polymicrobial (19–22). Sapico and coworkers (20) investi-gated quantitative deep tissue cultures of feet that had been amputated from patients with moderately severe to severe diabetic foot infections, while metic-ulously avoiding potentially colonized open ulcers during the collection of specimens for culture. An average of five species per specimen were isolated, with anaerobes and aerobes almost equally represented. Of the 32 specimens studied, 25 yielded both aerobes and anaerobes, six yielded only aerobes, and one yielded only anaerobes. Anaerobes, when present, produced growth of a heavier density in culture than did aerobes. Table 32.1 shows the most com-mon isolated representative species in the order of approximate frequency. However, a special situation exists with osteomyelitis associated with puncture wounds, particularly when it occurs during the wearing of rubber sneakers. In these cases, *P. aeruginosa* has been isolated with remarkable frequency (23).

Appropriate material must be submitted for culture if the results are to be accurate. In the case of infected ulcers, the necrotic tissue that overlies the base of the ulcer needs to be removed surgically, and culture specimens must be taken from the underlying tissue. Specimens taken with a dermal curette or tissue removed with a scalpel are the preferred specimens. Abscesses need to be drained completely by aspiration, and the pus must be sent for culture. Specimens for culture also may be obtained at the time of surgery, and anaer-obic transport media must be used for the culture of anaerobes.

Diagnosis

Diabetic patients with foot infections require a thorough examination that in-cludes evaluation of the patient's vascular and neurological status. The pa-tient should be asked about foot symptoms (e.g., burning, tingling, numbness, pain, coldness), nocturnal pain (or pain while at rest, especially if relieved by dependency of the foot), and intermittent claudication.

Table 32.1 Species Isolated from Deep Tissue Cultures of Moderate to Severe Diabetic Foot Infections*

Aerobes	Anaerobes
Gram-negative bacilli	**Gram-negative bacilli**
Proteus mirabilis	Bacteroides fragilis
Escherichia coli	B. ovatus
Pseudomonas aeruginosa	B. ureolyticus
Enterobacter aerogenes	Other Bacteroides species
Other organisms	**Gram-positive cocci**
Gram-positive cocci	Peptostreptococcus magnus
Enterococcus species	P. anaerobius
Staphylococcus aureus	Other Peptostreptococcus species
Streptococcus group B	**Gram-positive bacilli**
Other organisms	Clostridium bifermentans
	Other Clostridium species

* Listed in descending order of frequency.
Republished with permission from Sapico FL, Witte JL, Canawati HN, et al. The infected foot of the diabetic patient: quantitative microbiology and analysis of clinical features. *Rev Infect Dis.* 1984;6(Suppl 1):171–6.

The evaluation for vascular compromise may be performed initially by noninvasive means. Doppler ultrasonography with waveform analysis is a time-honored procedure that has shown good reliability in evaluating blood flow. However, always remember that noncompliant sclerotic arteries can produce ratios of lower- to upper-extremity flow that exceed 0.45, despite significant circulatory impairment in the legs and feet. Alternative studies include transcutaneous oximetry and magnetic resonance angiography. Contrast arteriograms are invasive and generally are reserved for patients who need vascular reconstruction.

Computed tomography may be valuable in assessing the extent of soft tissue involvement in diabetic foot infections in which edema and gas accumulation may be seen along the fascial planes, such as in necrotizing fasciitis. However, early osteomyelitis may not be detected readily with computed tomography. Triple-phase bone scans are very sensitive but lack specificity in the diagnosis of osteomyelitis. Gallium-67 scans and Indium-111–labeled white blood cell scans are sometimes insufficiently sensitive, especially when the bone infection is chronic. Sequential bone and Gallium-67 scans show better specificity than do bone scans alone, but the results do not seem to be as good as those with magnetic resonance imaging, which has a sensitivity of approximately 98% and a specificity of approximately 80% (24–26). Although false-positive magnetic resonance imaging results may occur in cases of neuropathic osteoarthropathy, especially if it is of relatively acute onset, this may still be the best single technique available for the evaluation of osteomyelitis.

Treatment

In managing infections in diabetic patients, the existing disordered metabolic state should be controlled promptly and aggressively. The effects of sepsis (e.g., hypotension) need to be controlled with intravenous hydration and, if necessary, with vasopressor drugs. The extent of tissue involvement, including the extent of cellulitis, tissue necrosis, and gangrene, has to be assessed. The adequacy of the patient's vascularity, severity of neuropathy, and presence and extent of underlying osteomyelitis must be determined. If the patient exhibits inadequate metabolic control of diabetes despite taking oral antidiabetic agents, the treatment should be replaced by insulin.

Surgical intervention is often necessary to control diabetic foot infections. A decision may have to be made about the need for ablative surgery. Infected ulcers may have to be debrided thoroughly. Early incision and drainage decreases the inoculum size of infecting microorganisms and may accelerate local healing. Before definitive surgery, a trial of appropriate antimicrobial therapy may be indicated to maximize control of cellulitis and to minimize the extent of infection at the intended surgical site. As much of the limb as is necessary must be preserved for future rehabilitation and ambulation, but not so much as to compromise control of the infectious state. Localized osteomyelitis often requires limited surgical ablation, such as toe amputation, ray resection, transmetatarsal amputation, or through-the-ankle (Syme's) amputation. Removal of the infected bone decreases the duration of need for antimicrobial therapy, hastens recovery, and decreases the incidence of relapse. Recent studies have shown that early and limited surgical intervention with aggressive antimicrobial therapy may reduce the number of days of hospitalization, the incidence of relapse, and the need for above-ankle amputation in cases of diabetic foot infection (27,28).

Initial empirical antimicrobial therapy for diabetic foot infections must be directed at the organisms most likely to be involved. Generally, severe infections call for broader-spectrum antimicrobial coverage. More severe infections are associated with extensive cellulitis, tissue necrosis, gas formation, gangrene, and/or bone involvement. Once a patient has begun antimicrobial therapy, it may be adjusted according to the results of culture and susceptibility testing. However, the clinician should be cautioned that isolation of anaerobic bacteria depends heavily on proper specimen collection, the use of anaerobic transport media, and the use of good anaerobic microbiology technique on the part of the clinical laboratory. If any of these criteria have not have been met and if the infectious process is likely to involve anaerobes (e.g., there is an associated foul smell, necrotic tissue is present, gangrene is evident), then coverage of anaerobes is strongly recommended despite the failure to isolate these organisms by culture (*see* Chapter 31).

Generally, milder infections—such as those that are superficial, have small, localized areas of cellulitis, exhibit minimal purulence, show no tissue necrosis or gangrene, are unlikely to involve bone or joint tissue, and show no concomitant signs of sepsis (e.g., high fever, chills, hypotension)—can be managed on an outpatient basis. For outpatient antimicrobial therapy, an oral agent (e.g., clindamycin, cephalexin, amoxicillin–clavulanate, trovafloxacin) may be used, depending on the results of culture. Subsequent culture and susceptibility-testing results may dictate changes in the treatment regimen, especially if there is no clinical response to the originally chosen drug. If hospitalization is required for other reasons (e.g., for control of the patient's metabolic state), parenteral therapy may be given with a first- or second-generation cephalosporin (e.g., cefazolin, cefuroxime).

More severe infections of the diabetic foot, especially limb-threatening infections, require coverage of a broader spectrum of potential pathogens. Recently, emphasis has been given to the use of cost-effective, single-drug regimens that provide broad-spectrum coverage. Antimicrobial agents for these regimens include ampicillin–sulbactam, ticarcillin–clavulanate, piperacillin–tazobactam, and imipenem (or meropenem)–cilastin (29,30). Another possible option is trovafloxacin, which has a very broad spectrum of antimicrobial coverage (including anaerobes) and can be given on a once-daily basis. Unfortunately, the significant liver toxicity of this agent sharply limits its use. Table 32.2 shows one possible approach to the choice of antimicrobial agents for treating diabetic foot infections.

Life-threatening infections, such as necrotizing fasciitis or nonclostridial myonecrosis, or infections associated with sepsis may warrant very broad-spectrum coverage. Piperacillin–tazobactam or imipenem (or meropenem) may be selected because of their superior activity against gram-negative and anaerobic pathogens. Vancomycin may be added, especially in institutions where methicillin-resistant *S. aureus* is a frequent clinical isolate (in community-acquired and other infections). Another possible option is to include an aminoglycoside in the treatment regimen, especially for synergistic activity against a variety of microorganisms; however, aminoglycosides should be used with the utmost caution in diabetic patients who have preexisting renal impairment.

Milder soft tissue infections of the diabetic foot may require no more than 10 to 14 days of antimicrobial therapy. More severe infections require longer therapy, especially if bone involvement is present. Limited ablative surgery to remove localized bone infection may decrease the duration of therapy and incidence of relapse. If bone infection is not ablated completely, prolonged therapy (involving a minimum of 4 weeks of intravenous or 10 weeks of combined intravenous and oral therapy) may be required (31,32).

Table 32.2 Working Guide to the Empirical Use of Antimicrobials for Diabetic Foot Infections*

Mild Infections[†]
 Parenteral Therapy[‡]
  Cefazolin
  Cefuroxime[§]
 Oral Therapy
  Clindamycin
  Cephalexin
  Amoxicillin–clavulanate
Severe Infections[¶]
  Ampicillin–sulbactam[**]
  Ticarcillin–clavulanate[††]
  Piperacillin–tazobactam
  Imipenem–cilastin
  Meropenem
Resistant Infections[‡‡]
  Vancomycin (for possible methicillin-resistant *Staphylococcus aureus*)
  Quinupristin–dalfopristin or linezolid (for vancomycin-resistant *Enterococcus* species)

---

* Selections can be adjusted according to results of antimicrobial susceptibility results.
[†] Those with localized cellulitis and without tissue necrosis, abundant purulence, gangrene, and foul smell.
[‡] If hospitalization is required.
[§] More stable to staphylococcal beta-lactamase than cefazolin.
[¶] Empirical broad-spectrum drug therapy.
[**] Ampicillin–sulbactam has the narrowest anti–gram-negative aerobic spectrum.
[††] Ticarcillin–clavulanate has borderline activity against enterococci.
[‡‡] When microorganisms resistant to the above antimicrobials are isolated or when life-threatening infections in hospitals where antimicrobial-resistant microorganisms are quite prevalent.

Prevention

The prevention of infection is the cornerstone of diabetic foot care (32). The basic principles of such prevention include good control of the diabetic state, weight reduction, smoking avoidance, and a diet low in fat and cholesterol. Appropriate footwear is of paramount importance, and special shoes and/or orthotic devices may have to be made for diabetic patients, especially if they have foot deformities.

Patients should take the primary responsibility for their own foot care, inspecting their feet at least once daily. Hand mirrors may be used for this, and the help of family members or friends should be solicited if the patient's vision is too poor for adequate self-examination. The feet should be washed daily with nonmedicated soap and tepid water whose temperature was first tested with the fingers (but only if significant sensory neuropathy does not exist in the upper extremities as well). The feet, including the interdigital areas, should be dried thoroughly after washing, and then a light coat of lubricating lotion or talcum powder may be applied. Woolen socks should be used when the feet feel cold; hot water bottles or heating pads should never be used to warm the feet. To prevent ingrown toenails, the toenails should be cut straight across with nail clippers, without rounding at the corners. Ingrown toenails should be discussed with the patient's primary care physician and/or podiatrist.

Diabetic patients should avoid walking barefoot, either indoors or outdoors. They also should refrain from removing corns or calluses without professional help and from using caustic chemicals on the feet. Open-toed footwear should be avoided.

Primary care physicians should be familiar with their responsibilities to the diabetic patient. Physical examination for vascular and neurological status should be performed at least twice yearly or more often if problems exist. Specialized examinations, such as Doppler studies, should be performed when indicated. Studies of shoe fitting and foot-loading patterns may be performed when necessary.

Summary

Total care of the diabetic patient requires the coordination of specialists in various fields of health care, including the primary care physician, podiatrist, orthopedist, shoe specialist, orthoses specialist, vascular surgeon, physical therapist, diabetologist and/or endocrinologist, dietician, neurologist, and infectious disease specialist.

Despite the knowledge gained and the progress made in diabetic foot care over the past several decades, considerable morbidity is still associated with diabetic foot infections. More effort should be given to preventing such infections, and education about the preventive aspects of diabetic foot care should be directed not only to the patient but also to the patient's primary care physician.

REFERENCES

1. **Levin ME, O'Neal LW.** Preface. In *The Diabetic Foot* 33rd ed. St. Louis: CV Mosby; 1983.
2. **Gibbons GW, Eliopoulos GM.** Infection of the diabetic foot. In Kozak BP, Hoar CS, Rowbotham JL, et al. (eds). *Management of Diabetic Foot Problems.* Philadelphia: WB Saunders; 1984:97–102.
3. **Lipsky BA, Pecoraro RE, Wheat LJ.** The diabetic foot: soft tissue and bone infection. *Infect Dis Clin North Am.* 1990;4:409–32.
4. **Bridges RM Jr, Deitch EA.** Diabetic foot infections: pathophysiology and treatment. *Surg Clin North Am.* 1994;74:537–55.

5. **Davidson MB.** An overview of diabetes mellitus. In Frykberg RG (ed). *The High Risk Foot in Diabetes Mellitus.* New York: Churchill Livingstone; 1991:1–22.

6. **Bagdade JD, Root RK, Balger RJ.** Impaired leukocyte function in patients with diabetes mellitus. *Diabetes.* 1974;23:9–15.

7. **Repine JE, Clawson CC, Goetz FC.** Bactericidal function of neutophils from patients with acute bacterial infections and from diabetes. *J Infect Dis.* 1980;142:869–75.

8. **Tan JS, Anderson JL, Watanakunakorn C, Phair JP.** Neutrophil dysfunction in diabetes mellitus. *J Lab Clin Med.* 1975;85:26–33.

9. **Bessman AN, Sapico FL, Tabatabai MF, Montgomerie JZ.** Persistence of polymicrobial abscesses in the poorly controlled diabetic host. *Diabetes.* 1986;35:448–53.

10. **Mahmoud AAF, Rodman HN, Mandel MG, Warren IS.** Induced and spontaneous diabetes mellitus and suppression of cell-mediated immunologic responses: granuloma formation, delayed dermal reactivity, and allograft rejection. *J Clin Invest.* 1976;57:362.

11. **Sapico FL, Bessman AN.** Diabetic foot infections. In Frykberg RG (ed). *The High Risk Foot in Diabetes Mellitus.* New York: Churchill Livingstone; 1991:197–211.

12. **Meade JW.** Major infections of the foot. *Med Times.* 1968;96:154–69.

13. **Bose K.** A surgical approach for the infected diabetic foot. *Int Orthop.* 1979;3:177–81.

14. **Todd WF, Armstrong DG, Liswood PJ.** Evaluation and treatment of the infected foot in a community teaching hospital. *J Am Podiatr Med Assoc.* 1996;86:421–6.

15. **Edmonds ME, Blundell MP, Morris HE, et al.** The diabetic foot: impact of a foot clinic. *Q J Med.* 1986;232:763–71.

16. **Grayson ML.** Diabetic foot infections: antimicrobial therapy. *Infect Dis Clin North Am.* 1995;9:143–61.

17. **Lipsky BA, Pecoraro RE, Larson SA, et al.** Outpatient management of uncomplicated lower-extremity infections in diabetic patients. *Arch Intern Med.* 1990;150:790–7.

18. **Leslie CA, Sapico FL, Ginunas VJ, Adkins RH.** Randomized controlled trial of topical hyperbaric oxygen for treatment of diabetic foot ulcers. *Diabetes Care.* 1988; 11:111–5.

19. **Louie TJ, Bartlett JG, Tally FP, Gorbach SL.** Aerobic and anaerobic bacteria in diabetic foot ulcers. *Ann Intern Med.* 1976;85:461–3.

20. **Sapico FL, Witte JL, Canawati HN, et al.** The infected foot of the diabetic patient: quantitative microbiology and analysis of clinical features. *Rev Infect Dis.* 1984;6(Suppl 1):171–6.

21. **Scher KS, Steele FJ.** The septic foot in patients with diabetes. *Surgery.* 1988;104: 661–6.

22. **Hughes CE, Johnson CC, Bamberger DM, et al.** Treatment and long-term follow-up of foot infections in patients with diabetes or ischemia: a randomized, prospective, double-blind comparison of cefoxatin and ceftizoxime. *Clin Ther.* 1987;10:36–49.

23. **Johnson PH.** *Pseudomonas* infections of the foot following puncture wounds. *JAMA.* 1968;204:170–2.

24. **Wang A, Weinstein D, Greenfield L.** MRI and diabetic foot infections. *Magn Reson Imaging.* 1990;8:805–9.

25. **Yul W, Carson J, Baraimewski H.** Osteomyelitis of the foot in diabetic patients: evaluation with plain film [99]Te-MDP bone scintigraphy and MR imaging. *Am J Roentgenol.* 1989;152:795–800.

26. **Beltran J, Campanini DS, Knight C.** The diabetic foot: magnetic resonance imaging evaluation. *Skeletal Radiol.* 1990;19:37–41.

27. **Tan JS, Friedman HM, Hazelton-Miller C, et al.** Can aggressive treatment of diabetic foot infections reduce the need for above-ankle amputation? *Clin Infect Dis.* 1996;23:286–91.

28. **Eckman MH, Greenfield S, Mackey WC, et al.** Foot infections in diabetic patients: decision and cost-effective analyses. *JAMA.* 1995;273:712–20.

29. **Grayson ML, Biggons GW, Habershaw GM, et al.** Use of ampicillin/sulbactam versus imipenem/cilastatin in the treatment of limb-threatening foot infections in diabetic patients. *Clin Infect Dis.* 1994;18:683–93.

30. **Tan JS, Wishnow RM, Talan DA, et al., and the Piperacillin/ Tazobactam Skin and Skin Structure Study Group.** Treatment of hospitalized patients with complicated skin and skin structure infections: double-blind, randomized, multi-center study group of piperacillin-tazobactam versus ticarcillin-clavulanate. *Antimicrob Agents Chemother.* 1993;37:1580–2.

31. **Bamberger DM, Dans GP, Berding DN.** Osteomyelitis in the foot of diabetic patients: long-term results, prognostic factors, and the role of antimicrobial and surgical therapy. *Am J Med.* 1987;83:653–60.

32. **Sapico FL.** Foot infections in patients with diabetes mellitus. *J Am Podiatr Med Assoc.* 1983;79:482–5.

33

Bite-Wound Infections

Joseph P. Myers, MD

A nimal and human bite wounds are common injuries to both adults and children and are responsible for an estimated 1% of all emergency department visits in the United States. It has been deduced that more than 1 million domestic animal bites are inflicted each year in the United States, and the true value may be significantly higher given that many of the more trivial injuries go unreported (1–5). Although many of these bites are innocuous, some may be serious. From 10 to 20 fatal animal bites are reported in the United States annually (6). Significant bite-wound morbidity may result from direct traumatic injury or from infectious complications, such as osteomyelitis, septic arthritis, tenosynovitis, cellulitis, and septicemia (7). The true incidence of human-bite wounds is uncertain, because many victims of these injuries conceal them for fear of embarrassment or legal ramifications (2,5,8). Wild-animal bites follow dog, cat, and human bites in frequency of occurrence and also may have infectious and noninfectious complications (2). This chapter concentrates on the infectious complications of dog-, cat-, and human-bite wounds, with occasional references to other types of bite wounds. Several excellent recent publications have reviewed the zoonotic diseases transmitted by both domestic and wild animals. The reader is referred to these publications for detailed information (6,9–12).

Epidemiology

Dog-Bite Wounds

Although fatalities from dog bites are rare (1,3), dog-bite wounds are common (2,13,14), accounting for up to 1% of all emergency department visits throughout the United States (2,3,13,14). Family or neighborhood dogs, as opposed to stray dogs, inflict the vast majority of dog-bite injuries (7,8). Dog-bite victims are commonly male (in a 2:1 predominance over females) and are usually under 16 years of age (3,6,7). It has been estimated that up to 20% of all children in the United States will be bitten by a dog at some point in their lives (7). Children are more likely than adults to be bitten by dogs; they are less intimidating to animals, more likely to be engaged in inadvertently provocative behavior, and less likely to recognize, and thereby to avoid, threatening behavior in animals (7). It is estimated that dog-bite wounds account for 70% to 93% of the mammalian bites seen in emergency departments throughout the United States (3,10). Young children 1) have a higher risk of being bitten and suffering fatal injury from dog bites than do either older children or adults; 2) are more likely to sustain bites to the head, face, and neck; and 3) are more likely to have the biting incident occur at home and be from by the child's own pet. Certain occupations have a high rate of job-related dog-bite injuries (3). Mail carriers are the victims of more than 30% of all occupationally related dog-bite injuries (3). Animal control officers and veterinarians also have a high incidence of bite injuries related to their animal-associated job duties (3).

Cat-Bite Wounds

Cats bite almost a half-million people each year in the United States (2,6). The incidence of cat bites is highest in people aged 21 to 35 years (3). Such bites are twice as common among women as men and occur primarily on the upper extremities (7). It has been estimated that cat bites constitute from 3% to 15% of all bite-wound cases presented to emergency departments throughout the United States (3). In one prospective study of cat bites seen in emergency departments, 45% of all such bites occurred to the hand, 22% were sustained on the arm above the hand, 13% occurred on the lower extremity, and the remaining 20% occurred on the head, neck, or trunk (15). In this same prospective study, the cat that inflicted the bite wound was a pet of the owner or was known to the owner in 55% of cases; the biting cat was a stray or a wild cat in 42% of cases (15). Only 3% of cat-bite wounds were inflicted by cats of unknown origin (15).

Human-Bite Wounds

Human-bite wounds are the third most common type of bite wound encountered in emergency departments (2) and generally can be classified into the three categories: self-inflicted paronychia, occlusional bite wounds, and clenched-fist injuries. Self-inflicted paronychia may be the result of nail biting, thumb sucking, or similar activities. Occlusional bite wounds are inflicted intentionally during a physical confrontation. Clenched-fist injuries are induced unintentionally to the hand of an offensive-minded pugilist (2,5,8,16). Human-bite wounds also may be sustained during passionate sexual activity (5). Bite wounds in children are often located on the scalp and face, whereas occlusional bite wounds are inflicted most commonly on the distal portion of the index or middle finger (2,5). The ear, nose, forearm, breasts, penis, scrotum, and vulva may be affected in adult bite wounds that result either from passionate or pugilistic activity (5). The clenched-fist injury usually produces a wound over the third, fourth, or fifth metacarpal head of the dominant hand (2). Any injury at this site should be presumed to be caused by an inadvertent human-bite wound until proven otherwise (2,17). Patients with clenched-fist injuries often provide the physician with false information about the exact circumstances of the injury because of fear of embarrassment or legal ramifications (2,5). Approximately 60% to 70% of all human-bite wounds are sustained on the hands and upper extremities, 15% to 20% on the head or neck, 10% to 20% on the trunk, and 5% on the lower extremities; other sites account for the remaining 5% to 10% of such wounds (18).

Classification

Bite wounds are classified as tears (avulsions), punctures, or scratches (2,13, 14,19). Tear wounds may have an associated component of crush injury (2) and are seen more commonly in dog-bite wounds (9). Puncture wounds are most common in cat bites (9), resulting from their sharp, piercing teeth, which usually puncture the skin and inoculate oral microflora into the subcutaneous tissue. Scratches from teeth or claws may occur with either dog- or cat-bite wounds; however, such scratch wounds are associated less frequently with infectious complications than are tear or puncture wounds because of the lower likelihood of organism inoculation during these more superficial injuries. Infections are more common after feline scratches than after canine scratches, probably because of the tendency of cats to lick their paws (and claws) during self-grooming and -cleaning rituals.

As noted previously, human-bite wounds are classified as self-inflicted, occlusional, or of the clenched-fist type (2,5,8,16). Self-inflicted bites tend to be relatively superficial; however, complicated paronychial infections may occur. Violent occlusional bite wounds often cause full-thickness injuries that result in deep soft tissue infection, osteomyelitis, and even traumatic amputation of a digit (2). Clenched-fist injuries, as previously noted, usually occur during pugilistic activity and may present a challenging diagnostic and therapeutic situation for the treating physician. The true diagnosis is often obscured by the victim's "cover-up" story, and the injury often causes serious infectious complications because of the injection of polymicrobial flora from the human mouth deep into the soft tissues of the hand. This deep inoculation may be compounded by extension into the fingers after the injury (5,20).

Clinical Presentation

Two distinct groups of patients eventually seek medical care for animal- and human-bite wounds. Members of the first group are seen within 8 hours of the original injury and usually present for immediate wound care or because of the fear of rabies or tetanus related to the bite wound. These patients may present without evidence of clinical infection and must be evaluated fully for risk factors for infection. The second group of patients presents more than 8 hours after the injury (often much later) and almost always after infection has been established. In these patients, a gray malodorous discharge may exude from the bite wound, with concomitant localized pain, tenderness, and erythema, for which a treatment strategy must be established immediately (2,13,14,19).

Risk Factors for Infection

In the evaluation and management of mammalian bites, knowing the species of the biting animal may help the physician to assess the most likely type of injury and the pathogenic organisms that may be associated with it. Cat-bite wounds are more likely than other bite wounds to become infected, probably because of the punctures normally inflicted by a cat's piercing teeth. A significant percentage of human-bite wounds subsequently develop active infectious complications (5,7). Dog-bite wounds are the least likely to become infected because the usual avulsion type injury produced in such bites allows open drainage at the wound site (7).

Factors that predispose to bite-wound infection include the passage of more than 12 hours before treatment, wounds on the hand or foot, clenched-fist injuries, and wounds that involve puncture alone (7). Victim factors that predispose to infection include age over 50 years, chronic alcohol abuse, diabetes mellitus, malignancy, and an immunocompromised state (e.g., from radiotherapy, chemotherapy, immunosuppressive medication, asplenism) (7). These factors should be explored carefully in the historical evaluation of patients with documented or potential bite-wound injuries. In bite-wound injuries that are evaluated within 8 hours after their occurrence and in which there is no definitive sign of clinical infection, the presence of any of predisposing factors suggests the need for the initiation of prophylactic antimicrobial therapy.

Meticulous wound care is more effective than antimicrobial prophylaxis in preventing bite-wound infection (7). In one study, debridement of devitalized tissue at the start of bite-wound management was found to reduce infection rates from 62% to 2% (7). Other studies have shown a significant increase in the infection rate when debridement is omitted from the management regimen (21). Irrigation of the wound decreases the rate of infection rate by 6- to 10-fold (7). Puncture wounds are prone to infection, at least in part because they are extremely difficult to debride and irrigate (7).

Microbiology

Most of the infections that complicate mammalian and human bite wounds are polymicrobial, with mixed aerobic and anaerobic microflora usually isolated in culture (3,5). Sources of infecting organisms include the oral and gingival microflora of the biting animal species, the skin of the bitten person, and the environmental microflora (e.g., water, soil) pertinent to the clinical situation in which the bite wound occurs (13,14). Aerobes commonly isolated from bite-wound infections include alpha-hemolytic streptococci, *Staphylococcus aureus*, *S. intermedius*, *Streptococcus pyogenes*, coagulase-negative staphylococci, *Capnocytophaga canimorsus*, *Pasteurella multocida*, bacteria that are alphanumerically designated according to the system of the Centers for Disease Control and Prevention (CDC) (e.g., EF-4, M-5), and multiple anaerobic microflora (2). A recent prospective study showed streptococci, staphylococci, and species of *Pasteurella*, *Neisseria*, *Corynebacterium*, and *Moraxella* as the most common aerobes isolated from dog- and cat-bite wounds (22).

Bacteriology of Dog Bites

The oral microflora of dogs includes up to 64 species of bacteria that may be potential human pathogens. Staphylococci, streptococci, *P. multocida* and other *Pasteurella* species, *Pseudomonas* species, other gram-negative aerobes, and multiple anaerobic species are isolated most commonly from infected dog-bite wounds (7,16,22). *Staphylococcus intermedius* is a coagulase-positive organism that is a normal component of the canine oral microflora; it can be mistaken for *S. aureus* and has been reported as a cause of infection in dog-bite wounds (16,23). *P. multocida* is isolated less frequently from infected dog-bite than from infected cat-bite wounds (2,7,22). *C. canimorsus*, formerly given the CDC alphanumeric designation DF-2, may be a normal component of the canine oral microflora; it can cause a devastating infectious illness in immunocompromised and asplenic patients (3,13,14).

Bacteriology of Cat Bites

The vast majority of infections in cat-bite wounds are caused by *P. multocida*, a facultatively anaerobic gram-negative organism that is a normal component of the oral flora of most feline species (7,15). Infections of cat-bite wounds are often polymicrobial, with staphylococci, streptococci, and aerobic enteric gram-negative bacilli frequently isolated (7,13,14). *Bartonella henselae*, the "cat-scratch" bacillus, is an unusual cause of infection that complicates cat bites or scratches but must be considered in certain clinical situations (2).

Bacteriology of Human Bites

The human mouth may harbor more than 40 species of bacteria under healthy circumstances, and almost 200 species of potentially pathogenic bacteria have been described in the presence of gingivitis and periodontal disease (7). More than 50% of infections in human-bite wounds contain mixed gram-negative and -positive bacteria (7,13,14). Anaerobes are found in more than 60% of human-bite wounds, and up to 100% of human-bite wounds are estimated to include anaerobic species (when sophisticated anaerobic culture techniques are used to identify these pathogens). The most common bacteria isolated from human-bite wounds are alpha-hemolytic streptococci (40%–95% of cases), staphylococci (25%–50%), and *Eikenella corrodens* (10%–35%) (7,8,16).

A detailed review of the microbiology of cat-, dog-, and human-bite wounds is provided in Tables 33.1 and 33.2 (2,7,8,13,14,18).

Bacteriology of Wild-Animal Bites

The medical literature is replete with isolated cases of bite-wound infections that occur after bites from exotic and/or wild animals, and infections caused by specific microorganisms have been associated with the bites of certain animals (3). These animal-microorganism associations are delineated in Table 33.3 (2,3,7,13,14,24).

Table 33.1   Bacteria Isolated from Domestic Animal Bite Wounds

Aerobes
Acinetobacter species
Actinobacillus actinomycetemcomitans
Aeromonas hydrophila
Alcaligenes species
Bacillus species
Capnocytophaga species (e.g., C. canimorsus, C. cynodegmi)
Chromobacterium species
Citrobacter freundii
Corynebacterium species*
EF-4a and EF-4b
Eikenella corrodens
Enterobacter species
Enterococcus species
Flavobacterium species
Flavimonas species
Gemella morbillorum
Haemophilus species (e.g., H. felis, H. influenzae, H. parainfluenzae)
Klebsiella pneumoniae
Micrococcus species
Moraxella species*
Neisseria species* (e.g., N. canis, N. weaveri [formerly M-5])
Pasteurella species* (e.g., P. cani, P. multocida, P. pestis, P. stomatis)
Proteus mirabilis

Pseudomonas species (e.g., P. aeruginosa, P. fluorescens)
Salmonella species
Staphylococcus species* (e.g., S. aureus, S. intermedius, coagulase-negative staphylococci)
Stenotrophomonas species
Stomatococcus species
Streptococcus species* (e.g., alpha-, beta-, and gamma-hemolytic species)
Weeksella zoohelcum
Other organisms

Anaerobes
Actinomyces species
Bacteroides species*
Clostridium species
Eubacterium species
Filifactor species
Fusobacterium species*
Lactobacillus species
Peptococcus species
Peptostreptococcus species
Porphyromonas species*
Prevotella species*
Propionibacterium species*
Veillonella species
Other organisms

* Denotes the most common isolates.
Adapted from references 2, 8, 13, and 18.

Pathophysiology

Animal-bite wounds may cause severe tissue injury and infection. Bites from large animals can generate pressure of up to 450 psi—a force more than sufficient to perforate lightweight sheet metal. This pressure may produce a severe crushing injury to human tissue (7,25). Edema and necrosis of crushed tissue in the area that surrounds a bite wound predispose the tissue to infection. Normal human cutaneous microflora and normal animal oral microflora may thrive in this necrotic, edematous tissue, thereby causing further predisposition to infection (7).

Table 33.2   Bacteria Isolated from Human Bite Wounds

Aerobes	Anaerobes
Acinetobacter species	Acidaminococcus species
Corynebacterium species	Actinomyces species
Eikenella corrodens*	Arachnia propionica
Enterobacter species (e.g., E. cloacae)	Bacteroides species*
Haemophilus species (e.g., H. influenzae,	Clostridium species
H. parainfluenzae*, H. aphrophilus)	Eubacterium species
Klebsiella pneumoniae*	Fusobacterium species*
Micrococcus species	Peptococcus species*
Moraxella species (e.g., M. catarrhalis)	Peptostreptococcus species*
Neisseria species	Prevotella species
Nocardia species	Veillonella species
Staphylococcus species (e.g., S. aureus*,	Other organisms
coagulase-negative staphylococci)	
Streptococcus species* (e.g., alpha-, beta-, and	
gamma-hemolytic streptococci)	
Other organisms	

* Denotes the most common isolates
Adapted from references 7, 8, 13, and 18.

Other Potential Infections Caused by Bite Wounds

Risk factors for tetanus and the bite victim's previous immunization status against *Clostridium tetani* must be evaluated in the treatment of every bite-wound injury. Standard CDC guidelines and protocols should be used to evaluate the adequacy of previous tetanus immunization (26). Table 33.4 provides detailed information on this subject (26).

All animal-bite wounds should be evaluated for the potential transmission of the rabies virus. The likelihood of the biting animal carrying the rabies virus should be evaluated on an individual basis, on the genus and species of the biting animal, and on local epidemiologic information about the potential transmission of the rabies virus. Again, standard CDC guidelines and protocols should be consulted to evaluate the need for rabies immunization (27). Tables 33.5 and 33.6 provide detailed information about this subject. (27)

Because monkeys are kept as pets, used in medical research, cared for in zoos, and encountered in the wild, their bites may be encountered more frequently in the medical care setting than may be anticipated. A review of infections in simian-bite wounds by Goldstein and colleagues (24) suggests a microbiological picture similar to that of infections in human-bite wounds. Additionally, antimicrobial therapy for simian bite wounds should include agents effective against *E. corrodens*. This study also documented that infection after a simian bite is common and that complications such as osteomyelitis

Table 33.3   Organisms Isolated in Unusual Bite Infections

Biting Animal	Microorganisms
Alligator	*Aeromonas hydrophila, Citrobacter diversus, Clostridium* species, *Enterobacter agglomerans, Pseudomonas* species, *Serratia* species
Coyote	*Francisella tularensis*
Cougar	*Pasteurella multocida*
Gerbil	*Streptobacillus moniliformis*
Hamster	*Acinetobacter anitratus*
Horse	*Actinobacillus lignieresii*
Lion	*Pasteurella multocida, Staphylococcus aureus, Escherichia coli*
Monkey	Herpes simiae (herpes B virus), *Streptococcus* species, *Staphylococcus* species, *Eikenella corrodens, Enterococcus* species
Opossum	*P. multocida*
Panther	*P. multocida*
Piranha	*Aeromonas hydrophila*
Pig	*Francisella tularensis, P. multocida, Streptococcus agalactiae, Streptococcus milleri, S. equisimilis, Proteus* species, *E. coli, Bacteroides* species
Rat	*S. moniliformis, Spirillum minor, Leptospira interrogans, P. multocida,* coagulase-negative staphylococci
Rooster	*Streptococcus bovis, Clostridium tertium, Aspergillus niger*
Seal	*Mycoplasma* species
Shark	*Vibrio carachariae*
Sheep	*Actinobacillus lignieresii*
Snake (venomous)	*C. perfringens,* other *Clostridium* species, *Bacteroides fragilis, Salmonella arizonae*
Squirrel	*F. tularensis*
Tiger	*P. multocida, Acinetobacter* species, *E. coli,* streptococci, staphylococci, corynebacteria (diptheroides)
Wolf	*P. multocida*

Adapted from references 2, 3, 13, and 24.

and flexion contractures of the hand are frequent (24). Of additional interest and medical significance is the transmission of herpesvirus simae (B virus) by Old World (*Macaca* species) monkeys. Therefore, information about the type of monkey implicated in a simian-bite wound is critical in evaluating the need for prophylactic acyclovir treatment in cases of such wounds (28).

Venomous snake bites pose a triad of potentially severe complications. The inoculated venom, which poses the most acute problem and may be fatal, must be neutralized as quickly as possible with species-specific antivenom. Soft tissue necrosis caused by the inoculated venom may be complicated by clostridial, pseudomonal, streptococcal, staphylococcal, or other infections. Puncture wounds also may predispose nonimmune individuals to tetanus and all of its potential complications.

Table 33.4   Tetanus Prophylaxis in Wound Management

History of Absorbed Tetanus Toxoid (No. of Doses)	Clean, Minor Wounds		All Other Wounds*	
	Td†	TIG	Td†	TIG
<3‡	Yes	No	Yes	Yes
≥3§	No¶	No	No**	No

DT = diphtheria and tetanus toxoids adsorbed for pediatric use; DTP = diphtheria and tetanus toxoids and pertussis vaccine adsorbed for pediatric use; Td = tetanus and diphtheria toxoids adsorbed for adult use; TIG = tetanus immunoglobulin.
* Including (but not limited to) wounds contaminated with dirt, feces, soil, and saliva; puncture wounds; avulsions; wounds from missiles, crushing, burns, and frostbite.
† For children <7 years of age, DTP (or DT if pertussis vaccine is contraindicated) is preferred to tetanus toxoid alone; for children >7 years of age and adults, Td is preferred to tetanus toxoid alone.
‡ Or unknown number of doses.
§ If only three doses of fluid toxoid have been received, then a fourth dose of toxoid (preferably an absorbed toxoid) should be given.
¶ Yes, but only if it has been >10 years since the patient's last dose.
** Yes, but only if it has been >5 years since the patient's last dose; more frequent boosters are not needed and can accentuate side effects.
Republished with permission from the Centers for Disease Control and Prevention. Diphtheria, tetanus, and pertussis: recommendations for vaccine use and other preventive measures: recommendations of the Immunization Practices Advisory Committee (ACIP). MMWR Morbid Mortal Weekly Rep. 1991;40:1–28.

Numerous other infectious diseases also may be transmitted by animal bites. Brucellosis (*Brucella* species), blastomycosis (*Blastomyces dermatitidis*), tularemia (*Francisella tularensis*), cat-scratch disease (*Bartonella henselae*), rat-bite fever (*Streptobacillus moniliformis* and *Spirillum minor*), bubonic plague (*Yersinia pestis*), leptospirosis (*Leptospira* species), erysipeloid (*Erysipelothrix rhusiopathiae*), and seal finger (possibly *Mycoplasma* species) are some of the other infections that may be transmitted by various domestic and wild animals (2,6–8,28,29).

Human-bite wounds should be evaluated on an individual basis for the potential transmission of infectious agents other than the usual bacterial pathogens that cause bite-wound infection. Hepatitis B virus, hepatitis C virus, HIV, *Treponema pallidum*, and *Mycobacterium tuberculosis* can be transmitted by human bites (2,19,30,31). The treating physician should ask the human-bite victim about the health and disease status of the assailant biter, if such information is available.

Complications

Infectious complications of bite wounds include cellulitis, wound infection, septic arthritis, osteomyelitis, tenosynovitis, lymphangitis, bacteremia, meningitis, brain abscess, sepsis, and disseminated intravascular coagulation (5,6,16). Noninfectious complications include peripheral neuropathy (either

Table 33.5   Rabies Postexposure Prophylaxis Guide

Animal Type	Evaluation and Disposition of Animal	Postexposure Prophylaxis Recommendations
Dogs, cats, and ferrets	Healthy and available for 10 days of observation	Should not begin prophylaxis unless the animal develops symptoms of rabies*
	Rabid or suspected rabid	Immediate vaccination
	Unknown (e.g., escaped)	Consult public health officials
Skunks, raccoons, bats, foxes, most other carnivores, and bats	Regarded as rabid unless geographic area is known to be free of rabies or until animal proven negative by laboratory tests†	Immediate vaccination
Livestock, small rodents, large rodents (e.g., woodchucks, beavers), lagomorphs (e.g., rabbits, hares), and other mammals	Consider individually	Consult public health officials; the bites of squirrels, hamsters, guinea pigs, gerbils, chipmunks, rats, mice, and other rodents and those of rabbits and hares almost never require antirabies treatment

* During the 10-day observation period, begin postexposure prophylaxis at the first sign of rabies in a dog, cat, or ferret that has bitten someone. If the animal exhibits clinical signs of rabies, it should be euthanized immediately and tested.
† The animal should be euthanized and tested as soon as possible; holding for observation is not recommended. Discontinue vaccine if immunofluorescence test results of the animal are negative.
Republished with permission from the Centers for Disease Control and Prevention. Diphtheria, tetanus, and pertussis: recommendations for vaccine use and other preventive measures: recommendations of the Immunization Practices Advisory Committee (ACIP). MMWR Morbid Mortal Weekly Rep. 1991;40:1–28.

direct or indirect), osseous crush injury and skeletal fracture, soft tissue crush injury, and cosmetic damage to skin and soft tissue (5,19). Delayed infectious complications may include tetanus, rabies virus infection, herpes simiae (B virus) infection, HIV infection, hepatitis B virus infection, and hepatitis C virus infection, etc. (2,7,26–28,30,31).

Diagnosis

History

Detailed information about the biting animal or human should be obtained in all cases of bite wounds. In animal bites, this information should include the

Table 33.6   Rabies Postexposure Prophylaxis Schedule

Vaccination Status	Treatment	Regimen*
Not previously vaccinated	Local wound cleansing	All postexposure treatment should begin with immediate cleansing of all wounds with soap and water. If available, a virucidal agent such as a povidone–iodine solution should be used to irrigate the wounds.
	RIG	20 IU/kg body weight. If anatomically feasible, the full dose should be infiltrated around the wounds and any remaining volume should be administered IM at an anatomical site distant from vaccine administration. Also, RIG should not be administered in the same syringe as vaccine. Because RIG may partially suppress active production of antibody, no more than the recommended dose should be given.
	Vaccine	HDCV, RVA, or PCEC 1.0 mL IM into deltoid area[†] on days 0, 3, 7, 14, and 28.
Previously vaccinated[‡]	Local wound cleansing	Same as if patient has not previously been vaccinated (see above)
	RIG	RIG should not be administered.
	Vaccine	HDCV, RVA, or PCEC 1.0 mL IM into deltoid area[†] on days 0 and 3.

HDCV = human diploid cell vaccine; IM = intramuscularly; RIG = rabies immunoglobulin; RVA = rabies vaccine adsorbed; PCEC = purified chick embryo cell vaccine.

*These regimens are applicable for all age groups, including children.

[†] The deltoid area is the only acceptable site of vaccination for adults and older children. For younger children, the outer aspect of the thigh may be used. Vaccine should never be administered in the gluteal area

[‡] Any person with a history of 1) preexposure vaccination with HDCV, RVA, or PCEC; 2) prior postexposure prophylaxis with HDCV, RVA, or PCEC; or 3) previous vaccination with any other type of rabies vaccine and a documented history of a response to the prior vaccination.

Republished with permission from the Centers for Disease Control and Prevention. Diphtheria, tetanus, and pertussis: recommendations for vaccine use and other preventive measures: recommendations of the Immunization Practices Advisory Committee (ACIP). MMWR Morbid Mortal Weekly Rep. 1991;40:1–28.

type of animal that inflicted the bite, whether or not the bite was provoked, the situation and/or environment in which the bite occurred, the exact time of the biting incident, and whether or not the source animal was captured and isolated for rabies observation. In human bites, as much information as possible should be obtained about the biting individual, the potential diseases he or she carries, and the exact circumstances under which the biting incident occurred (including the time elapsed). Important patient-related information includes antibiotic allergies; current medications, including immunosuppressive therapy; a history of previous splenectomy, mastectomy, or chronic liver disease; and any self-administered treatment given before the patient sought medical assistance (2,3). Important aspects of the patient history are delineated in Table 33.7 (2,3).

Table 33.7   History To Be Obtained in Bite-Wound Injury

Questions About the Biting Animal

What is the type and breed of the animal involved?
What is the immunization status of the animal?
Do you know the health status and behavior of the animal?
When did the biting incident occur (exact date and time)?
What were the exact circumstances of the bite wound?
Was the bite provoked or unprovoked?
Was the biting animal captured? If so, where is the animal being detained at this time?

Questions About the Biting Human

Do you know the person who bit you?
Does the biting person have:
  Any known medical illnesses?
  Hepatitis B infection?
  Hepatitis C infection?
  Syphilis?
  Recurrent oral *Herpes simplex* infection?
  Human immunodeficiency virus infection?
  Any other infectious illnesses?
What were the exact circumstances of the biting incident?
When did the biting incident occur (exact date and time)?

Questions About the Biting Victim

Did you receive or self-administer:
  Any pre-hospital care for the bite wound?
  Local wound care?
  Antibiotic therapy?
  Any other therapy, including home remedies?
What is your current immunization status?
When was your last tetanus immunization?
Have you completed a full series of tetanus immunization?
Do you have any allergies to medications? Specifically, do you have any allergies to any
  antibiotics?
Are you currently taking any medications?
Are you currently receiving any immunosuppressive therapy of any kind?
Have you had a previous splenectomy?
Have you had a previous mastectomy?
Do you have a history of chronic liver disease?
Have you received antibiotic therapy of any kind during the past month?

Physical Examination

The number, type, depth, and anatomical site of all bite wounds should be recorded in exquisite detail. Diagrams of such wounds should be included in the patient's medical record along with photographic documentation, if available. Other factors that should be recorded include the joint's range of motion adjacent to the injury, information about the possibility of joint penetration, the presence of edema or crush injury, nerve and tendon function, the clinical extent of infection (e.g., erythema, purulent drainage, necrotic tissue). The odor of any exudate also should be recorded (2,3,7,15,26). Table 33.8 provides a checklist of pertinent physical findings in cases of bite wounds (2,3,7,15,26).

Microbiological Culture

If possible, cultures for aerobic and anaerobic organisms should be made from all bite wounds. Some deep puncture wounds may not have drainage that is accessible to culture. Viral, mycobacterial, and fungal cultures should be made when clinical, environmental, or epidemiologic data dictate these.

Radiography

If a fracture or a bone or joint penetration is a consideration in a bite wound, the involved area should be examined radiographically. The resulting radiographs can be compared with subsequent radiographs in the event that osteomyelitis of the affected area is later suspected. More detailed radiographic testing, with computed axial tomography or magnetic resonance imaging, may be indicated in complicated infections (7,13,14).

Table 33.8   Physical Examination in Bite-Wound Injury: Important Points for Observation and Recording

Number of wounds	Crush injury
Type of wounds	Nerve damage
Puncture	Tendon damage
Avulsion (tear)	Necrotic tissue
Scratch	Malodorous exudate
Depth of wounds	Range of motion of involved joints
Tissue edema	Evaluation for joint penetration from bite
Tissue erythema	Detailed diagram of wounds in medical record
Purulent drainage	Photograph or videotape of wounds, if available

Treatment

Irrigation

All bite wounds should be irrigated with copious amounts (~200 mL) of normal saline. If possible, puncture wounds should be irrigated with a high-pressure jet of water, using a 20-mL syringe and an 18-gauge needle or catheter tip to access the wound. However, some puncture wounds are tiny and relatively inaccessible to irrigation (7,13,14). Appropriate wound irrigation may produce a 6- to 10-fold lower rate of bite-wound infection than it would without irrigation (7).

Debridement

The single most common error made in treating bite wounds is the failure to debride and irrigate the wound adequately (7). Devitalized or necrotic tissue should be debrided cautiously, and foreign bodies and all other debris should be removed fastidiously from the wound. Appropriate and adequate anesthesia should be provided to make the procedure tolerable for the patient (2,3,7, 13,14). Proper debridement decreased rates of bite-wound infection from 62% to 2% in one study (32) and by 2.5-fold in another published series (21).

Wound Closure

Primary wound closure may be indicated for some uninfected bite wounds, especially facial wounds. However, closure of other types of bite wounds is usually not indicated. Wound edges should be approximated with adhesive strips in certain cases, and healing by secondary intention or by delayed closure may be indicated after infectious complications have been addressed (13,14).

Antimicrobial Therapy

If a bite wound shows signs of active infection (e.g., cellulitis, purulent drainage, evidence of deep tissue infection), appropriate antimicrobial therapy should be initiated immediately. The antibiotics chosen should be directed against the usual oral pathogens of the biting animal, the usual human cutaneous pathogens, and pertinent environmental pathogens. These organisms include *Staphylococcus aureus*, *Streptococcus pyogenes*, and the oral microflora of dogs, cats, or humans (e.g., alpha-hemolytic streptococci, multiple anaerobic species). Ampicillin–sulbactam may be given intravenously to hospitalized patients. Other combinations of penicillins and beta-lactamase–inhibitors (e.g., ticarcillin–clavulanate, piperacillin–tazobactam) and carbapenems (e.g., imipenem, meropenem) also provide excellent broad-spectrum antimicrobial coverage of the microorganisms commonly isolated from severe bite-wound infections. However, these significantly more expensive antimicrobial agents are generally no more effective than ampicillin–sulbactam.

Amoxicillin–clavulanate is an excellent selection for the oral therapy of bite-wound infections (14,18,33). Patients who are allergic to penicillin or other beta-lactam antibiotics may be treated with a combination of clindamycin plus a fluoroquinolone (e.g., ciprofloxacin, levofloxacin) or with clindamycin plus trimethoprim–sulfamethoxazole. Recently published data confirm the excellent antimicrobial activity of trovafloxacin, a newer fluoroquinolone antibiotic, against both aerobic and anaerobic bite-wound pathogens (34). Therefore, trovafloxacin may be useful as single-agent therapy in the antibiotic management of bite-wound infections; however, concern about the toxicity of trovafloxacin has restricted its use to hospitalized or severely ill patients. Use of the newer broad-spectrum fluoroquinolones for single-agent therapy of bite-wound infections awaits further in vitro investigation and clinical study. Cefoxitin can been given intravenously for treating bite-wound infections in patients with non–life-threatening reactions to penicillin. Other antimicrobial agents are available for the treatment of less commonly encountered bacterial pathogens. Once culture results are available, antimicrobial therapy should be tailored to the most cost-effective regimen for the pathogens isolated. Table 33.9 provides detailed information about the antimicrobial susceptibility patterns of microorganisms that are commonly implicated as pathogens in bite-wound infections (2,6,13,14,34).

The duration of antibiotic therapy for a bite wound depends on the severity of the infectious process. Osteomyelitis and septic arthritis generally require longer courses of antibiotic therapy than do cellulitis and soft tissue infection and also may require concomitant surgical intervention.

A more difficult decision for the treating physician is whether or not to use antibiotics prophylactically for a bite wound that is not yet clinically infected. Few prospective studies have addressed this issue. Prophylactic antibiotic therapy is actually presumptive treatment of microbially contaminated tissue at the site of the bite wound. It should be instituted when clinical circumstances predict a high likelihood of infection after a bite-wound injury. These circumstances include:

- Moderate to severe injury less than 8 hours old, especially if edema or crush injury is present
- Documentation of or high suspicion for bone or joint penetration and pathogen inoculation
- Any hand wound
- Any foot wound
- A bite wound in any immunocompromised patient, especially in the setting of mastectomy, chronic liver disease, or corticosteroid or other immunosuppressive therapy

- A bite wound immediately adjacent to a prosthetic joint
- A bite wound in the genital area

Amoxicillin–clavulanic acid, clindamycin plus a fluoroquinolone, clindamycin plus a tetracycline, and clindamycin plus trimethoprim–sulfamethoxazole are all reasonable oral treatment regimens in the clinical setting of a presumptively infected bite wound (2,3,7,13,14). Table 33.9 provides further detailed information about the antimicrobial susceptibility patterns of pathogenic microorganisms commonly encountered in infected bite wounds (13,14, 34,35). Table 33.10 provides specific antibiotic recommendations for prophylaxis within 12 hours of a bite injury and for the presumptive treatment of a clinically established infection.

Immunization

A thorough history of the bite victim's previous immunization status should be obtained immediately after his or her presentation for treatment. Standard

Table 33.9   Antimicrobial Agent Activity Versus Selected Bite-Wound Pathogens

Antimicrobial Agents	Anaerobes	Capnocyto- phaga canimorsis	Eikenella corrodens	Haemo- philus species	Pasteurella multocida	Staphylo- coccus aureus	Staphylo- coccus intermedius
Amoxicillin– clavulanate	+	+	+	+	+	+	+
Ampicillin– sulbactam	+	+	+	+	+	+	+
Azithromycin	±	+	±	+	+	+	ND
Cefoxitin	+	+	+	±	+	+	ND
Cefuroxime	–	ND	±	+	+	+	ND
Cephalexin	–	ND	–	–	–	+	+
Ciprofloxacin	–	+	+	+	+	±	+
Clarithromycin	±	+	±	+	±	+	ND
Clindamycin	+	+	–	–	–	+	+
Dicloxacillin	±	ND	–	–	–	+	+
Erythromycin	–	+	–	–	–	+	+
Levofloxacin	±	+	+	+	+	+	+
Moxifloxacin	+	+	+	+	+	+	+
Penicillin	±	+	+	–	+	–	±
Tetracycline	±	+	+	–	+	+	ND
TMP-SMX	–	±	+	+	+	+	ND
Trovafloxacin	+	+	+	+	+	+	+

ND = no data available; TMP-SMX = trimethoprim–sulfamethoxazole; "+" = good antimicrobial activity (85%–100% of strains susceptible); "±" variable antimicrobial activity (50%–84% of strains susceptible); "–" = poor antimicrobial Activity (0%–49% of strains susceptible).

Table 33.10   Antimicrobial Therapy of Infected Bite Wounds

Type of Bite	Administration Route	Regimen	Dosage
Dog or cat	Intravenous	Ampicillin–sulbactam	1.5–3.0 g q6h
		Ticarcillin–clavulanate	3.1 g q6h
		Piperacillin–tazobactam	3.375 g q6h
		Imipenem	500 mg q6h
		Meropenem	1 g q8–12h
		Clindamycin + ciprofloxacin	600–900 mg q8h + 400 mg q12h
		Clindamycin + TMP-SMX	600–900 mg q8h + 160/800–320/1600 mg q8h
Dog or cat	Oral	Amoxicillin–clavulanate	500/125 mg tid or 875/125 mg bid
		Clindamycin + ciprofloxacin	300 mg qid + 500–750 mg bid
		Clindamycin + TMP-SMX	300 mg qid + 160/800 mg bid or tid
		Cefuroxime axetil + metronidazole	500 mg bid + 250–500 mg tid
Human	Parenteral	Ampicillin–sulbactam	1.5–3.0 g q6h
		Cefoxitin	2 g q6h
		Ticarcillin–clavulanate	3.1 g q6h
		Piperacillin–tazobactam	3.375 g
		Imipenem–cilastatin	500–750 mg q6h
		Meropenem	1 g q8–12h
		Clindamycin + ciprofloxacin	600–900 mg q6h + 400 mg q12h
		Clindamycin + TMP-SMX	600–900 mg q8h + 160/800–320/1600 mg q8h
Human	Oral	Amoxicillin–clavulanate	500/125 mg tid to 875/125 mg bid
		Clindamycin + ciprofloxacin	300 mg qid + 500–750 mg bid
		Clindamycin + TMP-SMX	300 mg qid + 160/800 mg bid or tid

TMP-SMX = trimethoprim–sulfamethoxazole

tetanus immunization guidelines should be followed in all circumstances, and appropriate vaccine or tetanus immunoglobulin should be given as required (26). All bite wounds carry a risk of tetanus. If information about the bite victim's primary tetanus immunization series is inadequate, the primary immunization series should be initiated immediately, and tetanus immunoglobulin should be given concomitantly. (*see* Table 33.4) (26).

All animal bites should be investigated for the risk of rabies virus infection. Standard protocols and local knowledge about the presence of the rabies virus in the animal population (both domestic and wild) should be used to evaluate the risk factors for rabies virus infection. Patients who are at significant risk for rabies virus exposure via a bite wound should receive human diploid cell rabies vaccine and rabies immunoglobulin, according to the standard protocol for each (*see* Tables 33.5 and 33.6) (27).

Hospitalization

A patient should be hospitalized for the treatment of a bite-wound injury if one or more of the following circumstances are present (2,7,13,14):

- A temperature over 100.5°F (38.1°C)
- Evidence of clinical sepsis
- Progressive cellulitis
- Clenched-fist injury
- Septic arthritis
- Osteomyelitis
- Failure of previous outpatient management
- Immunocompromised status
- Infection that has spread across a joint
- Hand or foot infection
- Severe crush injury
- Tendon or nerve injury
- Tenosynovitis
- Suspected or documented noncompliance with the therapeutic regimen

Consultation

Consulting the appropriate general, orthopedic, hand, or plastic surgeons or infectious disease, rehabilitative, and other appropriate specialists in the ongoing care of patients with bite wounds should be initiated according to the severity and nature of the bite wound injuries (7,18).

Elevation and Immobilization

Elevating the extremity affected by a bite-wound infection alleviates edema and prevents the spread of infection in the immediate vicinity of the wound

(13,14,19). Failure of the patient to elevate the involved extremity appropriately is a common cause for treatment failure in cases of bite-wound infections. Bite wounds to the hand should be immobilized with a splint that allows the hand to remain in the functional position (13,14,17).

Surgical Management

Surgical intervention is often required during the management of bite-wound infections. Irrigation and debridement of the bite wound should be part of the standard management protocol when the patient initially seeks medical care. Further surgical treatment may be required for therapeutic evacuation of purulent drainage, for therapeutic relief of tissue tension, for decompression to prevent peripheral nerve injury and neuropathy, and for the diagnostic recovery of microorganisms from the site of a closed-space infection (e.g., septic arthritis, osteomyelitis, tenosynovitis). Other indications for surgery include repair of vascular, muscular, or neurological tissue and cosmetic repair of soft tissue injuries and disfigured skin (3,13,14,17).

Follow-Up

The appropriate management of bite wounds on an outpatient basis requires that the patient be seen in a follow-up visit at 24 hours (possibly at 48 hours) after the initial evaluation. During the follow-up visit, the patient should be evaluated fully for both infectious and noninfectious complications of the original injury and for side effects of antibiotics or other medications prescribed at the initial visit (5,16).

Perils and Pitfalls of Bite-Wound Management

As noted previously, the single most common error made in the management of bite wounds is the failure to irrigate and debride the wound adequately. Other common mistakes include the failure to dress the wound with bulky dressings, failure to elevate the extremity for 24 to 48 hours after treatment of the wound, failure to recognize a clenched-fist injury as a human-bite wound, failure to recognize wounds to the genitalia as human-bite wounds, failure to obtain appropriate cultures during initial evaluation of the patient, and failure to recognize wounds that are not responding to oral antimicrobial therapy (7). Additionally, incorrect selection of antimicrobial agents, insufficient duration of antimicrobial therapy, inappropriately low doses of antimicrobial agents, antibiotic-resistant microbial isolates, and overlooking the presence of abscess, osteomyelitis, or pyarthrosis can be causes of therapeutic failure in patients with bite-wound infections (13,14,19).

Medicolegal Considerations

Reporting Bite Wounds

Local governmental regulations may require physicians to report bite wounds to the jurisdictional health department. In the absence of local reporting requirements, appropriate consultation with the local health department still may be necessary to ascertain the likelihood of rabies virus transmission by domestic and wild animal species in the geographic area in which a bite occurs (7,13,14).

Documenting Bite Wounds

Because animal bites often result in civil litigation against the owner of the biting animal, it is prudent to document thoroughly all injuries associated with a bite wound and all diagnostic and therapeutic regimens used for the wound. Although detailed diagrams and drawings are certainly appropriate, photographs or videotapes are extremely useful adjuncts to both the initial evaluation and to the follow-up documentation of bite-wound injuries (3–5,7,13, 14,19). They also provide graphic evidence of the exact nature of the injuries associated with a wound and may help clarify issues about the extent and severity of such injuries in the event that litigation occurs. The medicolegal ramifications of disease transmission by a human bite are extremely complex and, so far, have been addressed sparsely in the legal literature (7).

Summary

Bite-wound injuries and infections are common. Dog, cat, and human bites are the most frequently encountered bite wounds in clinical practice. Bite-wound injuries are underreported, and some bites (especially human bites) are actively concealed.

The cornerstones of bite-wound management include scrupulous irrigation and debridement with surgical care appropriate to the individual case. Antimicrobial therapy should be instituted in cases of active infection. In cases in which there is no evidence of clinical infection, empirical broad-spectrum antimicrobial therapy is often appropriate as a prophylactic measure when the likelihood of infection is high. Immunization for tetanus and rabies virus should be provided as required by the standard CDC protocols (26,27). Special circumstances (e.g., bites from monkeys, venomous snake bites, and known HIV-infected individuals) may dictate the initiation of specialized evaluation and treatment protocols (28,36). A detailed assessment for bite-wound complications should be undertaken in every patient who has sustained a bite injury. Judicious and expedient follow-up is essential for an optimal clinical outcome after a bite injury.

REFERENCES

1. **Weiss HB, Friedman DI, Coben JH.** Incidence of dog bite injuries treated in emergency departments. *JAMA.* 1998;279:51–3.

2. **Goldstein EJC, Talan DA.** Bite wounds. In Hoeprich PD Jordan MC (eds). *Infectious Diseases: A Treatise of Infectious Processes,* 5th ed. Philadelphia: JB Lippincott; 1994: 1420–3.

3. **Weber DJ, Hansen AR.** Infections resulting from animal bites. *Infect Dis Clin North Am.* 1991;5:663–80.

4. **McDonoug JJ, Stern PJ, Alexander JW.** Management of animal and human bites and resulting human infections. *Curr Clin Top Infect Dis.* 1987;8:11–36.

5. **Wahl RP, Eggleston J, Edlich R.** Puncture wounds and animal bites. In Tintinalli JE, Ruiz E, Krome RL (eds). *Emergency Medicine: A Comprehensive Study Guide,* 4th ed. New York: McGraw-Hill; 1996:317–22.

6. **Bowman MJA.** Animal bites in infants and children: an approach to diagnosis and treatment. *Pediatr Emerg Med Rep.* 1999;4:53–62.

7. **Newton E.** Mammalian bites. In Schwartz GR et al. (ed). *Principles and Practice of Emergency Medicine,* 3rd ed. Philadelphia: Lea & Febiger; 1992:2750–61.

8. **Goldstein EJC, Richwald GA.** Human and animal bite wounds. *Am Fam Physician.* 1987;36:101–9.

9. **Chretien JH, Garagusi VF.** Infections associated with pets. *Am Fam Physician.* 1990;41:831–45.

10. **Tan JS.** Human zoonotic infections transmitted by dogs and cats. *Arch Intern Med.* 1997;157:1933–43.

11. **Plaut M, Zimmerman EM, Goldstein RA.** Health hazards to humans associated with domestic pets. *Annu Rev Public Health.* 1996;17:221–45.

12. **Weber DJ, Weinberg AN.** Animal-associated human infections. *Infect Dis Clin North Am.* 1991;5:1–181.

13. **Goldstein EJC.** Bites. In Mandell GL, Bennett JE, Dolin R (eds). *Principles and Practice of Infectious Diseases,* 4th ed. New York: Churchill Livingstone; 1995:2765–9.

14. **Goldstein EJC.** Bites. In Mandell GL, Bennett JE, Dolin R (eds). *Principles and Practice of Infectious Diseases,* 5th ed. New York: Churchill Livingstone; 2000:3202–6.

15. **Dire DJ.** Cat bite wounds: risk factors for infection. *Ann Emerg Med.* 1991;20:973–9.

16. **Moran GJ, Talan DA.** Hand infections. *Emerg Med Clin North Am.* 1993;11:601–619.

17. **McGrath MH.** Infections of the hand. In McCarthy JG, May JWJ, Littler JW (eds). *The Hand. Plastic Surgery,* vol 8. Philadelphia: WB Saunders; 1990:5529–56.

18. **Brook I.** Human and animal bite infections. *J Fam Pract.* 1989;28:713–8.

19. **Goldstein EJC.** Human and animal bites. In Schlossberg D (ed). *Current Therapy of Infectious Disease.* St. Louis: Mosby Year Book; 1996:66–8.

20. **Edlich RF, Spengler MD, Rodeheaver GT.** Mammalian bites. *Compr Ther.* 1983;9: 41–7.

21. **Callaham ML.** Treatment of common dog bites: infection risk factors. *JACEP.* 1978; 7:83–7.

22. **Talan DA, Citron DM, Abrahamian FM, et al.** Bacteriologic analysis of infected dog and cat bites. *N Engl J Med.* 1999;340:85–92.

23. **Talan DA.** *Staphylococcus intermedius*: clinical presentation of a new human dog bite pathogen. *Ann Emerg Med.* 1989;18:410–3.

24. **Goldstein EJC, Pryor EP III, Citron DM.** Simian bites and bacterial infection. *Clin Infect Dis.* 1995;20:1551–2.

25. **Chambers GH, Payne JF.** Treatment of dog bite wounds. *Minn Med.* 1969;52: 427–30.

26. **Centers for Disease Control and Prevention.** Diptheria, tetanus, and pertussis: recommendations for vaccine use and other preventive measures: recommendations of the Immunization Practices Advisory Committee (ACIP). *MMWR Morbid Mortal Weekly Rep.* 1991;40:1–28.

27. **Centers for Disease Control.** Human rabies prevention–United States, 1999: recommendations of the Advisory Committee on Immunization Practices (ACIP). *MMWR Morbid Mortal Weekly Rep.* 1999;48:1–21.

28. **Holmes GP, Chapman LE, Stewart JA et al.** Guidelines for the prevention and treatment of B-virus infections in exposed persons. *Clin Infect Dis.* 1995;20:421–39.

29. **Baker AS, Ruoff KL, Madoff S.** Isolation of *Mycoplasma* species from a patient with seal finger. *Clin Infect Dis.* 1998;27:1168–70.

30. **Vidmar L, Poljak M, Tomazic J, et al.** Transmission of HIV-1 by human bite. *Lancet.* 1996;347:1762.

31. **Anonymous.** HIV infection by a human bite. *Infect Control Hosp Epidemiol.* 1996;17:707.

32. **Callaham ML.** Prophylactic antibiotics in common dog bite wounds: a controlled study. *Ann Emerg Med.* 1980;9:410–4.

33. **Goldstein EJC, Reinhardt JF, Murray PM, et al.** Animal and human bite wounds, a comparative study: augmentin vs. a penicillin + dicloxacillin. *Postgrad Med J.* 1984; (Suppl):105–10.

34. **Goldstein EJC, Citron DM, Hudspeth M, et al.** Trovafloxacin compared with levofloxacin, azithromycin, and clarithromycin against unusual aerobic and anaerobic human and animal bite-wound pathogens. J Antimicrob Chemother 1998;41:391–6.

35. **Goldstein EJC.** Animal bite infections. In Stevens DL (ed). *Skin, Soft Tissue, Bone, and Joint Infections.* Philadelphia: Churchill Livingstone; 1995:4.1–4.16.

36. **Centers for Disease Control.** Public Health Service guidelines for the management of health-care worker exposures to HIV and recommendations for postexposure prophylaxis. *MMWR Morbid Mortal Weekly Rep.* 1998;47:1–34.

34

Viral Exanthems

Blaise L. Congeni, MD

B
ecause the skin is the largest of the body's organs, it is not surprising that skin involvement is seen in the course of a variety of infectious diseases. This is especially the case for viral infections. An exanthem, eruption, or rash may be the only manifestation of an infection and the only reason that a patient may seek medical care. Furthermore, frequently the physician is able to arrive at a diagnosis from the dermatologic manifestation of an infection purely on clinical grounds. By paying careful attention to the characteristics of the exanthem, the physician can at least develop a differential diagnosis (before laboratory results are available). Common viral exanthems are listed in Table 34.1.

Measles (Rubeola)

Measles was one of the earliest viral exanthems to be recognized. An accurate diagnosis of this disease can be made on the basis of the rash and associated symptomatology alone. Traditionally, measles has been distinguished from another childhood disease called rubella, or German measles. Both derive their name from the Latin *ruber*, meaning red or reddish. Generally, immunization for both diseases is given simultaneously; however, the significance of both infections is quite different. Measles causes significant morbidity and even occasional mortality through its complications; in the prevaccine era, measles killed more people than did polio.

Table 34.1   Viral Exanthems

Disease	Common Name	Etiologic Agent
Rubeola	Measles	Morbillivirus
Rubella	German measles	Rubella virus
Mononucleosis	Mononucleosis	EBV, CMV
Exanthem subitum	Roseola	HHV-6, HHV-7
Erythema infectiosum	Fifth disease	Parvovirus B-19
Varicella	Chicken pox	Varicella–zoster virus
Boston exanthem	Roseola	Echovirus 16, 25
	Petechiae	Coxsackie; A49; B2-4; echovirus 4,7,9
Hand–foot–mouth disease		Coxsackie, echovirus, enterovirus

CMV = cytomegalovirus; EBV = Epstein–Barr virus; HHV = human herpesvirus.

In the prevaccine era, virtually all children became infected with the measles virus. After widespread immunization became available in 1963, the incidence of measles steadily declined until 1983 (1). The number of reported cases then steadily increased, and numerous outbreaks occurred in school children and college students (2). Approximately one half of these cases occurred in unvaccinated preschool children and the other half in previously vaccinated students between the ages of 5 and 24 years (3). For this reason, a two-dose vaccination strategy was adopted in the early 1990s, and subsequently the incidence of measles has been very low (4).

Etiology

Measles virus (Morbillivirus) is a member of the Paramyxovirus family. Other members of this family include respiratory syncytial virus, parainfluenza virus, influenza virus, and mumps virus. The measles virus contains a single-stranded RNA genome with a lipid envelope. The hemagglutinin of the virus is a surface protein that facilitates its attachment to cells. In contrast with the influenza virus, the measles virion lacks a neuraminidase. Only one antigenic type of the virus exists, and, because humans are the only hosts, measles seems to be an excellent candidate for worldwide eradication following universal immunization.

Clinical Manifestations

Measles is a highly contagious infection, with approximately 90% of susceptible exposed individuals becoming infected. In contrast to most viral infections, subclinical disease seems to occur infrequently in measles virus infection.

After an incubation period of 8 to 12 days, the individual exposed to the measles virus develops symptoms of a common cold. This prodrome lasts 2 to 4 days, with fever, cough, conjunctivitis, photophobia, and coryza being prominent. A faint scarlatinal rash that quickly fades may then be seen. Then Koplik's spots, which are pathognomonic for measles and look like small grains of sand on an erythematous base, appear on the buccal mucosa. The Koplik's spots disappear within 12 to 18 hours, and the characteristic exanthem of measles appears within 1 to 2 days thereafter. This rash is first noted on the face, neck, and behind the ears, later spreading down the body. It may start as a macular rash, becoming maculopapular and then finally coalescing, especially on the trunk. Within 2 to 3 days the rash begins to fade and takes on a darker color, which is when desquamation may occur. Additionally, the rash can have a hemorrhagic appearance.

Complications of measles (e.g., otitis media, pneumonia) are primarily secondary to bacterial infection. However, pneumonia may be caused by the measles virus itself. Encephalitis is the most feared complication of measles, occurring in 1 to 2 cases per 1000, with a mortality rate as high as 10% and a substantial number of survivors suffering sequelae.

Atypical Measles

Children who received the killed measles vaccine between 1963 and 1968 and who later either received live vaccine or were exposed naturally to measles virus frequently developed atypical measles (5). The clinical disease seen in these children was more severe than what is usually seen, and approximately three fourths of them required hospitalization. Koplik's spots were notably absent, and the rash developed after a fever of abrupt onset. Prodromal symptoms were less conspicuous than the typical manifestation. The exanthem was noted to include papules and vesicles and was observed to start distally, in contrast with typical measles. Additionally, peripheral edema, cough, and pulmonary complications were noted more commonly.

Diagnosis

The diagnosis of measles is usually made on clinical grounds alone. A history of exposure, the presence of prodromal symptoms (e.g., cough, conjunctivitis, coryza, Koplik's spots), and the typical rash are sufficient to make the diagnosis. Symptoms in previously vaccinated patients may be mild.

Cultivating the measles virus from nasopharyngeal secretions, conjunctiva, blood, or urine is seldom done. Serology is used more often to confirm the diagnosis in suspected cases. The presence of IgM antibody or a fourfold rise in acute and convalescent antibody titers also confirms the diagnosis. The serologic tests generally used for measles are complement fixation, hemagglutination inhibition, or enzyme immunoassay. Neutralization assays are less likely to be available and are more difficult to perform.

Treatment

The treatment of measles is primarily supportive. Appropriate antibiotic therapy is indicated for any of the bacterial complications that may occur, such as otitis media or pneumonia. Low serum concentrations of vitamin A have been associated with severe measles. Consequently, vitamin A therapy should be considered for children diagnosed as having measles under the following circumstances:

- Children from countries associated with vitamin A deficiency
- Children 6 to 12 months of age hospitalized with measles
- Children older than 12 months of age with the risk factors of immunodeficiency, ophthalmologic evidence of vitamin A deficiency, incomplete intestinal absorption of vitamin A, moderate to severe malnutrition, or recent immigration from countries known to have high measles-related mortality rates

Measles is susceptible to ribavirin in vitro. Controlled studies that have documented a clinical benefit of ribavirin in immunosuppressed or other patients are unavailable.

Prevention

Since the mid-1960s, the prevention of measles has been accomplished with a live measles virus vaccine. Several significant changes have occurred since 1963 concerning the recommendations for the initiation of measles immunization. Currently, it is recommended that all children receive measles vaccine after their first birthday unless there are contraindications. Usually, the first dose is given as a part of the standard measles, mumps, and rubella vaccine at the age of 12 to 15 months (6). A second dose of measles vaccine is given on entry into school at an age of 4 to 6 years, but this dose can be given as early as 1 month after the initial dose. All children should have their immunization records reviewed at 11 to 12 years of age.

Rubella

The rash and clinical features of rubella were initially described early in the 19th century. The importance of diagnosing rubella was thought to derive primarily from the ability to distinguish it from rubeola (measles) and scarlet fever, two illnesses known to be associated with significant morbidity. The notion that rubella was a trivial disease continued until 1941, when Australian ophthalmologist Norman Gregg observed congenital cataracts in 58 infants in association with maternal rubella early in pregnancy (7). Congenital heart disease and failure to thrive also were seen in many of these infants. Within a few years, it became apparent that microcephaly, deafness, and mental retardation were a part of the congenital rubella syndrome as well.

Throughout the first half of the 20th century, rubella was noted to occur in epidemics in 7- to 10-year cycles. The last major epidemic in the United States occurred in 1964 and resulted in 20,000 infants born with congenital defects and perhaps as many fetal deaths (8,9). The first of a number of live vaccines for rubella was introduced in 1969, and its widespread use was achieved within a year (10). Since then, the number of cases of congenital rubella syndrome has declined steadily.

Etiology

The rubella virus is a member of the Togavirus family and is the only member of the Rubivirus genus. It is an enveloped, spherical virion that measures 60 nm in diameter and has a single-stranded RNA genome. There is only one serotype. Humans are usually the only natural hosts of the virus, but other species have been infected, including monkeys and ferrets.

Clinical Manifestations

In most patients with rubella, clinical disease is mild or unapparent. Patients with clinically recognizable disease are noted to have a mild prodrome of malaise and low-grade fever after an incubation period of 14 to 21 days. Swelling of lymph nodes in the suboccipital and postauricular region is then noted, which may be followed by mild, transient conjunctivitis. The lymph nodes remain swollen. Within a few days, a rash—most often described as a fine, discrete, maculopapular eruption starting on the face and trunk—is noted. By the second day, the rash spreads to involve the arms and trunk and then may become confluent. In another day, the rash begins to fade. Within 3 to 4 days of its onset, the rash is gone.

As in children, adults with rubella often have clinically unapparent disease. At times, however, the disease in adults may be more severe and prolonged, especially in women in whom rubella may be associated with polyarthralgia or even arthritis. Complications are rare but include encephalitis or thrombocytopenia.

Diagnosis

As with measles, the diagnosis of rubella is almost always based on clinical grounds alone. Although rubella virus can be cultured from the throat, blood, urine, cerebrospinal fluid, and cataracts, most clinicians rely on serology to confirm the diagnosis when confirmation is necessary (11). Growing the virus in tissue cultures is time consuming and not performed routinely but is generally available by special request.

Rubella virus grows well in a variety of primary and continuous cell lines, including monkey kidney cells. This has no cytopathic effect, but after several days the culture is challenged with a picornavirus and inhibition of growth is seen.

Traditionally, the hemagglutination inhibition antibody test has been used for serologic testing for rubella; however, more recently, a variety of other assays have replaced this test in most clinical laboratories. These newer tests include passive hemagglutination, latex agglutination, fluorescent immunoassay, and enzyme immunoassay. A fourfold rise in titer or a positive rubella-specific IgM-antibody test is needed to confirm the diagnosis.

Treatment and Prevention

Treatment for rubella is supportive, and specific antiviral chemotherapy is unavailable.

Rubella immunization is now accomplished with a live vaccine in a two-dose regimen. The vaccine is given as a part of the standard measles, mumps, and rubella vaccine. Generally, the first dose is administered at 12 to 15 months of age and the second dose at 4 to 6 years of age. Primary vaccine failures have not been a significant problem with the rubella vaccine, but the addition of a second dose has added a measure of safety.

Because the primary target population for immunization against rubella consists of women of childbearing age, the immunization of susceptible postpubertal individuals (e.g., college students, military recruits, health care workers) remains a priority. Contraindications to immunization with the live rubella virus vaccine include pregnancy, immunodeficiency, and having received intravenous gammaglobulin or blood products within the previous 3 to 4 months, depending on the dose of gammaglobulin.

The care of an individual with rubella, especially a pregnant woman, primarily involves confirming the diagnosis. If serologic testing indicates that the exposed individual is susceptible to rubella, a second serum specimen should be examined in 3 to 4 weeks to check for seroconversion.

Vaccination after exposure to rubella does not prevent infection, and the administration of immune serum globulin after exposure generally is not recommended. Studies have suggested that immune serum globulin may modify or attenuate the course of disease but that it does not necessarily prevent viremia or fetal infection.

Infectious Mononucleosis

Infectious mononucleosis (IM) is an illness characterized by fever, pharyngitis, and adenopathy. The 20th century saw the gradual emergence of the association of IM with atypical lymphocytes, heterophilic antibodies, and the Epstein-Barr virus (EBV).

Infections with EBV occur commonly during childhood; however, primary infection in children is usually either mild or asymptomatic (12,13). Consequently, 50% of college freshmen in the United States already have antibodies to EBV. Approximately 10% to 20% of the susceptible population are expected to seroconvert every year during college. Most of these infections, however, tend to be asymptomatic (14).

Etiology

Epstein-Barr virus is the responsible agent in approximately 90% of patients who present with typical IM. Cytomegalovirus (CMV) infection is responsible for most of the remaining patients. Both of these closely related viruses are members of the herpes family. The virion of EBV is 110 nm in diameter and has a genome of double-stranded DNA. EBV infects cells of the lymphoreticular system exclusively.

Clinical Manifestations

The onset of IM is often heralded by constitutional complaints, including headache, chills, myalgia, and cough, followed within a week by sore throat and dysphagia. Sweats associated with fever are common. These symptoms frequently last 7 to 10 days and are followed by malaise, fatigue, and anorexia that persist from several days to weeks (Table 34.2).

Between 83% and 100% of IM patients have abnormal liver function studies, but the serum bilirubin level is invariably below 5 mg/dL. Thirty percent of these patients have an associated positive throat culture for group A streptococci.

Table 34.2   Clinical Features of Infectious Mononucleosis

Symptoms	Frequency
Adenopathy	100%
Malaise and fatigue	90%–100%
Sweats	80%–95%
Anorexia	50%–80%
Nausea	50%–70%
Chills	40%–60%
Fever	80%–95%
Pharyngitis	65%–85%
Splenomegaly	50%–60%

Skin manifestations occur in approximately 3% to 10% of IM cases (15,16). In the vast majority of these patients, a macular or maculopapular or morbilliform rash is seen, which generally involves the trunk but also may involve the extremities and palms and soles. Occasionally, this rash has been described as petechial, erythema multiforme, or even papulovesicular or urticarial (17,18).

Because IM patients often have a sore throat and a positive throat culture for group A streptococci, antibiotics are commonly prescribed. Patients who are treated with antibiotics are much more likely to develop a rash, and 69% to 100% of patients who receive ampicillin and 14% of those treated with either penicillin or tetracycline have been noted to develop a rash (15). One fourth of patients also have an enanthem, which is most often described as palatal petechiae. A variety of complications can be seen with IM (Table 34.3); other clinical manifestations of IM may not be obvious, and patients may lack heterophilic antibodies (19).

Generally, patients with IM caused by CMV who are negative for heterophilic antibodies are slightly older than those with IM caused by EBV. Additionally, pharyngitis and adenopathy are often not as striking, and a rash also may be a part of this syndrome.

Often, primary infection with perinatally acquired CMV also is associated with an erythematous and maculopapular rash. However, the rash of congenital CMV acquired in utero is most often petechial and a consequence of thrombocytopenia.

Diagnosis

Physicians frequently arrive at a tentative diagnosis of IM on the basis of fever, marked adenopathy, pharyngitis, and splenomegaly. Confirming a diagnosis of IM rests primarily on serologic methods. EBV culture is technically difficult and not generally available. The presence of atypical lymphocytosis often can be helpful, especially in children under 5 years of age, who often

Table 34.3   Complications of Infectious Mononucleosis

Neurological	Liver
Guillain–Barré seizures	Necrosis
Meningoencephalitis	Cirrhosis
Peripheral neuritis	
Bell's palsy	**Cardiac**
	Myocarditis
Hematologic	Pericarditis
Hemolytic anemia	
Thrombocytopenia	**Spleen**
Aplastic anemia	Splenic rupture

lack heterophilic antibodies (18). The presence of heterophilic antibodies is documented with the Paul-Bunnell test or the slide agglutination (Monospot) test. Although these tests are not very sensitive in children under 5 years of age, their sensitivity approaches 90% in older children and adults (20).

A variety of specific serologic tests are available to document EBV infection. Tests for both IgG and IgM antibody to the viral capsid antigen are readily available. The presence of IgM antibody suggests an acute, recent infection. Antibody to early antigen also suggests an acute or recent infection and may be helpful in the diagnosis. Occasionally, antibody to EBV nuclear antigen can be identified in a patient whose other antibody test results are confusing relative to the time of infection occurrence. Because antibody to EBV nuclear antigen develops at a late stage and is not present during an acute infection, its absence would be consistent with other serologic findings that indicate acute infection. This specific EBV test should be performed only when the Monospot test is negative.

Patients who present with IM in the absence of serologic evidence for EBV infection may be infected with CMV. CMV can be cultured readily from the throat and from urine. Serologic methods are used less often to confirm infection with CMV than they are with EBV.

Treatment and Prevention

The treatment of IM is primarily supportive. Antiviral chemotherapy for EBV is ineffective. Steroids are probably used more often than indicated. In severe IM caused by EBV, the use of steroids shortens the duration of fever (21). Additional indications for steroid use include impending airway obstruction, hemolytic anemia, and thrombocytopenia. Possible indications for steroids include neurological complications of IM, pericarditis, and myocarditis.

Neither active nor passive immunization is currently available to prevent EBV-associated IM.

Roseola (Exanthem Subitum)

Roseola is a common pediatric exanthematous illness that occurs in children between the ages of 3 months and 3 years. It has often been overdiagnosed by physicians who care for children, many of whom typically assign this diagnosis to any child with an acute febrile illness who develops a rash after defervescence. Subsequent to the identification of the causative agent-human herpesvirus 6 (HHV-6)-a better understanding of the clinical disease has emerged (22). Primary infection has been reported occasionally in adults who presented either with hepatitis or mononucleosis syndrome. Infection also has been reported in immunocompromised patients (e.g., transplant recipients,

HIV-infected individuals, patients with malignancy). The role of HHV-6 in the manifestations of the diseases seen in these patients is often unclear.

Few children escape infection with HHV-6 during the first 2 years of life (23,24). Acquisition of antibody to the virus occurs at an age earlier than with either CMV or EBV. Within the first 6 months of life, the titer of maternal antibody to HHV-6 decreases, and the illness caused by the virus becomes common. By the age of 2 years, few children have experienced recognizable disease, yet virtually all of them have acquired antibody to HHV-6.

Etiology

As with other members of the herpesvirus family, HHV-6 is enveloped and has a double-stranded DNA genome and demonstrates tropism to T lymphocytes, especially activated CD4 cells. Two serogroups of the virus (A and B) have been identified.

Clinical Manifestations

Primary infection with HHV-6 is a major cause of undifferentiated febrile illness in children under 2 years of age. In a recent study, 14% of acutely ill febrile children under 2 years of age who presented to an emergency department had documented HHV-6 infection (23). Although a wide variety of clinical manifestations were seen, rash was present in only 18% of the patients. Fever in excess of 40°C, malaise, irritability, inflamed tympanic membranes, and nasal congestion were observed in most patients. On the other hand, febrile seizures occurred in only 1 of 34 (3%) patients. The average white blood cell (WBC) count was lower in HHV-6-infected patients than in control subjects.

An exanthem was noted in only 18% of the patients in the study described above; it most often involved the face and trunk and was defined as macular or maculopapular (23). In slightly more than half of patients with the rash it was noted to have appeared after fever had abated. Therefore, it seems that the characteristic rash of roseola occurs infrequently in HHV-6-infected patients and even less often after the fever has disappeared. Infection with HHV-7, a closely related virus, is also universal but generally occurs slightly later than does infection with HHV-6. Primary infection with HHV-7 is believed to result in an acute, undifferentiated, febrile illness that occasionally is accompanied by a rash similar to that seen with HHV-6.

Diagnosis

Confirmation of roseola is not readily available. A reduction in the total WBC count, especially the presence of lymphocytosis in a child who presents with a typical clinical picture, is helpful in suggesting the diagnosis. Growth in tissue culture of HHV-6 remains investigational.

A variety of serologic assays are available for identifying HHV-6 infection, including an indirect immunofluorescent antibody assay and enzyme immunoassay. The presence of maternal antibody, viral reactivation, and cross-reacting antibody occasionally may make serologic results difficult to interpret.

Treatment and Prevention

Treatment for roseola remains supportive, and neither passive nor active immunization is available.

Erythema Infectiosum (Fifth Disease)

For more than 100 years, physicians have recognized a distinct syndrome named erythema infectiosum (EI) and have endeavored to distinguish it from rubella. At around the turn of the 20th century, six common childhood exanthems were described in detail and were numbered. EI was the fifth such disease described and thus received its common name, Fifth disease. In 1975, investigators identified a virus designated parvovirus (B19), which in 1983 was identified as the cause of EI (25,26).

Etiology

Parvovirus B19, a member of the Parvoviridae family, is a small (20-25 nm in diameter) enveloped virus. A recent study has demonstrated five separate genotypes of B19, but no clinical significance has been attached to this finding.

Clinical Manifestations

Erythema infectiosum is seen most commonly in children aged 5 to 15 years. Ten percent of cases occur in children under 5 years of age, and 20% occur in adults (26a). Because approximately half of all adults have antibody to parvovirus B19 and because few recall having had characteristic disease, it can be assumed that a substantial proportion of primary cases of EI are asymptomatic (26a). Two studies of EI found that 17% to 25% of infections were asymptomatic (25,26b).

The incubation period of EI is 4 to 14 days. Approximately half of patients with the disease experience mild prodromal symptoms including malaise, sore throat, coryza, and low-grade fever. A characteristic rash then appears on the

cheeks. The cheeks appear erythematous and warm, with an associated circu-
moral pallor. In the second phase of the illness, the rash spreads to the extremities and is usually morbilliform, annular with central clearing, or
reticular. The rash is less likely to involve the trunk, palms, or soles. In this
phase of the illness, the rash occasionally is described as petechial or purpuric.
In the final phase of the illness, which may last for several weeks, the rash re-
mits and recurs with stress, exercise, or bathing.

Associated symptoms in patients with EI vary, but most children feel well.
A variety of other symptoms have been described and include coryza, vomiting, diarrhea, adenopathy, conjunctivitis, and arthritis. Arthralgia, arthritis,
and myalgia are seen occasionally in children with EI, but these symptoms occur in half of all infected adults. The role of parvovirus B19 in causing disease
in other hosts is summarized in Table 34.4.

Diagnosis

The demonstration of parvovirus B19 by culture or polymerase chain reaction remains investigational. Confirmation of infection or documentation of
immunity rests on serologic methods. Assays for serum IgG and IgM antibodies to the virus are available.

Treatment and Prevention

No specific antiviral chemotherapy or vaccine is currently available for EI.
Exposure of women of childbearing age to EI is a problem that is encountered
not infrequently in clinical practice. Approximately half of all adults are already immune, and immune status can be evaluated in the exposed individual. From 30% to 50% of susceptible exposed individuals become infected,
and the risk of fetal death in a pregnant woman (even with primary infection)
is approximately 10%. On the basis of these figures, an exposed, susceptible
pregnant woman can anticipate an upper-limit risk of fetal death of 1.5% to
2.5% (27).

Table 34.4   Associated Clinical Syndromes in Parvovirus Infection

Host	Syndrome
Chronic hemolytic anemia	Transient aplastic anemia
Pregnancy	Spontaneous abortion
Immunodeficiency	Chronic anemia
Adults	Arthritis
Children	Encephalitis, Henoch–Schönlein purpura, pneumonitis

On the basis of currently available information and of the difficulty in obtaining serologic data for EI, it does not seem reasonable to recommend the screening of all pregnant women for susceptibility to the disease. Certain teachers and day care personnel have an increased risk of acquiring EI (28), and physicians must deal with issues of occupational exposure on an individual basis (29).

Varicella and Zoster (Chicken Pox and Shingles)

Chicken pox (varicella) is a vesicular exanthematous illness that few children escape unless they are vaccinated against it. Asymptomatic disease occurs rarely, if ever (30), and repeated infection is documented rarely in a normal host. Ninety-five percent of adults are immune to varicella even if they have a negative history for the disease.

Varicella is extremely contagious, with 90% of susceptible household contacts developing the disease. Infectivity rates are lower with less-intense exposure, such as in the school setting. Interestingly, cases caused by household exposure are more severe. Adults, neonates born to nonimmune mothers, and immunocompromised patients also have more severe disease.

After the resolution of clinical disease, the varicella zoster virus (VZV) remains latent in cells of the dorsal root ganglia. Reactivation may occur later in life, and shingles (zoster) represents a secondary infection with VZV.

Etiology

The VZV that causes both chicken pox and shingles is a member of the herpes virus family, is closely related to herpes simplex virus, and has a double-stranded DNA genome. (CMV and EBV are also members of the herpes virus family.)

Clinical Manifestations

After an incubation period of 10 to 21 days, patients with varicella develop mild prodromal symptoms of a low-grade fever, headache, and malaise. The characteristic skin lesions are noted within 24 to 48 hours, usually on the trunk, face, or scalp. The lesions start as papules but rapidly become vesicular, with clear, fluid-filled lesions noted on an erythematous base—the so-called "tear drop on a rose petal." These lesions progress to the pustular and then crusted stages. New crops of lesions occur with a centrifugal spread. As new crops of lesions become apparent, papules, vesicles, and pustules all may be present at the same time. Involvement by lesions of mucous membranes, including those of the mouth and eyes, is frequent. The lesions in these sites are intensely pruritic and may become secondarily infected, with a resultant increase in surrounding erythema. The patient may continue to have new lesions for up to 7 days.

Besides the pruritus of varicella, patients with the disease are likely to have fever (occasionally as high as 106°C), malaise, and anorexia that are most pronounced during the first few days of illness.

As with varicella, the characteristic skin lesions of shingles (zoster) are also vesicular and occur in a dermatomal distribution, involving one or more adjacent dermatomes. New lesions appear for up to 7 days. Zoster in children is milder than that which is seen in adults and is accompanied less often by neuritis or postherpetic neuralgia. The most common complications are related to bacterial coinfection. Severe cellulitis, fasciitis, and toxic shock syndrome caused by *Streptococcus pyogenes*, when seen in children, frequently follow infection with VZV (31). Other complications of infections with VZV include various hematologic or neurological manifestations, especially ataxia and, rarely, Reye's syndrome.

Diagnosis

Usually, the diagnosis of VZV is made on clinical grounds alone. The appearance of the typical exanthem in a susceptible host occurring after exposure and an appropriate incubation period usually suggests the diagnosis. Identification of the virus in tissue culture with specimens of vesicular fluid can be used to confirm the diagnosis. More rapid confirmation is possible by scraping material from the base of a vesicle and looking for multinucleated giant cells or by the direct immunofluorescence using a monoclonal antibody to VZV. Cytologic methods lack sufficient sensitivity and fail to distinguish VZV from herpes simplex virus infections.

Serology with enzyme immunoassay methods is used primarily to assess susceptibility to varicella in adults. These results can help the physician make decisions about active versus passive immunization after exposure to VZV (30). IgM-antibody techniques are generally not useful outside the research setting.

Treatment

In certain clinical situations, VZV infections are treated with acyclovir. Generally, VZV infections in immunocompromised hosts require intravenous therapy (32). In all patients, it is imperative to initiate treatment as early as possible. Recommendations for treating VZV infection are listed in Table 34.5 (33).

Table 34.5   Therapy for Varicella and Zoster Infections

Patient Group	Treatment Options*
Varicella	
Immunocompetent persons	
Neonates	Intravenous acyclovir for 10 days
Children <12 years of age	Symptomatic care only; consider 5 days of oral acyclovir
Adolescents and adults	Oral valacyclovir,† famciclovir,† or acyclovir for 5 days
Women in last trimester of pregnancy	Oral acyclovir for 5 days
Patients with pneumonitis or other severe infection	Intravenous acyclovir for 7–10 days
Immunocompromised persons	
Corticosteroid therapy, continuous or intermittent high dose	Oral valacyclovir,† famciclovir,† or acyclovir for 7 days
Low-dose daily cytotoxic drug use†	Oral valacyclovir,† famciclovir,† or acyclovir for 7 days
HIV-infected	Intraenous acyclovir for 7 days or longer, or oral valacyclovir,† famciclovir† or acyclovir for 7–10 days if symptoms are mild
Hematologic or solid-organ malignant conditions or transplant recipient	Intravenous acyclovir for 7–10 days
Acyclovir-resistant lesions	Intravenous foscarnet† for 14 days or longer (until healing)
Zoster	
Immunocompetent persons	
Age <50 years with mild pain	Symptomatic care only
With ophthalmic rash	Oral famciclovir, valacyclovir, or acyclovir for 7 days; ophthalmologic assessment
Age ≥50 years or moderate to severe pain	Oral famciclovir, valacyclovir, or acyclovir for 7 days; consider corticosteroids§
Immunocompromised persons	
Corticosteroid therapy, continuous or intermittent high dose	Oral famciclovir, valacyclovir, or acyclovir for 7 days
Low-dose daily cytotoxic drug use‡	Oral famciclovir, valacyclovir, or acyclovir for 7 days
HIV-infected	Oral valacyclovir, famciclovir, or acyclovir for 7–10 days
Hematologic or solid-organ malignant conditions or transplant recipient	Intravenous acyclovir or oral valacyclovir or famciclovir for 7–10 days
Disseminated disease	Intravenous acyclovir for 10 days
Acyclovir-resistant lesions	Intravenous foscarnet† for 14 days or longer (until healing)

*Standard dosages are oral acyclovir, 20 mg/kg five times daily for children or 800 mg five times daily for adults; intravenous acyclovir, 500 mg/m² every 8 hours for children or 10 mg/kg every 8 hours for adults; oral valacyclovir, 1000 mg three times per day; oral famciclovir, 500 mg three times per day; intravenous foscarnet, 40 mg/kg every 8 hours.
†Not approved by the Food and Drug Administration for this indication.
‡Examples include daily oral cyclophosphamide, methotrexate, azathioprine, and 6-mercaptopurine.
§Oral prednisone, 30 mg twice per day for 7 days, 15 mg twice per day for 7 days, and 7.5 mg twice per day for 7 days.
Republished with permission from Cohen JI, Brunell PA, Strauss SE, Krause PR. Recent advances in Varicella–Zoster Virus Infection. Ann Intern Med. 1999;130:922–932.

Prevention

A cell-free, attenuated, live-virus vaccine for varicella has been available in the United States for 6 years. This vaccine is highly effective in preventing serious disease but has been underutilized in the United States (34). Occasional recipients develop a rash, and in rare cases there is transmission of the vaccine strain of the virus to susceptible individuals. The duration of immunity conferred by vaccination seems to be excellent, and the subsequent development of shingles actually occurs less frequently than in individuals otherwise infected with virus. Contraindications for this vaccine are similar to those seen with other live vaccines and include moderate to severe febrile illness, immunocompromise, current steroid therapy in children, pregnancy, recent treatment with immunoglobulin, use of salicylates, or allergy to vaccine components.

Passive protection against varicella is possible after exposure to VZV through the use of immune serum globulin, intravenous gammaglobulin, or varicella-zoster immunoglobulin (VZIG) (35). VZIG is preferred and indicated for susceptible individuals after a significant exposure. Individuals for whom VZIG should be considered include immunocompromised patients, newborn infants whose mothers had chicken pox between 5 days before to 2 days after delivery, premature infants of more than 28-weeks' gestation and whose mothers have no history of chicken pox, and premature infants of less than 28-weeks' gestation regardless of the maternal history. For additional details, consult the Report of the Committee on Infectious Diseases, 24th edition (35a).

Enteroviruses

Enteroviruses (EVs) are ubiquitous agents that are responsible for a wide variety of diseases, of which poliomyelitis is the best known. EVs are spread by the fecal-oral route, and their activity in more temperate climates is most marked in the late summer and early fall (although they occur throughout the year). The exanthems associated with enteroviral disease vary from maculopapular to petechial to vesicular, and consequently these diseases must be included in the differential diagnosis of any disease that causes fever and rash in a child (36).

Clinical Manifestations

Infants and children are infected with EV most often. As with poliomyelitis, most disease is clinically unapparent. Infections with EV are often seen as part of outbreaks. Patients with symptomatic disease have a wide range of clinical manifestations that range from mild, nonspecific, febrile disease to more severe disease with associated paralysis or fatal myocarditis.

Prodromal symptoms of EV infection include fever, nausea, vomiting, conjunctivitis, or eye irritation. The clinical illness caused by EV is often biphasic, and several associated features help the clinician arrive at the diagnosis. Some patients have an enanthem characterized by the development of vesicular and/or papular lesions (*herpangina*) in the posterior pharynx or on the soft palate. Aseptic meningitis is a common feature of EV infection.

Rash associated with EV disease is most often described as maculopapular, macular, or morbilliform. As in rubella and rubeola, the EV rash starts on the face and neck and spreads downward to involve the trunk and extremities. The rash is rarely vesicular but can be confused with varicella under these circumstances. A petechial rash is not uncommon, especially in cases of infection with echovirus 9, and can be confused with the skin manifestations of meningococcemia.

Exanthematous disease, which is associated with at least two echoviruses (types 16 and 25) has occurred as part of well-defined outbreaks of EV disease, with a rash that appears in many of these patients after defervescence (as occurs with roseola). These patients with Boston or Pittsburgh exanthem exhibit features common to EV disease. Aseptic meningitis is a frequent occurrence. The rash of roseola lasts from 1 to 7 days, and an enanthem of papules or vesicles in the posterior pharynx is not uncommon.

Hand, Foot, and Mouth Disease

As with other diseases caused by EV, hand, foot, and mouth (HFM) disease is more often seen in the summer and early autumn. After a short incubation period of 2 to 6 days, a brief prodrome of low-grade fever, sore throat, and anorexia appears; within another day, involvement of the oral cavity and/or skin is noted.

Generally, the enanthem of HFM disease is thought to be the most common manifestation and is estimated to occur in 90% of patients. The lesions of the enanthem are most often vesicular and are found, in decreasing order of frequency, on the buccal mucosa, tongue, palate, uvula, and/or anterior pillars. These enanthema can be confused with herpetic stomatitis or aphthous ulcers.

An exanthem is seen in more than half of patients with HFM disease, with involvement of the hands (52%), feet (31%), and buttocks (31%) noted in one study (36). Lesions on the hands and feet consist of small vesicles and last from 2 to 7 days.

Although Coxsackie A16 virus is recovered most often from patients with HFM disease, other Coxsackie viruses of both types A and B have been recovered occasionally.

Diagnosis

Confirmation of EV disease usually depends on identification of the virus in tissue culture. Fibroblasts or primary monkey kidney cells are used, and virus is identified in 2 to 10 days. Identification in "shell vial" culture can be made within 72 hours. Suitable specimens for culture include cerebrospinal fluid, vesicle and pericardial fluid, and blood. Identification of EV in the throat or in stool can be suggestive of disease; however, because of the frequency of asymptomatic shedding of EV (especially in the summer and autumn), these specimens are not preferred. Serology is generally not useful because of the large number of serotypes of EV that are potentially involved in causing disease. Recently, the polymerase chain reaction test has been applied to several clinical specimens, especially cerebrospinal fluid, in cases of EV disease. Polymerase chain reaction in a limited number of studies that used cerebrospinal fluid has provided more timely and sensitive results than other assay methods. The diagnosis is confirmed through culture of infected material, which usually is indicated only to distinguish EV disease from other, more serious illnesses that require specific therapy (e.g., meningococcemia, bacterial meningitis).

Treatment and Prevention

No specific antiviral chemotherapy is yet available for EV disease. Immune serum globulin has been used in selected immunocompromised patients and has been found to modify the course of disease. Neither active immunization or passive protection with immune serum globulin is now feasible for individuals exposed to nonpolio enteroviruses.

REFERENCES

1. **Hinman AR, Eddins DL, Kirby CD, et al.** Progress in measles elimination. *JAMA.* 1982;247:1592–5.
2. **Gustafson TL, Levens AW, Brunell PA, et al.** Measles outbreak in a fully immunized secondary-school population. *N Engl J Med.* 1987;316:771–4.
3. **Emonson MB, Addiss DG, McPherson JT, et al.** Mild measles and secondary vaccine failure during a sustained outbreak in a highly vaccinated population. *JAMA.* 1990;263:2467–71.
4. **Measles prevention: Recommendations of the immunization practices advisory committee (ACIP).** *MMWR Morbid Mortal Wkly Rep.* 1989;38:1–18.
5. **Fulginiti VA, Eller JJ, Downie AW, Kempe CH.** Altered reactivity to measles virus. *JAMA.* 1967;202:101–6.
6. **American Academy of Pediatrics, Committee on Infectious Diseases.** Recommended childhood immunization schedule. *Pediatrics.* 1998;101:134–5.

7. **Gregg N, McA TR.** Congenital cataract following German measles in the mother. *Ophthalmol Soc Aust.* 1941;3:35.

8. **Lamprecht C, Schauf V, Warren D, et al.** An outbreak of congenital rubella in Chicago. *JAMA.* 1982;247:1129–33.

9. **Orenstein WA, Greaves WL.** Congenital rubella syndrome: a continuing problem. *JAMA.* 1982;247:1174–5.

10 . **JF, Brandling-Bennett AD, Witte JJ, et al.** A review of five-years͏ experience with rubella vaccine in the United States. *Pediatrics.* 1975;55:20–8.

11. **Ziring PR, Florman AL, Cooper LZ.** The diagnosis of rubella. *Pediatr Clin North Am.* 1971;18:87–97.

12. **Sumaya CV.** Primary Epstein-Barr virus infections in children. *Pediatrics.* 1977;59:16–20.

13 . **D, Benderly A, Levy J, et al.** Infectious mononucleosis and Epstein-Barr virus in childhood. *Pediatrics.* 1974;53:330–5.

14. **Andiman WA.** The Epstein-Barr virus and EB virus infections in childhood. *J Pediatr.* 1979;95:171–82.

15. **Patel BM.** Skin rash with infectious mononucleosis. *Pediatrics.* 1967;40:910–1.

16. **McCarthy JT, Hoagland RJ.** Cutaneous manifestations of infectious mononucleosis. *JAMA.* 1964;187:153–4.

17. **Africk, JA, Halprin KM.** Infectious mononucleosis presenting as urticaria. *JAMA.* 1969;209:1524–5.

18. **Sumaya CV, Ench Y.** Epstein-Barr virus infectious mononucleosis in children. Part I: Clinical and general laboratory findings. *Pediatrics.* 1985;75:1003–9.

19. **Grose C, Henle W, Henle G, Feorino PM.** Primary Epstein-Barr virus infections in acute neurologic diseases. *N Engl J Med.* 1975;292:392–6.

20. **Sumaya CV, Ench Y.** Epstein-Barr virus infectious mononucleosis in children. Part II: Heterophil antibody and viral-specific responses. *Pediatrics.* 1985;75:1011–9.

21. **Bender, CE.** The value of corticosteroids in the treatment of infectious mononucleosis. *JAMA.* 1967;199:97–9.

22. **Yamanishi K, Shiraki K, Kondo T, et al.** Identification of human herpesvirus-6 as a causal agent for exanthem subitum. *Lancet.* 1988;1:1065–7.

23. **Pruksananonda P, Hall CB, Insel RA, et al.** Primary human herpesvirus 6 infection in young children. *N Engl J Med.* 1992;326:1445–50.

24. **Hall CB, Long CE, Schnabel KC, et al.** Human herpesvirus-6 infection in children: a prospective study of complications and reactivation. *N Engl J Med.* 1994;331:432–8.

25. **Plummer FA, Hammond GW, Forward K, et al.** An erythema infectiosum-like illness caused by human parvovirus infection. *N Engl J Med.* 1985;313:74–9.

26. **Thurn J.** Human parvovirus B19: historical and clinical review. *Rev Infect Dis.* 1988;10:1005–11.

26a. **Anderson LJ.** Role of parvovirus B19 in human disease. *Ped Infect Dis J.* 1987;6:711–8.

26b. **Chorba T, et al.** The role of parvovirus B19 in aplastic crisis and erythema infectiosum (fifth disease). *J Infect Dis.* 1986;154:383–93.

27. **Risks associated with human parvovirus B19 infection.** *MMWR Morb Mortal Wkly Rep.* 1989;38:81–94.

28. **Gillespie SM, Cartter ML, Asch S, et al.** Occupational risk of human parvovirus B19 infection for school and daycare personnel during an outbreak of erythema infectiosum. *JAMA.* 1990;263:2061–5.

29. **Pickering LK, Reves RR.** Occupational risks for child-care providers and teachers. *JAMA.* 1990;263:2096–7.

30. **Gerson AA, Krugman S.** Seroepidemiologic survey of varicella: values of specific fluorescent antibody test. *Pediatrics.* 1975;56:1005–8.

31. **Smith EWP, Garson A, Boyleston JA, et al.** Varicella gangrenosa due to group A B-hemolytic streptococcus. *Pediatrics.* 1976;57:306–10.

32. **Shepp DH, Dandliker PS, Meyers JD.** Treatment of varicella-zoster infection in severely immunocompromised patients: a randomized comparison of acyclovir and vidarabine. *N Engl J Med.* 1986;314:208–18.

33. **Cohen JI, Burnell PA, Strauss SE, Krause PR.** Recent advances in varicella-zoster virus infection. *Ann Intern Med.* 1999;130:922–32.

34. **Plotkin SA.** Varicella vaccine: a point of decision. *Pediatrics.* 1986;78:705–7.

35. **Ross AH, Lenchner E, Reitman G.** Modification of chicken pox in family contacts by administration of gamma globulin. *N Engl J Med.* 1962;627:369–76.

35a. **Pickering LK (ed).** *Red Book 2000: Report of the Committee on Infectious Diseases,* ed 25. Elk Grove Village, IL: American Academy of Pediatrics; 2000.

36. **Cherry JD.** Newer viral exanthems. In Schulman I (ed). *Advances in Pediatrics,* vol 16. Chicago: Year Book; 1969:233–86.

35

HIV Infection

Denise J. Signs, MD, MS

Investigation in the early 1980s into the cause of profound immunodeficiency in previously healthy, young, homosexual men who developed unusual occurrences of *Pneumocystis carinii* pneumonia and Kaposi's sarcoma (1) led to the discovery of HIV (HIV-1) (2). The disease caused by the virus has become a pandemic issue that, despite well-defined means of preventing its transmission, continues to rage like a wildfire fed by ignorance, irrational biases, and apathy even within the health care community.

Care of the HIV-infected population is becoming overwhelmingly complex, and data suggest that patient survival is affected by the extent of HIV-treatment experience of the patient's physician (3). Although not every internist can be an HIV-care specialist, every practicing clinician should be able to do the following:

- Screen patients with risk factors for HIV infection and provide patient counseling about HIV testing
- Recognize symptoms of the acute retroviral syndrome, clinical manifestations of HIV infection, and presenting symptoms of common opportunistic infections
- Understand tests used to evaluate the degree of immunodeficiency and viremia in HIV-infected people
- Be familiar with general HIV treatment principles, medication side effects, and drug-drug interactions

Appreciating the basic virology, pathogenesis, and epidemiology of HIV infection is fundamental to understanding this disease.

Virology

HIV-1 is classified in the Lentivirus genus of the Retroviridae family, along with HIV-2 and the visna and maedi viruses. The most striking feature of these nontransforming, cytopathic, *slow* lentiviruses is their persistence within infected host cells despite the host's immune response (4). Originally called human T lymphocyte virus 3, the virus was renamed HIV-1 in 1986.

HIV-1 has subtypes, called *clades*, that display substantial heterogeneity (5). They are classified into the following three major groups:

- **Group M:** contains 10 genetically distinct subtypes (A–J) subdivided on the basis of their 15% to 30% genetic variation
- **Group O:** outliers, which show up to 50% genetic variability from M types of the virus
- **Group CPZ:** described in Cameroon and is genetically similar to the simian immunodeficiency virus

Subtype B predominates in the Americas and Europe, but the non-B subtypes predominate in the rest of the world. Investigation into possible differences in infectivity among the non-B subtypes of HIV-1, as well as their sensitivity to currently used antiretroviral drugs, is under investigation.

HIV-2 causes an infection similar to that caused by HIV-1 but usually with less severe destruction of the host immune system and characterized by a less-rapid disease progression and less-efficient sexual (threefold less than HIV-1) and vertical (10-fold less than HIV-1) transmission (6).

Because HIV is a retrovirus, its RNA is packaged with a reverse transcriptase (RT) enzyme that provides transcription of the viral genome into DNA, along with the core protein (p24) of the virus. Transmembrane proteins (gp 41) are embedded within the lipid envelope surrounding the core of the virion, with external glycoproteins (gp 120) protruding from this envelope. The gp 120 serves as the attachment site to a host cell receptor. The CD4 receptor present on T-helper lymphocytes and macrophages has been the most widely recognized target of HIV-1. However, it is now established that there are other cell coreceptors involved with viral cell attachment. Seven transmembrane G-protein–coupled chemokine coreceptors have been described. Coreceptors are involved with the cell attachment of viral strains that are tropic for either T cells or macrophages (i.e., M-tropic). Replication of HIV in patients who are newly infected with the virus is almost always associated with M-tropic strains. The CCR5 coreceptor is crucial for infection with M-tropic strains of the virus, and fusin (the CXCR4 coreceptor) is required for cell fusion with the envelope protein of T-cell–tropic viral strains (7). Individuals who are heterozygous for the CCR5-delta 32 allele, a common mutational variant, can be infected with HIV but tend to have an asymptomatic period that averages 2 to 4 years longer than usual. Homozygotes for the CCR5-delta 32 allele are genetically resistant to HIV infection (8,9).

After viral infection of the host cell, the RNA of HIV is transcribed by the RT enzyme, with integration of the resulting linear double-stranded DNA into host genetic material, thereby establishing lifelong latent infection. The RT enzyme has been a target of antiretroviral therapy with nucleoside analogue drugs (nucleoside reverse-transcriptase inhibitors [NRTIs]) and nonnucleoside reverse-transcriptase inhibitors (NNRTIs) that directly inhibit the RT enzyme. The complex gene processing and packaging of HIV is regulated by a large number of viral genes (*tat, rev, nef, vif, vpr, vpu*). The formation of new virus from infected cells requires the assembly of the translated proteins and viral RNA and viral budding from the host cell. Viral proteases must provide proteolytic cleavage of the gag and gag-pol proteins to activate the newly formed virus. Protease-inhibitor drugs have been powerful tools in the drug treatment of HIV infection.

Pathogenesis

After experimental vaginal infection with HIV-1, the virus enters Langerhans cells and macrophages in the lamina propria that underlie the epithelium. Within 2 days, these infected cells migrate to the T-cell–dependent sections of regional lymph nodes. Infected T cells and free virus leave the lymph nodes and can be detected in peripheral blood within 5 days of exposure (10). Therefore, there is a limited window of opportunity for attempting to prevent the establishment of infection after an exposure.

HIV-1 infection is a dynamic process, in which new rounds of viral infection and replication that produce billions of virions per day occur in susceptible cells, resulting in the killing of HIV-infected CD4-positive T cells by HIV-specific CD8 cytotoxic lymphocytes. Despite the loss of billions of cells per day, CD4 lymphocyte counts decline at approximately only 50–70 cells/mL/year because of increased CD4 cell production in infected patients. Even before significant depletion of CD4 lymphocytes, there is dysfunction of the cellular immune system, despite the observations that only 1 per 1000 to 100,000 CD4 cells may be infected in early-stage disease and 1 per 100 CD4 cells may be infected in advanced disease (11). The strain of virus and the type of cell infected determine whether cell death, latent intracellular infection, or active virus production results. Long-lived viral reservoirs, particularly resting-memory CD4 T lymphocytes, present an obstacle to eliminating HIV. Although present at approximately 16 per million peripheral blood mononuclear cells, infected resting-memory T cells evade antiretroviral drug therapy, which affects only actively replicating virus (12).

The balance between viral production and destruction in HIV infection depends on multiple factors, including the virulence of the viral strain, the viral inoculum, and the integrity of the immune system. Genetics and comorbidities, including other infections, variably affect the immune system and its ability to combat HIV infection (13). A study of rates of HIV disease progression in 43 infection chain clusters that had been infected with the same HIV strain versus rates of disease progression in patients infected with different strains concluded that host factors outweigh the differences among viral strains in determining HIV progression (14). An exception to this observation is an extensively studied series of cases in Australia, in which a donor and seven recipients infected with HIV from 1982 to 1984 did not have overt manifestations attributable to the virus for up to 13 years (15). Documentation of a deletion in a regulatory nef region of the HIV genome was believed to have rendered the virus in these cases less virulent.

The average duration after HIV infection before the development of advanced immunodeficiency and AIDS is 10 to 12 years in an untreated patient (16). If the balance of virus against the host shifts in favor of viral replication and destruction of the immune system (rapid progressors), advanced immunodeficiency may occur an average of 4 years after infection. A small percentage of patients, ranging from 6% to 9%, do not experience a decline in their CD4 cell counts or detectable HIV viremia (nonprogressors), sometimes for as long as 10 years after HIV infection. Before the advent of techniques to measure the amount of virus in the blood, predicting the rate of disease progression in an individual was difficult. Plasma viral load is relatively constant in a stable patient after approximately 4 to 6 months of HIV infection and can predict disease progression (17). In the Multicenter Aids Cohort Study, untreated patients who had viral loads of fewer than 10,000 copies/mL had a median survival of more than 10 years compared with 7.5 years for those with viral loads of 10,000–30,000 copies/mL and 4.4 years for those with viral loads greater than 30,000 copies /mL (18).

After the institution of antiretroviral therapy in HIV-infected patients, CD4 cell counts initially increase, primarily because of redistribution of memory T cells, followed by a slow (after 3–6 months) repopulation with newly produced naive T cells (19). The integrity of the reconstituted immune system in patients given antiretroviral therapy for HIV is under intense study. However, the proven safety of stopping prophylactic drugs against such opportunistic infections as *Pneumocystis carinii* pneumonia and *Mycobacterium avium* complex once CD4 cell counts rise above critical levels (200 cells/mm^3 and 100 cells/mm^3, respectively) is encouraging (20).

Untreated patients with ongoing viral replication develop natural mutational virus variants because of the lack of replicational integrity of HIV's RT enzyme. Patients subjected to less than a completely suppressive antiretroviral therapy develop drug-resistant variants of the virus. These mutational viruses, arising naturally or under drug pressure, may pose obstacles to drug-therapy regimens.

Epidemiology

Data suggest that HIV-1 originated in Africa, with the oldest recognized case traced to an adult Bantu man in the Democratic Republic of the Congo in 1959 (21), and that the disease had spread to the United States by 1968 (22). Initially endemic at low levels in the 1970s in remote areas of rural sub-Saharan Africa, HIV has disseminated throughout the world in pandemic proportions. Assessing the true numbers of infected people has been difficult because of the lengthy subclinical stage of HIV infection, underdiagnosis, and inaccurate reporting (23). Silent spread of infection has occurred among sexually active populations in developing countries. In these settings the spread of infection has been primarily heterosexual, heavily involving female prostitutes and their clients. In industrialized countries, the spread of HIV infection has primarily been among homosexual men and injection-drug users, but has been increasingly recognized in heterosexuals in recent years. The United Nations Program on HIV/AIDS (UNAIDS) estimates that 34.3 million people are currently infected with HIV, with only 1 in 10 infected people having been tested and their disease documented (24). An estimated 16,000 new HIV infections occur in the world each day, with 10% occurring in children under 15 years of age. Over 40% of new cases are in women of childbearing age, most of them between 15 and 24 years old. Approximately 90% of the world's HIV cases occur in developing nations, with an estimated 24.5 million (two thirds of the total) in sub-Saharan Africa, 5.6 million in Southeast Asia, and 1.3 million in Latin America.

In the United States, heterosexual transmission of HIV is showing an alarming increase. Sub-populations experiencing the greatest increases include women (now 22% of all AIDS cases), people of color, especially African-American men and women, and adolescents. With extensive education directed at preventing the disease, there was a marked decrease from 1987 to 1997 in cases of HIV infection among men who had sex with men, from 65% to 35% of all cases, at the same time that an increase from 17% to 25% was seen among injection-drug users (25). Unfortunately, a second wave of infection among young men who had sex with men has been recently recognized, along with increasing rates of gonorrhea and syphilis in men who had sex with men in San Francisco. At the beginning of the epidemic of HIV infection, the vast majority of women acquired the virus from injection-drug users, but currently 50% of newly infected women list sex with a heterosexual man as their HIV risk factor. Women of color are disproportionately infected, with African-American women 15-fold and Hispanic women 10-fold more likely to have AIDS than white women (26).

A 25% decline in AIDS deaths from 1995 to 1996 was not associated with a parallel decline in new HIV cases, which rose by 11% (27). Further declines in AIDS deaths since 1996 reflect the greater use of highly active anti-retroviral therapy (HAART) (28). Lesser declines have been seen in African-Americans and Hispanics than in white people, which is in part attributable to access to medication and issues related to compliance with treatment (28).

Transmission

Transmission of HIV occurs through exposure to infected blood or body fluids. The larger the amount of virus entering the body (viral inoculum), the greater the risk of transmission. Blood titers of HIV seem to be highest during primary retroviral infection and in the advanced stage of disease, when the immune system can no longer contain the infection.

Throughout the world, sexual transmission is the most common means of spread of HIV. The risk of sexual transmission of HIV is highly variable per sexual encounter, and depends on the disease stage, type of sexual encounter, presence of concurrent sexually transmitted diseases (STDs), genital trauma occurring during the encounter, and use of barrier or virucidal protection (and its efficacy). Studies have shown a higher risk of transmission with receptive rectal intercourse than with receptive vaginal intercourse (infected man, uninfected female recipient) and lower rates with insertive penile intercourse (infected woman, uninfected man) (29) (Table 35.1). Unprotected oral sex is not without risk, especially when performed by an uninfected man on an infected man. Rare reports of the spread of HIV infection through cunnilingus performed on an infected woman raise the concern of disease transmission with noninsertive sexual practices. The issue of transmission through deep kissing became an irrational concern with the advertisement of the salivary HIV test because of public misconception that virus, instead of antibody, was being tested. The amount of HIV present in saliva is negligible, and the rare case reports of HIV transmission by kissing involved unusual circumstances, with contamination of blood through oral ulcers or bleeding gums (30).

Sexually transmitted diseases that lead to breaks in the mucosal barrier and an influx of inflammatory cells enhance HIV transmission (31). HIV levels in semen were reduced eightfold after the treatment of urethritis (32). It has been estimated that urethritis and cervicitis increase the risk of acquiring HIV infection by threefold, whereas genital ulcer disease increases the risk of transmission by eightfold. Considerable effort has been made to investigate

Table 35.1   Risk of Transmitting HIV

Type of Sexual Exposure	Risk of Infection
Receptive anal intercourse	0.08%–0.32%*
Receptive vaginal intercourse	0.08%–0.2%*
Insertive vaginal intercourse	0.03%–0.09%*
Receptive oral intercourse	Rare but possible
Performing cunnilingus on infected woman	Rare but possible
Blood transfusion in U.S.	1 per 493,000 units
Shared injection-drug equipment	0.67%
Health care worker blood exposure	0.3%
Vertical transmission	25%–40%
Vertical transmission with zidovudine	5%–8%
Vertical transmission with zidovudine and caesarean section	2%–5%
Breast feeding	~15%

* Risk per sexual encounter.

methods of preventing STDs as well as HIV transmission with male and female condoms and various vaginal virucidal agents. It is difficult to define the failure of male condoms to prevent HIV transmission, although failure of these devices to prevent pregnancy occurs in 3% to 12% of situations. Studies of thousands of couples in which only one is infected with HIV have reported HIV transmission despite the absence of condom breakage, but most couples fall short of 100% compliance (33). Female condoms have an estimated contraceptive failure rate of approximately 5%, and are often more acceptable to men than are male condoms. Rectal use of the female condom is widespread, although U.S. Food and Drug Administration approval for this use of the device is lacking (34). In the macaque monkey model, subcutaneous progesterone implants increased HIV infection by eightfold (35). However, controversy exists over differences in susceptibility to HIV transmission according to human female hormone levels, with most studies failing to show such differences even in pregnancy.

HIV can also be transmitted in the transfusion of infected blood (36) and through mother-to-child (vertical) transmission (37), breast feeding, exposure to contaminated drug-treatment equipment (38), and through exposure of health care workers (HCW) to infected blood or body fluids (39). The highest risk of HCW transmission involves blood from a patient with advanced immunodeficiency (a high viral inoculum) that is injected into deep tissue, especially a blood vessel (40).

Vertical transmission of HIV infection will have resulted in 600,000 newly infected infants in 2000 (24). Developed countries that can comply with prevention strategies (*see* section on Prevention of HIV Infection) have achieved marked decreases in the transmission of HIV infection, from levels of 25% or more to 2% to 5%, with the lowest rates of 2% achieved with azidothymidine (AZT) (Zidovudine [ZDV]) prophylaxis plus cesarean section (41). Breast feeding probably also contributes as much as an additional 15% risk of HIV transmission, and should be avoided when alternative means of infant nutrition are feasible. This issue was hotly debated at the 13th International AIDS Conference in Durban, South Africa, where safe bottle-feeding practices are clearly less of an option than in societies with more advanced systems of health care delivery, as supported by data from the Nairobi bottle feeding study. (42)

Clinical Manifestations

The signs and symptoms of HIV infection vary during infection, normally increasing as the immunodeficiency caused by the disease advances. The most recent HIV staging system proposed by the Centers for Disease Control and Prevention (CDC), in 1993 (43), designates disease stage by CD4 cell count and the presence of symptoms defining HIV infection or of AIDS. Viral load testing has made this staging system seem inadequate at capturing the probability of disease progression, but no further staging guidelines are available.

Primary Infection

Primary Infection with HIV may be an asymptomatic event, without clinical symptoms to alert the affected individual, or with a range of manifestations from a mild, viral-like illness with nonspecific symptoms of swollen glands and fatigue to a severe symptomatic illness resembling infectious mononucleosis, the so-called *acute retroviral syndrome.*

Rarely, acute disease evolves rapidly into advanced immunodeficiency with death. Many HIV infections go undocumented because of the nonspecific nature of symptoms and failure of the patient to seek medical attention. Physicians continue to fail to diagnose primary conversion because the diagnosis is not considered or because of inappropriate use of laboratory procedures.

The period between HIV infection and antibody development varies on the basis of a number of factors, including the viral inoculum. The average incubation time ranges from 3 weeks to 3 months, with a small proportion of individuals requiring up to 6 months to develop antibody, and rare cases of seroconversion occurring after more than a year (44). Antibody may not be formed at the time a patient presents with symptoms. Culturing for HIV virus or obtaining an HIV gene probe test may be necessary to make a rapid diagnosis.

Prospective studies suggest that most individuals have a variety of symptoms following HIV infection (45). The time from exposure to the onset of symptoms varies, but in a study of sexual transmission, symptoms occurred from as early as 5 days to more than 30 days after exposure (46). Signs, symptoms, and physical findings during primary HIV infection are listed in Table 35.2. Skin involvement may consist of a maculopapular rash on the palms and soles, or disseminated urticaria. Mucous membrane ulcers are common. The constellation of fever, a maculopapular skin rash, and ulcers with lymphadenopathy should be a warning to consider primary HIV infection. Neurological symptoms are common, especially aseptic meningitis with photophobia and nuchal rigidity (24%), as well as hypoasthesias, transverse myelitis, cranial neuropathies, and seizures (47).

Laboratory abnormalities seen during the acute retroviral syndrome are typical of the mononucleosis syndrome, including neutropenia (34.8%), thrombocytopenia (73.9%), and anemia (26.1%). The total lymphocyte count is reduced, the erythrocyte sedimentation rate increased, the heterophile antibody test negative, and transaminase enzymes and alkaline phosphatase levels increased (48).

The average duration of symptoms in primary infection with HIV is 2 to 3 weeks, but patients may report symptoms of fatigue for several months. In a study of primary HIV infection in a large university hospital, only 5 of 19 (26%) physicians considered HIV infection as a diagnosis during a medical visit with a patient undergoing seroconversion syndrome (47). The differential diagnosis at the time of admission in 31 cases of documented, acute, symptomatic HIV infection are listed in Table 35.3.

After the acute phase of infection, HIV infection progresses through successive stages, with the average patient remaining asymptomatic or mildly symptomatic for 10 to 12 years before the occurrence of advanced destruction

---

Table 35.2   Acute Retroviral Syndrome: Common Signs and Symptoms

Fatigue (90%)	Diarrhea (32%–49%)
Fever (87%–94%)	Aseptic meningitis (24%)
Rash (32%–68%)	Cranial neuropathies
Headache (39%–56%)	Transverse myelitis
Exudative pharyngitis (48%–70%)	Thrush
Weight loss (13%–59%)	Oral ulcerations
Lymphadenopathy (50%)	Genital and rectal ulcerations
Night sweats (49%)	Splenomegaly
Vomiting (23%–36%)	

Adapted from Kinloch-de Loes S, de Saussure P, Saurat J, et al. Symptomatic primary infection due to HIV-1: review of 31 cases. *Clin Infect Dis.* 1993;17:59–65; and Schacker T, Collier A, Hughes J, et al. Clinical and epidemiologic features of primary HIV infection. *Ann Intern Med.* 1996;125:257–34.

Table 35.3   Differential Diagnosis of the Acute Retroviral Syndrome

Epstein–Barr virus	Rubella
Cytomegalovirus	Hepatitis
Toxoplasmosis	Syphilis
Influenza	

of the immune system with wasting syndrome, opportunistic infections, and malignancies.

Early-Stage Human Immunodeficiency Virus Disease

A number of problems may occur in patients with CD4 counts above 200 cells/mm^3, especially consisting of oral and dermatologic diseases (Table 35.4). Kaposi's sarcoma attributed to infection by human herpes virus-8, has been described throughout all stages of HIV infection in the form of skin macules/papules, erosive lesions, extensive lymphedema, oral lesions, and visceral organ involvement especially of the lung or gastrointestinal tract. Periodontal disease is a common problem with HIV infection. Generalized lymphadenopathy, with involvement of lymph nodes in two or more noncontiguous extrainguinal sites, is common in untreated patients, and is best established by examination of the anterior and posterior cervical and axillary lymph nodes (49). Dementia is a late complication of neurological involvement by HIV, and complaints of problems with memory and comprehension in early-stage disease may be a consequence of depression or anxiety. Neurological symptoms should not be ignored at any stage of HIV disease, since progressive multifocal leukoencephalitis, central nervous system lymphomas, syphilis, and bacterial meningitis all fail to respect the CD4 cell count and can occur before the onset of advanced immunodeficiency. Peripheral neuropathies of the feet/legs and hands may be caused by HIV infection, but should also be evaluated as possible side effects of anti-retroviral therapy (especially with didanosine and stavudine), as well as possible effects of diabetes, thyroid disease, and vitamin B$_{12}$ deficiency. AIDS-defining illnesses such as non-Hodgkin's lymphoma and tuberculosis can also occur at a CD4 count above 200 cells/mm^3, and should be considered in patients with prolonged fevers.

Advanced Immunodeficiency

Advanced immunodeficiency occurs at CD4 counts of 200 cells/mm^3 or fewer. Although many patients have no HIV-related symptoms even with

Table 35.4   Oral and Dermatologic Findings in HIV-Infected Individuals

Recurrent oral and genital herpetic disease	Pruritic popular rashes
Aphthous stomatitis	Fungal skin infections (e.g., jock itch, ring-
Periodontal disease	worm, and seborrheic dermatitis)
Oral and cutaneous papillomavirus	Eosinophilic folliculits
Oral and cutaneous Kaposi's sarcoma	Shingles
Oral and vaginal candidiasis	Molluscum contagiosum
Fungal nail infections	

CD4 counts below 50 cells/mm^3, further symptoms may occur as the immune system becomes progressively weakened, with depletion of immune cells. Common problems of advanced HIV-induced immunodeficiency include anorexia, weight loss despite a high calorie intake, diarrhea, fatigue, thrush, night sweats, hairy leukoplakia, and alopecia. Lymph nodes scar down with destruction of the immune system, and manifest lymphadenopathy disappears. The wasting syndrome in advanced HIV-related disease, which may also result from an active opportunistic infection, especially *Mycobacterium avium* complex, is remarkable for weight loss exceeding 10% of lean body mass, muscle wasting, and progressive weakness. Recently, losses of bone density and aseptic hip necrosis have been increasingly recognized in people with advanced HIV disease, but whether these are effects of HIV or side effects of medication is uncertain.

A list of AIDS-defining conditions is found in Table 35.5. Different opportunistic infections seem to occur at different levels of immunodeficiency, with *Pneumocystis carinii* pneumonia occurring after CD4 counts drop below 200 cells/mm^3 (or 14% of total lymphocytes). At CD4 counts below 100 cells/mm^3, toxoplasmosis and cryptococcal disease as well as other disseminated fungal diseases, such as histoplasmosis and blastomycosis, begin to become manifest. It is unusual to see *Mycobacterium avium* complex disease at a CD4 count above 75 cells/mm^3, or cytomegalovirus disease at a CD4 count above 50 cells/mm^3 (*see* Chapter 36).

Testing

Tests for Human Immunodeficiency Virus

Testing for anti-HIV antibody became available in March 1985. Since then, several additional tests have been developed to access the degree of immune integrity of HIV-infected individuals, evaluate the activity of HIV (viral load testing), and evaluate for viral resistance to currently available antiviral drugs (Table 35.6).

Table 35.5   AIDS-Defining Illnesses

Candidiasis of bronchi, trachea, or lungs
Candidiasis, esophageal
Cervical cancer, invasive
Coccidioidomycosis, disseminated or
    extrapulmonary
Cryptococcosis, extrapulmonary
Cryptosporidiosis, chronic intestinal
    (>1-month's duration)
Cytomegalovirus disease (other than liver,
    spleen, nodes)
Cytomegalovirus retinitis with loss of vision
Chronic herpes simplex ulcers >1-month's
    duration or herpes simplex bronchitis,
    pneumonitis, or esophagitis
Histoplasmosis, disseminated or
    extrapulmonary
HIV-related encephalopathy

Isosporiasis, chronic intestinal (>1-month's
    duration)
Kaposi's sarcoma
Lymphoma, Burkitt's, immunoblastic, or
    primary brain
Mycobacterium avium complex or *M. kansasii*
    infection, disseminated or extrapulmonary
Mycobactrium tuberculosis infection
Pneumocystis carinii pneumonia
Pneumonia, recurrent
Progressive multifocal leukoencephalopathy
Salmonella septicemia, recurrent
Toxoplasmosis of brain
Wasting syndrome (involuntary weight loss
    >10% with diarrhea or weakness and fever)

Table 35.6   Some Causes of False-Positive HIV ELISA Tests

Autoimmune diseases
Recent vaccine inoculation, especially
    influenza
Recent viral infections
Alcoholic liver disease
Primary biliary cirrhosis
Sclerosing cholangitis

Rapid plasma reagin positive serum
Hematologic malignancies
Lymphoma
Antibodies against class II HLA leukocyte
    antigens
Chronic renal failure

ELISA = enzyme-linked immunosorbent assay.

The current standard test for HIV is the screening enzyme linked immunoassay (ELISA), which can be performed on blood, urine, and gingival salivary specimens. The test uses recombinant viral proteins and peptides of HIV antigen fixed to a solid phase to bind to anti-HIV antibodies in a patient's blood specimen. If antibody is present, it is labeled with an anti-human antibody and subjected to a colorimetric enzymatic reaction that can be quantified in a spectrophotometer. The screening ELISA is relatively inexpensive and relatively rapid to perform. Its drawback is that it can give false-positive results (50), which may cause undue anxiety until confirmatory testing can be performed (Table 35.7). The ELISA is approximately 99% sensitive, but because of false-positive results, a repeatedly positive ELISA is subjected to Western blot (WB) analysis for confirmation. A rapid test (SUDS, Abbott Di-

Table 35.7   HIV Tests

Detection of HIV Infection	Ease of Use	Sensitivity	Specificity
Antibody Tests			
Screening: ELISA	++++	+++	+
Confirmation: Western blot	++	++++	+++
Antigen Tests			
P24 antigen	++	+	+++
Qualitative PCR	+	+++	+++
Viral culture	+	+	++++
Determination of Immunologic Healthiness			
CD4 Count	+++	+++	++
Anergy testing	++	++	+++
Measurement of Viral Activity			
Viral Load Testing			
RNA-PCR	+		
Branched-chain DNA	+		
NASBA	++		
Drug Resistance Monitoring			
Genotypic assays		NE	NE
Phenotypic assays		NE	NE

ELISA = enzyme-linked immunosorbent assay; NASBA = nucleic acid–sequence base amplification; NE = not established; PCE = polymerase chain reaction test; + = reasonable; ++ = good; +++ = very good; ++++ = excellent.

agnostics) gives results in 10 to 15 minutes, with good specificity (99.6%) and excellent sensitivity (99.9%). The gingival fluid salivary test (Orasure Test System, Epitope, Beaver, OR) involves collecting saliva, which normally has far higher IgG levels than plasma, with a small sponge that is inserted between the cheek and gum, left for 2 minutes to collect the specimen, and then placed in a transport vial. This test has become the preferred mode of testing for HIV in many public health departments because of the stability of samples (several weeks), avoidance of blood drawing, low cost ($24), and ability to perform a WB on samples positive for HIV by ELISA. The urine test (Calypte HIV-1 Urine EIA, Seradyn, Inc.) must be performed and, if positive, one must have blood drawn for a confirmatory WB (51).

The WB is a protein electrophoretic immunoblot technique that in the case of HIV infection identifies specific antibodies to HIV proteins and glycoproteins. It is highly sensitive and specific, but is labor intensive and impractical for screening. The temporal course of the appearance of serum antibodies to HIV begins with appearance of the anti-gp160/120 antibody at approximately 2 weeks after infection, followed by the anti-p24 antibody after day 24 and the anti-gp41 antibody shortly thereafter. The CDC guidelines for the laboratory diagnosis of HIV infection require that two of the three bands for these antibodies be present for a positive test (51a). The presence of one band is considered indeterminate. Blood donors without risk factors for HIV infection, who had an indeterminate WB test and were followed with subsequent testing, were found to be negative for HIV (52). However, patients at risk for HIV who have an indeterminate WB result should be followed with serial antibody tests or with viral gene probes. Viral gene probes with amplification of the signal can be done by various techniques, including the polymerase chain reaction (PCR) and the branched-chain deoxyribonucleic acid (bDNA) test for both qualitative detection of HIV and quantitation of the viral load. Reports suggest that PCR assays give twice the number of copies of plasma RNA given by the branched-chain DNA assay (18). Before the advent of quantitative PCR, neonatal testing was problematic because of the persistence of maternal antibody to HIV for up to 15 to 18 months, and because of rather insensitive tests to detect the core (p24) antigen of the virus. A negative PCR at 6 months correlates highly with the absence of perinatal transmission of HIV. Indications for ordering non-antibody HIV tests are given in Table 35.8.

Viral culture is also sensitive for HIV, but is labor intensive, and has been replaced in the clinical setting by gene amplification techniques.

Evaluation and Management of Human Immunodeficiency Virus-Infected Patients

Patients with a diagnosis of HIV infection should be evaluated through a complete history and physical examination, CD4 cell count, and measurement of the plasma HIV viral load, as well as additional testing discussed in the following sections. The history should attempt to capture high-risk behaviors, and previous STDs or infections that might be latent or difficult to eradicate in an immunocompromised individual, such as syphilis, tuberculosis,

Table 35.8   Indications for Ordering Nonantibody HIV Tests

- To test the newborn child of an HIV-infected mother
- Because maternal IgG antibodies may be present in the child's blood up to 15 months post-partum
- Because P24 antigen detection is not as sensitive
- To test an individual with suspected acute retroviral syndrome when insufficient time may have elapsed for antibody development
- To evaluate an indeterminate Western blot in a person at risk of HIV infection
- To test a health care worker, rape victim or other HIV-exposed individual for which acute antiretroviral PEP therapy may affect the subsequent disease course

IgG = immunoglobulin G; PEP = postexposure prophylaxis.

fungal infections (e.g., histoplasmosis, coccidioidomycosis, blastomycosis, cryptococcosis), parasitic diseases (e.g., toxoplasmosis, giardiasis), and viral infections (especially hepatitis B and C, papillomavirus infection, and herpes virus infections). Substance use should be explored, and a psychological history and assessment should be done. Because of the enormous costs of HIV care, a social worker should be available for patients with financial needs. The Ryan White Act has provided funding to each state for emergency services and assistance in medication costs for HIV-infected patients. The local case managers for the Ryan White Act can be extremely useful in resolving psychosocial/financial issues.

CD4 Cell Counts

Normally exceeding 500 cells/mm^3, the CD4 count decreases with the progressive activity of HIV infection, and determining the CD4 cell count therefore helps in the staging of HIV disease. The CD4 cell count can vary considerably among laboratories, and is subject to seasonal variations and diurnal changes (lowest at noon and highest at approximately 8 P.M.), as well as variation with surgery and acute infections. The CD4 percent is the percentage that CD4 cells represent of all lymphocytes, and is more reflective of immune status than the CD4 cell count itself, because it is less subject to variation (a CD4 count >500 cells/mm^3 corresponds to a CD4 cell percent >29%; a CD4 count <200 cells/mm^3 CD4 corresponds to a CD4 cell percent <14%). Moreover, the standard CD4 cell test merely quantifies the number and percent of CD4 cells, and does not reflect the qualitative cell changes that begin with the onset of infection. A CD4 count of fewer than 200 cells/mm^3 is an AIDS-defining condition. Although CD4 cell counts most commonly rise in response to HAART, patients with low pre-therapy CD4 counts of fewer than 50 cells/mm^3, who then had an increase in counts to more than 200 cells/mm^3, were shown to have a moderately high risk for disease progression as compared with people who never had profound immunodeficiency (53). This finding emphasizes the need to prevent the development of advanced immunodeficiency (53). In stable patients, CD4 cell counts should be monitored every 3 or 4 months.

Monitoring of Viral Load

The amount of virus present in plasma varies among patients with HIV infection, but in a stable situation in a given individual is relatively constant by 4 to 6 months after infection (18). The term *viral set point* has been coined to describe an individual patient's baseline viral load. Because many factors can cause transient increases in viral load, including acute infections, relapses of herpes virus infections, or vaccinations, testing of the viral load should be delayed to 4 to 6 weeks after an illness or vaccination. A significant change in viral load is a change of 0.5 log or more in the value of the load, since the test itself has as much as 0.3 log variability. After treatment of HIV is begun, measurement of the viral load should be repeated at 2 to 8 weeks, with the expectation of at least a 1 log (10-fold) decrease in the load, and then again at 16 to 20 weeks, when the load should be under the limit of detection (<50 copies/mL) (54). The rate of decline in the viral load is affected by the degree of immunodeficiency, presence of co-infections, patient adherence to the treatment regimen, and potency of the regimen.

The viral load should be monitored every 3 to 4 months to assess the ongoing effectiveness of treatment, and to monitor for an increasing load in people who defer therapy. Of current interest are the *viral blips* that are seen to transiently occur in patients who reach a viral load of fewer than 50 copies/mL and in whom the load may then rise to <400 copies/mL. These blips are thought to result from a number of factors, including changes in antiviral drug levels as a result of non-compliance with treatment, pharmacokinetic factors, or concomitant infections. Follow-up studies suggest that such blips do not have a negative prognostic significance (55).

Viral Resistance Assays

Viral genotyping and phenotyping are tools to evaluate viral drug resistance in patients in whom anti-retroviral drug regimens prove ineffective. Genotyping is readily available, with turnaround times of 1 to 4 weeks, but is highly expensive. Genotyping assays detect point mutations in the RT and protease amino acid sequences of HIV that have been associated with resistance to various anti-retroviral drugs. However, the complex interpretation of multiple mutations limits the usefulness of this test. Phenotyping assays measure the ability of a patient's virus to grow in various concentrations of anti-retroviral drugs, but do not give information about viral growth in the presence of drug combinations. These assays are even more expensive than genotyping assays and their interpretation is surrounded by even more controversy.

Although drug resistant mutations of HIV typically develop under drug pressure, drug resistant virus may be seen even in newly infected individuals who have not been previously exposed to anti-retroviral drugs. The significance for future drug treatment of resistant mutations of HIV in naive patients is uncertain, and resistance testing is not routinely recommended unless a particular drug regimen is failing for a patient. Once anti-retroviral drugs are discontinued, the original wild-type virus usually predominates, with suppression of the resistant virus, with the result that resistance assays may give false information unless performed while the patient is actively receiving medication. Several large studies (VIRADAPT) and a study of the short-term effects of antiretroviral management based on plasma genotypic antiretroviral resistance testing [GART]) have compared genotyping with physicians' clinical decision-making in effecting changes in drug therapy for patients for whom existing antiretroviral drug regimens were failing (56,57). Short-term virologic responses were greater in the groups of patients who had genotyping-guided changes in their regimens. Long-term benefits and the utility of genotyping for patients in whom multiple treatment regimens have failed remains to be seen. The virtual phenotype is a genotype with quantitative phenotype analyses (VIRCO Central Virological Laboratory, Dublin, Ireland). It has a fast turnaround time of approximately 10 days and is less expensive than a phenotype. Preliminary studies suggest that it may be equivalent to the phenotype in predicting drug failure and may be superior to the genotype (57a). Descriptions of additional tests and their indications are given in Table 35.9 (54).

Treatment

The most recent Guidelines for the Use of Antiretroviral Agents developed by the Panel on Clinical Practices for Treatment of HIV Infection were published

Table 35.9   Additional Testing for HIV-Infected Individuals

Test	Reason for Test	Retesting Interval
CBC	Evaluate for anemia, leukopena, and thrombocytopenia secondary to HIV or medication adverse effect	3–6 months
Serum chemistry	Screen for LFT abnormalities secondary to hepatitis or medication adverse effect; rule out renal insufficiency especially in black patients; baseline cholesterol and triglycerides in patients to start protease inhibitors	3–6 months
Syphilis serology	High rates of coinfection	Annually
PPD skin test	Screen for latent tuberculosis	Annually if negative
Toxoplasma serology	Screen for toxoplasmosis	
Pap smears	Higher risk of cervical cancer in HIV infected women	6 months if negative
Chest radiography	Baseline for patient at risk of pulmonary disease and for detection of asymptomatic tuberculosis	As needed
Hepatitis serology	If abnormal liver function tests	As needed

CBC = complete blood count; LFT = liver function tests; PPD = purified protein derivative.
Adapted from the Panel on Clinical Practices for Treatment of HIV Infection. *Guidelines for the Use of Antiretroviral Agents in HIV Infected Adults and Adolescents.* Washington, DC: U.S. Department of Health and Human Services; 2001.

by the Department of Health and Human Services (DHHS) in February of 2001 (54). They recommend that treatment should be offered to all patients with acute retroviral syndrome, those who have undergone seroconversion for HIV infection within the previous 6 months, and all patients with symptomatic HIV disease (Table 35.10). It had previously been recommended that symptomatic patients take therapy if their CD4 counts were under 500 cells/mm^3 or their plasma HIV viral load was greater than 10,000 copies/mL by the bDNA assay or 20,000 copies/mL by the RT-PCR assay. Under the new guidelines, therapy need not be started until CD4 cell counts drop below 350 cells/mm^3 or if the plasma viral RNA exceeds 30,000 copies/mL (bDNA assay) or 55,000 copies/mL (RT-PCR assay) in the context of the patient's willingness to take medication, adherence to treatment, and the rate of disease progression. The major rationale for reducing the treatment requirements for HIV infection has to do with the balance of risks and benefits of therapy. Although earlier therapy may preserve immune function, prolong disease-free survival, and decrease the risk of viral transmission, concern is growing about the long-term toxicities of antiretroviral drugs, adherence problems leading to drug resistance and the future possibility of fewer treatment options, and the unknown durability of currently available therapies.

The optimal goal of HAART is to suppress viral load to undetectable (<50 copies/mL), which is idealistically an achievable goal for up to 80% of patients naive to all HIV medications and who are given a potent drug-treatment regimen and show >95% adherence to treatment. However, in a meta-analysis of 18 clinical trials, durable suppression after 24 weeks of therapy was actually achieved in approximately only 50% of treatment-naive patients. (58). Further goals include improvement in quality of life, restoration and/or preservation of immunologic function, and reduction of HIV-related morbidity. The slope of the decay in plasma HIV viral load after treatment is begun crudely predicts the probability of achieving a viral load of fewer than 50 copies/mL. A 1.5 to 2 log decrease in viral load should be seen at 4 weeks; by 12 weeks the viral load should be <500 copies/mL, and by 16 to 24 weeks it should be <50 copies/mL.

The available anti-retroviral drugs currently fall into four major classes, as follows: 1) NRTIs, 2) NNRTIs, 3) protease inhibitors (PIs), and 4) nucleotide reverse transcriptase inhibitors. (It is beyond the scope of this chapter to discuss each of these drug classes in detail, but a more extensive discussion of them can be found in the literature [54,59], and in Tables 35.12–35.15.) Guidelines for the use of anti-retroviral agents have been published by a panel of the National Institutes of Health (NIH) (60), as well as by the panel convened by the Department of Health and Human Services (54). The NIH guidelines are based on principles (Table 35.11) that assume that ongoing viral replication leads to immune-system destruction, and that antiretroviral therapy can suppress viral replication and may delay disease progression.

Table 35.10   Indications for Initiating Antiretroviral Therapy

Treatment Recipients
- All patients with the acute retroviral syndrome
- All patients diagnosed with 6 months of HIV seroconversion
- All patients with symptoms related to AIDS (e.g., thrush, weight loss, unexplained fever)
- Asymptomatic patients*

Treatment Goals
- Maximal and durable supression of the viral load
- Restoration and/or preservation of immunologic function
- Improvement of quality of life
- Reduction of HIV-related morbidity and mortality.

Treatment Recommedations
Strongly Recommended Regimens†‡

Column A	Column B
Efavirenz	Stavudine + didanosine
Indinavir	Stavudine + lamivudine
Nelfinavir	Zidovudine + didanosine
Ritonavir + indinavir	Zidovudine + lamivudine
Ritonavir + lopinavir	
Ritonavir + saquinavir (SGC or HGC)	

Alternative Regimens‡

Column A	Column B
Abacavir	Didanosine + lamivudine
Amprenavir	Zidovudine + zalcitabine
Delavirdine	
Nelfinavir + saquinavir SGC	
Nevirapine	
Ritonavir	
Saquinavir SGC	

Not recommended§
Saquinavir HGC
All monotherapies
Stavudine + zidovudine
Zalcitabine + didanosine
Zalcitabine + lamivudine
Zalvitabine + stavudine

No Recommendations¶
Hydroxyurea
Ritonavir + amprenaivir
Ritonavir + nelfinavir

*Asymptomatic HIV patients are defined as those whose CD4-positive T cell count is <350 cells/mm³ or those whose HIV RNA levels exceed 30,000 copies/mL by DNA assay or 55,000 copies/mL by reverse transcriptase–polymerase chain reaction assay. The strength of the recommendation to treat asymptomatic patients should be based on the willingness and readiness of the individual patient to begin therapy, the potential benefits and risks of initiating therapy in the asymptomatic individual, and the probability of drug adherence based on appropriate counseling and education.
† There is strong evidence that these treatments show clinical benefit and/or sustained suppression of plasma viral load.
‡ Start treatment with one choice each from columns A and B.
§ There is evidence against the use of these drugs, they are virologically undesirable, or they have overlapping toxicities.
¶ There are insufficient data for these regimens.
Adapted from the Panel on Clinical Practices for Treatment of HIV Infection. *Guidelines for the Use of Antiretroviral Agents in HIV Infected Adults and Adolescents.* Washington, DC: U.S. Department of Health and Human Services; 2001.

Table 35.11 Principles of HIV Therapy Strategies

- Ongoing HIV replication leads to immune system damage and progression to AIDS. HIV infection is always harmful, and long-term survival that is free of clinically significant dysfunction is unusual.
- Plasma HIV RNA levels indicate the magnitude of HIV replication and its associated rate of CD4 T-cell destruction, whereas CD4 T-cell counts indicate the extent of HIV-induced immune damage already suffered. Regular periodic measurements of plasma HIV RNA level and CD4 T-cell count are necessary to determine the risk of disease progression in an HIV-infected individual and to determine when to initiate or modify antiretroviral treatment regimens.
- Because the rate of disease progression differs among patients, treatment decisions should be individualized by the level of risk indicated by plasma HIV RNA levels and CD4 T-cell counts.
- The use of potent combination antiretroviral therapy to suppress HIV replication below the detection levels of sensitive plasma HIV RNA assays limits the potential for selecting antiretroviral drugs to inhibit virus replication and to delay disease progression. Therefore, the maximum achievable suppression of HIV replication should be the goal of therapy.
- The most effective route to the durable suppression of HIV replication is the simultaneous initiation of combinations of effective anti-HIV drugs with which the patient has not been previously treated and that are not cross-resistant with antiretroviral agents with which the patient *has* been previously treated.
- Each of the antiretroviral drugs that are used in combination therapy regimens should always be used according to optimum schedules and doses.
- The available effective antiretroviral drugs are limited in number and mechanism of action, and cross-resistance between specific drugs has been documented. Therefore, any change in antiretroviral therapy may increase future therapeutic constraints.
- Women should receive optimal antiretroviral therapy regardless of pregnancy status.
- The same principles of antiretroviral therapy apply to both HIV-infected children and adults; however, the treatment of HIV-infected children involves unique pharmacologic, virologic, and immunologic considerations.
- Individuals with acute primary HIV infections should be treated with combination antiretroviral therapy to suppress virus replication to levels below the limit of detection of sensitive plasma HIV RNA assays.
- HIV-infected individuals, even those with viral loads below detectable limits, should be considered infectious and should be counseled to avoid sexual and drug-use behaviors that are associated with the transmission or acquisition of HIV and other infectious pathogens.

Nucleoside Reverse-Transcriptase Inhibitors

The first class of drugs introduced for treating HIV infection were the NRTIs, with AZT (ZDV) entering clinical trials in 1986. Years of controversy surrounded the issue of whether or not monotherapy with very-high-dose ZDV (250 mg every 4 hours) prolonged the duration of asymptomatic disease and decreased mortality. In retrospect, conflicting study results were probably due in part to the inability of clinicians to distinguish between patients with high viral loads and those with moderate or low viral loads merely from their CD4 cell counts. Additionally, these patients would gain little benefit from monotherapy with an agent that would decrease their viral load only marginally (~0.7 log). This was probably responsible for the approximately 3- to 6-month prolongation of disease in some patients treated with ZDV as opposed to the disease prolongation of more than 1 year seen in others.

With newer NRTI drugs, such as didanosine (dideoxyinosine [ddI]), stavudine (D4T), and zalcitabine (dideoxycytosine [ddC]), trials of sequential monotherapy showed far better results with concomitant or dual-NRTI therapy than with monotherapy, with the ability to decrease viral load by 1.2 to 1.5 log with some combinations, especially ZDV plus lamivudine (3TC) and ddI plus D4T. Yet even with dual-NRTI therapy, less than 25% of patients had their viral loads reduced to less than detectable levels. An important lesson of the failures of NRTI therapy was the ability of HIV to mutate and thereby escape the effects of one NRTI after another, especially in individuals with high viral loads, and the diminishing returns of HAART therapy in patients with heavy NRTI treatment experience. The newest NRTI, abacavir (Ziagen), is as potent as dual-NRTI therapy, and is now available together with two additional NRTIs, ZDV and 3TC, in a triple NRTI combination (Trizivir). This PI- and NNRTI-sparing regimen has reasonable utility in naive patients with moderate to low baseline viral loads.

As a class, NRTIs show relatively low drug toxicity (Table 35.12), except for the peripheral neuropathy seen with ddI and D4T, and a hypersensitivity syndrome seen in approximately 5% of patients starting abacavir. However, metabolic concerns, and especially depletion of mitochondrial DNA with mitochondrial toxicity, lactic acidosis, pancreatic failure, liver failure, and bone marrow failure, are under investigation. Vitamin supplementation with riboflavin, L-carnitine, and co-enzyme Q is being prescribed to decrease these toxicities, but has not been studied in controlled trials. (61).

No other class of drugs has revolutionized the care of HIV-infected individuals and effected such drastic changes in disease mortality and the occurrence of opportunistic infections as the PIs (62). As a class, the PIs share the basic obstacles of high cost, a large number of drug–drug interactions, gastrointestinal distress, and rapid development of resistance when medication is stopped for even short periods (Table 35.13). When used as monotherapy, the PIs can be met by viral resistance within 6 weeks to 3 months. In the same vein, there is little use in adding a PI to a failing dual-NRTI regimen. As compared with naive patients, patients previously treated with NRTIs have less success with PIs even when the NRTIs are changed. Cross-resistance among PIs depends on their specific resistance patterns, and tremendous controversy surrounds the question of which PI is the safest one with which to begin treat-

Table 35.12   Nucleoside Reverse-Transcriptase Inhibitors

Drugs	Dosage	Major Side Effects	Advantages	Concerns
Zidovudine (Azidothymidine)*	300 mg PO q12h	Hematologic, especially anemia; dose-dependent and idiopathic nausea, headaches	Convenient dosing	Cannot be combined with stavudine; monitor CBC; do not restart if severe anemia occurs
Didanosine (Videx)	200–250 mg PO q12h or 400 mg/d†	Pancreatitis (7% per year, especially in alcohol abusers), peripheral neuropathy (9%)	Probably the most potent NRTI available (ACTG 175)	Monitor amylase level if pancreatitis symptoms develop; neuropathy is usually reversible if dose is reduced or if drug is discontinued
Dideoxycytidine (HIVID)	0.375–0.750 mg PO tid	Peripheral neuropathy		Not widely used because of its weak antiviral effect
Stavudine (Zerit)	30–40 mg PO q12h	Peripheral neuropathy	Low side-effect profile, ease of administration, reasonable potency	Neuropathy is usually reversible if dose is reduced or if drug is discontinued; do not combine with zidovudine
Lamivudine (Epivir)	150 mg PO q12h	Hepatic dysfunction (rare)	Low side-effect profile, ease of administration	Not to be used as monotherapy because of a rapid emergence of resistance
Abacivir (Ziagen)	300 mg PO bid	Severe systemic drug reaction during the first 2 weeks of treatment (5%)	Low side effects with long-term use	Continuation of drug in patient with a severe drug reaction may be fatal
Trizivir (Combivir and Ziagen)	1 PO bid	Same toxicities as the AZT, Epivir, and Ziagen	Convenience	If side effects occur, one must change drug regimen rather than just one drug.

CBC = complete blood count; ACTG = AIDS Clinical Trial Group; NRTI = nucleoside reverse-transcriptase inhibitors; PO = orally.
* Also available in a combination with lamivudine called Combivir.
† The 400-mg/d dosage of didanosine is commonly used but has not yet received approval from the Food and Drug Administration for use in the United States.

ment (i.e., to permit a regimen that will leave other therapeutic options open if this PI fails). New concerns include the possible long-term consequences of PIs on blood cholesterol and triglyceride levels, as well as the increased incidence of lipodystrophy with buffalo humps, protease paunches (protuberant abdomens), and lipomas, in addition to an increased incidence of insulin resis-

Table 35.13   Protease Inhibitors

Drug	Dosage	Major Side Effects	Concerns
Indinavir (Crixivan)	800 mg PO q8h (as 200- or 400-mg caplets)	Renal stones, asymptomatic hyperbilirubinemia, hepatic dysfunction, diarrhea, GI intolerance, lipodystrophies, diabetes, drug interactions	Must be taken with a low-fat meal; drug holidays are not allowed; drink at least 48 oz of water daily to help prevent renal sludging
Ritonavir (Norvir)	600 mg PO q12h*	Perioral paresthesias, diarrhea, bloating, liver dysfunction, hyperglycemia, drug interactions, lipodystrophies, diabetes, GI intolerance	Medication must be refrigerated; should be taken with a fatty meal; use in patients with chronic liver disease
Nelfinavir (Viracept)	750 mg PO tid (as 250-mg tablets)†	Diarrhea, hepatic dysfunction, drug interactions, lipodystrophies, diabetes	Take with food (meal or light snack)
Saquinavir (Invirase, Fortovase)	Fortovase: 1200 mg PO tid (as 200-mg caplets) Invirase: 400 mg PO bid with ritonavir	Liver dysfunction, GI intolerance, hyperglycemia, headache	Bioavailability only 4% with Invirase, not increased 10 times with Fortovase; should be taken with a meal; is taken more popularly as 400 mg bid in combination with Ritonavir 400 mg bid
Amprenavir (Agenerase)	150 mg 8 po bid	GI intolerance, possibly less lipodystrophy	Pill burden; GI complaints
Lopinavir/ ritonavir (Kaletra)	3 caplets 133.3 mg/ 33.3 mg PO bid with food	Minor GI complaints, pancreatitis, hyperlipidemia lipodystrophy,‡ drug interactions, hyperglycemia	Use in patients with liver disease, especially chronic hepatitis

GI = gastrointestinal; PO = orally.
* Start with three 100-mg pills q12h, building up to six 100-mg pills q12h by day 14 of therapy. Norvir comes in 100-mg caplets or in a 600-mg/7.5-mL solution.
† Alternative regimen: 50 mg/g powder or five tablets PO bid.
‡ Drug interactions with lovastatin, simvastatin, St. John's wort (*Hyperium perforatum*) and rifampin.

tance with use of these drugs (63). Those patients unable to comply with treatment involving a PI and who develop cross-resistance to other drugs in this class have been at a considerable disadvantage.

Therapy after the failure of an initial PI is referred to as *salvage* or *rescue* therapy. Dual-PI therapy, with or without an NNRTI and two new NRTIs, is often used in salvage therapy, but produces durable suppression of the viral load in only 25% to 40% of patients.

The NNRTIs, consisting of nevirapine (Viramune), delavirdine (Rescriptor), and efavirenz (Sustiva), are becoming popular for PI-sparing regimens, when added to NRTIs (Table 35.14). Like the PIs, the NNRTIs cannot be used as monotherapy because of rapid emergence of viral resistance. As a group, however, they have demonstrated usefulness in patients with advanced disease (Efavirenz), in patients with moderately advanced disease without the need for extensive NNRTI use (nevirapine), and in salvage regimens. The unique property of delavirdine of enhancing PI levels instead of decreasing them, as do efavirenz and nevirapine, has given it a unique role in multi-drug regimens involving PIs. The NNRTIs share the common side effect of a pruritic, generalized drug rash, which commonly occurs during the second week of therapy. The high rate of occurrence of this rash with nevirapine has been reduced to approximately 17% by dose escalation over a 2-week period of therapy. Patients taking NNRTIs should be warned about the possibility of Stevens-Johnson syndrome. Efavirenz has disturbing CNS toxicity for some patients, with agitation, insomnia, and night terrors. Fortunately, these symptoms abate for the majority of patients over the first 2 to 6 weeks of therapy. When compared directly with PIs (indinavir and nelfinavir), efavirenz has produced a clearly superior response (64).

Success with an antiretroviral drug regimen is associated with a number of factors, chief among them patient adherence to the regimen. Adherence is negatively associated with substance abuse, and especially alcoholism, as well as with depression and with complex drug regimens that are poorly tolerated. More attention has been given to drug pharmacokinetics and the correlation of drug resistance with subtherapeutic drug levels (65). In addition, data indicate that improved patient outcomes with HIV care depend on the experience of the treating physician. (3). Previous patient drug experience with single- or dual-NRTI therapy is associated with a decreased response to HAART (66). Failure of therapy (the inability to suppress viral load, or the occurrence of a

Table 35.14   Non-Nucleoside Reverse-Transcriptase Inhibitors

Drugs	Dosage	Major Side Effects
Nevirapine (Viramune)	200 mg PO qd for 14 days, then 200 mg PO bid (as 200-mg tablets)	Rash, elevated liver enzymes, hepatitis
Delaviridine (Rescriptor)	400 mg PO tid (as 100-mg tablets)	Rash, headache
Sustiva (Efavirenz)	3 pills at bedtime	Nightmares (27%), insomnia, agitation, rash

PO = orally.

rising viral load) should prompt a change of regimen. Patients should be highly encouraged to adhere closely to their initial regimen, since a smaller percentage of subsequent regimens are successful in suppressing viral load. Drug changes should be guided by a careful drug treatment history and drug resistance testing. Guidelines for changing a patient's antiretroviral regimen, modified from the DHHS Guidelines of April 2000, are an excellent reference for making such changes (59).

Much interest is currently focused on the issue of structured treatment interruptions for HIV infection. Several small studies have examined the issue of scheduled cyclic treatment interruptions of 2 weeks or longer, followed by reinstitution of the regimen used before interruption (66a). The advantages of decreased drug costs and presumably decreased drug side effects with such interrupted therapy are weighed against the risk of the development of drug resistance. A perceived immunologic advantage would be auto-immunization through temporary resurgence of the patient's HIV viral load, which might boost cellular immunity. At present, treatment interruptions should be made only in a research setting.

Information on the only nucleotide reverse transcriptase inhibitor is listed in Table 35.15.

Prevention

Education is the cornerstone of control of HIV infection, and abstinence remains the surest way to prevent infection. Given that most individuals are not amenable to this option, access to information about safe sexual practices, transmission barriers such as male and female condoms and dental dams, and promotion of HIV status disclosure to sexual partners allows interpersonal negotiation for safer sexual activity.

Current approaches to decreasing the sexual transmission of HIV infection include monogamous partnerships, delay of first intercourse, barrier precautions, and use of vaginal virucidal agents. Circumcision has been shown to be protective against transmitting HIV (67).

Table 35.15   Nucleotide Reverse-Transcriptase Inhibitors

Drugs	Dosage	Major Side Effects	Advantages	Concerns
Tenofovir	300 mg/d PO	Not known	Convenient once-daily dosing, often useful for patients resistant to AZT	Nephrotoxicity not seen as with earlier nucleotides (adefovir)

Guidelines for prophylaxis after sexual exposure have been proposed for people subject to rape and for instances in which a condom breaks, but not for people repeatedly engaging in risky behavior (68). Interestingly, when 376 victims of rape were evaluated, and 213 were offered post-exposure prophylaxis, only 32.4% chose to initiate such therapy, and only 12% returned to complete the 4 week course of treatment (69).

The success of the NIH-sponsored AIDS Clinical Trial Group 076 (ACTG 076) study, in which treatment with ZDV decreased the vertical transmission of disease from 25% to 8% in HIV-infected pregnant women (70) (Table 35.16), brought recognition of the need to identify pregnant women infected with the virus. Laws prohibit mandatory testing of all pregnant women for HIV, and practitioners often mistakenly fail to offer HIV tests to pregnant women on the assumption that they have no HIV risk factors. All pregnant women should be encouraged to have an HIV test.

Studies in which the ACTG 076 protocol has been aggressively instituted show declines in HIV transmission to less than 5%, and European data for cesarean section along with ZDV therapy show transmission rates of less than 3% (71). The benefit of cesarean section in patients who already have an undetectable viral load at delivery remains dubious.

Because most of the vertical transmission of HIV occurs in the developing world, where cultural barriers exist to HIV testing, disease disclosure, and acceptance of therapy, and drug access is a problem even for shortened treatment protocols, greater barriers exist in this part of the world to eliminating the vertical transmission of HIV. Discouraging breastfeeding in developed countries, given its ability to double the risk of HIV transmission, has not posed a major problem because of the ready access to infant feeding formulas. In Third World countries, considerable controversy surrounds this issue, especially when powdered formulas may be mixed with contaminated water or may be overly diluted because of short supply, creating more disease and nutritional issues (37)

The overall risk of HIV transmission to HCW after percutaneous exposure ranges from 0.3% to 0.09% with mucous membrane exposure. The risk is higher with exposure to a larger volume of blood; with exposure through a

Table 35.16   Guidelines to Prevent Vertical HIV Transmission

Women

Zidovudine 200 mg PO tid or 300 mg bid beginning at week 14 of pregnancy
Zidovudine 2 mg/kg bolus IVPB, then 1 mg/kg/h during labor

Infants

Zidovudine 2 mg/kg PO every 6 hours for 6 weeks beginning 8–12 hours after birth

IVPB = intravenous piggyback; PO = orally.

hollow-bore needle than through a suture needle or other sharp object; and with a deep injection, especially if it is into a blood vessel.(72).

The status of the source patient's viremia is important in establishing the risk of HIV infection, but a case of seroconversion in an HCW has been reported after exposure to a patient with a plasma viral load below the level of detection (73). In addition to blood, blood-contaminated secretions, semen,

Table 35.17   Postexposure Prophylaxis for Health Care Workers

Step 1: Determine the Exposure Code (EC)
Determine whether the source material involved contaminated blood, bloody fluid, or other potentially infectious material or instruments. No postexposure prophylaxis (PEP) is needed if exposure was to intact skin only.
EC-1: Volume small—a few drops, short-duration exposure to mucus membrane or skin with compromised integrity
EC-2: Volume large—several drops, major blood splash, longer duration (i.e., several minutes) to mucus membrane or nonintact skin, or percutaneous exposure with a solid needle or superficial scratch
EC-3: Severe percutaneous exposure—exposure via large-bore hollow needle, deep puncture, device on which there is visible blood, or needle used in a source patient's artery or vein
Step 2: Determine the HIV Status Code (SC)
If the source is HIV negative, no PEP is required.
SC-1: HIV-positive source with low titer exposure (e.g., asymptomatic patient with low viral load and/or high CD4 count)
SC-2: HIV-positive source with higher titer exposure (e.g., patient with advanced AIDS, primary HIV infection, high viral load, or low CD-4 count)
SC-Unknown
Step 3: Determine the PEP Recommendation
EC-1, SC-1: PEP may not be warranted; exposure type does not pose a known risk for HIV transmission; whether the risk for drug toxicity outweighs the benefit of PEP should be decided by the health care worker (HCW) who has been exposed and his or her treating clinician
EC-1, SC-2: Consider basic PEP regimen*; exposure type poses a negligible risk for HIV transmission; a high HIV titer in the source may justify consideration of PEP; whether the risk for drug toxicity outweighs the benefit of PEP should be decided by the HCW who has been exposed and his or her treating clinician
EC-2, SC-1: Recommend basic PEP regimen*; most HIV exposures are in this category; although no increased risk for HIV transmission has been observed, PEP is believed to be appropriate
EC-2 or 3, SC-1 or 2: Recommend expanded PEP regimen†; exposure type represents an increased risk of HIV transmission

---

* Basic PEP regimen: zidovudine plus lamivudine for 4 weeks.
† Expanded PEP regimen: Basic regimen plus either oral indinavir 800 mg q8h or oral nelfinavir 750 mg q8h.
Adapted from Centers for Disease Control and Prevention. Public Health Service guidelines for the management of health-care worker exposure to HIV and recommendations for post exposure prophylaxis. MMWR Morb Mortal Wkly Rep. 1998;47(RR-7):1–33.

and vaginal fluid, other fluids believed to be infectious include cerebrospinal fluid and synovial, pleural, pericardial, and amniotic fluid.

In a study of 51 HCW who seroconverted to HIV positivity after exposure, 81% had a primary HIV seroconversion syndrome, occurring a median of 25 days after exposure. Seroconversion occurred at a median of 46 days after exposure, with three instances of delayed seroconversion occurring beyond 6 months but at less than 12 months (72).

Few data exist on the efficacy of post-exposure prophylaxis after a significant exposure to a known HIV-infected source, but in a retrospective case-control study, the risk of transmission was reduced by 81% among HCW who began treatment with ZDV (47). Failure of postexposure prophylaxis has been documented in 14 cases, with possible reasons including a delay in starting anti-retroviral therapy, drug resistance to ZDV, and exposure to a large viral inoculum, as well as poor compliance with drug treatment (74). Guidelines have been published for the management of an exposed HCW (Table 35.17), with recommendations for two- to three-drug therapy based on concerns about resistance to ZDV and the observation that greater reductions in viral load occur with dual- and triple-drug therapies. In view of the additional toxicities, cost, and expense, the decision to use three-drug instead of two-drug therapy must be weighed against the additional potency of the three-drug regimen in cases of high-risk exposure. Because of concerns about drug resistance, a high-risk exposure to a heavily drug-pretreated patient should prompt consultation with an HIV specialist to individualize the post-exposure prophylaxis regimen for the exposed individual.

REFERENCES

1. **Gottlieb M, Schroff R, Schawker H, et al.** *Pneumocystis carinii* pneumonia and mucosal candidiasis in previously healthy homosexual men: Evidence of a new acquiried cellular immunodeficiency. *N Engl J Med.* 1981;305:1425–31.

2. **Gallo, R, Sarin, P, Gelmann E, et al.** Isolation of human T cell leukemia virus in acquired immunodeficiency syndrome (AIDS). *Science.* 1983;220:865.

3. **Hecht F, Wilson I, Wu A, et al.** Optimizing care for persons with HIV infection. *Ann Intern Med.* 1999;131:136–43.

4. **Murray P, Baron E, Pfaller M, et al.** *Manual of Clinical Microbiology, 6th Ed.* Washington, DC: ASM Press (American Society for Microbiology); 1995.

5. **Myers G, Korea B, Wain-Hobson S, et al.** *Human Retroviruses in AIDS.* Los Alamos, NM: Los Alamos National Laboratory; 1995.

6. **Weiss S, Lombard J, Michaels J, et al.** AIDS due to HIV-2 infection in New Jersey. *MMWR Morb Mortal Wkly Rep.* 1988;259:969–72.

7. **Alkhatib G, Broder C, Berger E.** Cell type-specific fusion cofactors determine human immunodeficiency virus type 1 tropism for T-cell lines vs. primary macrophages. *J Virol.* 1996;70:5487–94.

8. **Lieu R, Paxton W, Choe S, et al.** Homozygous defect in HIV-1 coreceptor accounts for resistance of some multiply-exposed individuals to HIV-1 infection. *Cell.* 1996;6: 367–77.

9. **Husman A, Koot, M, Cornelissen M, et al.** Association between CCR5 genotype and the clinical course of HIV-1 infection. *Ann Intern Med.* 1998;127:882–90.

10. **Spira A, Marx P, Patterson B, et al.** Cellular targets of infection and route of viral dissemination after an intravaginal inoculation of simian immunodeficiency virus into rhesus macaques. *J Exp Med.* 1996;183:215–25.

11. **Cohen O, Cicala C, Vaccarezza M, Fauci A.** The immunology of human immunodeficiency virus infection. In *Principles and Practice of Infectious Diseases, 5th Ed.* Philadelphia: Churchill Livingstone; 2000.

12. **Finzi D, Hermankova M, Pierson T, et al.** Identification of a reservoir for HIV-1 in patients on highly active antiretroviral therapy. *Science.* 1997;278:1295.

13. **Coffin J.** HIV population dynamics *in vivo*: implications for genetic variation, pathogenesis, and therapy. *Science.* 1995;267:483.

14. **Operskalski, E, Busch M, Mosley J, et al.** Comparative rates of disease progression among persons infected with the same or different HIV-1 strains. *J AIDS Hum Retrovirol.* 1997;15:145–50.

15. **Learmont J, Cook L, Dunckley H, et al.** Update on long-term symptomless HIV type 1 infection in recipients of blood products from a single donor. *AIDS Res Hum Retroviruses.* 1995;11:1.

16. **Enger C, Graham N, Peng Y, et al.** Survival from early, intermediate, and late stages of HIV infection. *JAMA.* 1996;275:1329–34.

17. **Mellors J, Rinaldo C, Gupta P, et al.** Prognosis in HIV-1 infection predicted by the quantity of virus in plasma. *Science.* 1995;272:1167–70.

18. **Mellors J, Munoz A, Giorgi J, et al.** Plasma viral load and CD4 lymphoctyes as prognostic markers of HIV-1 infection. *Ann Intern Med.* 1997;126:946–54.

19. **Pakker N, Notermans D, deBoer R, et al.** Biphasic kinetics of peripheral blood redistribution and proliferation. *Nat Med.* 1998;4:208.

20. **Schneider M, Borleffs J, Stol R, et al.** Discontinuation of prophylaxis for PCP in HIV-1 infected patients treated with highly active antiretroviral therapy. *Lancet.* 1999;53:201–3.

21. **Zhu T, Karber B, Nahmias A, et al.** An African HIV-1 sequence from 1959 and implications for the origin of the epidemic. *Nature.* 1998;391:594–7.

22. **Garry R, Witte M, Gottlieb A, et al.** Documentation of AIDS virus infection in the United States in 1968. *JAMA.* 1988;260:2085.

23. **Quinn T.** Global burden of the HIV pandemic. *Lancet.* 1996;348:99–106.

24. **Joint United Nations Program on HIV/AIDS.** *Report on the Global HIV/AIDS Epidemic.* Geneva, Switzerland: UNAIDS; June 2000.

25. **Centers for Disease Control and Prevention.** Increases in unsafe sex and rectal gonorrhea among men who have sex with men: San Francisco, CA 1996–97. *MMWR Morb Mortal Wkly Rep.* 1999;48:45–8.

26. **Centers for Disease Control and Prevention.** AIDS among racial/ethnic minorities: United States 1993. *MMWR Morb Mortal Wkly Rep.* 1994;43:644–55.

27. **Palella F, Moorman A, Delaney K et al.** *Dramatically Declining Morbidity and Mortality in an Ambulatory HIV Infected Population* [Abstract]. Presented at the Fifth Conference on Retroviruses and Opportunistic Infections. 1998, p 98.

28. **Decock K.** Sharp reductions reported in deaths from AIDS. *Retrovirus Update.* 1998; 3:2–3.

29. **Downs A, DeVincenzi I.** Probability of heterosexual transmission of HIV: relationship to the number of unprotected sexual contacts. *J Acquir Immune Defic Syndr Hum Retrovirol.* 11:388–95,1996.

30. **Rothenberg R, Scarlett M, del Rio C, et al.** Oral transmission of HIV. *AIDS.* 1998;12:2095–105.

31. **Cohen M.** Sexually transmitted diseases enhance HIV transmission: no longer an hypothesis. *Lancet.* 1998;358(Suppl 3):S5–S7.

32. **Cohen M, Hoffman I, Royce R, et al.** Reduction of concentration of HIV-1 in semen after treatment of urethritis: Implications for prevention of sexual transmission of HIV-1. *Lancet.* 1997;349:1868–73.

33. **Schechtal J.** Risky business. *AIDS Care.* 1997;1:25–38.

34. **Lawrence J.** Preventing AIDS by targeting other STDs. *AIDS Patient Care STD.* 1997; 11:217–22.

35. **Marx P, Spira A, Gettie A, et al.** *Nature Med.* 1996;2:1084–9.

36. **Holland P.** Viral infections and the blood supply. *N Engl J Med.* 1996;334:1734–5.

37. **Mofenson L, McIntyre J.** Advances and research directions in the prevention of mother to child HIV-1 transmission. *Lancet.* 2000;355:2237–44.

38. **Kaplan E, Hemier R.** Model-based estimate of HIV infectivity via needle sharing. *J AIDS.* 1992;5:1116–8.

39. **Centers for Disease Control and Prevention.** Case-control study of HIV seroconversion in heath care workers after percutaneous exposure to HIV infected blood-France, United Kingdom, and the United States. *MMWR Morb Mortal Wkly Rep.* 1995;44:929–33.

40. **Cardo D, Culver D, Ciesielski C, et al.** A case-control study of HIV seroconversion in health care workers after percutaneous exposure. *N Engl J Med.* 1997;337:1485–90.

41. **The European Mode of Delivery Collabortion.** Elective cesarean-section versus vaginal delivery in prevention of vertical HIV-1 transmission: a randomized clinical trial. *Lancet.* 1999;353:1035–39.

42. **Ndauti R.** *The Nairobi Breastfeeding Study* [Abstract]. Presented at The Second Conference on Global Stategies for the Reduction of Mother-to-Child Transmission of HIV. Montreal, Canada; September 1999;47.

43. **Centers for Disease Control and Prevention.** 1993 revised classification system for HIV infection and expanded surveillance case definition for AIDS under adolescents and adults. *MMWR Morb Mortal Wkly Rep.* 1992;41:1–19.

44. **Wolinsky S, Rinaldo C, Kwok S, et al.** Human immunodeficiency virus type 1 infection a median of 18 months before a diagnostic Western Blot: evidence from a cohort of homosexual men. *Ann Intern Med.* 1989;111:961–72.

45. **Tindall B, Barker B, Donovan B, et al.** Characterization of the acute clinical illness associated with HIV infecton. *Arch Intern Med.* 1988;148:945–9.

46. **Kinloch-de Loes S, de Saussure P, Saurat J, et al.** Symptomatic primary infection due to HIV-1: review of 31 cases. *Clin Infect Dis.* 1993;17:59–65.

47. **Schacker T, Collier A, Hughes J, et al.** Clinical and epidemiologic features of primary HIV infection. *Ann Intern Med.* 1996;125:257–34.

48. **Niu M, Stein D, Schmittman S.** Primary HIV-1 infection: Review of pathogenesis and early treatment intervention in human and animal retrovirus infections *J Infect Dis.* 1993;168:1490–501.

49. **Kaslow R, Phair J, Friedman H, et al.** Infection with the human immunodeficiency virus: clinical manifestations and their relationship to immune deficiency. *Ann Intern Med.* 1987;104:474–80.

50. **Bylund D, Ziegner U, Hooper D.** Review of testing for HIV. *Clin Lab Med.* 1992; 12:305–33.

51. **Bartlett J, Gallant J, Laboratory Tests.** In *Medical Management of HIV Infection.* Baltimore, MD: Port City Press; 2000.

51a. **Centers for Disease Control and Prevention.** Interpretation and use of the Western Blot assay for serodiagnosis of HIV-1 infections. *MMWR Mortal Wkly Rep.* 1989;38:1–7.

52. **Sherman M, Dock N, Ehrlich G, et al.** Evaluation of HIV type 1 Western blot-indeterminate blood donors for the presence of human or bovine retroviruses. *AIDS Res Hum Retroviruses.* 1995;11:409–14.

53. **Miller V, Mocroft A, Reiss P, et al.** Relations among CD4 lymphocyte count nadir, antiretroviral therapy and HIV-1 disease progression: results from the EuroSIDA Study. *Ann Intern Med.* 1999;130:569–77.

54. **Panel on Clinical Practices for Treatment of HIV Infection.** *Guidelines for the Use of Antiretroviral Agents in HIV Infected Adults and Adolescents.* Washington, DC: U.S. Department of Health and Human Services; February 2001.

55. **Ward D, Sklar P.** *The Significance of Low-Level Viremia in Patients with Previously "Undetectable" HIV-1 RNA levels.* [Abstract]. Presented at the XIII International Aids Conference. Durban, South Africa; July 2000:1450.

56. **Durant J, Clevenbergh P, Halfon P, et al.** Drug-resistance genotyping in HIV-1 therapy: the VIRADAPT randomised controlled trial. *Lancet.* 1999;353:2195–9.

57. **Baxter J, Mayers D, Wentworth D, et al.** and the CPCRA 046 Study Team. *A Pilot Study of the Short-Term Effects of Antiretroviral Management Based on Plasma Genotypic Antiretroviral Resistance Testing (GART) in Patients Failing Antiretroviral Therapy* [Abstract]. Presented at The Sixth Conference on Retroviruses and Opportunistic Infections. Chicago; 1999:LB8.

57a. **Graham.** Buenos Aires International AIDS Conference. July 8–11, 2001 [Abstract 125].

58. **Bartlett J, Demasi R, Quinn J, et al.** *Meta-analysis of Efficacy of Triple Combination Therapy in Antiretroviral-Naive HIV-1-Infected Adult* [Abstract]. Presented at The Seventh Conference on Retroviruses and Opportunistic Infections. San Francisco; January 2000.

59. **Bartlett J, Gallant J.** *Medical Management of HIV Infection: Antiretroviral Therapy.* Baltimore: Port City Press; 2000:52–5.

60. **Centers for Disease Control and Prevention.** Report of the NIH panel to define principles of therapy of HIV infection and guidelines for use of antiretroviral agents in HIV-infected adults and adolescents. *MMWR Morb Mortal Wkly Rep.* 1998;47:1–41.

61. **Brinkman K, Smeitink J, Romijn J, et al.** Mitochondrial toxicity induced by nucleoside-analogue reverse transcriptase inhibitors is a key cofactor in the pathogenesis of antiretroviral-therapy-related lipodystropy. *Lancet.* 1999;354:1112–5.

62. **Center for Disease Control.** Update–Trends in AIDS incidence: United States 1996. *MMWR Morb Mortal Wkly Rep.* 1996;46:861–67.

63. **Safrin S, Gunfeld C.** Fat distribution and metabolic changes in patients with HIV infection. *AIDS.* 1999;13:2493–505.

64. **Staszeski S, Morales-Ramierez J, Godofsky E, et al.** *Longer Time to Treatment Failure and Durability of Response with Efavirenz +Zdv +3TC: First Analysis of Full 1266 Patient Cohort from Study 006.* Presented at the 39th ICAAC. 1999.

65. **Powderly W, Saag M, Chapman S, et al.** Predictors of optimal virological response to potent antiretroviral therapy. *AIDS.* 1999;13;1873–80.

66. **Swiss Cohort study.** *Lancet.* 1999;353:863.

66a. **Fanci A.** Buenos Aires International AIDS Conference. July 8–11, 2001. [Abstract PL4].

67. **Van Howe R.** Circumcision and IV infection: review of the literature and meta-analysis. *Int J STD AIDS.* 1999;10:8–16.

68. **Katz M, Gerberding J.** Postexposure treatment of people exposed to the human immunodeficiency virus through sexual contact or injection drug use. *N Engl J Med.* 1997;336:1097–1100.

69. **Myles J, Hirozawa A, Katz M, Bamberger J.** *Postexposure Prophylaxis (PEP) After Sexual Assault: San Francisco* [Abstract]. Presented at The XIII International AIDS Conference. Durban, South Africa; July 2000:1450.

70. **Sperling R, Shapiro D, Coombs R, et al.** Maternal viral load, zidovudine treatment, and the risk of transmission of HIV-1 from mother to infant: Pediatric AIDS Clinical Trials Group Protocol 076 Study Group. *N Engl J Med.* 1996;335:1621–9.

71. **The European Mode of Delivery Collaboration.** Elective cesarean-section versus vaginal delivery in prevention of vertical HIV-1 transmission: a randomized clinical trial. *Lancet.* 1999;353:1035–9.

72. **Centers for Disease Control and Prevention.** Case-control study of HIV seroconversion in health care workers after percutaneous exposure to HIV-infected blood–France, United Kingdom, and the United States: Jan 1988-Aug 1994. *MMWR Morb Mortal Wkly Rep.* 1995;44:929–33.

73. **Centers for Disease Control and Prevention.** Public Health Service guidelines for the management of health-care worker exposure to HIV and recommendations for post exposure prophylaxis. *MMWR Morb Mortal Wkly Rep.* 1998;47(RR-7):1–33.

74. **Jochemsen E.** Failure of zidovudine post-exposure prophylaxis. *Am J Med.* 1997; 102(Suppl 5B):52–55.

36

Opportunistic Infections in Patients with AIDS

Amy S. Indorf, MD

AIDS is the clinical syndrome that represents the late stage of infection with human immunodeficiency virus type 1 (HIV-1). Infection with HIV-1, over time, causes a progressive decline in the number of CD4 T lymphocytes and an accompanying, progressive deterioration of all aspects of cell-mediated immunity. This immunosuppression eventually leaves the host susceptible to serious opportunistic infections and neoplasms.

The initial AIDS surveillance case definition was based primarily on the presence of an opportunistic infection or neoplasm, in the absence of other evident immunosuppression, that was felt to be specifically related to and therefore diagnostic of AIDS. Modifications to the case definition were made in 1985 and 1987, and most recently in 1993 (1). These modifications reflected the advent of serologic testing for HIV-1 in 1985, the recognition of additional clinical entities that were associated with HIV-1 infection, and the evolution of clinical management of infected patients. Most notable in the 1993 AIDS surveillance case definition was the inclusion of HIV-infected people with CD4 T-lymphocyte counts below 200 cells/mm^3, pulmonary tuberculosis, recurrent pneumonia, and invasive cervical cancer. AIDS-defining diagnoses are listed in Table 36.1 (1).

A comprehensive review of all AIDS-associated opportunistic infections is beyond the scope of this chapter. Rather, this chapter provides an overview of some of the most common and significant AIDS-associated opportunistic infections. The chapter will address the clinical manifestations and diagnosis, treatment, and prevention issues for each of these infections.

Table 36.1   Conditions Included in the 1993 AIDS Surveillance Case Definition

Bacterial infections, multiple or recurrent*
Candidiasis of bronchi, trachea, or lungs
Candidiasis, esophageal
Cervical cancer, invasive†
Coccidioidomycosis, disseminated or extrapulmonary
Cryptococcosis, extrapulmonary
Cryptosporidiosis, chronic intestinal (>1-month duration)
Cytomegalovirus disease (other than liver, spleen, or nodes)
Cytomegalovirus retinitis (with loss of vision)
Encephalopathy, HIV-related
Herpes simplex, chronic ulcer (>1-month duration), bronchitis, pneumonitis, or esophagitis
Histoplasmosis, disseminated or extrapulmonary
Isosporiasis, chronic intestinal (>1-month duration)
Kaposi's sarcoma
Lymphoid interstitial pneumonia and/or pulmonary lymphoid hyperplasia*
Lymphoma, Burkitt's (or equivalent term)
Lymphoma, immunoblastic (or equivalent term)
Lymphoma, primary, of brain
Mycobacterium avium-intracellulare or *M. kansasii*, disseminated or extrapulmonary
M. tuberculosis, any site (pulmonary† or extrapulmonary)
Mycobacterium or other species (or unidentified species), disseminated or extrapulmonary
Pneumocystis carinii pneumonia
Pneumonia, recurrent†
Progressive multifocal leukoencephalopathy
Salmonella septicemia, recurrent
Toxoplasmosis of brain
Wasting syndrome caused by HIV infection

* Children under 13 years of age.
† Added in the 1993 expansion of the AIDS surveillance case definition for adolescents and adults.

Pneumocystis carinii Pneumonia

Before the early 1980s, *Pneumocystis carinii* pneumonia (PCP) was seen only sporadically in immunocompromised patients. It then became a common clinical problem with the advent of the AIDS epidemic, occurring early in the epidemic in up to 75% of patients at some point in their illness. *Pneumocystis* infection occurs most commonly in patients with a CD4 count of fewer than 200 cells/mm^3; the use of prophylactic regimens in this population has significantly decreased the incidence of this opportunistic infection. PCP was the AIDS-defining diagnosis in 47% of patients in 1988, falling to 25% in 1991 after the introduction of PCP prophylaxis in the at-risk patient population (2).

Organism and Etiology

P. carinii has been varyingly categorized by taxonomists since its initial discovery in 1909. It was long considered a protozoan because of its morphologic features and response to some antiprotozoal drugs. More recently, it has been classified as a fungus based on biochemical and molecular biological assays that have shown homology with fungal organisms. However, the organism does not grow on fungal culture media and does not respond to antifungal therapy; therefore, some controversy still exists about its correct taxonomy.

The environmental source or natural reservoir of *P. carinii* is unclear. Animal studies have shown that the organism can be transmitted by airborne routes. It is generally believed that humans are exposed to *P. carinii* early in life and that the organism exists as a commensal within the respiratory tract until immunosuppression allows it to reactivate and cause overt infection. Deficiency of cell-mediated immunity is the most significant predisposing factor for *P. carinii* infection.

Clinical Manifestations

A patient with PCP most commonly presents with symptoms of fever, cough (often without significant sputum production), dyspnea, and chest pain. The clinical course is often subacute, with symptoms gradually worsening for several weeks before diagnosis, but can be fulminant. Auscultation of the lungs may reveal rales, rhonchi, or wheezes, but is often normal. Pneumothorax occurs in a small percentage of patients. PCP is the most common opportunistic infection of AIDS associated with pneumothorax, and the presence of pneumothorax should indicate a presumptive diagnosis of PCP unless proven otherwise (3). Extrapulmonary sites of infection can also occur; the most common are lymph nodes, bone marrow, spleen, and liver.

Diagnosis

The most common radiologic appearance of PCP is of diffuse bilateral interstitial infiltrates. Other findings may include focal infiltrates, nodular infiltrates, cavitation, pneumothorax, blebs, bullae, and cyst formation. The chest radiograph may be normal. Hilar adenopathy and pleural effusions are uncommon.

Laboratory evaluation of a patient with suspected PCP includes previous and current CD4 cell counts. PCP is unlikely to occur in a patient with a CD4 count above 200 cells/mm^3. Arterial blood gas measurement may reveal hypoxemia or an increased alveolar-arterial (A-a) oxygen gradient. The serum lactate dehydrogenase level is increased in as many as 90% of patients with PCP, but is relatively nonspecific, since it can also be increased as a result of other pulmonary processes or lymphoma (4). Because of this high sensitivity and often low specificity, a normal serum lactate dehydrogenase level makes PCP unlikely.

Establishing a diagnosis of PCP primarily involves the identification of characteristic cyst forms in respiratory specimens stained with Gomori's methenamine silver stain, toluidine blue, or periodic acid-Schiff stain. Expectorated sputum alone is often an unsatisfactory specimen; induced sputum specimens may have sensitivities of 55% to 95% (5). Bronchoscopy with bronchoalveolar lavage is often the preferred method for obtaining deep respiratory specimens and optimizing the diagnostic yield for this infection.

Treatment

Treatment options for PCP are outlined in Table 36.2 (5–8). Adjunctive corticosteroid therapy is recommended for patients with moderate to severe PCP (PO2 <70 mm Hg or A-a gradient >35 mm Hg). This should preferably be started at the initiation of anti-PCP therapy or within the first 72 hours of treatment. This strategy has been shown to improve survival and decrease the occurrence of respiratory failure in the patient population with PCP (9,10). The recommended regimen is prednisone (or an intravenous equivalent) at 40 mg twice daily for 5 days, followed by 40 mg daily for 5 days and then by 20 mg daily for 11 days or until PCP therapy is completed (7,10).

Prevention

Prophylaxis for PCP in HIV-infected individuals is indicated for the following: 1) CD4 count below 200 cells/mm^3; 2) oropharyngeal candidiasis, 3) unexplained fever for more than 2 weeks, and 4) a prior episode of PCP. Options for preventing PCP are outlined in Table 36.3 (11,12).

Cerebral Toxoplasmosis

Cerebral toxoplasmosis is the most common mass lesion of the central nervous system (CNS) in patients with AIDS. It occurs in up to 40% of patients with advanced immunosuppression (most commonly with a CD4 count <100 cells/mm^3) and latent *Toxoplasma gondii* infection (13).

Organism and Etiology

T. gondii is a protozoan most commonly acquired in adults by exposure to oocysts in cat feces or ingestion of tissue cysts in undercooked meat. The sero-

Table 36.2 Drug Therapies for *Pneumocystis carinii* Pneumonia

Drug	Dosage	Route	Adverse Effects
Mild to Moderate Disease*			
First-line therapy			
TMP-SMX	TMP 15–20 mg/kg/d in 3–4 divided doses for 21 days	Oral	Rash, fever, bone marrow suppression, hepatotoxicity
Alternative therapies			
TMP + dapsone	TMP 15–20 mg/kg/d in 3–4 divided doses	Oral	TMP: rash
	Dapsone 100 mg/d for 21 days		Dapsone: hemolysis (especially in G6PD deficiency), methemoglobinemia
Clindamycin + primaquine	Clindamycin 300-450 mg q6–8h	Oral	Clindamycin: diarrhea, *Clostridium difficile* colitis
	Primaquine base 15 mg/d for 21 days		Primaquine: hemolysis (G6PD deficiency), methemoglobinemia
Atovaquone	750 mg bid for 21 days	Oral, suspension	Rash, fever, GI disturbance, hepatotoxicity
Moderate to Severe Disease†			
First-line therapy			
TMP-SMX	TMP 15–20 mg/kg/d in 3–4 divided doses for 21 days	IV	Rash, fever, bone marrow suppression, hepatotoxicity
Alternative therapies			
Pentamidine	4 mg/kg/d for 21 days	IV	Hypotension, hypoglycemia, hyperglycemia, pancreatitis, neutropenia, nephrotoxicity, cardiac arrhythmias
Clindamycin + primaquine	Clindamycin 600–900 mg q8h	IV, oral	Clindamycin: diarrhea, *Clostridium difficile* colitis
	Primaquine base 15–30 mg/d for 21 days		Primaquine: hemolysis (G6PD deficiency), methemoglobinemia
Trimetrexate	45 mg/m^2 (with leucovorin 20 mg/m^2 qid) for 21 days	IV	Bone marrow suppression

GI = gastrointestinal; G6PD = glucose-6-phosphate-dehydrogenase; IV = intravenous; pO$_2$ = partial pressure of oxygen; TMP-SMX = trimethoprim–sulfamethoxazole.

* Defined as not acutely ill, able to take oral medications, room air pO$_2$ >70 mm Hg.

† Defined as acutely ill and room air pO$_2$ <70 mm Hg.

Table 36.3   Prophylaxis for *Pneumocystis carinii* Pneumonia

Drug	Dosage	Route
First-line prophylaxis		
TMP-SMX	I DS daily	Oral
	I SS daily	Oral
Alternative prophylaxis		
TMP-SMX	I DS three times weekly	Oral
Dapsone	50 mg twice daily	Oral
	100 mg daily	Oral
Dapsone +	Dapsone 50 mg daily	Oral
Pyrimethamine +	Pyrimethamine 50 mg weekly	
Leucovorin	Leucovorin 25 mg weekly	
	or	
	Dapsone 200 mg weekly	Oral
	Pyrimethamine 75 mg weekly	
	Leucovorin 25 mg weekly	
Aerosolized pentamidine	300 mg monthly	Respirgard II nebulizer
Atovaquone	1500 mg daily	Oral

DS = double strength; SS = single strength.

prevalence of *T. gondii* infection varies widely geographically, in some countries being as high as 90%; in the United States it ranges from approximately 10% to 40% (14). Once acquired, the organism establishes latent infection in body tissues and can reactivate when immunosuppression occurs. The high incidence of multicentric lesions and the occurrence of choroid plexus infections suggest hematogenous dissemination from reactivated infection in systemic organs, rather than reactivation of latent infection within the CNS (14).

Clinical Manifestations

A patient with AIDS-associated cerebral toxoplasmosis may manifest generalized or focal CNS abnormalities. In one large series the most common symptoms were headache (55%), confusion (52%), fever (47%), lethargy (43%), and seizures (29%) (15). Focal neurological signs were present in 69% of patients; the most common were hemiparesis, ataxia, and cranial nerve palsies (15).

Diagnosis

Cranial computed tomography (CT) in cerebral toxoplasmosis typically reveals single or multiple enhancing lesions, usually with a ring-enhancing morphology. Gadolinium-67-enhanced magnetic resonance imaging (MRI) is often more sensitive than CT for cerebral toxoplasmosis, revealing lesions not evident on an initial CT scan (14,15). Because of the greater sensitivity of

MRI, it is generally advisable to either do MRI initially if toxoplasmosis is suspected, or to do MRI in addition to CT if no lesions or only one lesion is seen on CT. The presence of multiple lesions is often more suggestive of cerebral toxoplasmosis, occurring in 73% of patients in one large series (15). This is in comparison with CNS lymphoma, which is often the other major diagnostic consideration for CNS mass lesions in HIV-infected patients.

Serum anti-*Toxoplasma* antibody, specifically IgG, is often present in cases of cerebral toxoplasmosis, and adds assurance to a presumptive diagnosis. However, anti-*Toxoplasma* antibodies may be absent in approximately 15% to 20% of patients, and the absence of detectable antibody does not exclude the diagnosis (15). Biopsy of CNS lesions is sometimes necessary to establish a diagnosis. Polymerase chain reaction testing of CSF may be a clinically applicable diagnostic tool in the future. In general, however, CSF studies are not helpful in cerebral toxoplasmosis, and lumbar puncture is often contraindicated in the presence of mass lesions or associated cerebral edema.

Treatment

Empiric therapy for cerebral toxoplasmosis is generally acceptable in a patient with a compatible CT or MRI scan and positive *Toxoplasma* serology. Biopsy should be considered if clinical improvement has not occurred within 1 to 2 weeks after empiric therapy is begun. Treatment options for cerebral toxoplasmosis are outlined in Table 36.4 (15–19).

Prevention

Options for preventing *Toxoplasma* infection are outlined in Table 36.5 (11). Patients who are HIV-infected and have a negative serologic result for anti-*Toxoplasma* IgG antibody should be counseled about avoiding potential exposures to *Toxoplasma* (11).

Cryptococcal Meningitis

Cryptococcal meningitis is one of the most significant opportunistic fungal infections in patients with AIDS. It occurs in approximately 5% to 10% of patients with advanced immunosuppression (most commonly a CD4 count <100 cells/mm^3) (20).

Organism and Etiology

Cryptococcus neoformans is an encapsulated yeast, 4 to 6 μm in diameter, that is ubiquitous in its geographic distribution. The most common source of infec-

Table 36.4   Drug Therapies for Cerebral Toxoplasmosis

First-Line Therapy
Pyrimethamine 100–200 mg PO (loading dose) then 50–100 mg/d PO
  plus Leucovorin 10 mg/d PO
  plus Sulfadiazine 1–2 g PO every 6 hours

Alternative Therapies
Pyrimethamine 100–200 mg PO (loading dose) then 50–100 mg/d PO
  plus Leucovorin 10 mg/d PO
  plus one of the following:
    Clindamycin 600–1200 mg IV every 6 hours or 300–450 mg PO every 6 hours
    Azithromycin 1200–1500 mg/d PO
    Clarithromycin 1 g PO twice daily
    Atovaquone 750 mg every 6 hours

Comments
Treatment duration is usually 4–6 weeks, followed by maintenance therapy to prevent
  relapse (see recommendations for secondary prophylaxis)
Corticosteroids are usually used adjunctively if significant edema or mass effect is present

IV = intravenously; PO = orally.

tion is soil contaminated with bird droppings, particularly those of pigeons, but also of other avian species as well. Infection is thought to occur via inhalation of organisms, with the small size of these organisms allowing their passage to the alveolar spaces. A compromised cell-mediated immune system allows dissemination of the organisms, with a predilection for infection of the meninges and CNS.

Clinical Manifestations

The clinical presentation of cryptococcal meningitis in AIDS patients is often indolent and subacute, with symptoms escalating over a period of several weeks. The most common symptoms are fever and headache, occurring in at least 60% of patients. Less common symptoms include photophobia, neck stiffness, altered mental status, focal neurological deficits, and seizures (20). Other sites involved in a disseminated infection may include the lung, skin, and eye. Asymptomatic infection of the prostate may act as a reservoir for relapses of disseminated infection.

Diagnosis

CT or MRI is often done initially in suspected cryptococcal meningitis to exclude other HIV-related infections or neoplasms. CNS cryptococcomas are

Table 36.5   Prophylaxis for *Toxoplasma* Infection

	Indication	First-Line Therapy	Alternative Therapies
Primary prophylaxis	IgG antibody to *Toxoplasma* species and CD4 count <100 cells/mm³	TMP-SMX 1 DS daily PO	TMP-SMX 1 SS daily PO Dapsone 50 mg/d PO + pyrimethamine 50 mg/wk PO + leucovorin 25 mg/wk PO
Secondary prophylaxis	Maintenance after therapy for acute disease	Pyrimethamine 25–75 mg/d PO + leucovorin 10–25 mg/d PO + sulfadiazine 500–1000 mg PO four times daily	Pyrimethamine 25–75 mg/d PO + leucovorin 10–25 mg/d PO + clindamycin 300–450 mg PO every 6–8 hours

DS = double strength; IgG = immunoglobulin G; PO = orally; SS = single strength; TMP-SMX = trimethoprim–sulfamethoxazole.

uncommon; they are usually seen as ring-enhancing lesions. Lumbar puncture, if not contraindicated, is the most direct diagnostic method. CSF indices may be normal or only mildly abnormal in the face of advanced immunosuppression. Abnormal indices may include an increased opening pressure, decreased glucose, increased protein, and lymphocytic pleocytosis. An India ink preparation may reveal the presence of encapsulated yeast organisms; the sensitivity of this test in the setting of HIV infection is 60% to 80% (20,21). Cryptococcal antigen detection by latex agglutination methodology applied to CSF is nearly 100% sensitive and specific for *C. Neoformans*, with the sensitivity of concomitant serum testing being at least 95% (21). Definitive diagnosis of cryptococcal meningitis, however, requires culture of the organism from CSF.

Treatment

Some controversy still exists about the best initial management of cryptococcal meningitis, the role of flucytosine and azole drugs in its initial treatment, and the duration of initial treatment. General treatment guidelines are outlined in Table 36.6 (22). Initial therapy with oral drugs should be reserved for patients with favorable prognostic factors, such as normal mental status, a CSF antigen titer below 1:1024, and a CSF white blood cell count above 20 cells/mm³. Increased intracranial pressure is associated with poor outcome, and requires specific management as well (23). Consultation with an infectious disease specialist experienced in the management of cryptococcal meningitis should be considered.

Table 36.6   Preferred Treatment Options for Central Nervous System Cryptococcal Infection

Induction and Consolidation

Amphotericin B 0.7–1.0 mg/kg/d + flucytosine* 100 mg/kg/d for 2 weeks, then fluconazole 400 mg/d for a minimum of 10 weeks

Amphotericin B 0.7–1.0 mg/kg/d + flucytosine* 100 mg/kg/d for 6–10 weeks

Amphotericin B 0.7–1.0 mg/kg/d for 6–10 weeks

Fluconazole 400–800 mg/d for 10–12 weeks

Itraconazole 400 mg/d for 10–12 weeks[†]

Fluconazole 400–800 mg/d + flucytosine* 100–150 mg/kg/d for 6 weeks

Lipid formulation of amphotericin B[†] (e.g., AmBisome 45 mg/kg, 3–6 mg/kg/d for 6–10 weeks)

Maintenance[‡]

Fluconazole 200–400 mg PO qd for life

Itraconazole 200 mg PO bid for life

Amphotericin B 1 mg/kg IV 1–3 times weekly for life

---

* For patients who have undergone prolonged (>2 weeks) administration of flucytosine, renal function should be monitored frequently and dose adjustments should be made via the use of a nomogram or, preferably, by monitoring serum flucytosine levels. Serum flucytosine levels should be measured 2 hours after each dose, with optimal levels between 30 and 80 μg/mL

[†] Not approved by the FDA.

[‡] Whether secondary prophylaxis may be discontinued in patients with prolonged success with highly active retroviral therapy is unclear.

Modified from Saag MS, Graybill RJ, Larsen RA, et al. Practice guidelines for the management of cryptococcal disease. *Clin Infect Dis.* 2000;30:710–18.

Prevention

Options for preventing cryptococcal infection are outlined in Table 36.7 (11,22). Although exposure cannot be completely avoided, patients who are HIV-infected should be counseled to avoid sites that are likely to be heavily contaminated with *Cryptococcus* (e.g., areas with pigeon or other bird droppings).

Cytomegalovirus

Cytomegalovirus (CMV) is one of the most common viral opportunistic pathogens in patients with AIDS. Its most serious clinical manifestations usually occur in patients with advanced immunosuppression (i.e., CD4 count <50 cells/mm³).

Organism and Etiology

Primary CMV infection occurs in most individuals by the end of childhood, through various routes; these include maternal or perinatal transmission

Table 36.7   Prophylaxis for Cryptococcal Meningitis

	Indication	First-Line Therapy	Alternative Therapies
Primary prophylaxis*	CD4 count <50 cells/mm³	Fluconazole 100–200 mg/d PO	Itraconazole 200 mg/d PO
Secondary prophylaxis	Maintenance after therapy for acute disease	Fluconazole 200 mg/d PO	Amphotericin B 0.6–1.0 mg/kg IV 1–3 times weekly Itraconazole 200 mg/d PO

* Not recommended for most patients; indicated for use only in selected circumstances.

and exposure to respiratory or urinary sources in the home or in day care settings. Later, most additional seroconversion results from sexual transmission of CMV in people who were not infected in childhood. As with other herpesviruses, CMV establishes latency, and it is mainly through reactivation of latent infection (or less often through superinfection with new CMV strains) that viremia and subsequent end-organ CMV disease occurs in AIDS patients.

Clinical Manifestations

The most common clinical manifestation (approximately 80%) of CMV in AIDS is retinitis. Virtually all cases occur in patients with CD4 counts fewer than 50 cells/mm³. The initial presentation of retinitis is often subtle, with painless unilateral scotomata, blurred vision, or a decrease in visual acuity. Screening in patients at high risk for infection can be achieved with Amsler grid testing or routine ophthalmologic examination. Fundoscopic examination reveals characteristic white necrotic patches with associated hemorrhage. If untreated, visual impairment can progress to blindness in several months, and the contralateral eye almost inevitably becomes infected.

Cytomegalovirus may cause gastrointestinal disease as well as disease in other organs. The most common gastrointestinal manifestations are esophageal ulceration (symptoms of dysphagia and odynophagia) and colitis (symptoms of abdominal pain and watery, often bloody diarrhea). Other gastrointestinal manifestations may include hepatitis, cholangitis, pancreatitis, and erosive gastritis.

Additional clinical manifestations of CMV infection may include neurological disease, in the form of encephalitis, polyradiculopathy, or multifocal neuropathy. CMV may also be detected in bronchoscopy specimens from

HIV-infected patients, but is thought to uncommonly be a primary pulmonary pathogen; it more often may be a co-infecting organism with pathogens such as *P. carinii* (24).

Diagnosis

Serology may help to establish CMV as a possible etiologic agent of disease in the appropriate clinical setting. A positive IgG antibody test indicates prior exposure to the virus and therefore latent infection. A positive IgM antibody test may be a manifestation of reactivation of a latent infection or may indicate an acute infection (which is usually less likely in the HIV-infected patient population) (24). Negative serologic findings make a diagnosis of CMV disease unlikely. Isolation of CMV from urine through intermittent shedding of the organism is common in the HIV-infected population, and is often not helpful diagnostically. Detection of CMV in peripheral blood cells by standard viral culture, the shell vial culture technique, or nucleic acid assays such as polymerase chain reaction testing may be more predictive of disseminated infection or end-organ involvement.

Specific organ involvement by CMV requires directed diagnostic efforts. As mentioned earlier, the diagnosis of retinitis is made fundoscopically by an experienced examiner who can detect the characteristic ophthalmologic findings. Diagnosis of alimentary tract lesions is best made by biopsy of involved areas, with histopathologic findings consistent with CMV disease. The diagnosis of neurological disease is often more difficult. CNS disease may be diagnosed by culture of CSF (generally of low yield) or detection of CMV in CSF through polymerase chain reaction testing.

Treatment

Treatment recommendations for CMV infection are outlined primarily for CMV retinitis, since this is the most common clinical manifestation of infection. There are included in Table 36.8 (25,26). Consultation with an infectious disease specialist should be considered, particularly for the best treatment option in a given clinical situation and for adverse effect monitoring and management. Patients with retinitis also require close ophthalmologic follow-up to detect a treatment response or disease progression.

Prevention

Prophylaxis for CMV is not recommended for most patients. It is generally indicated only in selected circumstances for patients with a CD4 cell count of

Table 36.8 Treatment Options for Cytomegalovirus Retinitis

Treatment	Dosage	Adverse Effects	Advantages	Disadvantages	Median Time to Retinitis Progression
IV ganciclovir	Induction: 5 mg/kg q12h for 14–21 days Maintenance: 5 mg/kg/d*	Neutropenia, thrombocytopenia	Systemic therapy, anti-HSV activity	Hematologic toxicity; requires daily infusions, indwelling catheter	47–104 days
IV foscarnet	Induction: 90 mg/kg q12h for 14–21 days Maintenance: 90–120 mg/kg/d (500–1000 mL 0.9% saline with each dose)*	Nephrotoxicity, electrolyte abnormalities, anemia, nausea, genital ulceration	Systemic therapy, anti-HSV activity (including acyclovir-resistant strains), anti-HIV activity	Nephrotoxicity; requires daily infusions, indwelling catheter; supplemental hydration, a prolonged infusion time, and infusion-pump/controlled-rate device	53–93 days
IV ganciclovir + IV foscarnet	**For prior ganciclovir:** Induction: ganciclovir 5 mg/kg/d for 14–21 days + foscarnet 90 mg/kg q12h for 14–21 days Maintenance: ganciclovir 5 mg/kg/d + foscarnet 90–120 mg/kg/d **For prior foscarnet:** Induction: ganciclovir 5 mg/kg q12h for 14–21 days + foscarnet 90–120 mg/kg/d for 14–21 days Maintenance: ganciclovir 5 mg/kg/d + foscarnet 90–120 mg/kg/d	Same as ganciclovir and foscarnet	Same as ganciclovir and foscarnet	Same as ganciclovir and foscarnet	129 days
IV ganciclovir + oral ganciclovir	Induction: 5 mg/kg q12h for 14–21 days Maintenance: 3000–6000 mg/d in 3 divided doses with food	Neutropenia, nausea, diarrhea	Systemic therapy, oral administration	Faster time to retinitis progression, poor oral bioavailability (6%)	29–53 days
Intraocular ganciclovir implant	Surgical implantation: 4.5 mg implant releasing 1 μg/h Duration: 6–8 months; replace every 5–8 months Recommended concomitant systemic therapy: ganciclovir 4500 mg/d PO in 3 divided doses	Surgical complications (e.g., transient blurred vision, infection, hemorrhage)	Longest time to retinitis progression in treated eye; no IV dosing or catheter required	Increased risk of disease in other eye and of extraocular disease	216–226 days
IV cidofovir	Induction: 5 mg/kg for 2 weeks Maintenance: 5 mg/kg every 2 weeks*†	Nephrotoxicity, neutropenia, uveitis, alopecia, hypotonia Probenecid's adverse effects: rash, fever, nausea, fatigue	Systemic therapy; no indwelling catheter required; infrequent dosing	Requires probenecid and IV hydration; probenecid toxicity, nephrotoxicity (may be prolonged)	64–120 days

HSV = herpes simplex virus; IV = intravenous; PO = orally.
* May require dosage adjustment for renal insufficiency.
† All doses given with probenecid and IV fluids.

fewer than 50 cells/mm^3 and positive serologic findings for CMV. The regimen for prophylaxis consists of oral ganciclovir at 1000 mg three times a day (11).

Mycobacterium avium Complex

Mycobacterium avium complex (MAC) infection, particularly when disseminated, is a common opportunistic bacterial infection in patients with AIDS. It may occur at a rate of approximately 20% per year in patients with advanced immunosuppression who do not receive prophylaxis; however, the overall incidence has declined since the advent of highly active antiretrovrial therapy (27,28). MAC infection is generally seen only in patients with advanced immunosuppression (i.e., CD4 counts <50 cells/mm^3 and often as low as <10 cells/mm^3).

Organism and Etiology

MAC consists of two closely related atypical mycobacterial species: *M. avium* and *M. intracellulare*. It was previously recognized primarily as a cause of pneumonia and chronic respiratory infection in patients with underlying lung disease. With the advent of the AIDS epidemic it was recognized as a cause of disseminated infection in these patients, with a high associated morbidity and mortality.

MAC is relatively ubiquitous in the environment, and can be found in diverse places, including water, soil, food, and animals. The environmental sources that present the greatest risk of infection is unclear, however, and it is difficult to avoid exposures to the organism. Most clinical infection with MAC is thought to occur after primary infection rather than after reactivation, as is more common with *M. tuberculosis* infection. MAC first colonizes the respiratory or gastrointestinal tract and then disseminates systemically in patients with severely compromised cell-mediated immunity.

Clinical Manifestations

Bacteremia with dissemination of MAC to areas including liver, spleen, bone marrow, and lymph nodes is the most common occurrence in MAC infection in AIDS patients. The most common signs and symptoms are fever, night sweats, diarrhea, abdominal pain, nausea and vomiting, weight loss, hepatosplenomegaly, and lymphadenopathy. Common laboratory abnormalities are anemia and increased alkaline phosphatase activity (28). Localized infections can also occur and may include pulmonary infection (though MAC isolation from sputum in the AIDS population is more commonly the result of colonization), CNS infections, skin and soft-tissue infections, and osteomyelitis.

Diagnosis

The most direct and definitive method of diagnosing MAC infection is mycobacterial blood culture. Bacteremia is often continuous in cases of MAC infection, and the yield of blood cultures is generally high; occasionally, however, transient bacteremia may occur, and negative blood cultures should be repeated if clinical suspicion remains high. Tissue from involved areas may also be sampled for diagnosis, with acid-fast staining and culture of these specimens. Characteristic granuloma formation may not be seen in tissues in the AIDS patient population with MAC infection. Positive cultures of sputum and stool usually represent colonization (but may support the suspicion of a disseminated MAC infection), and are not diagnostic in and of themselves.

Treatment

Although there is no definitive treatment regimen of choice for MAC infection, multiple studies have provided general treatment principles. An initial treatment regimen should include at least two drugs, one of these drugs being either clarithromycin at 500 mg twice daily or azithromycin 500 mg/d. The preferred second agent in most cases of MAC is ethambutol at 15 mg/kg/d. Other active agents that may be used in three- or four-drug regimens include rifabutin at 300 mg/d, ciprofloxacin at 750 mg twice a day, or amikacin given intravenously at 10–15 mg/kg/d (28,29). The efficacy of clofazimine has recently been called into question, and this drug should probably not be part of an initial treatment regimen. As with most other opportunistic infections in AIDS, lifelong maintenance therapy is required to prevent relapse of MAC infection.

Prevention

Prophylaxis is generally recommended for patients with MAC infection who have CD4 counts of fewer than 50 to 75 cells/mm^3. First-line regimens for prophylaxis are clarithromycin at 500 mg twice daily or azithromycin at 1200 mg weekly. An alternative regimen is rifabutin at 300 mg/d (11); care must be taken to ensure that coexistent *M. tuberculosis* infection is not present, since use of rifabutin alone in this circumstance may promote rifamycin-resistant tuberculosis.

REFERENCES

1. **Centers for Disease Control and Prevention.** 1993 Revised classification system for HIV infection and expanded surveillance case definition for AIDS among adolescents and adults. *MMWR Morb Mortal Wkly Rep.* 1992;41(RR-17):1–19.

2. **Hoover DR, Saah AJ, Bacellar H, et al.** Clinical manifestations of AIDS in the era of *Pneumocystis* prophylaxis. *N Engl J Med.* 1993;329:1922–26.

3. **Sepkowitz KA, Telzak EE, Gold JWM, et al.** Pneumothorax in AIDS. *Ann Intern Med.* 1991;114:455–59.

4. **Zaman MK, White DA.** Serum lactate dehydrogenase levels and *Pneumocystis carinii* pneumonia. *Am Rev Respir Dis.* 1988;137:796–800.

5. **Santamauro JT, Stover DE.** *Pneumocystis carinii* pneumonia. *Med Clin North Am.* 1997;81:299–318.

6. **Fishman JA.** Treatment of infection due to *Pneumocystis carinii*. *Antimicrob Agents Chemother.* 1998;42:1309–14.

7. **Bartlett JG, Gallant JE.** *Medical Management of HIV Infection.* Baltimore: Port City Press; 2000:99.

8. **Safrin S, Finkelstein DM, Feinberg J, et al.** Comparison of three regimens for treatment of mild to moderate *Pneumocystis carinii* penumonia in patients with AIDS. *Ann Intern Med.* 1996;124:792–802.

9. **Gagnon S, Boota AM, Fischl MA, et al.** Corticosteroids as adjunctive therapy for severe *Pneumocystis carinii* pneumonia in the acquired immunodeficiency syndrome. *N Engl J Med.* 1990;323:1444–50.

10. **Bozzette SA, Sattler FR, Chiu J, et al.** A controlled trial of early adjunctive treatment with corticosteroids for *Pneumocystis carinii* pneumonia in the acquired immunodeficiency syndrome. *N Engl J Med.* 1990;323:1451–57.

11. **USPHS/IDSA Prevention of Opportunistic Infections Working Group.** 1999 USPHS/IDSA guidelines for the prevention of opportunistic infections in persons infected with human immunodeficiency virus. *Clin Infect Dis.* 2000;30:S29–65.

12. **Fishman JA.** Prevention of infection due to *Pneumocystis carinii*. *Antimicrob Agents Chemother.* 1998;42:995–1004.

13. **Luft BJ, Remington JS.** Toxoplasmic encephalitis. *J Infect Dis.* 1988;157:1–6.

14. **Luft BJ, Remington JS.** Toxoplasmic encephalitis in AIDS. *Clin Infect Dis.* 1992; 15:211–22.

15. **Porter SB, Sande MA.** Toxoplasmosis of the central nervous system in the acquired immunodeficiency syndrome. *N Engl J Med.* 1992;327:1643–48.

16. **Dannemann B, McCutchan JA, Israelski D, et al.** Treatment of toxoplasmic encephalitis in patients with AIDS. *Ann Intern Med.* 1992;116:33–43.

17. **Bartlett JG, Gallant JE.** *Medical Management of HIV Infection.* Baltimore: Port City Press; 2000:108.

18. **Murray HW.** Toxoplasmosis. In Dolin R, Masur H, Saag MS, eds. *AIDS Therapy.* Philadelphia: Churchill Livingstone; 1999:315–19.

19. **Torres RA, Weinberg W, Stansell J, et al.** Atovaquone for salvage treatment and suppression of toxoplasmic encephalitis in patients with AIDS. *Clin Infect Dis.* 1997;24:422–29.

20. **Powderly WG.** Cryptococcal meningitis and AIDS. *Clin Infect Dis.* 1993;17:837–42.

21. **Powderly WG.** Cryptococcosis. In Dolin R, Masur H, Saag MS, eds. *AIDS Therapy.* Philadelphia: Churchill Livingstone; 1999:403.

22. **Saag MS, Graybill RJ, Larsen RA, et al.** Practice guidelines for the management of cryptococcal disease. *Clin Infect Dis.* 2000;30:710–18.

23. **Denning DW, Armstrong RW, Lewis BH, Stevens DA.** Elevated cerebrospinal fluid pressures in patients with cryptococcal meningitis and acquired immunodeficiency syndrome. *Am J Med.* 1991;91:267–72.

24. **Drew WL.** Cytomegalovirus infection in patients with AIDS. *Clin Infect Dis.* 1992; 14:608–15.

25. **Whitley RJ, Jacobson MA, Friedberg DN, et al.** Guidelines for the treatment of cytomegalovirus diseases in patients with AIDS in the era of potent antiretroviral therapy. *Arch Intern Med.* 1998;158:957–69.

26. **Jacobson MA.** Treatment of cytomegalovirus retinitis in patients with the acquired immunodeficiency syndrome. *N Engl J Med.* 1997;337:105–14.

27. **Horsburgh CR.** Epidemiology of *Mycobacterium avium* complex disease. *Am J Med.* 1997;102(5C):11–15.

28. **Benson CA.** *Mycobacterium avium* complex and other atypical mycobacterial infections. In Dolin R, Masur H, Saag MS, eds. *AIDS Therapy.* Philadelphia: Churchill Livingstone; 1999:375–85.

29. **Bartlett JG, Gallant JE.** *Medical Management of HIV Infection.* Baltimore: Port City Press; 2000:114–15.

37

Infections in the
Immunocompromised Host

Jason W. Chien, MD
Robert A. Salata, MD

Paradoxically, advances in medicine since the 1980s have contributed significantly to the frequency of infection in immunocompromised patients. Developments such as bone-marrow transplantation, new and more intensive chemotherapeutic and immunosuppressive agents, and an increased number of solid organ transplants have created more challenging and significant states of immunosuppression. Technological advances such as long-term indwelling catheters or ports, and more sophisticated methods of monitoring and ventilation, have also created a milieu in which infections are a major complication. Furthermore, many intravenous therapies are now being undertaken in the ambulatory setting. These developments have increased the number of immunosuppressed patients dramatically, and brought them to the outpatient arena. Consequently, primary-care physicians now more frequently see immunocompromised patients. Beyond this, the advent of HIV infection has brought about the emergence of new opportunistic infections as well as the resurgence of old diseases. Thus, it is essential to be able to recognize, diagnose, and treat infections occurring in the immunocompromised patient.

This chapter will first detail the nature of the immune defects in immunocompromised patients, an understanding of which can help prioritize infectious agents and syndromes in this patient population. Thereafter, the discussion will focus on selected types of immunocompromised patients frequently encountered in primary care practice, and will detail the epidemiology, etiology, and approaches to the diagnosis and management of associated infections in this group. A discussion of HIV-related infections is beyond the scope of this chapter; however, HIV-related infections are covered in Chapter 35, HIV Infection, and Chapter 36, Opportunistic Infections in Patients with AIDS.

Host-Defense Mechanisms

The type and extent of immunosuppression can often predict the spectrum of organisms that cause infections in immunocompromised patients. Hence, it is important to first become familiar with the types of immunodeficiencies and the defects they cause in host-defense mechanisms. These mechanisms include 1) mechanical defense barriers, 2) humoral immunity (HI), 3) cell-mediated immunity (CMI), and 4) cellular host defense. Once the type of an immunodeficiency is established, the most likely causes of infections can be established and the approach to diagnosis and management of these infections can then be more specifically directed.

Mechanical Defense Barriers

The skin and mucosal surfaces, in conjunction with many other nonspecific mechanisms of defense, such as ciliary activity, gastric acid, and intestinal motility, are considered the primary mechanical defense barriers (1). In a normal host, brief disruption of these mechanisms rarely results in infection. However, when the secondary mechanisms of defense, such as cell-mediated and humoral immunity, are impaired, even transient disruptions of mechanical barriers may result in morbidity and mortality. These disruptions can be secondary to invasive procedures such as surgery, trauma, burns, the use of long-term intravenous catheters, or local destruction of the mucosa by infections (e.g., influenza or oral herpes simplex) and cytotoxic chemotherapeutic agents (e.g., cytarabine, the anthracyclines, methotrexate, 6-mercaptopurine, and 5-fluorouracil). Since various bacteria such as coagulase-negative staphylococci and *Staphylococcus aureus* colonize the skin and mucosal surfaces, disruptions in these barriers can provide a port of entry for these colonizing organisms. Unfortunately, in patients who have had prolonged or multiple hospital stays, or who have been treated with broad-spectrum antibiotics (e.g., carbapenems, anti-pseudomonal beta-lactam drugs, new fluoroquinolones), the skin flora may be replaced by more resistant and less common organisms, thus subjecting these patients to infections that are more challenging to diagnose and more difficult to eradicate. In these situations, effective therapy often requires appropriate antibiotic drug use and resolution of the source of infection (1). The latter usually refers to a definitive surgical procedure, such as removal of a long-term catheter, repair/drainage of a site of infection, or removal/treatment of the cause of mucosal breakdown.

Cell-Mediated Immunity

Cell-mediated immunity involves a complex series of interactions between T lymphocytes and other effector cells (2). Through different mechanisms, antigen-specific T cells can either act directly on target cells or can secrete cytokines that recruit other, less specific cells such as macrophages and natural killer cells to act on the target cell. A defect in this system can result either from a primary (congenital immunodeficiency) or secondary process. Because CMI is responsible for the control of a number of types of infections, a deficiency in this type of immunity increases the risk of certain bacterial, fungal, viral, and parasitic infections (Table 37.1).

Primary disorders of CMI commonly involve both B- and T-cell abnormalities (3). This is often a result of congenital diseases such as severe combined immunodeficiency disease, Wiskott-Aldrich syndrome, ataxia-telangiectasia, and certain purine pathway enzyme deficiencies. As expected with congenital diseases, infections in cases of such primary disorders of CMI often appear early and are recurrent throughout the first few years of life. Since depression of humoral immunity is commonly also involved, these early infections are often caused by encapsulated organisms. However, because of their T-cell abnormalities, these hosts are at risk for opportunistic infections by organisms such as *Pneumocystis carinii* and *Candida* species, and for various human herpes virus infections.

Later in life, secondary processes, including malignant and nonmalignant hematologic diseases such as hairy-cell leukemia, Hodgkin's and non-Hodgkin's lymphoma, T-cell malignancies such as mycosis fungoides and lymphoma, and other advanced solid tumors, such as lymphoma, can result in defects of CMI. Often, treatment of these underlying diseases with chemotherapeutic agents or radiation worsens the immunologic defects, resulting in a more severe and generalized immunocompromised state.

A number of infectious diseases can compromise CMI. The infection that causes the most severe such compromise is HIV infection. A number of other infections have also been associated with varying degrees of CMI deficiency; these include measles, varicella, cytomegalovirus, Epstein-Barr virus, respiratory syncytial virus, hepatitis B, influenza, tuberculosis, histoplasmosis, coccidioidomycosis, typhoid fever, syphilis, and a number of parasitic infections (malaria, filariasis), as well as infections related to vaccines (mumps, measles, rubella) (1,3). Fortunately, the resultant defect in CMI is short lived because the majority of these infections are either self-limited or readily treatable. Non-

Table 37.1   Causes of Cell-Mediated Immunity and Related Infections

Causes	Bacterial infections	Fungal infections	Viral infections	Other infections
Congenital	*Mycobacterium*	*Histoplasma*	Cytomegalovirus	*Toxoplasma*
Severe combined	*tuberculosis*	*capsulatum*	Varicella–zoster	*gondii*
immunodeficiency	Nontuberculous	*Coccidioides*	virus	*Cryptosporidium*
Wiskott-Aldrich	mycobacteria	*immitis*	Herpes simplex	*parvum*
syndrome	*Listeria mono-*	*Cryptococcus*	virus	*Leishmania*
Ataxia-telangiectasia	*cytogenes*	*neoformans*	Human	*donovani*
Chronic mucocutaneous	*Nocardia* species	*Candida* species	herpesvirus-6	*Giardia lamblia*
candidiasis	*Legionella*	*Pneumocystis carinii*	Human	*Strongyloides*
DiGeorge syndrome	*pneumophilia*	*Aspergillus*	herpesvirus-8	*stercoralis*
X-linked agamma-	*Salmonella* species	*Zygomycetes*		
globulinemia	*Streptococcus pneu-*			
Nezelof's syndrome	*moniae*			
Malignancies				
Hairy-cell leukemia,				
Hodgkin's lymphoma				
Non-Hodgkin's				
lymphoma				
Mycosis fungoides				
T-cell lymphomas				
Other solid tumors				
Infections				
HIV				
Cytomegalovirus				
Epstein–Barr virus				
Respiratory syncytial				
virus				
Varicella–zoster virus				
Measles				
Syphilis				
Malaria				
Typhoid fever				
Filariasis				
Tuberculosis				
Histoplasmosis				
Leprosy				
Drugs				
Corticosteroids				
Methotrexate				
Cyclophosphamide				
6-Mercaptopurine				
Azathioprine				
Tacrolimus				
Miscellaneous				
Protein-calorie				
malnutrition				
Diabetes mellitus				
Sarcoidosis				
Renal and hepatic failure				
Cushing's disease				
Radiation therapy				

infectious causes of deficiency in CMI are more common and generally not as severe. These include chronic protein-calorie malnutrition, diabetes mellitus, sarcoidosis, and renal failure.

Corticosteroids are the most notable pharmacologic agents associated with abnormalities of CMI (1). Corticosteroid therapy is commonly used to treat various disorders and conditions, such as chronic obstructive pulmonary disease, refractory asthma, autoimmune diseases, inflammatory bowel disease, malignancies, organ transplants, dermatologic conditions, and adrenal insufficiency. Therefore, the potential for immune deficiency among an average patient population is actually larger than expected, and this should be contemplated whenever the use of prolonged corticosteroid therapy is considered (e.g., treatment with 30 mg/d prednisone for 3 weeks). A number of cytotoxic agents or radiation therapy used in the treatment of malignancy, organ transplantation, and autoimmune diseases also impair CMI. The cytotoxic agents include methotrexate, cyclophosphamide, 6-mercaptopurine, azathioprine, and tacrolimus (1). The degree of immunosuppression caused by these drugs, as with corticosteroid use, correlates with the dose and duration of therapy.

Humoral Immunity

The antibody response produced by cells of the B lymphocyte lineage is the most important component of HI. Depending on whether the stimulating antigen is a protein or a nonprotein, such as a polysaccharide or lipid, the humoral immune response can be classified as either T-cell dependent or independent. T-cell–dependent antibodies produced in response to protein antigens are usually more specialized, with long-lived memories, whereas T-cell–independent responses to nonprotein antigens are mediated largely by low-affinity IgM and some IgG, with little generation of memory cells (2).

T-cell–dependent antibody responses occur as either primary or secondary responses (2). Primary responses result in activation of naive B cells after the initial exposure to an antigen, such as a vaccine. A repeat exposure to that same antigen results in a secondary response, which involves the stimulation of previously stimulated, already expanded clones of memory B cells. This adaptive mechanism enables the secondary response to develop more rapidly and result in larger amounts of antigen-specific antibodies than are produced in the primary response (2).

The most common T-cell–independent antigens are bacterial cell-wall polysaccharides, glycolipids, and nucleic acids. Although they are not recognized by helper T cells, these antigens can activate B cells directly by initially eliciting an IgM antibody response, followed by an IgG response (2). Individuals with a congenital or acquired deficiency in HI, such as common variable immunodeficiency, chronic lymphocytic leukemia, lymphosarcoma, multiple myeloma, nephrotic syndrome, major burns, asplenia or a functional asplenic state, and protein-losing enteropathy are therefore at high risk for life-threatening infections by encapsulated organisms such as *Streptococcus pneumoniae*, *Neisseria meningitidis*, and *Haemophilus influenzae* (Table 37.2).

Another important component of the humoral immune system is the complement system, which is largely considered an effector mechanism of HI as well as a means of amplification of antibody responses. Complement deficiencies can be present in either the classic or alternate pathway (2). Deficiencies of the early classic complement components (C1, C2, and C4) have been described. Although unexplained, C2 and C4 deficiencies are observed in more than 50% of patients with systemic lupus erythematosus (SLE) (2). Surprisingly, infection rarely occurs in individuals with early classic complement component deficiencies, most likely because the alternate pathway of complement activation remains intact.

In contrast, individuals with inherited deficiencies of C3 and C5 and Chediak-Higashi syndrome have significant impairment of opsonization that leads to defective neutrophil chemotaxis, aggregation, and phagocytosis. This can result in severe infections by encapsulated organisms, enteric gram-negative bacteria, and staphylococci, illustrating the importance of these complement components in bacterial lysis. Deficiencies of the late complement components (C5b, C6, C7, C8, and C9) are most common. Because they prevent development of a membrane attack complex for lysing foreign organisms, these

Table 37.2   Causes of Humoral Immune Deficiency and Common Associated Infections

Causes	Organisms
Common variable hypogammaglobulinemia	*Streptococcus* species
Nezelof's syndrome	*Staphylococcus* species
Ataxia telangiectasia	*Salmonella* species
Wiskott–Aldrich syndrome	*Neisseria meningitidis*
Chédiak-Higashi syndrome	*N. gonorrhoeae*
Chronic lymphocytic leukemia	*Haemophilus influenzae*
Lymphosarcoma	
Multiple myeloma	
Asplenia or hyposplenia	
Systemic lupus erythematosus	
Sickle cell disease	
Major burns	
Nephrotic syndrome	
Protein-losing enteropathy	
C1-9 deficiencies	

deficiencies are associated with infections by *N. meningitidis* and *N. gonorrhoeae* (2). Anyone with recurrent *Neisseria* infections should be investigated for complement deficiency.

One of the most common clinical conditions causing deficient HI is asplenia or hyposplenia. Since the spleen is a major source of antibody production, these states result in an immunoglobulin-deficient state that puts the patient at unusually high risk for infection by encapsulated organisms (4). This is especially true for patients with sickle cell anemia because not only are these patients hyposplenic and antibody deficient, but they are also complement deficient because complement is depleted by the stroma of the sickled erythrocytes (5). This impairs effective opsonization of encapsulated organisms such as *S. pneumoniae*, *H. influenzae*, and *Salmonella* species. Infections and their management in asplenic or hyposplenic patients will be discussed in detail later in this chapter.

Polymorphonuclear Leukocytes

Polymorphonuclear leukocytes (PMNLs; neutrophils) represent the most important component of the cellular host defense system against bacterial and selected fungal infections. Both quantitative and qualitative abnormalities in PMNLs can lead to a predisposition to recurrent infections (1). Conditions that can cause such abnormalities are numerous (Table 37.3).

Many diseases impair neutrophil function, including myelodysplasia, paroxysmal nocturnal hemoglobinuria, chronic granulomatous disease, and Job's syndrome. These cause neutrophil dysfunction through a number of mechanisms. For instance, chronic granulomatous disease and myeloperoxidase deficiency both result in an intrinsic defect of the neutrophil (1). The defective neutrophils lack essential components required for oxidative metabolism, which results in their failure to generate an oxidative burst in response to certain pathogenic organisms. This burst is essential for the killing of catalase-producing organisms such as staphylococci, *Serratia*, *Nocardia*, and *Aspergillus*. Depending on its dose and duration, corticosteroid therapy can also impair neutrophil chemotaxis, phagocytosis, microbicidal activity, and antibody-dependent cytotoxicity. In these settings, although the circulating neutrophil count may be normal or increased, the neutrophils are considered dysfunctional and inadequate for effective phagocytosis.

Infections in Patients with Neutropenia

Neutropenia, defined as an absolute neutrophil count of fewer than 500 cells/μL, is among the most important risk factors for life-threatening infections. Most

Table 37.3   Causes of Decreased Function or Numbers of Polymorphonuclear Cells and Common Associated Infections

Causes	Organisms
Myelodysplasia	*Streptococcus* species
Paroxysmal nocturnal hemoglobinuria	*Staphylococcus* species
Chronic granulomatous disease	*Serratia* species
Job's syndrome	*Pseudomonas aeruginosa*
Chédiak-Higashi syndrome	*Escherichia coli*
Myeloperoxidase deficiency	*Klebsiella* species
Peroxidase deficiency	*Enterobacter* species
G-6-PD deficiency	*Nocardia*
"Lazy" leukocyte syndrome	*Aspergillus*
Aplastic anemia	*Candida* species
Hypersplenism	
Felty's syndrome	
Sarcoidosis	
Circulating immune complexes	
Alcohol	
Corticosteroids	
Immunosuppressive and chemotherapeutic agents	

commonly, it is caused by malignancies and their treatment with cytotoxic agents, especially in conjunction with bone marrow or peripheral stem cell transplantation. The classic study by Bodey and coworkers demonstrated a direct correlation between the degree and duration of neutropenia and the likelihood of infection (6). The risk of infection begins to increase significantly when the granulocyte count falls below 1000 cells/µL. This is even more pronounced when the granulocyte count is below 100 cells/µL, with the result that if this degree of neutropenia persists for 6 weeks, 100% of these patients will develop an infectious complication. Hence, when dealing with a neutropenic patient, it is important to first consider the absolute granulocyte count, the duration of neutropenia, and whether the neutrophil count is rising or decreasing. Other risk factors associated with infection include immune defects caused by the patient's underlying disease and alterations in the integrity of physical defense barriers by mucositis, indwelling catheters, or invasive procedures.

Epidemiologic Resistance Patterns

Neutropenia primarily predisposes patients to bacterial and fungal infections. Over the past several decades, the typical pathogens associated with neutropenia have shifted with the rapid development of different antibiotic resistance patterns. In the 1960s, gram-positive organisms such as *Staphylococcus aureus* were the predominant infecting organisms. In the 1970s, however, this shifted largely to gram-negative organisms (*Escherichia coli, Klebsiella* species, *Pseudomonas aeruginosa, Enterobacter* species), most likely in relation to the use of broad-spectrum antimicrobial drugs and newer, more aggressive chemotherapy (7). Most recently, both gram-positive and gram-negative organisms have become problematic, owing to the changing resistance patterns to a large percentage of the antimicrobial drugs now on the market.

Treatment

Despite the traditional, rigorous recommendation of giving narrow-spectrum antibiotic therapy to most neutropenic patients, the febrile neutropenic patient represents an exception. Because a high percentage of neutropenic patients can develop fulminant, life-threatening infections, it is recommended that all febrile neutropenic patients or afebrile neutropenic patients with signs or symptoms suggestive of infection initially receive empirical therapy with a broad-spectrum antimicrobial regimen (8). Selection of an empirical antibiotic regimen depends on a number of factors. The cause of infection in the neutropenic patient with a secondary infection depends on the extent and duration of neutropenia, the status of the patient's cellular and humoral immune system, the underlying illness, alteration of physical defense barriers, the patient's endogenous microbial flora (hospital or community), and the frequency and resistance patterns of pathogens encountered in the treating institution (1).

Eighty percent of organisms causing infections of neutropenic hosts are part of the microbial flora that colonize the gastrointestinal tract and oropharynx (9). The major organisms causing infections in the neutropenic host are both gram-positive and gram-negative bacteria (1). In particular, this includes *E. coli, K. pneumoniae, P. aeruginosa, Streptococcus* species, and *S. aureus*. Under certain conditions the patient is predisposed to infection by certain organisms. For instance, a vascular access device (subcutaneous ports, indwelling central line) provides a port of entry for organisms that are part of the skin flora, such as *S. aureus* and coagulase-negative staphylococci. In these circumstances, an attempt to sterilize the vascular access device can be made with a trial of antibiotic therapy administered through the ports. However, if the bacteremia fails to clear after 72 hours of antibiotic administration, and/or the patient remains persistently febrile, has a tunnel infection or local cellulitis, develops a pulmonary complication (septic or bland pulmonary emboli), has evidence of endocarditis, develops central septic thrombophlebitis, or has an infection of fungal etiology, removal of the prosthesis must be pursued (9). Investigation with ultrasound or angiography is helpful for diagnosing suppurative complications.

Pulmonary infiltrates in the febrile, neutropenic patient require immediate and special attention. Although noninfectious etiologies must be considered for such infiltrates (hemorrhage, radiation- or drug-induced pneumonitis, fluid overload, thromboembolic disease), a lobar infiltrate is most likely to be pyogenic. Depending on the duration and trend of the neutropenia and the patient's antibiotic regimen, a number of infectious agents must be considered. Among the most common and virulent organisms are gram-negative bacteria, which are of major concern and should be well covered by empiric antimicrobial therapy (9). Timing of the development of a pulmonary infiltrate is also important; pulmonary infiltrates appearing during granulocyte recovery may not represent a new infection. In contrast, new and progressive pulmonary infiltrates that develop during antibiotic therapy and prolonged neutropenia are likely to have a fungal etiology (9). Ideally, a diagnostic open-lung biopsy should be done early in the clinical course of disease, when the patient is stable. This will help establish the diagnosis and guide the duration of therapy. Nevertheless, empiric antifungal therapy should be instituted if a biopsy is not a feasible option and a fungal infection is strongly suspected.

Many broad-spectrum antibiotics with similar efficacy and different side-effect profiles are currently available. Because of the high likelihood of resistant gram-negative organisms, combination antibiotic coverage has been the standard treatment for patients with infections complicating neutropenia. However, the most recent recommendations of the Infectious Diseases Society of America (IDSA) are for any of three general schemes for empiric antibiotic therapy, one of which includes monotherapy (8). In most cases, a single broad-spectrum antimicrobial agent with anti-pseudomonal activity is adequate (ceftazidime, carbapenems, or extended-spectrum penicillins), especially if the degree of neutropenia is not profound and the expected duration of neutropenia will be short. If a resistant gram-negative organism is suspected as the pathogen, an aminoglycoside or fluoroquinolone can be added. If methicillin-resistant S. aureus is also of concern, vancomycin should be added. However, with the emergence of vancomycin-resistant enterococcus as a significant nosocomial pathogen, vancomycin should be reserved for clear indications.

Duration of Therapy

The duration of antimicrobial therapy for infections in neutropenic patients is not well defined. Regardless of whether the patient is febrile or afebrile, it is recommended that at minimum, a 5- to 7-day course of antimicrobial therapy be completed (8). Since the single most important determinant of duration of therapy is recovery of the neutrophil count, it is safe to stop intravenous antibiotic administration 3 or 4 days after the neutrophil count reaches 500 cells/mL. If no discernible infection is found and the patient is afebrile, the 7-

day course can be completed with oral therapy. However, if profound neutropenia is persistent. and there are continuous signs of possible infection (tachycardia, tachypnea, hypotension, and mucous membrane lesions) after 3 days of intravenous antibiotic therapy, a meticulous evaluation for alternative causes of fever must be undertaken and the antibiotic therapy should be continued throughout the neutropenic period. Alternative causes of infection to be considered include a bacterial infection resistant to the antibiotic drug(s) in use; a second infection (bacterial, fungal, or viral); inadequate dosing of antibiotics; drug fever; or alternate sites of infection (abscesses or catheter-associated infection). Unfortunately, infection is clinically documented in only 48% to 60% of febrile episodes (8).

Treatment of Refractory Infection

If fever persists after 4 to 7 days of antimicrobial therapy and reassessment does not yield a cause, the clinician must decide whether to continue with the initial antimicrobial drugs, change or add antimicrobial drugs, or add antifungal therapy (8). The latter two approaches are recommended because the likelihood of a second or of multiple infections increases as the duration of neutropenia increases. The most notable of these infections are invasive mycoses such as candidiasis and aspergillosis. Studies have indicated that up to 33% of febrile neutropenic patients who do not respond to a 1-week course of antimicrobial therapy will have systemic fungal infections. For invasive mycoses, amphotericin B is probably the drug of choice, but fluconazole is an acceptable option, so long as fluconazole resistance is not prevalent at that treating institution (1,9,10). Although no formal recommendations exist for the use of antifungal prophylaxis, studies have shown that the frequency of some invasive fungal infections can be dramatically decreased with the use of empiric antifungal therapy (11,12). Therefore, in profoundly neutropenic patients who have persistent fever despite broad-spectrum antimicrobial therapy, empiric antifungal therapy with either fluconazole or amphotericin B is reasonable. No indication now exists for empiric antiviral therapy unless there is documented herpes simplex virus, varicella-zoster virus, or cytomegalovirus infection in a persistently febrile individual.

Colony-Stimulating Factors

At present, the routine use of colony-stimulating factors (e.g., granulocyte colony-stimulating factor [G-CSF]) is not recommended by the IDSA because the outcome for typical febrile neutropenic episodes is good with standard antimicrobial therapy (8). However, in conditions in which a delay is expected in the recovery of the bone marrow, or a worsening course is predicted, administration of G-CSF until the neutrophil count stabilizes at more than 500–1000 cells/µL can be beneficial. Granulocyte transfusions are not routinely recommended unless the documented cause of infection is not responsive to optimal antibiotic therapy plus administration of G-CSF.

Infections in Patients with Diabetes Mellitus

Recent data provide compelling evidence that tight glucose control can delay or prevent diabetic microvascular complications such as retinopathy, microalbuminuria, renal insufficiency, and neuropathy. Although data about hyperglycemia and its effects on the immune system are not as extensive, there is reason to suspect that poor glucose control can lead to an increased incidence of infection. It is well established that diabetic patients are prone to certain types of infections, such as with *S. aureus*, chronic osteomyelitis of the foot, rhinocerebral mucormycosis, emphysematous cholecystitis, pyelonephritis, and soft-tissue infections (13). However the reason for this increased incidence is not completely clear. Although hyperglycemia and acidosis, along with microvascular compromise, predispose diabetic patients to infection, it is suspected that these patients also have an underlying compromise of the immune system.

Since the late 1970s, it has been shown *in vitro* that granulocytes from patients with poorly controlled diabetes have abnormalities in adherence, chemotaxis, phagocytosis, and microbicidal function (14). *In vitro* studies of PMNLs from healthy subjects have shown significant reductions in respiratory burst activity after 30 minutes of exposure to high glucose concentrations (15,16). These functions improve significantly when glucose concentrations are normalized. The same investigations have also demonstrated that a hyperglycemic state may disrupt complement function through the formation of a complement-glucose bond that prevents the complement from binding to bacteria (15,16). An interesting effect of hyperglycemia on *Candida albicans* has also been noted (15,16): the hyperglycemic state induces the expression of a surface protein on the yeast that can impair its phagocytic recognition and promote adherence of the yeast to endothelial surfaces. Clinical studies found that hyperglycemia within 3 days before the isolation of *C. albicans* was the most important risk factor for *Candida* infection in hospitalized diabetic patients. Other clinical evidence for an association of hyperglycemia and infection includes the increased incidence of catheter-related infections among intensive-care-unit patients receiving total parenteral nutrition compared with enterally fed patients (17).

Except for *S. aureus* and *Mucor*, no organisms occur more often in diabetic patients than in the general population. The increased rate of infection with *S. aureus* is partly attributed to higher rates of skin and mucosal staphylococcal colonization in diabetic patients. Several studies found that diabetic patients who were regular injection-insulin users had the highest colonizing rates of *S. aureus* (18,19). This supports studies showing diabetes as an underlying disease in 8% to 36% of patients with staphylococcal bacteremia. Patients who develop chronic renal failure from diabetic nephropathy, and who require hemodialysis, have a high rate of vascular infection and bacteremia caused by repetitive manipulation (20). Again, *S. aureus* is frequently found, causing 40% to 70% of cutaneous and intravenous-infusion-related bacteremias (19). Rhinocerebral mucormycosis is a condition well known to be associated with poorly controlled diabetes marked by recurrent episodes of diabetic ketoacidosis (13). This is because the relatively acidic environment in such disease is ideal for the growth of mucormycosis. The peripheral vascular disease and neuropathy observed in most chronically diabetic patients make foot ulcers a common infectious complication in this population. (*See* Chapter 32 for recommendations for medical and surgical management of diabetic foot infections).

At present, no published recommendations exist for the management of infections in diabetic patients. On the basis of available data, it would be prudent to maintain glycemic control as tightly as possible and to maintain a vigilant watch for signs of infections, as well as to conduct regular podiatric examinations and regular sensory and vascular evaluations when indicated. In dealing with a possibly infected diabetic patient, it is important to remember that immune compromise may result in a physiologic response to infection that is not typical of a normal host. Diagnostic investigations should be directed toward the most common sites of infection. In choosing an antimicrobial regimen, strong consideration should be given to the probable pathogens.

Infections in Patients with Asplenia

Overwhelming post-splenectomy infection (OPSI) in children was initially described in 1952 (21). Since then, it has been recognized that the asplenic patient represents a unique compromised immunologic state, involving nearly all aspects of host defense (4,22). The spleen plays a critical role in host defense through several mechanisms. Its microcirculation facilitates mechanical clearance of organisms (bacteria and parasites) that have been ineffectively opsonized by components of complement. It also plays an important role in the synthesis and regulation of soluble mediators such as antibodies, complement components, and tuftsin, which are critical in the defense against organisms with polysaccharide capsules. IgM, which is responsible for the early antibody response and overall peripheral blood mononuclear cell response, has also been reported to be subnormal in asplenic individuals, most likely because the spleen is a primary site for IgM synthesis.

Asplenia can be the result either of auto-splenectomy (sickle cell disease, congenital asplenia, splenic atrophy) or surgical splenectomy. The latter is usually performed as part of the staging process for malignant disease (Hodgkin's disease) or as a therapeutic intervention for disorders such as autoimmune diseases, thalassemia, spherocytosis, and splenic rupture from trauma or viral infection. The incidence of septicemia, pneumonia, or meningitis in asplenic individuals ranges from 2% to 8% (22). It is unclear when, after splenectomy, the risk of infection begins to increase, when this risk peaks, and when the risk becomes negligible. The present consensus is that the risk of infection is greatest in the first few years after splenectomy. Thereafter, the cumulative incidence is linear for approximately 7 years, after which the occurrence of infection begins to decrease significantly (4). However, it is important to note that cases of OPSI have been reported 40 years after splenectomy.

The major pathogen associated with asplenia is *S. pneumoniae*, which accounts for 50% to 90% of the cases of such infection in some series (4,22). This can result in pneumococcal bacteremia, endocarditis, meningitis, and pneumonia. Other frequently observed organisms in asplenic individuals are listed in Table 37.4. Worth noting is the fastidious organism *Capnocytophaga canimorsus*. Although this organism rarely causes sepsis in the normal host, it was recently recognized as a cause of infection after dog bites in asplenic people (4). There are insufficient data about other infectious agents such as viruses, fungi, and parasites (e.g. malaria, *Babesia*) to determine whether asplenia or asplenia predisposes to infection with them.

Clinical Manifestations

The initial clinical presentation of infection in an asplenic individual can be subtle and nonspecific (4,22). Symptoms suggesting a viral illness, such as fever, sore throat, myalgia, diarrhea, and malaise, are common. Clinical clues to absent or impaired splenic function include an abdominal scar suggesting a

Table 37.4   Common Bacterial Causes of Infection in Asplenic Patients

Streptococcus pneumoniae	*Pseudomonas* species
Haemophilus influenzae	*Neisseria* species
Staphylococcus aureus	*Proteus* species
Clostridium species	*Serratia* species
Escherichia coli	*Acinetobacter* species
Group B and D *Streptococcus*	*Bacteroides* species
Klebsiella species	*Salmonella* species
Enterobacter species	*Capnocytophaga canimorsus*

previous splenectomy, or the presence of Howell-Jolly bodies in the peripheral blood smear, indicating impaired splenic function. After the prodrome, the majority of cases of OPSI progress to a sudden and rapidly fulminant course, often resulting in bacteremia, meningitis, pneumonia, or overwhelming sepsis. Refractory hypotension, respiratory distress, disseminated intravascular coagulation, peripheral gangrene, Waterhouse-Friederichsen syndrome, hypofibrinogenemia, and hypocomplementemia can be complications (13). Despite appropriate and aggressive antibiotic therapy accompanied by intensive medical management, the mortality rate remains extremely high, ranging from 50% to 75% (4).

Treatment

Given the large number of possible etiologic organisms of infection in hyposplenic or asplenic individuals, it is recommended that empirical antimicrobial therapy be directed toward the most likely organisms, such as pneumococcus and other encapsulated organisms (22). In addition, because the clinical course of infection can be rapidly fatal, the liberal use of early empirical antibiotic therapy can be of significant benefit to the asplenic or hyposplenic patient. In most instances, high-dose penicillin, ampicillin, or a third-generation cephalosporin is adequate, with the latter two choices providing additional coverage for gramnegative organisms. Unfortunately, the development of penicillin-resistant pneumococcus and resistant gram-negative organisms mandates that consideration be given to the antimicrobial resistance pattern and the incidence of these organisms in the community and hospital when choosing a treatment regimen for infection in the asplenic patient. If resistant pathogens are possible infecting organisms, initial antimicrobial coverage may be broadened to include vancomycin, new-generation fluoroquinolones, broad-spectrum penicillins, carbapenems, and anti-pseudomonal third-generation cephalosporins. Once the infectious agent is identified and its antibiotic susceptibility pattern is determined, treatment should be modified appropriately.

Prophylaxis

Efforts aimed at decreasing morbidity and mortality in the patient at risk for OPSI have focused on antibiotic prophylaxis and vaccination. Prophylactic antibiotic use has been suggested as a method of reducing the incidence of infection. However, short-term and long-term drug adherence issues are almost always encountered, especially since the risk of infection has been known to persist for up to 40 years after splenectomy. In addition, the issue of antibiotic resistance becomes significant when the asplenic individual develops a lifethreatening infection despite antibiotic prophylaxis. Nevertheless, good experience exists for the use of antibiotic prophylaxis in children with sickle cell disease (5). Multiple studies have shown that in these children, who have a 6% to 8% lifetime chance of developing bacterial meningitis, which in 70% to 90% of cases is caused by *S. pneumoniae*, monthly prophylactic intramuscular penicillin injections can reduce the rate of infection to 50% to 84% (23,24).

A more realistic and cost-effective approach to preventing infection in the asplenic individual is through the use of vaccination, such as with a pneumococcal, meningococcal, and *H. influenzae* type B vaccine. These confer the most protection when administered before splenectomy, and should be recommended to all patients who expect a splenectomy. The Advisory Committee on Immunization Practices of the American Medical Association recommends administration of the vaccines at least 2 weeks before elective splenectomy whenever possible (25). Although data suggest that there is suboptimal antibody production in splenectomized individuals, these vaccines still confer some protective effect even when given after splenectomy (4). However, because these vaccinations do not confer 100% protection, OPSI must still be considered in an acutely ill asplenic patient who has been previously vaccinated.

Infections and Corticosteroid Use

As mentioned earlier, corticosteroids are commonly used for a number of medical conditions. It has long been known that corticosteroids affect the immune response through impairment of both T-cell and phagocytic function (13). Corticosteroids impair neutrophil chemotaxis, phagocytosis, microbicidal effects, and antibody-dependent cytotoxicity. The degree by which these functions are depressed depends strongly on the dose and duration of corticosteroid therapy. For instance, chronic low-dose corticosteroid therapy (<20 mg/d prednisone) is unlikely to have a significant impact on T-cell function. However, split doses of high-dose steroids given for prolonged periods (>40–60 mg/d prednisone) have been shown to cause significant impairment of T-cell–mediated immunity.

Because corticosteroids can profoundly depress cell-mediated immunity, the patient receiving prolonged high-dose corticosteroid therapy is at risk for a spectrum of infections that can include bacterial, fungal, viral, and mycobacterial infections (13). A significant relationship also exists between chronic corticosteroid use and atypical presentations of infections. In particular, viral infections, such as with cytomegalovirus and herpes simplex virus, as well as *M. tuberculosis* and fungal infections, can present in a disseminated fashion. Classic *Pneumocystis carinii* pneumonia (PCP) often presents shortly after the discontinuation or during the tapering of steroid therapy because removal of the immunosuppressive drug permits an enhanced inflammatory response to the organism (26,27). Interestingly, corticosteroids often play an important role in the treatment of certain severe infections. For instance, the outcome of severe PCP in HIV-infected patients is dramatically improved when a corticosteroid is added to the treatment regimen (28). This is because corticosteroids blunt the inflammatory response to the high concentration of lysed organisms. This is also true for certain forms of *M. tuberculosis* infection, such as meningitis, pericarditis, and overwhelming pneumonitis, in which treatment of the infection may increase inflammatory response to tubercular antigens (29).

Infections in Patients with Multiple Myeloma

Since 1953, a high incidence of bacterial infection has been noted in myeloma patients, accounting for 20% to 50% of deaths in this patient population (30). This observation prompted investigations of the immune response in these patients, which demonstrated that multiple myeloma was associated with several defects in immune function (30). The first demonstrated abnormality was of the humoral immune system. Patients with multiple myeloma mounted a weak or absent primary antibody response to immunization with various bacterial and viral antigens, and had decreased levels of normal immunoglobulins. Defects in cell-mediated immunity in these patients have been less clear. Patients with myeloma seem to have suppressed development of delayed-type hypersensitivity to various antigens, such as those of *Candida*, mumps, and tubercle bacillus. However, these findings are far from conclusive. There has also been a high level of suspicion that complement components are affected by myeloma. This is because infections in myeloma patients seem to be predominantly caused by encapsulated organisms (31). Although no consistent pattern of complement deficiency has been demonstrated, *in vitro* studies have shown that most myeloma patients demonstrate decreased complement activity, even in the absence of identifiable decreases in complement components (30). Granulocyte function has also been found to be defective in patients with myeloma. It has been shown that granulocytes from myeloma patients have decreased receptors for IgG and C3b (30). However, these abnormalities did not correlate with the incidence of infection.

Despite the advances in relatively nontoxic chemotherapy for myeloma, from 20% to 50% of patients with the disease still die as a result of complicating infections (30). These infections are predominantly bacterial (32). Between 1953 and 1963, the most common site of infection was the lower respiratory tract, with infection related to *S. pneumoniae*, followed by urinary tract infection (UTI) with *E. coli*. Since then, the frequency of gram-positive infections has shown little change. More recently, the frequency of gram-negative infections (Enterobacteriaceae and *P. aeruginosa*) has risen significantly, mainly in patients with advancing, refractory disease (31). This is reflected by the significant increase in the incidence of hospital-acquired gram-negative pneumonia in myeloma patients. It has been postulated that this increase is an effect of previous antibiotic therapy, instrumentation, immobilization, and colonization with hospital flora (31).

The risk of infection appears to increase during three specific phases of myeloma (32). The first phase is in the first 3 months after diagnosis, during initial chemotherapy. It is during this period that viral and fungal infections are more likely to occur. The second phase is the stable-disease phase, which is mainly associated with bacterial infection as a result of the persistence of dysfunctional HI. The last phase is during relapses of myeloma, when additional chemotherapy is given. This usually signifies a progression of the disease and is complicated by infections with a wide variety of organisms, suggesting a more generalized dysfunction of the entire immune system.

Prophylaxis

Interventions intended to prevent infection in patients with multiple myeloma have largely been directed at vaccination, with the best-studied vaccine being the pneumococcal vaccine. Unfortunately, a number of studies have found that patients with multiple myeloma have subnormal post-immunization titers of anti-pneumococcal antibody (30). In only a single animal study has it been demonstrated that pneumococcal immunization prevented fatal pneumococcal sepsis. Nevertheless, because its possible benefits significantly outweigh the minimal cost and toxicity, the pneumococcal vaccine is recommended for all myeloma patients. Reimmunization may also be of benefit because secondary antibody responses have been determined to be normal in myeloma patients. Since myeloma patients can experience a rapid decrease in antibody titer as early as 18 months after immunization, it has been hypothesized that reimmunization every 3 to 5 years may provide more effective protection against pneumococcal infection (30). Whether this is true requires future study. Although the use of prophylactic antimicrobial therapy has been considered for preventing infection in patients with myeloma, it is not currently recommended. Although prophylactic antibiotic use may be reasonable for the patient who develops recurrent infections with the same organism, general use of such treatment is not recommended because of the high likelihood of its leading to infection with resistant organisms (33). Empiric antibiotic therapy for an infected patient should be directed against the most likely source of infection.

More recently, intravenous immune globulin therapy has been shown to prevent life-threatening infections and reduce the risk of recurrent infections in patients with myeloma (34). In a randomized, placebo-controlled trial, Chapel and coworkers (32) demonstrated that all members of a group of myeloma patients who received monthly intravenous immune globulin therapy experienced a significantly lower incidence of serious and recurrent bacterial infections. Individuals who had a poor pneumococcal IgG antibody response to pneumococcal vaccine benefited most from monthly intravenous immune globulin therapy.

Infections in Patients with Systemic Lupus Erythematosus

From before the advent of immunosuppressive therapy more than 50 years ago, infection has been recognized as a major cause of morbidity and mortality in patients with SLE (13,33,35,36). This increased rate of infection reflects the extensive immunologic dysregulation that is the hallmark of SLE. The use of corticosteroid and immunosuppressive agents has been found to be the strongest correlate with death from infection in patients with SLE (33). As a result, the lupus patient is at an extraordinary risk for various types of opportunistic infections that may ultimately prove fatal.

It is important to first understand the immune defects associated with SLE (33). Both macrophage and neutrophil defects have been documented. The macrophage defects are multiple. These include diminished phagocytic activity of lupus monocytes, decreased superoxide generation by phagocytes, and decreased production of tumor necrosis factor, all of which may predispose to bacterial infections. The neutrophil defects are multifaceted as well. Neutropenia, a common finding in SLE, correlates with the presence of complement-activating anti-neutrophil antibodies. Defective phagocytosis and chemotaxis has also been documented in untreated individuals. Excessive concentrations of circulating immune complexes, which are present during the active phase of the disease, result in persistent activation of neutrophils, which in turn causes subsequent defective responses to secondary stimuli. Defects in CMI most commonly result in CD4 lymphopenia and decreased *in vitro* production of various cytokines important for T-cell–mediated cytolytic activity. This has been demonstrated by significantly reduced delayed-type hypersensitivity responses in the skin. Defects of HI seem largely to come from nonspecific polyclonal B-cell activation and hypergammaglobulinemia. This is accompanied by significant deficiency of complement components, which may be due to the consumption of complement proteins by circulating and tissue-fixed immune complexes. Although it is uncommon, functional asplenia, with a high incidence of bacterial septicemia, has also been reported in SLE (37).

The most common infections seen in lupus patients are infections of the central nervous system (CNS), pneumonia, skin and soft-tissue infections, and UTIs (13,35). The diagnostic possibilities in each of these organ systems depend on whether the patient is receiving corticosteroid or immunosuppressive therapy, which determines the spectrum of likely pathogens (Table 37.5) (35).

Urinary tract infections are by far the most common cause of fever in lupus patients. Common organisms causing UTI include *E. coli*, *Proteus mirabilis*, and to a lesser extent enterococci and *Staphylococcus saprophyticus*. It is important to remember that sepsis syndrome is a common complication for UTI in the lupus patient. Skin and soft tissue infections, although more common in lupus patients, are caused largely by common organisms such as *S. aureus* and *Streptococcus* species. Treatment for these infections should be the same as for normal hosts. Lupus patients who are receiving corticosteroid or immunosuppressive therapy may not manifest typical signs and symptoms of infections. In such circumstances, common infectious problems, such as UTIs or soft-tissue infections, may develop a rapidly progressive course if not promptly recognized and treated with appropriate antimicrobial drugs. Fungal UTIs with *Candida*, and chronic fungal skin infections (histoplasmosis, *Cryptococcus*), should also be considered when the lupus patient is receiving immunosuppressive therapy

Infections of the CNS are difficult to diagnose in lupus patients. This is because there are multiple causes of CNS disease in this population. Lupus cerebritis is often confused with meningitis. Patients with cerebritis usually do not have signs of meningeal irritation. However, severe headache with fever and meningismus is common, and mandates that a diagnosis of cerebritis be considered only after an infectious etiology has been excluded. The only reliable way to rule out a CNS infection is with analysis of cerebrospinal fluid (CSF). Patients with lupus cerebritis may have hypoglycorrhachia accompa-

Table 37.5   Common Microorganisms Causing Infection in Systemic Lupus Erythematosus

No Immunosuppressive Therapy	On Immunosuppressive Therapy
Staphylococcus aureus	Herpes zoster
Escherichia coli	Cytomegalovirus
Streptococcus pneumoniae	*Mycobacterium tuberculosis*
Haemophilus influenzae	*Listeria monocytogenes*
Mycoplasma pneumoniae	*Pneumocystis carinii*
Salmonella species	*Cryptococcus neoformans*
Neisseria species	*Nocardia* species
Klebsiella pneumoniae	Disseminated *Aspergillus*
Pseudomonas aeruginosa	*Candida* species
Enterobacter species	*Toxoplasma gondii*
Legionella pneumophila	*Histoplasma capsulatum*

nied by mild pleocytosis with PMNLs predominance. However, the Gram stain and a culture obtained before antimicrobial therapy is begun should be negative. A reliable but not readily available test is for the CSF C4 level, in which a depressed C4 level is confirmatory of lupus cerebritis (35). Radiologic imaging with MRI may also be helpful in differentiating the diagnosis.

Pathogens causing infectious meningitis in lupus patients are determined by whether the patient is receiving corticosteroids and/or immunosuppressive therapy (35). In the untreated patient, the pathogens causing meningitis are the same as those found in normal hosts. These primarily include *S. pneumoniae*, *N. meningitidis*, and *H. influenzae*. In the patient receiving corticosteroid and/or immunosuppressive therapy, the spectrum of organisms that can cause CNS infections is different. These include *Listeria monocytogenes*, *M. tuberculosis*, *C. neoformans*, *Toxoplasma gondii*, cytomegalovirus, and herpes simplex virus (encephalitis). Because empiric therapy to cover all of these organisms is not generally practical, empiric therapy should be aimed at the more likely organisms based on clinical presentation and local epidemiology. In addition, it is advised that an aggressive approach be taken to diagnosis. A clue to *Listeria* meningitis is the presence of red blood cells in the CSF. *Listeria* can also be seen as gram-positive bacilli on a Gram-stained smear, with cultures often being positive for these organisms. Cryptococcal meningitis is typically associated with hypoglycorrhachia and can be diagnosed by demonstration of *Cryptococcus* in an India ink preparation of the CSF and increased cryptococcal antigen titers in the CSF. Tuberculous meningitis is a difficult diagnosis to make because its symptoms are often chronic and the CSF evaluation often reveals hypoglycorrhachia and an increased protein concentration, which resembles what is found in other infectious etiologies. Diagnosis of tuberculous meningitis should be based on the clinical history, demonstration of acid-fast bacilli by smear, or culture of the CSF. Toxoplasmosis commonly presents as a mass lesion. Clinically, this may result in a focal neurological deficit or seizures. Demonstration of an increased CSF titer of anti-*Toxoplasma* IgM antibody is diagnostic. Imaging with computed tomography or MRI is helpful when ring-enhancing lesions are demonstrated (*see* Chapter 2).

Identifying the cause of pneumonia in a lupus patient also depends on whether corticosteroid and/or immunosuppressive therapy has been instituted (35). In the untreated lupus patient, SLE pneumonitis must be a diagnosis of exclusion. SLE pneumonitis typically presents in the form of migratory, non-segmental/lobar pulmonary infiltrates accompanied by a nonproductive cough, chest pain, and/or small pleural effusions. The lack of fever and chills is in favor of lupus pneumonitis. Community-acquired pneumonia in untreated lupus patients is caused by the same pathogens found in other hosts. This includes both the typical pathogens, such as *S. pneumoniae* and *H. influenzae*, and atypical pathogens such as *Mycoplasma*, *Chlamydia*, and *Legionella*. In the lupus patient receiving corticosteroid and/or immunosuppressive therapy, the spectrum of agents of infection is as wide as that found with meningitis. Possible causes include *P. carinii*, cytomegalovirus, *Toxoplasma*, and *C. neoformans*. Since the clinical syndromes associated with these organisms are similar, a definite diagnosis almost always requires the assistance of bronchoscopy with bronchoalveolar lavage and/or transbronchial biopsy, unless blood culture is positive. *P. carinii* pneumonia (PCP) should always be considered first if the patient has been receiving chronic high-dose corticosteroid therapy. PCP often becomes clinically apparent when the dose of corticosteroid is tapered. The clinical course of PCP is similar to that found in HIV infection, with subacute symptoms, a dry cough, fever, shortness of breath, hypoxemia, and diffuse bilateral infiltrates. Treatment should always be organism-specific to minimize antimicrobial resistance, since it is highly likely that future infections will occur with the same organism.

Summary

Infections in the immunocompromised host are difficult to diagnose. Immunocompromising conditions may be associated with multiple defects in host defenses that predispose to infections. These defects lead to characteristic infections that are not typical of a normal host. Therefore, a general understanding of the immune system and its possible defects in any given patient are essential to the diagnosis and treatment of infection in immunocompromised hosts. This should be accompanied by a high index of suspicion, especially since infections in the immunosuppressed hosts often have an atypical clinical course. Whenever feasible, the diagnosis of infection should be pursued aggressively, because of the importance to outcome of establishing a definitive cause of infection. Prophylaxis against future infections should focus on measures such as immunization and, in some patients, the selected use of prophylactic antimicrobial drugs.

REFERENCES

1. **Pizzo PA.** The compromised host. In Wyngaarden J, Smith L, Bennett J, eds. *Cecil Textbook of Medicine, 19th Ed.* Philidelphia: WB Saunders; 1992:1537–48.
2. **Abbas A, Lichtman A, Pober J.** *Cellular and Molecular Immunology, 3rd Ed.* Philadelphia: WB Saunders; 1997:195–6, 335–7.
3. **Alvarez S.** Infections in the compromised host. *Med Clin North Am.* 1992;76:1135–42.
4. **Styrt B.** Infection associated with asplenia: risks, mechanisms, and prevention. *Am J Med.* 1990; 88:33–42N.
5. **Wong WY, Overturf GD, Powars DR.** Infection caused by *Streptococcus pneumoniae* in children with sickle cell disease: epidemiology, immunologic mechanisms, prophylaxis, and vaccination. *Clin Infect Dis.* 1992;14:1124–36.

6. **Bodey GP, Rodriguez V, McCredie KB, Freireich EJ.** Neutropenia and infection following cancer chemotherapy. *Int J Radiat Oncol Biol Phys.* 1976;1:301–4.

7. **Pizzo PA.** Management of fever in patients with cancer and treatment-induced neutropenia. *N Engl J Med.* 1993;328:1323–32.

8. **Hughes WT, Armstrong D, Bodey GP, et al.** 1997 Guidelines for the use of antimicrobial agents in neutropenic patients with unexplained fever: Infectious Diseases Society of America. *Clin Infect Dis.* 1997;25:551–73.

9. **Pizzo PA, Commers J, Cotton D, et al.** Approaching the controversies in antibacterial management of cancer patients. *Am J Med.* 1984;76:436–49.

10. **Philpott-Howard J.** Infections in neutropenic patients. *Curr Opin Infect Dis.* 1995: 234–40.

11. **Goodman JL, Winston DJ, Greenfield RA, et al.** A controlled trial of fluconazole to prevent fungal infections in patients undergoing bone marrow transplantation. *N Engl J Med.* 1992;326:845–51.

12. **Pizzo PA, Robichaud KJ, Gill FA, Witebsky FG.** Empiric antibiotic and antifungal therapy for cancer patients with prolonged fever and granulocytopenia. *Am J Med.* 1982;72:101–11.

13. **Cunha BA.** Infections in nonleukopenic compromised hosts (diabetes mellitus, SLE, steroids, and asplenia) in critical care. *Crit Care Clin.* 1998;14:263–82.

14. **McMahon MM, Bistrian BR.** Host defenses and susceptibility to infection in patients with diabetes mellitus. *Infect Dis Clin North Am.* 1995;9:1–9.

15. **Hostetter MK, Lorenz JS, Preus L, Kendrick KE.** The iC3b receptor on *Candida albicans*: subcellular localization and modulation of receptor expression by glucose. *J Infect Dis.* 1990;161:761–8.

16. **Hostetter MK.** Handicaps to host defense. Effects of hyperglycemia on C3 and *Candida albicans. Diabetes.* 1990;39:271–5.

17. **Moore FA, Feliciano DV, Andrassy RJ, et al.** Early enteral feeding, compared with parenteral, reduces postoperative septic complications: the results of a meta-analysis. *Ann Surg.* 1992;216:172–83.

18. **Chow JW, Yu VL.** *Staphylococcus aureus* nasal carriage in hemodialysis patients: its role in infection and approaches to prophylaxis. *Arch Intern Med.* 1989;149:1258–62.

19. **Breen JD, Karchmer AW.** *Staphylococcus aureus* infections in diabetic patients. *Infect Dis Clin North Am.* 1995;9:11–24.

20. **Ifudu O.** Review articles: care of patients undergoing hemodialysis. *N Engl J Med.* 1998;339:1054–1062.

21. **King H, Shumacker HBJ.** Splenic studies. Part I: Susceptibility to infection after splenectomy performed in infancy. *Ann Surg.* 1952:239–42.

22. **Cole JT, Flaum MA.** Postsplenectomy infections. *South Med J.* 1992;85:1220–6.

23. **Buchanan GR, Smith SJ.** Pneumococcal septicemia despite pneumococcal vaccine and prescription of penicillin prophylaxis in children with sickle cell anemia. *Am J Dis Child.* 1986;140:428–32.

24. **Gaston MH, Verter JI, Woods G, et al.** Prophylaxis with oral penicillin in children with sickle cell anemia: a randomized trial. *N Engl J Med.* 1986;314:1593–9.

25. **Leads from the MMWR.** Recommendations of the Immunization Practices Advisory Committee: pneumococcal polysaccharide vaccine. *JAMA.* 1989;261:1265–7.

26. **Sepkowitz KA, Brown AE, Telzak EE, et al.** *Pneumocystis carinii* pneumonia among patients without AIDS at a cancer hospital. *JAMA.* 1992;267:832–7.

27. **Yale SH, Limper AH.** *Pneumocystis carinii* pneumonia in patients without acquired immunodeficiency syndrome: associated illness and prior corticosteroid therapy. *Mayo Clin Proc.* 1996;71:5–13.

28. Consensus statement on the use of corticosteroids as adjunctive therapy for *Pneumocystis* pneumonia in the acquired immunodeficiency syndrome: the National Institutes of Health–University of California Expert Panel for Corticosteroids as Adjunctive Therapy for *Pneumocystis* Pneumonia. *N Engl J Med.* 1990;323:1500–4.

29. **Dooley DP, Carpenter JL, Rademacher S.** Adjunctive corticosteroid therapy for tuberculosis: a critical reappraisal of the literature. *Clin Infect Dis.* 1997;25:872–87.

30. **Jacobson DR, Zolla-Pazner S.** Immunosuppression and infection in multiple myeloma. *Semin Oncol.* 1986; 13:282–90.

31. **Doughney KB, Williams DM, Penn RL.** Multiple myeloma: infectious complications. *South Med J.* 1988;81:855–8.

32. **Chapel HM, Lee M.** The use of intravenous immune globulin in multiple myeloma. *Clin Exp Immunol.* 1994;97(Suppl 1):21–4.

33. **Iliopoulos AG, Tsokos GC.** Immunopathogenesis and spectrum of infections in systemic lupus erythematosus. *Semin Arthritis Rheum.* 1996;25:318–36.

34. **Chapel HM, Lee M, Hargreaves R, et al.** Randomised trial of intravenous immunoglobulin as prophylaxis against infection in plateau-phase multiple myeloma: the UK Group for Immunoglobulin Replacement Therapy in Multiple Myeloma. *Lancet.* 1994;343:1059–63.

35. **Cunha BA.** Infections in SLE. *Infect Dis Pract.* 1997:41–6.

36. **Hellmann DB, Petri M, Whiting-O'Keefe Q.** Fatal infections in systemic lupus erythematosus: the role of opportunistic organisms. *Medicine.* 1987;66:341–8.

37. **Piliero P, Furie R.** Functional asplenia in systemic lupus erythematosus. *Semin Arthritis Rheum.* 1990;20:185–9.

38

Herpes Virus Infections

Gary I. Sinclair, MD

Charles H. King, MD

Herpes viruses are large (150–250-nm), DNA-containing, enveloped viruses. At present, there are approximately eighty known members of the herpesvirus family, which infect a broad range of animal species. Nine of the herpes viruses are pathogenic for humans. Herpes simplex virus type 1 (HSV-1) or human herpes virus type 1 (HHV-1) and HSV-2 or HHV-2 cause genital and oral ulcers. These are discussed in detail in Chapters 13 and 34. This chapter describes varicella zoster virus (VZV or HHV-3), the cause of chickenpox and shingles, Epstein-Barr virus (EBV or HHV-4), the cause of infectious mononucleosis, and cytomegalovirus (CMV or HHV-5), a cause of both localized and systemic illness in immunocompetent and immunosuppressed patients. Not discussed are the viruses HHV-6, HHV-7, and HHV-8, which seem to cause severe disease only in immunocompromised individuals. HHV-6 and HHV-7 cause the short-lasting pediatric syndrome known as exanthem subitum (roseola), and in rare cases cause meningoencephalitis or mononucleosis syndromes. HHV-8 has been identified in cells from Kaposi's sarcomas in HIV-infected patients. Its role in the pathogenesis of this sarcoma remains uncertain. The ninth human herpesvirus pathogen, Herpes B virus, is primarily a simian virus that causes a rare zoonotic illness in humans working with or caring for primates.

Varicella Zoster Virus Infection

Two distinct clinical syndromes are associated with VZV infection: chickenpox (primary varicella) and herpes zoster (shingles).

Epidemiology

Chickenpox

Chickenpox (primary varicella) is a highly contagious and therefore extremely common disease. It is caused by primary infection with VZV and is manifested by febrile illness with a diffuse vesicular rash. Humans are the only known reservoir of VZV. Spread of the virus occurs through respiratory droplets as well as through the inhalation of particles aerosolized from new crops of chickenpox or zoster lesions. Early viral replication occurs in the nasopharynx and upper respiratory tract, and is followed by viremia and subsequent skin and neural infection. Although the disease is ubiquitous, clusters or *epidemics* of chickenpox occur in late winter and early spring. In the United States the annual incidence of chickenpox is 3 to 4 million cases per year—a figure approximately the same as the national birth rate (1). The median age of onset of chickenpox is less than 3 years, but 5% to 10% of patients will escape infection and will still be susceptible to VZV when they reach adulthood (1). More than half a million visits to physician offices each year are related to chickenpox infection, and 250 people die each year because of chickenpox (1). The risk of dying from chickenpox is 2 in 100,000 for healthy children, but increases by a factor of 15 for adults (1).

Herpes Zoster

After resolution of primary varicella infection, VZV persists in latent form in the dorsal root ganglia. Later, localized viral activation and replication may occur if the balance between viral factors and host immunity is altered. Disease caused by reactivation of the virus occurs in 20% of infected individuals at some point in life (1). The annual incidence of herpes zoster ranges from 0.4 to 1.6 cases per 1000 people among healthy people under the age of 20 years, and as high as 4.5 to 11 cases per 1000 people among those 80 years of age and older (2). Most commonly, patients with herpes zoster are over the age of 55 (30% in one study of a managed care population, in which patients over the age of 55 constituted only 8% of all patients) (3). The risk of a second attack is as high as the risk of a first (2), however, three or more episodes should raise concern about occult immunosuppression. Notably, nonimmune individuals can contract primary varicella by exposure to the lesions of herpes zoster. Because these lesions can be aerosolized, patients with herpes zoster in medical facilities should be placed in private rooms to avoid risking exposure to nonimmune healthcare workers and immunocompromised patients.

Pathophysiology

The pathophysiology of the pox in both chickenpox and herpes zoster is similar. Vesicles involve the corium and the dermis. The vesicular fluid is initially clear and centered on an erythematous base, thus giving the classic *dewdrop on a rose petal* appearance. The fluid becomes cloudy as polymorphonuclear leukocytes infiltrate, local cells degenerate, and fibrin collects in the vesicle. The pustule then breaks down, crusts over with scab, and eventually heals (4).

Clinical Manifestations

Chickenpox

The typical course of chickenpox involves rash, low-grade fever, listlessness, pruritus, and malaise. Body temperature ranges from 100 to 103°F (37.7°–39.4° C), and the fever lasts for 3 to 5 days (1). It takes approximately 14 days to develop the rash of chickenpox after exposure, with a range of 10 to 20 days (1). The infectious period starts approximately 48 hours before the appearance of lesions and lasts until approximately 4 or 5 days thereafter, when the lesions have crusted over (1). The initial rash is usually localized to the trunk and face. Successive crops of pox appear for 2 to 4 days, spreading to the periphery and scalp, and may be found anywhere, including the oropharynx and the vagina (1). Crusts generally fall off after 1 to 2 weeks, leaving slight depressions in the skin (1,2). Secondary bacterial infection of pox lesions may lead to local scarring.

A number of unusual and serious complications may result from chickenpox, and the primary-care physician should be aware of these. A study done in the early 1990s estimated that the 30-day rate of reported complications ranged from 167 to 249 cases for every 10,000 cases of primary varicella—a rate much higher than reported in similar previous studies done in the 1970s (5). In the recent study, complications included central nervous system (CNS) disease, varicella pneumonia, skin superinfection, and Reye's syndrome. Fetal and neonatal infection also represent complicated cases of varicella.

Central nervous system complications of chickenpox include acute cerebellar ataxia, varicella encephalitis, transverse myelitis, and aseptic meningitis. Acute cerebellar ataxia occurs in approximately 1 in every 4000 children under the age of 15 years (1). Symptoms appear from several days before to 2 weeks after the appearance of rash, and usually resolve within 2 to 4 weeks without additional treatment (6). Mortality has been estimated to be between 0 and 5%, and is usually associated with the development of other complications of varicella, such as pneumonia (6). Varicella encephalitis occurs with an incidence of 0.1% to 0.2% (1). It is characterized by depressed consciousness, headache, vomiting, altered thought patterns, high fever, and seizures. Symptoms may occur from 11 days before to several weeks after the onset of the rash (6). Mortality estimates for varicella encephalitis range from 0% to 35% (1,6). Rare cases of both transverse myelitis and aseptic meningitis caused by VZV have been reported, usually with complete recovery as the outcome (6). CNS complications in the course of chickenpox usually merit expert consultation, since patients may benefit from treatment with antiviral medications and/or corticosteroids, although the data on this remain somewhat ambiguous (6).

Varicella pneumonia is another serious complication of chickenpox. It is more common in adults, with clinical pneumonia developing in 0.3% to 1.8% of cases, and radiologic changes occurring even more frequently (7). Varicella pneumonia is probably the most common severe complication of chickenpox, accounting for 27.6% of varicella-related deaths (7). Cigarette smoking is a risk factor for such pneumonia; rates of 42% to 47% have been reported for varicella pneumonia among smokers (7). Tachypnea, cough, and dyspnea are prominent presenting features, beginning 3 to 5 days into the illness (1). Nodular or interstitial patterns can be seen on chest radiography. Mortality of untreated varicella pneumonia is estimated at 11% in otherwise healthy adults (7), and from 35% to 44% in pregnant women (7,8). Expert consultation is warranted for such pneumonia, since aggressive treatment, including antiviral medication, has been proven to decrease morbidity and mortality resulting from it (8).

Varicella infection during pregnancy is a complex management problem. In addition to an increased severity of the disease and its complications for the mother owing to her suppressed immunity, two distinct risks are posed to the baby. First, when primary varicella occurs early in pregnancy, there is an increased risk of congenital abnormalities (occurring in 1% to 2% of infants of infected mothers), including skin scarring, hypoplastic extremities, eye abnormalities, and mental retardation (1). Second, a high perinatal infant death rate (30% for infants of untreated mothers) is noted when pregnant women develop chickenpox during the period from 5 days before to 48 hours after delivery (9). This period of fetal/neonatal vulnerability is most likely related to the absence of protective transplacental antibodies from the mother, who at this time is in an early stage of infection and has not yet developed protective anti-VZV antibodies. Multiple systemic complications may occur in the affected infant, and expert consultation is mandatory. Because of these significant risks of chickenpox in pregnancy, a pregnant woman exposed to chickenpox who has no history of prior infection or immunization should be given passive immunization (*see* discussion of varicella zoster immunoglobulin in the Passive Immunization section). Acyclovir should be given when chickenpox develops during pregnancy (*see* the Treatment sections in this chapter).

Reye's syndrome is a hepatic and systemic disorder that occurs in some patients with chickenpox who take aspirin for symptom relief. The syndrome is characterized by vomiting, restlessness, increased blood ammonia levels, hyperglycemia, and increased transaminase activity (1).

Other potential complications of chickenpox include skin superinfections, necrotizing fasciitis (particularly with Group A streptococci)(10), myocarditis, nephritis, a bleeding diathesis, and hepatitis (1).

Herpes Zoster

The lesions of varicella zoster or shingles most commonly occur in the thoracic or lumbar dermatomal distributions but can occur in any dermatome (1). Pain in the dermatomes precedes the appearance of lesions by 48 to 72 hours. The lesions are vesicular on an erythematous base, much like those of primary varicella. New lesions appear for 3 to 7 days, and pain usually lasts for approximately 2 weeks. Complete healing of the skin can take as long as a month (1).

In addition to the effects just discussed, isolated involvement of divisions of the fifth cranial nerve can be seen in cases of zoster. When the ophthalmic branch of the trigeminal nerve (V1) is involved, eyelid involvement, keratitis, iridocyclitis, secondary glaucoma, and zoster ophthalmicus can occur (1). Ocular involvement mandates ophthalmologic consultation. When any of the branches of the fifth cranial nerve are involved, mucous membrane and tonsillar lesions also can be seen. Involvement of the geniculate ganglion leads to the Ramsay-Hunt syndrome, with pain and vesicles occurring in the external auditory meatus; additionally, loss of taste can occur in the anterior two thirds of the tongue, and ipsilateral facial palsy can occur (1).

Extracutaneous manifestations of zoster are rare. Meningoencephalitis, a painful motor paralysis (which is distinctive, since most paralysis syndromes are associated with anesthesia), Guillain-Barré syndrome, transverse myelitis, and myositis have all been reported. In the immunosuppressed patient, dissemination of VZV, with pneumonitis, hepatitis, and encephalitis, is more common, and the syndrome may affect multiple dermatomes for a prolonged period (1).

Perhaps the most significant complication of herpes zoster is post-herpetic neuralgia. Although rare in children, it occurs in 27%, 47%, and 73% of zoster patients who are over 55, 60, and 70 years of age, respectively (2). The neuralgia is generally defined as pain in a dermatome previously affected by zoster and which lasts longer than 1 month. Early treatment with antiviral agents and corticosteroids may play a role in reducing this feared complication (*see* the Treatment section below) (2).

Diagnosis

The diagnoses of both chickenpox and varicella zoster are largely clinical and are based on the appearance of the rash and the usual natural history of the disease as outlined above. Disseminated HSV infection may be mistaken for varicella. Viral culture is more sensitive for HSV than for VZV, which grows slowly and unreliably *in vitro* (11). Late pustules and crusted lesions can be confused with impetigo, and individual pox lesions may actually be superinfected with *Staphylococcus aureus* and/or Group A beta-hemolytic streptococci (10). A Gram stain may be helpful in distinguishing VZV from bacterial pustules or impetigo. A Tzanck preparation can also be performed, but is only helpful when classic multinucleated giant cells are identified (Fig. 38.1). Serum titers of anti-VZV IgG antibody are of little benefit in acute disease, but are helpful in determining the immune status of exposed people without a clear history of clinical varicella (11).

The most sensitive confirmatory test for herpes zoster or chickenpox is the VZV-specific direct fluorescence monoclonal antibody test (DFA) performed on scrapings taken from the base of an unroofed pox lesion during an episode of either condition (*see* Fig. 38.1). In one study in which clinical diagnoses of chickenpox and herpes zoster were used as the gold standard, sensitivity and negative predictive value were estimated at 97%, and specificity was 100%. By contrast, the sensitivity and negative predictive value of VZV culture were estimated at 49% and 60%, respectively. Discordance between results of the DFA test and culture was associated with acyclovir treatment, with testing of lesions more than 5 days old, and with testing of lesions less than 1 day old. Notably, only two cases were found in which culture was positive and the DFA test was negative. Both of these cases involved pox lesions less than 1 day old. Had the DFA test been repeated later in these cases, more cells may have been expressed viral antigen and the discordance in diagnostic results may have been eliminated (12). We recommend using the DFA test for diagnostic confirmation whenever there is clinical doubt. Coxsackie virus, enterovirus, and HSV infections can all present with vesicular rashes, and each of these entities requires a different therapeutic approach.

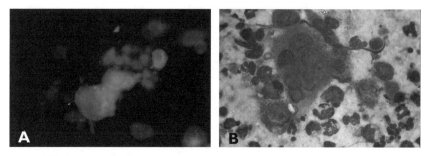

Figure 38.1   A, The results of a direct fluorescent monoclonal antibody stain of cells scraped from the base of a pox lesion. The green staining cells are expressing varicella viral antigens. Picture courtesy of Anne Morrissey and Scott Hite, Department of Microbiology, University Hospitals of Cleveland. **B,** A Tzanck smear, which is prepared by performing a Wright, Giemsa, or methylene blue stain of scrapings taken from the base of an unroofed pox lesion. Note the multinucleated giant cell. (Courtesy Dr. Robert Salata.)

Treatment

Chickenpox

For chickenpox in small children, the traditional approach to care has been to control symptoms and maintain hygiene by bathing, astringent soaks, and aluminum acetate soaks (1). Pruritus is eased by the use of topical lotions or oral antihistamines. Acetaminophen should be used instead of aspirin because of aspirin's association with Reye's syndrome.

The American Academy of Pediatrics recommends treatment with acyclovir for all adults and adolescents, and for children with other underlying disease, especially those with immunosuppression, because of their increased risk of developing severe disease (1,11). For chickenpox, the oral pediatric dose of acyclovir is 20 mg/kg given four times per day for 5 days. The oral adult dose is 800 mg given five times per day for 5 to 7 days (1,11). Ideally, the first dose should be given within 24 hours of the onset of symptoms. Oral acyclovir is not recommended for healthy children with uncomplicated chickenpox. The newer anti-herpes agents valacyclovir and famciclovir have yet to be adequately tested in children.

We recommend acyclovir for all women who contract varicella during pregnancy. Acyclovir is now listed as a Class B teratogen. Though no definitive controlled trials have been done to assess adverse outcomes of its use in pregnancy, a registry of 1117 prenatal exposures to acyclovir failed to show an increased incidence of prenatal complications and/or birth defects (personal communication on September 17, 1998, with Glaxo-Wellcome) (7,8). Studies have shown decreased maternal and fetal morbidity and mortality with acyclovir (7,8). Most experts agree that the potential benefits of acyclovir outweigh the risks of using it. Valacyclovir is also in Category B during pregnancy, but is less well studied than acyclovir. The safety of famciclovir in pregnancy is currently being assessed by its manufacturer, SmithKline-Beecham.

Intravenous acyclovir (500 mg/m2 every 8 hours or 10-12 mg/kg every 8 hours) and aggressive supportive care should be given to anyone exhibiting severe local or systemic complications of chickenpox (such as pneumonitis or CNS disease). Intravenous acyclovir should also be used for anyone whose illness is severe enough to require hospitalization.

Herpes Zoster

Treatment of herpes zoster is a problem more common to the primary care physician than to other practitioners. Corticosteroid therapy has been recommended both for alleviating symptoms of acute neuritis and for decreasing the incidence of post-herpetic neuralgia, but the data for its efficacy are somewhat controversial (1,2). Oral acyclovir, as well as the newer anti-herpes agents valacyclovir and famciclovir, has clearly been proven to accelerate healing and to decrease symptoms if given within 72 hours of the onset of rash (13–16). The efficacy of the three drugs seems to be equivalent. Meta-analyses demonstrate a decreased incidence of post-herpetic neuralgia in patients who have received antiviral medications (13–16). We recommend that an oral antiviral agent be routinely given to all patients presenting within 72 hours of the onset of symptoms of zoster if they have no contraindications to such drugs. Decisions about which of the three drugs to use should be based on cost and ease of administration for the individual patient. The dosage for acyclovir is the same as would be used for chickenpox (800 mg given five times per day for 7 days). The dosage of famciclovir for zoster is 500 mg every 8 hours for 7 days, and the dosage of valacyclovir is 1 g every eight hours for 7 days. Because of a paucity of data, the decision to use corticosteroids and/or to treat patients outside of the 72-hour framework must be individualized. Acute pain should be managed with analgesic agents, including narcotics if necessary. Chronic pain, which may occur in up to 50% of older patients, is managed with tricyclic antidepressants, anticonvulsant medications (usually carbamazepine), and agents that deplete substance P (capsaicin cream), as in other chronic pain syndromes (2).

Prevention

Isolation
Hospitalized patients who contract VZV infection or exhibit zoster lesions must be isolated until all lesions have crusted over to protect the infection of non-immune and immunocompromised individuals. Non-immune patients and health care workers who are significantly exposed to chickenpox and/or zoster should be considered infectious from day 8 to day 21 after exposure, and should be isolated or relieved of duty as appropriate. "Non-immune" is defined as having low or negative titers of anti-VZV IgG antibody (<1.0 Index Units by enzyme-linked immunosorbent assay), or having a negative clinical history of chickenpox if titer results are pending. Significant exposures include residence in the same household as the index patient, face-to-face indoor play with the patient, occupying an adjacent bed to the patient in a multipatient room or ward, and touching or hugging the index patient (9).

Passive Immunization
Varicella zoster immunoglobulin (VZIG) is indicated for all nonimmune pregnant women who sustain significant exposure to VZV. The dose of VZIG is 125 units given intramuscularly for every 10 kg of body weight, up to a maximum of 625 units (9). A 125-unit dose should be given to all infants whose

mothers developed primary varicella at any time from 5 days before delivery to 48 hours postpartum (9). VZIG can also be considered for immunocompromised patients who sustain significant contacts with VZV-infected people. Ideally, VZIG should be given within 96 hours of exposure (9). Its efficacy after VZV disease has become manifest is unproven.

Active Immunization

Vaccination against chickenpox is currently recommended for all immunocompetent children and adolescents unless they have a clear clinical history of chickenpox and are therefore immune (17). Vaccination of nonimmune adults is strongly encouraged, but not currently recommended by the Centers for Disease Control and Prevention. It should be given to all nonimmune health care or day care workers because of the high risk of exposure to VZV in these professions (17). A reliable history of having had clinical chickenpox is adequate for establishing immune status. For adults who do not recall having had chickenpox, assaying titers of anti-VZV IgG antibody is likely to be cost effective, since 71% to 93% of these people will prove to be immune (17).

The vaccine for chickenpox is a cell-free preparation of live, attenuated VZV of the wild OKA strain. It contains trace quantities of Neosporin and gelatin, to which a small minority of patients may have an allergic reaction. A single dose in children 12 months to 12 years of age results in a 97% rate of seroconversion (17). Two doses given over an interval of 4 to 8 weeks seem to be necessary for effecting immunity in people over 13 years of age (17). Studies in Japan, where the vaccine has been licensed since the 1970s, suggest that it confers protective immunity for at least 20 years (17). Vaccination is protective against severe VZV disease in 95% of vaccinees, and protective against all disease in 70% (17). Within 1 month of vaccination, 7% to 8% of vaccinees will develop a mild maculopapular or vesicular rash (17).

A zoster-like syndrome has been seen in 18 cases per 100,000 person years in vaccinated children followed for 7 years. Because the estimate for zoster occurring after natural infection is 77 cases per 100,000 person years, immunization does not seem to increase the risk of zoster (17).

Vaccination against chickenpox is contraindicated for immunocompromised individuals. This includes patients receiving systemic corticosteroid therapy (except in the case of adrenal replacement therapy), pregnant women, patients with HIV/AIDS, and patients with lymphoproliferative malignancies (except for children with acute lymphoblastic leukemia in remission, for whom ongoing studies suggest that vaccination against chickenpox is beneficial) (17). Inhaled corticosteroid therapy is not a contraindication to vaccination (17). Patients who have not received systemic corticosteroids for 3 months may also be vaccinated safely (17). Whenever possible, vaccinees should avoid contact with immunocompromised people for 3 weeks after vaccination. Plasma, whole blood, intravenous immune globulin, and VZIG may theoretically interfere with the antibody response to varicella vaccine for approximately 5 months (17). Vaccination has not yet been proven beneficial as a prophylactic measure after exposure to VZV, and should not be used instead of VZIG (*see* previous section on Passive Immunization) (17).

Epstein-Barr Virus and Infectious Mononucleosis

Epidemiology

Infection with EBV causes a ubiquitous febrile syndrome occurring in 90% to 95% of most populations tested for serologic evidence of such infection (18,19). In western countries, approximately 50% of seroconversions for EBV infection occur before the age of 5 years, and a second peak occurs during the second decade of life (18,19). Symptomatic infectious mononucleosis (IM) is more common when infection occurs in the second decade (18,19). Low titers of anti-EBV antibody are present in throat washings of people with IM (18). Virus persists in the oropharynx for up to 18 months after acute EBV infection. It can be cultured from the oropharynx of 10% to 20% of immunocompetent adults at any time. Susceptible college roommates of people with EBV infection experience seroconversion no more often than the general susceptible college population. For these reasons, precautions for isolating EBV-infected individuals in the community are neither advisable nor feasible (18). The primary mode of transmission is through saliva transferred by various means including kissing. Transfused blood can also transmit EBV disease (18).

Pathogenesis

In tissue culture, EBV can be grown only in B cells and in epithelial tissues of the nasopharynx (18). Primary inoculation is believed to be through the nasopharynx. A 30- to 50-day incubation period ensues (19). Viral replication starts in the lymphoid tissue of the pharynx and spreads throughout the entire lymphoreticular system. Disease is almost always self-limiting, although intermittent shedding of virus occurs for the remainder of life (18).

Clinical Manifestations

Although generally a benign, self-limiting illness, IM can have a clinical presentation that seems out of proportion to the true severity of illness. IM can mimic leukemia, streptococcal pharyngitis, and acute viral hepatitis. Table 38.1 provides signs and symptoms of IM.

Table 38.1 Signs and Symptoms of Acute Epstein-Barr Virus (Infectious Mononucleosis)

Symptoms and Signs	Percent of Patients with Symptom
Sore throat	82%
Malaise	57%
Headache	51%
Anorexia	21%
Myalgias	20%
Chills	16%
Nausea	12%
Abdominal discomfort	9%
Cough	5%
Arthralgias	2%
Lymphadenopathy	94%
Pharyngitis	84%
Fever	76%
Splenomegaly	52%
Hepatomegaly	12%
Palatal exanthem	11%
Jaundice	9%
Rash	10%

Adapted from Schooley RT. Epstein-Barr virus (infectious mononucleosis). In Mandell GL, Bennett JE, Dolin R, eds. *Principles and Practice of Infectious Diseases, 4th Ed.* New York: Churchill Livingstone; 1995:1364–77.

The likelihood of symptomatic infection with EBV increases with age. Pediatric infections are likely to be asymptomatic, whereas in military recruits, 90% of infections have been found to be clinically apparent (18). Signs and symptoms of infection generally last 2 to 3 weeks, though fatigue can last somewhat longer (18). Sore throat is maximal for 3 to 5 days. Fever tends to last for 10 to 14 days (18). Administration of ampicillin, which frequently occurs when the syndrome is mistaken for acute streptococcal pharyngitis, produces a pruritic maculopapular eruption in 90% to 100% of cases and is contraindicated (18). However, development of such a rash should not cause a patient to be labeled as penicillin-allergic (19). Initial suggestions that EBV is the causative agent of chronic fatigue syndrome are no longer supported by most reviewers (20,21).

Complications

EBV infection may be attended by a number of hematologic complications. Autoimmune hemolytic anemia occurs in 0.5% to 3% of cases and is associated with cold agglutinins of the IgM class. Hemolysis usually starts in the second or third week of illness and can persist for 1 to 2 months. Cortico-steroids may hasten recovery (18). A mild thrombocytopenia, with platelet counts below 140,000 cells/mm^3, has been noted in 50% of cases of IM (18). Severe cases are rare but have been reported, and responses of such cases to corticosteroids and splenectomy have been documented (18). Mild neutrope-nia is frequent in IM, although severe cases of EBV infection leading to sepsis have been reported (18).

Splenic rupture is a rare complication of IM, with the highest incidence oc-curring between the fourth and twenty-first days of illness (18,19). It is esti-mated to occur in 1 or 2 of every 1000 cases (19). Since abdominal pain is not a striking feature of mononucleosis, its appearance warrants investigation for splenic rupture. Occasionally, splenic rupture can be the presenting symptom of IM. The abdominal catastrophe can alter the differential blood count, and affected patients may paradoxically have an increased granulocyte count. Ap-proximately one half of splenic ruptures are attributable to trauma, and con-tact sports should be avoided for at least the first 3 weeks after diagnosis of such rupture (18). Overly vigorous physical examination should also be avoided (19).

Neurological syndromes occur in fewer than 1% of cases of primary EBV infection, but are occasionally the only manifestation of such infection (18,19). They include encephalitis, meningitis, myelitis, Guillain-Barré syndrome, op-tic neuritis, retrobulbar neuritis, cranial nerve palsies, mononeuritis multiplex, brachial plexus neuropathy, seizures, subacute sclerosing panencephalitis, transverse myelitis, psychosis, demyelination, and hemiplegia. One unusual syndrome is called metamorphopsia, or *Alice in Wonderland syndrome.* It involves deficits in perception of size, shape, and spatial orientation (19). Neurological complications are actually the most frequent cause of death in acute EBV in-fection in otherwise healthy individuals (22). However, the course of such in-fection is usually benign, and most patients recover completely. A 1970 review (covering the pre-acyclovir era) revealed only 20 documented EBV- associ-ated deaths (22). EBV infection is associated with Burkitt's lymphoma and with nasopharyngeal carcinoma (18).

Severe upper airway obstruction occurs in 1 of every 100 to 1000 cases of EBV infection. It can occur at any age but is more common in young children for anatomic reasons. Airway obstruction is considered an indication for steroid therapy, but the clinician must remain aware of the possibility of a con-current bacterial pharyngitis (19).

Diagnosis

The diagnosis of syndromic acute EBV infection is generally straightforward and is based on typical manifestations as described earlier, the presence of atypical lymphocytosis, and a positive monospot test. Infectious agents that cause syndromes that resemble mononucleosis include adenovirus, CMV, hepatitis A, HHV-6, HIV-1 (in acute infection), rubella virus, and *Toxoplasma* (in acute infection) (19). Medications such as phenytoin and sulfa drugs can also cause symptoms resembling those of IM, including fever and lymphadenopathy (19). Lymphoma and leukemia are sometimes initially mistaken for mononucleosis. A variety of processes can produce "false positive" monospot tests. These include mumps, malaria, rubella, serum sickness, and lymphoma. However, these conditions tend to produce much lower titers of heterophile antibodies than does acute EBV infection (19).

Laboratory Findings

In 70% of cases of IM, a 60% to 70% mononuclear lymphocytosis with a white blood cell count of approximately 15,000 will be seen, thus imparting the name *infectious* mononucleosis to the syndrome (18). Atypical lymphocytes are usually seen, but their numbers can range from almost none to more than 90% of the total lymphocyte count (18). It should be noted that atypical lymphocytes can also be seen in CMV and HIV infections, viral hepatitis, toxoplasmosis, rubella, mumps, roseola, and drug reactions (19). Atypical lymphocytes are large and heterogeneous, and have a vacuolated cytoplasm and lobulated, eccentric nucleus. This is in contrast to the more uniform appearance of lymphoblasts as seen in acute leukemia (Fig. 38.2).

The classic heterophile antibody test is performed by reporting the highest serum dilution capable of agglutinating sheep erythrocytes after adsorption of a test serum by guinea pig kidney. A titer of 40 or greater is strong evidence for IM (18).

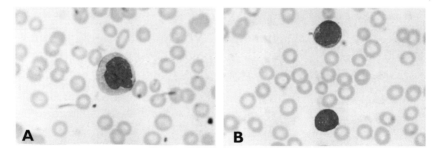

Figure 38.2 An atypical lymphocyte from a patient with infectious mononucleosis (*part A*) compared with lymphoblasts from a patient with acute lymphoblastic leukemia (*part B*). Note the paucity of cytoplasm, the large relatively homogeneous nucleus, and the prominent nucleolus typical of blasts. The atypical lymphocytes have large, lobulated, eccentric nuclei and vacuolated cytoplasm. (Courtesy of Dr. Phyllis Fersky.)

Classic agglutination tests, which took 24 hours to perform, have been modified to create commercially available monospot tests whose sensitivity and specificity are similar to those of agglutination tests even though they can be performed in 2 minutes (19).

The time at which heterophile antibody tests become positive in IM is variable, with pediatric cases tending to develop heterophile antibody positivity later or not at all, whereas most adolescent and young adult cases are heterophile antibody-positive at presentation (18). As a rule of thumb, heterophile antibodies are present in 60% to 70% of patients in the first week of symptoms and in 80% to 90% by the third and fourth weeks. The heterophile antibody usually disappears after 3 months, but can persist for up to a year (19). Overall, rapid monospot kits are estimated to have sensitivities ranging from 63% to 84% and specificities ranging from 84% to 100% (19).

A panel of Epstein-Barr virus-related antibodies is shown in Table 38.2 (23). This sort of analysis should be reserved for situations in which heterophile antibody tests are negative (suspected *monospot-negative mononucleosis*), a definitive diagnosis is critical, the presentation is atypical, and/or the phase of EBV infection must be known (19). The estimated 1997 cost of a monospot test was $16, whereas an EBV panel can cost over $80 (19).

Treatment

Treatment of IM is largely supportive, since 95% of cases recover uneventfully (18). Corticosteroids decrease the period of febrility and hasten the resolution of constitutional symptoms in IM, but should be reserved for severe complications. Indications for their use are impending airway obstruction, severe thrombocytopenia, hemolytic anemia, CNS involvement, myocarditis,

Table 38.2   Serum Epstein-Barr Virus Antibodies as a Function of Infection Status

Infection Status	Anti-VCA IgG	Anti-VCA IgM	Anti-VCA EA	Anti-VCA EBNA
No previous infection	O	O	O	O
Acute infection (0-3 months)	+	+	+/O	O
Recent infection (3-12 months)	+	+/O	+/O	O
Past infection (>12 months)	+	O	O	+

Anti-VCA IgG = IgG class antibody to viral capsid antigen; Anti-VCA IgM = IgM class antibody to viral capsid antigen; EA = early antigen; EBNA = Epstein-Barr nuclear antigen; O = <1:10 (<1:2 for EBNA); + = >1:10 (>1:2 for EBNA).

severe pneumonitis, and pericarditis (18,24). The recommended dosing schedule is 30 to 40 mg of prednisone twice daily, tapered over a period of 1 to 2 weeks (18). Controlled trials of acyclovir in EBV infection have shown decreased viral shedding but no clear-cut clinical benefit (18,25). The use of acyclovir in complicated cases of IM and in patients with malignancies associated with immunocompromise is under investigation.

Prevention

Isolation is not indicated for patients with IM, since the infection is ubiquitous and requires intimate contact for transmission. People with IM should consider abstaining from blood donation for 6 months after acute infection (18).

Cytomegalovirus Infection

A brief discussion of CMV is included here for comparative purposes. However, CMV infection in the immunocompetent host is rarely associated with significant disease, and is thus not usually an issue related to primary-care practice.

Epidemiology

The prevalence of CMV infection varies, depending on the population surveyed, from 40% to 100% (26). People in developing countries and those of lower socioeconomic background tend to have higher prevalence rates. One peak of seroconversion is noted in the perinatal period and the second is noted in the reproductive years. The virus has been isolated from blood, cervical secretions, breast milk, semen, and, particularly in children, urine and respiratory tract secretions (26,27). Seroconversion after blood transfusion and/or transplantation has also been documented, presumably from latent virus stored in leukocytes and other tissues. In contrast to the case with EBV, immunocompetent adults do not routinely shed CMV in throat secretions, blood, respiratory secretions, or urine, but patients who are recovering from an acute systemic illness may shed CMV for several months (26). Women have been noted to carry CMV persistently in cervical secretions, and homosexual men have been noted to carry it persistently in their semen (27).

Horizontal transmission of CMV infection is frequent. In daycare centers, excretion rates of the virus are estimated at 70% (27). Children can pass the virus to each other and to nonimmune adult providers through saliva and urine. Adolescents and young adults can pass the virus through sexual activity and kissing.

Vertical transmission of CMV can occur through transplacental passage of the virus, through contact with the cervix at birth, and postnatally through ingestion of breast milk (27). One percent of live-born infants excrete CMV at birth (27). *In utero* infection can result either from primary maternal infection or through maternal reactivation disease, but serious sequelae are much more likely to be the result of primary maternal infection (27). From 10% to 20% of infants whose *in utero* infections result from primary maternal infection with CMV will have mental retardation or deafness (27). Infection *in utero* seems to be much more dangerous than infection in the birth canal or infection from breast milk, neither of which is likely to be associated with clinical disease (27).

Clinical Manifestations

Congenitally acquired CMV can cause jaundice, hepatosplenomegaly, a petechial rash, CNS malformation, and multiple organ involvement in the affected newborn. The course of this syndrome can be devastating, but its management is beyond the scope of this chapter. Neonatal infection with CMV has been associated with subtle learning disabilities and with interstitial pneumonia (27).

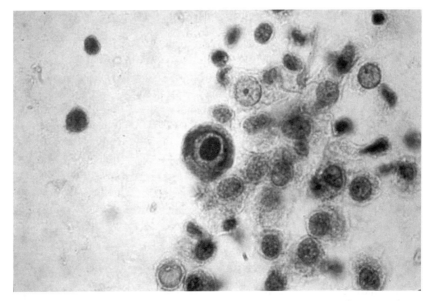

Figure 38.3 A cell with an intranuclear inclusion body, indicating infection with cytomegalovirus. Note the "owl's eye" appearance of the cell. (Courtesy Dr. Robert Salata.)

After the newborn period, CMV tends to cause a mononucleosis-like syndrome. CMV-induced mononucleosis can be clinically hard to distinguish from its EBV-associated counterpart. It is part of the differential diagnosis of monospot-negative mononucleosis. It also can occur postoperatively through the transfusion of blood containing CMV, and is sometimes the cause of late-onset (2-4 weeks) post-operative fevers. The probability of being infected with CMV by a unit of blood is less than 3% (26). Although the syndrome of acute CMV infection is usually benign and self-limiting, a number of complications have been reported. These include interstitial pneumonitis, hepatitis, granulomatous hepatitis, Guillain-Barré syndrome, meningoencephalitis, myocarditis, thrombocytopenia, and hemolytic anemia (26,28).

Diagnosis

Proof of congenital infection with CMV requires obtaining blood specimens within 3 weeks of birth (27). Isolation of CMV in culture and/or a strongly positive CMV IgM titer are considered proof of congenital infection (27).

In adults, culture of CMV from affected organs, detection of virus with the polymerase chain reaction, the presence of CMV-related inclusion bodies in affected cells (Fig. 38.3), and a fourfold increase in anti-CMV antibody titers are all used as evidence of active infection (27).

Prevention

Because of the ubiquitous nature of CMV infection, and because of prolonged viral shedding in the urine of infected children, no specific screening or isolation precautions for the disease have proven feasible. Hand washing and routine hygienic measures are recommended when caring for all children (27). Severely immunosuppressed individuals should be isolated from known cases of CMV infection, and consideration should be given to using CMV-negative blood products (27). At present, no specific guidelines for avoiding CMV infection are available to pregnant women, other than hand washing and good hygiene (27). Intravenous CMV immune globulin has been used with some efficacy in transplant recipients, but has not yet been adequately tested in other populations (27).

Treatment

No standard guidelines are available for treating immunocompetent patients with complications of CMV infection because of the rarity of such cases. Treatment of CMV and other infections in patients with AIDS and in the immuno-compromised host is covered in Chapters 36 and 37, respectively. CMV is resistant to acyclovir, but ganciclovir, foscarnet, and cidofovir all have activity against it. All three drugs have major toxicities associated with them, and their use in treating the immunocompetent individual, even in those rare cases in which serious CMV disease has manifested, has yet to be proven (28).

REFERENCES

1. **Whitley RJ.** Varicella-zoster virus. In Mandell GL, Bennett JE, Dolin R, eds. *Principles and Practice of Infectious Diseases, 4th Ed.* New York: Churchill Livingstone; 1995: 1345–50.

2. **Kost RG, Straus SE.** Postherpetic neuralgia-pathogenesis, treatment, and prevention. *N Engl J Med.* 1996;335:32–42.

3. **Donahue JG, Choo PW, Manson JE, Platt R.** The incidence of herpes zoster. *Arch Intern Med.* 1995;155:1605–9.

4. **Plotkin SA.** Clinical and pathogenetic aspects of varicella-zoster. *Postgrad Med J.* 1985;61(Suppl.4):7–14.

5. **Choo PW, Donahue JG, Manson JE, Platt R.** The epidemiology of varicella and its complications. *J Infect Dis.* 1995;172:706–12.

6. **Barnes DW, Whitley RJ.** CNS diseases associated with varicella zoster virus and herpes simplex virus infection: pathogenesis and current therapy. *Neurol Clin.* 1986;4:265–83.

7. **Haake DA, Zakowski PC, Haake DL, Bryson YJ.** Early treatment with acyclovir for varicella pneumonia in otherwise healthy adults: retrospective controlled study and review. *Rev Infect Dis.* 1990;12:788–98.

8. **Broussard RC, Payne DK, George RB.** Treatment with acyclovir of varicella pneumonia in pregnancy. *Chest.* 1991;99:1045–7.

9. **American Academy of Pediatrics.** Varicella-zoster infections. *1997 Red Book: Report of the Committee on Infectious Diseases,* 27th ed. Elk Grove Village, IL: American Academy of Pediatrics; 1997:573–5.

10. **Wilson GJ, Talkington DF, Gruber W, et al.** Group A streptococcal necrotizing fasciitis following varicella in children: case reports and review. *Clin Infect Dis.* 1995;20:1333–8.

11. **Erlich KS.** Management of herpes simplex and varicella-zoster virus infections. *Western J Med.* 1997;166:211–5.

12. **Coffin SE, Hodinka RL.** Utility of direct immunofluorescence and virus culture for detection of varicella-zoster virus in skin lesions. *J Clin Microbiol.* 1995;33:2792–5.

13. **Wood MJ, Kay R, Dworkin RH, et al.** Oral acyclovir therapy accelerates pain resolution in patients with herpes zoster: a meta-analysis of placebo controlled trials. *Clin Infect Dis.* 1996;22:341–7.

14. **Tyring S, Barbarash RA, Nahlik JE, et al. and the Collaborative Famciclovir Herpes Zoster Study Group.** Famciclovir for the treatment of acute herpes zoster: effects on acute disease and postherpetic neuralgia: a randomized, double-blind controlled trial. *Ann Intern Med.* 1995;123:89–96.

15. **Perry CM, Faulds D.** Valaciclovir. A review of its antiviral activity, pharmacokinetic properties and therapeutic efficacy in herpesvirus infections. *Drugs.* 1996;52:754–72.

16. **Jackson JL, Gibbons R, Meyer G, Inouye L.** The effect of treating herpes zoster with oral acyclovir in preventing postherpetic neuralgia: a meta-analysis. *Arch Intern Med.* 1997;157:909–12.

17. **Centers for Disease Control and Prevention.** Prevention of varicella: recommendations of the Advisory Committee on Immunization Practices. *MMWR Morb Mortal Wkly Rep.*1996;45(RR-11):1–32.

18. **Schooley RT.** Epstein-Barr virus (infectious mononucleosis). In Mandell GL, Bennett JE, Dolin R, eds. *Principles and Practice of Infectious Diseases, 4th Ed.* New York: Churchill Livingstone; 1995:1364–77.

19. **Hickey SM, Strasburger VC.** What every pediatrician should know about infectious mononucleosis in adolescents. *Pediatr Clin North Am.*1997;44:1541–56.

20. **Ablashi DV.** Summary: viral studies of chronic fatigue syndrome. *Clin Infect Dis.* 1994;18(Suppl 1):S130–3.

21. **Bell DS.** Chronic fatigue syndrome update. *Postgrad Med.* 1994;96:73–81.

22. **Penman HG.** Fatal infectious mononucleosis: a critical review. *J Clin Pathol.* 1970;23:765–71.

23. **American Academy of Pediatrics.** Epstein-Barr virus infections (infectious mononucleosis). *1997 Red Book: Report of the Committee on Infectious Diseases, 27th Ed.* Elk Grove Village, IL: American Academy of Pediatrics; 1997:199–201.

24. **Haller A, VonSegesser L, Baumann PC, Krause M.** Severe respiratory insufficiency complicating Epstein-Barr virus infection: case report and review. *Clin Infect Dis.* 1995;21:206–9.

25. **Andersson J, Ernberg I.** Management of Epstein-Barr virus infection. *Am J Med.* 1988;85(Suppl 2a):107–15.

26. **Ho M.** Cytomegalovirus. In Mandell GL, Bennett JE, Dolin R, eds. *Principles and Practice of Infectious Diseases, 4th Ed.* New York: Churchill Livingstone; 1995:1351–64.

27. **American Academy of Pediatrics.** Cytomegalovirus infection. *1997 Red Book: Report of the Committee on Infectious Diseases, 27th Ed.* Elk Grove Village, IL: American Academy of Pediatrics; 1997:187–91.

28. **Eddleston M, Peacock S, Warrell DA.** Severe cytomegalovirus infection in immunocompetent patients. *Clin Infect Dis.* 1997;24:52–6.

39

Lyme Disease

Sharon B. Weissman, MD

Kathleen T. Jordan, MD

Definition and Etiology

Lyme disease is a multisystem illness caused by the spirochete *Borrelia burgdorferi*. The disease usually manifests as an expanding skin lesion, erythema migrans (EM), accompanied by symptoms that resemble those of a viral disease. Within several days to weeks, the spirochete spreads hematogenously to many different sites, resulting in protean manifestations of disease that include secondary rashes, fatigue, musculoskeletal aches, arthralgias, and meningismus. Organs involved include the skin and the musculoskeletal, cardiac, and nervous systems. Untreated Lyme disease can resolve without sequelae but, in most patients, progresses to cause intermittent or chronic arthritis and occasionally chronic neurological or cardiac manifestations. To assist with epidemiologic surveys, the Centers for Disease Control and Prevention (CDC) has established a case definition of Lyme disease (Table 39.1), which can be useful to the clinician making treatment decisions (1).

Lyme disease was first described in 1975 after a number of children with oligoarticular arthritis was reported in three Connecticut towns, including Old Lyme, Connecticut, from which the disease gets its name (2). Decades before Steere and coworkers (2) first described this epidemic, a similar syndrome had been recognized in Europe. In the European syndrome, the EM rash was attributed to the bite of the tick *Ixodes ricinus* (3). Recognition of the relationship between the arthritis and the characteristic EM rash linked the U.S. illness to the disease seen in Europe, and a tick-borne vector was sought. *B. burgdorferi,*

**Table 39.1   Centers for Disease Control and Prevention's Case
Definition of Lyme Disease**

Clinical Case Definition

Erythema migrans (EM) or at least one late manifestation and laboratory confirmation of
infection

Laboratory Criteria

Isolation of *Borrelia burgdorferi* from a clinical specimen

or

Demonstration of diagnostic immunoglobulin (Ig)M or IgG antibodies to *B. burgdorferi* in
serum or cerebrospinal fluid (CSF); a two-step approach using a sensitive enzyme immunoassay or immunofluorescence antibody followed by Western blot is recommended

Clinical Criteria

Erythema Migrans

Defined as a skin lesion that typically begins as a red macule or papule and expands over a
period of days to weeks to form a large round lesion, often with partial central clearing. A
single primary lesion must reach ≥5 cm in size. Secondary lesions also may occur. Annular
erythematous lesions occurring within several hours of a tick bite represent hypersensitivity reactions and do not qualify as EM. (EM does not require serological confirmation).

Late Manifestations

Musculoskeletal System

Recurrent, brief attacks (weeks or months) of objective joint swelling in one or a few
joints, sometimes followed by chronic arthritis in one or a few joints. Manifestation
not considered as criteria for diagnosis include symmetrical polyarthritis. Additionally,
arthralgia, myalgia, or fibromyalgia syndromes alone are not criteria for musculoskeletal involvement

Nervous System

Any of the following, alone or in combination: lymphocytic meningitis; cranial neuritis,
particularly facial palsy (may be bilateral); radiculoneuropathy; or, rarely, encephalomyelitis. Encephalomyelitis must be confirmed by demonstration of antibody production against *B. burgdorferi* in the CSF, evidenced by a higher titer antibody in CSF
than in serum. Headache, fatigue, paresthesia, or mild stiff neck alone are not criteria
for neurologic involvement.

Cardiovascular System

Acute onset of high-grade (second or third degree) atrioventricular conduction defects
that resolve in days to weeks and are sometimes associated with myocarditis.
Palpitations, bradycardia, bundle branch block, or myocarditis alone are not criteria for
cardiovascular involvement.

Exposure

Defined as having been in wooded, brushy, or grassy areas in a county in which Lyme
disease is endemic within 30 days of onset of erythema migrans. A history of tick bite is
not required.

Endemic Area

A county in which at least two confirmed cases of Lyme disease have been previously
acquired or in which established populations of a known tick vector are infected with
B. burgdorferi.

the spirochete responsible for Lyme disease, was first isolated in 1982 (4). This discovery definitively linked the American and European illnesses (3).

The vectors of Lyme borreliosis are the deer ticks known as *I. scapularis* (previously named *Ixodes dammini*) in the Northeast and Midwest United States and *I. pacificus* on the West Coast (5–7). In Europe, *I. ricinus* is the primary vector (3). The immature nymph stage of the tick is primarily responsible for transmitting the spirochete; however, all stages of the tick can be infected with the spirochete and can feed on humans (8). The tick needs to be attached for at least 24 hours for transmission of the spirochete (9–11). Nymphs of the tick feed primarily on the white-footed mouse, and the adult tick feeds on the white-tailed deer. These animals are important for maintaining the life cycle of the tick and, thus, that of the Lyme spirochete (12).

The clinical picture of an intermittent, chronic monoarticular or oligoarticular arthritis (usually of large joints, such as the knee) in an area endemic for Lyme disease has remained the classic clinical presentation of the disease; however, this represents only a small percentage of cases in the broad spectrum of Lyme disease. Since the 1970s, the typical course and variety of manifestations have been better elucidated, including classifications of *early* and *late* disease.

Although much has been learned about Lyme disease in the past two decades, there remains a significant amount of confusion about the disease among patients as well as physicians. Probably the most widely held misconception about Lyme disease is that it is difficult to treat and always results in chronic symptoms and recurrences. Several studies have shown that children and adults with a history of Lyme disease have a higher incidence of arthralgias and memory impairment (13–16), but other studies have not shown evidence of long-term sequelae (17,18). The discrepancy between these results may be due to differences in the stage of Lyme disease when the diagnosis was made and treatment begun. The disease seldom has long-term sequelae when treated in its early stages, whereas treatment after a prolonged course of illness may be followed by residual impairments (13).

Epidemiology

Lyme disease has become the most common tick-borne illness in the United States (5). It has been reported in all 48 states in the continental United States, as well as in Europe, Australia, China, and Japan. In 1996, 16,455 cases of Lyme disease were reported to the CDC, a 41% increase from 1995 (Fig. 39.1). The overall incidence of Lyme disease in 1996 was of 6.2 cases per 100,000 population. Ninety-one percent of these cases were reported from eight states: Connecticut, Rhode Island, New York, New Jersey, Delaware, Pennsylvania, Maryland, and Wisconsin (19) (Fig. 39.2).

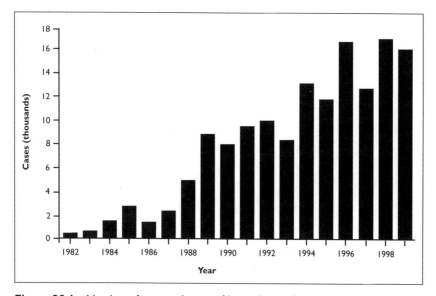

Figure 39.1   Number of reported cases of Lyme disease by year in the United States from 1982 to 1999. (Adapted from Lyme disease—United States, 1999. *MMWR Morb Mortal Wkly Rep.* 2001;50:181-5.)

Since January 1991, Lyme disease has been a reportable disease. The CDC case definition is required for reporting purposes (*see* Table 39.1). A definitive diagnosis of Lyme disease is often difficult to make. In addition, many definitive cases go unreported, with the result that the reported incidence and prevalence of Lyme disease are likely to be underestimates (20).

Lyme disease is most prevalent in areas with significant populations of white-tailed deer and the deer tick vectors *Ixodes scapularis* and *Ixodes pacificus*, with the highest prevalence across the Northeastern United States, extending from Maine to Maryland. (Fig. 39.3). Other endemic areas include the upper Midwest (Wisconsin), northern California, and the southeastern United States (19).

In New England and the upper Midwest, Lyme-disease borreliosis usually occurs during the during the summer months, when the tick population, and particularly the nymph form of the tick, is at its peak. Less commonly, adult ticks can transmit disease when they feed during the fall. In California and the Pacific Northwest, infection is more common between January and May. Both early and late disease have been reported throughout the year (21).

Approximately 15% to 30% of the *I. scapularis* nymphs in New England are infected with *B. burgdorferi* (22,23). In some hyperendemic areas, such as Shelter Island, New York, more than 60% of ticks are infected (4). The reforesta-

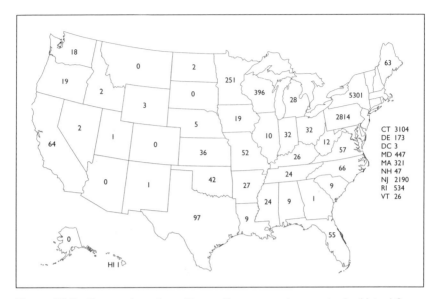

Figure 39.2   Reported number of Lyme disease cases by state in the United States during 1996. (Courtesy of the Centers for Disease Control and Prevention.)

tion of lands across the United States, and the increasing population of white-tailed deer in the Midwest and South, are likely to increase and change the distribution of Lyme disease across the United States (12).

Clinical Manifestations

Lyme disease is a multisystem disease that has both early and late manifestations. Early localized infection (also referred to as Stage 1 EM), begins shortly after a bite by one of the species of *Ixodes* that are vectors for the disease, with an expanding annular erythematous lesion starting from the site of the bite. The rash is often accompanied by nonspecific flu-like symptoms (24). Because the nymph of the *Ixodes* tick is small, the tick bite often goes unnoticed (Fig. 39.4). Furthermore, the classic rash is seen in only 60% to 80% of patients (25,26). Early dissemination (also referred to as Stage 2 EM) begins days to weeks after EM, at which time the Lyme disease spirochete is hematogenously spread to many sites in the body. Secondary EM lesions can develop on the skin, and fevers, myalgias, migratory arthralgias, headaches, and fatigue are common. Early dissemination can result in mild symptoms or a more profound presentation with cranial nerve palsies, heart block, and meningitis. Often, symptoms will ease or resolve with time even in cases of

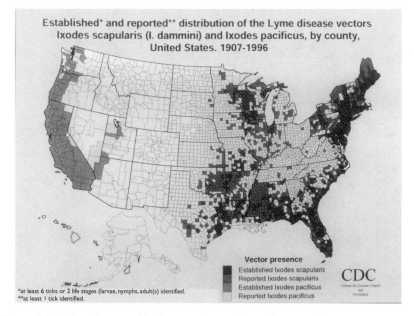

Figure 39.3   Distribution of *Ixodes scapularis* and *I. pacificus* ticks from 1907 to 1996. (Courtesy of the Centers for Disease Control and Prevention.)

untreated infection. However, Lyme disease can progress and present with late manifestations if the infection is left untreated (3). Late or persistent infection (also referred to as Stage 3 EM) begins from months to years after the initial infection. Late manifestations include a variety of nonspecific symptoms of arthritis, myalgias, memory impairment, and fatigue. Arthralgias can progress to joint swelling, with waxing and waning effusions without erosive arthritis, but approximately 60% of untreated patients eventually develop frank arthritis (27). Chronic neurological infection can result in chronic radiculopathies or in subtle encephalopathy with mild confusion, memory impairment, and mood changes. Rarely, more severe neurological sequelae occur (14,28). These late manifestations probably offer the most difficult diagnostic challenge, since they are variable and overlap with an array of clinical syndromes such as depression, chronic fatigue syndrome, rheumatoid arthritis, and syphilis (29,30).

Although attempts have been made to characterize different *stages* of Lyme infection, there is significant variation in the individual course of disease. Some individuals present only with later manifestations, whereas others never develop effects beyond the early manifestations of disease.

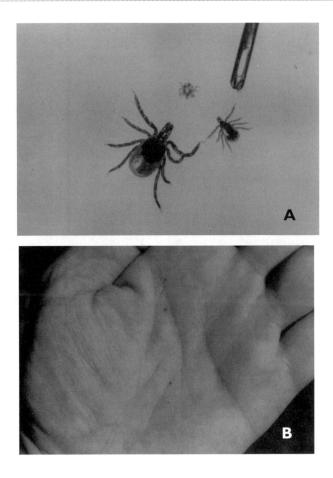

Figure 39.4   A, The three stages of the deer tick *Ixodes scapularis* (clockwise from the top): larvae, nymph, and mature adult compared in size with the head of a needle. **B,** Two nymphal ticks in the palm of a human hand. (Courtesy of the American Lyme Disease Foundation.)

Dermatologic Manifestations

The hallmark rash of Lyme disease is EM, also called erythema chronicum migrans (Fig. 39.5). It occurs in 60% to 80% of patients with Lyme disease (25,26), beginning as an erythematous macule or papule that enlarges centrifugally to roughly 15 cm. The rash is warm but painless. The center of the lesion sometimes becomes crusted and necrotic (25,26). The rash develops

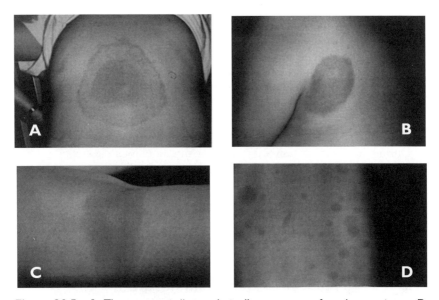

Figure 39.5   A, The concentric "target lesion" appearance of erythema migrans. **B,** Central clearing begins to appear on erythema migrans in the axilla. **C,** The rash as a single erythematous patch behind the knee. **D,** Erythema migrans as multicentric erythematous macules. (*Parts A* and *B* republished with permission from Barbour A, Fish D. *The Biological and Social Phenomenon of Lyme Disease,* vol 260. Washington, DC: American Association for the Advancement of Science; 1993:1610-6. *Part C* courtesy of Dr. D. Fish. *Part D* courtesy of Dr. A. MacDonald.)

from days to 1 month after a tick bite (median: 7–10 days) (25,26,31). An erythematous rash with swelling that occurs within hours of a bite is more likely to be due to a hypersensitivity reaction to a bite than to EM from Lyme infection. The classic central clearing that is described for EM occurs later, as the lesion expands. Only 37% of lesions present for less than 1 to 2 weeks have central clearing (25). The EM rash fades, without treatment, within a median of 1 month (31).

A history of outdoor activities, in a community endemic for Lyme disease and from 1 to 4 weeks before a rash typical of the disease, suggests the existence of EM. A history of a tick bite is seldom obtained, since the nymph of the tick is hard to see. Furthermore, transmission is most likely to result when the tick can remain attached to the skin and feed for days without being noticed. Bites and EM rashes often occur in poorly visualized areas of the body such as the popliteal fossa, buttocks, axillae, back, or groin (26). The absence of EM does not exclude Lyme disease.

The differential diagnosis of EM includes hypersensitivity reactions to insect bites (such as the common mosquito bite), tinea corporis (ringworm), urticaria, erythema multiforme, and cutaneous lupus erythematosus (Table 39.2). Contact dermatitis from plants such as poison ivy or sumac should also be considered in people returning from wooded areas, but this is usually intensely pruritic, distinguishing it from EM. The most distinguishing characteristic of EM is its association with systemic complaints of fatigue (54%), myalgia (44%), arthralgia (44%), headache (42%), or fever and chills (39%) (24).

During the dissemination phase of Lyme infection, multiple secondary EM lesions may appear. These secondary lesions resemble the initial lesion but are smaller, less erythematous, and do not expand (26). In Europe, a late skin manifestation of Lyme disease has been described. The lesion in this condition, named *acrodermatitis chronica atrophicans*, is a violaceous patch that becomes sclerotic. *B. burgdorferi* has been cultured from these lesions (3).

Musculoskeletal Manifestations

Early in the clinical phase of Lyme disease, migratory arthralgias and myalgias are common. Pain usually affects one or two joints in an asymmetric pattern. Symptoms are intermittent, lasting a few hours to days. Rarely, myositis occurs, with increases in muscle enzymes (32). Chronic arthritis is uncommon when treatment is initiated in early disease (17,18).

During later stages of clinically manifest Lyme disease, joint involvement can progress to joint swelling and frank arthritis. The typical pattern for late disease consists of intermittent attacks of oligoarthritis, particularly in large joints such as the knees. Attacks can last weeks to months, with episodes becoming longer in the second or third year of illness. Joints are swollen and hot but rarely red. Synovial fluid will contain from 500 to 110,000 white cells per cubic millimeter, with a predominance of polymorphonuclear cells (3). The Lyme spirochete is rarely cultured from joint fluid (33). In severe cases, arthritis can lead to erosions of cartilage and bone.

In a study of 55 patients with untreated Lyme disease, 20% had no further symptoms, 18% had brief periods of joint pain, 51% had intermittent attacks of arthritis, and 11% developed chronic synovitis with erosions and joint deformities. The incidence of Lyme arthritis declines with each year of illness (27), and some patients cease to have arthritic symptoms after the first few years of illness. It is believed that the host immunologic response to the Lyme disease spirochete accounts for these differences in disease course. There is evidence that people with more chronic arthritis have a more vigorous immune response with higher titers of IgG and IgM antibodies (16).

Table 39.2   Differential Diagnosis of Erythema Migrans

	Erythema Migrans of Lyme Disease	Insect Bite Hypersensitivity Reaction	Tinea corporis "Ringworm"	Urticaria	Erythema Multiforme	Subacute Cutaneous Lupus Erythematosus
Pruritis	None or mild	Intense	Often, mild	Intense	Sometimes	None
Rash distribution	Anywhere (commonly on thighs, groin, or axilla)	Exposed surfaces	Anywhere	Anywhere	Anywhere	Sun-exposed areas
Rash appearance	Erythematous, rapidly enlarging lesion; expands to 3–68 cm (median diameter 15 cm)	Papular ± central punctum	Scaly papule or plaque	Edematous papules or plaques	Targetoid; bullous lesions	Scaly annular or psoriasiform
Central clearing	Usual (more common if lesion is several weeks old)	Never	Usual	Sometimes	Sometimes	Sometimes
Rash duration	5–6 weeks	Days to weeks	Weeks to months	Fleeting (lasts <24 hours)	1–3 weeks	Chronic
Associated illness or symptoms	Fatigue, myalgias, arthralgias, fever	None	None	Angioedema	Infections (especially HSV)	Systemic lupus erythematosus
Diagnostic test	Serology or culture of B. burgdorferi from leading edge of rash	Clinical or biopsy	KOH scraping of leading edge of rash	None	Skin biopsy	Skin biopsy; SS-A(Ro) and SS-B(La) antibodies
Treatment	Oral antibiotics	Antihistamines, topical steroids	Antifungals	Antihistamine	Treat infection or remove inciting drug	Antimalarials; sunscreen

HSV = herpes simplex virus; KOH = potassium hydroxide; SS-A = Sjörgen's syndrome A; SS-B = Sjörgen's syndrome B.

Neurological Manifestations

The nervous system tends to be affected early in Lyme disease. Symptoms of headache, neck pain, and neck stiffness can occur while EM is present. The symptoms are intermittent, with a fluctuating intensity. The headaches can be excruciating, and episodes of headaches and neck pain may last for hours. In the first weeks of illness, a cerebrospinal fluid (CSF) pleocytosis and objective neurological deficits are often missing (3); however, as the disease progresses, objective laboratory and clinical findings of neurological involvement may appear (28,34).

Subtle encephalitis with symptoms of forgetfulness, sleep disturbances, irritability or emotional lability (28,34), and aseptic meningitis are common during the second stage of Lyme disease, with 15% of untreated patients developing aseptic meningitis. Symptoms are often indolent, with waxing and waning headaches, fatigue, and neck stiffness. With early treatment, these subtle neurological symptoms should be less frequent (14,17,35). When neurological symptoms are present, the CSF is abnormal, with a lymphocytic pleocytosis (~100 cells/mm^3) and mildly increased protein concentration (34,36). CSF assays for antibodies to *B. burgdorferi* are positive (3), but the organism has only rarely been cultured from CSF (37). The CSF pleocytosis disappears quickly with antimicrobial therapy, and persistent pleocytosis suggests a diagnosis other than Lyme disease (34,36).

Cranial neuritis, and especially facial nerve (Bell's) palsy, is the most common and earliest clinical manifestation of nervous system invasion by *B. burgdorferi*. Cranial neuritis may present concomitantly with EM or a few months after the rash resolves (35), and usually occurs simultaneously with meningitis or peripheral radiculopathies. A small number of patients will have bilateral facial nerve palsy. Cranial nerves III, IV, and VI are the next most frequently involved cranial nerves (28). In the European variant of Lyme disease, a syndrome of chronic aching, radicular pain (especially in the shoulders and back) with CSF pleocytosis (Bannwarth's syndrome) is a common neurological manifestation (28).

Late neurological manifestations of Lyme disease are rare but can be severe. There have been reports of severe encephalomyelitis, with demyelination (mimicking multiple sclerosis) and progressive dementia. This rare complication occurs in less than 0.1% of patients (28,38).

Cardiac Manifestations

Cardiac abnormalities occur in 4% to 10% of untreated patients with Lyme disease (39), and may be observed at any stage of disease or as a sole manifestation of Lyme disease. Cardiac manifestations include pericarditis, pancarditis, and conduction abnormalities. Valvular damage does not occur (40). The most common cardiac abnormality is conduction system delay, particularly in the atrioventricular node, resulting in first-degree to complete heart block. A temporary pacemaker may be needed when complete heart block develops. However, a permanent pacemaker is not required because of the self-limited nature of the blocks (41). There are reports of patients with Lyme disease developing acute myocarditis, left ventricular dysfunction, cardiomegaly, and rarely fatal pancarditis (42–44). Carditis is usually mild, rarely causing any significant myocardial damage (40). Myocardial biopsy reveals a lymphocytic infiltration, and the Lyme spirochete has been isolated from myocardium (43,45). In treated Lyme disease, persistent cardiac abnormalities are unlikely (46).

Ocular Manifestations

Ocular manifestations of Lyme disease are rare. The most common is a neurotrophic keratitis caused by seventh cranial nerve (Bell's) palsy (34). A nonspecific follicular conjunctivitis has been reported in up to 10% of patients during early Lyme disease (47). *B. burgdorferi* has been isolated from the vitreous and the iris in patients with vitritis or uveitis. Lyme disease is a rare cause of optic neuritis and interstitial keratitis (47).

Congenital Infection

Transplacental transmission of *B. burgdorferi* has been reported in three infants whose mothers had Lyme disease during pregnancy. All three of the mothers acquired the disease during the first trimester, and the infants in all three cases died within the first 5 days of life. Two of the infants had cardiac abnormalities and the third had cerebral edema. Spirochetes were seen in multiple organs in autopsy specimens (48–50). In one retrospective study of 19 women with Lyme disease during pregnancy, there seemed to be an association between maternal Lyme disease and adverse pregnancy outcomes (51). This association has not been confirmed in larger prospective studies (52,53), although maternal infection may be associated with a slightly increased risk of spontaneous abortion (54). Because transplacental transmission of *B. burgdorferi* seems to be rare, routine serologic testing of pregnant women is not indicated.

Chronic Lyme Disease

A widely held misconception, both in the lay and medical community, is that Lyme disease is commonly a chronic, incurable condition resulting in lifelong physical and psychological impairments. This belief has led to misdiagnosis and overtreatment of Lyme disease (18,55). Part of the reason for the mistaken belief in the incurability of Lyme disease is that approximately one fourth of patients with both early and late features of the disease do not have immediate resolution of symptoms with treatment. Often, symptoms do not resolve until weeks or months after treatment is completed (55). The first studies of Lyme disease described myriad chronic symptoms. Most of these earlier reports were of patients in whom Lyme disease was diagnosed before appropriate treatment was defined. These patients often had not received prompt or optimal antimicrobial therapy. Those patients who received early treatment, before chronic symptoms developed were much less likely to have persistent problems. It is now clear that early treatment of Lyme disease reduces the incidence of chronic symptoms (13,17,18).

Nevertheless, persistent symptoms can occur in some patients with Lyme disease. This is rarely due to an ongoing active infection (30,31); it is usually due to an advanced stage of disease at the time of diagnosis and treatment, an inflammatory response to dead organisms, or permanent tissue damage. Other possible causes of persistent symptoms include inadequate treatment, an inadequate period for resolution of symptoms, and chronic problems unrelated to Lyme disease (Table 39.3). Further antimicrobial therapy does not hasten recovery except in the rare person who has a truly ongoing active infection (30,31).

Diagnosis

The diagnosis of Lyme disease should be based on characteristic clinical findings in a person from an endemic area. Serologic tests can confirm a diagnosis, but should not be used as the sole basis for making a diagnosis of Lyme

---

Table 39.3   Questions To Consider When Searching for Possible Causes of Persistent Symptoms After Lyme Disease Treatment

- Is the diagnosis of Lyme disease correct?
- Did the patient complete an adequate course of antibiotics? If so, was the patient compliant?
- Are chronic problems unrelated to Lyme disease contributing to the symptoms (e.g., fibromyalgia, sleep disorders, depression or anxiety)?
- Is there evidence of an active, ongoing infection?
- Has there been adequate time between the diagnosis and treatment of Lyme disease and the current presentation to expect a resolution of symptoms (up to 2 years for neuropathies)?
- Is this consistent with a post–Lyme disease immune reaction?

Republished with permission from Sigal LH. Persisting complaints attributed to chronic Lyme disease: possible mechanisms and implications for management. Am J Med. 1994;96:365–374.

disease. Several laboratory tests are available to aid in the diagnosis of Lyme disease (3,8). However, none of these tests is highly accurate, and all are liable to false-positive and false-negative results (Table 39.4). Furthermore, inter-laboratory and intra-laboratory reliability of these tests is poor, and standardization for the tests has not been developed (56–59).

The use of serologic tests for the diagnosis of Lyme disease has recently been extensively reviewed (59). The American College of Physicians has developed guidelines for the use of laboratory evaluation in diagnosing Lyme disease (Table 39.5). These guidelines can help the clinician with treatment and testing decisions.

Table 39.4 Diagnostic Laboratory Studies for Lyme Disease

Test	Test Specimen	Advantages	Disadvantages
Culture	Serum, skin aspirate, synovial fluid, CSF, biopsy specimen	100% specific; distinguishes live from dead spirochetes (33,36a,42,44,47,48,49)	Rarely positive except when cultures are taken from the perimeter of an EM lesion; not available in most laboratories (24,58,59)
ELISA (IgG)	Serum, CSF	In experienced laboratories, sensitivity approaches 100% (range 40%–100%) (57,58); a CSF:serum ratio of >1 is useful for diagnosing neurological involvement (8,58)	Significant intra- and interlaboratory variability exists (57,58); false-negative results are possible in early disease when EM lesions are present; false-positive results are common (see text); IgG remains positive after treatment, so ELISA can not distinguish between previous and active infections (3,21,55–58,60)
ELISA (IgM)	Serum, CSF	May be positive in early disease with EM when tests for IgG antibodies are still negative (8)	Only transiently elevated in early disease (8)
IFA	Serum	Similar sensitivity and specificity as ELISA (58)	More difficult to automate and interpret than ELISA (58)
Western blot (IgG or IgM)	Serum	More specific than ELISA; useful as a confirmatory test especially when ELISA results are indeterminate (58)	Similar to ELISA but with better specificity; thus, fewer false-positive results (58)
PCR	Serum, CSF, synovial fluid	Specificity approaches 100% (58,61a,61b)	Costly; investigational; *Boriella burgdorferi* is present only transiently in the bloodstream 2 weeks after the tick bite, so PCR is usually negative by the time the patient presents for evaluation; sensitivity is only 25%–35%; it can not distinguish between live and dead organisms (58,61a,61b,62,63)

CSF = cerebrospinal fluid; ELISA = enzyme-linked immunosorbent assay; EM = erythema migrans; IFA = immunofluorescence assay; IgG = immunoglobulin G; IgM = immunoglobulin M; PCR = polymerase chain reaction.

Table 39.5   American College of Physicians–American Society of Internal Medicine's Guidelines for the Use of Serologic Testing in Suspected Lyme Disease

Pretest Probability of Lyme Disease*	Testing	Interpretation
Low pretest probability (<0.2)[†]	Serologic testing for Lyme disease not recommended	If ELISA is performed, a positive result is likely to be falsely positive and does not warrant treatment; a negative result confirms that Lyme disease is not present.
Intermediate pretest probability (0.2–0.8)[‡]	Two-test protocol: ELISA (or IFA) followed by Western blot on specimens with indeterminate ELISA results.	A positive result increases the probability of disease sufficiently to warrant antibiotic treatment; a negative result sufficiently reduces the probability of disease to warrant investigations for other causes of the symptoms.
High pretest probability (>0.8)[§]	Empirical treatment without serologic testing is recommended	If ELISA is performed, a positive result increases the likelihood of disease; a negative result reduces the probability of disease only by a small increment; because the patient is still likely to have the disease, empirical treatment is recommended.

ELISA = enzyme-linked immunosorbent assay; IFA = immunofluorescence assay.

* Probability should be based on clinical findings and a knowledge of the incidence of Lyme disease in the population.

[†] Patients who present with nonspecific complaints (e.g., arthralgias, myalgias, headaches, fatigue, palpitations) without objective signs of Lyme disease; even in areas endemic for Lyme disease, the pretest probability for patients who present with nonspecific symptoms is <0.2.

[‡] Patients who present with a vague history of a rash, no history of a tick bite, and recurrent attacks of joint swelling from an area moderately endemic for Lyme disease.

[§] Patients who present with an erythema migrans rash (or a history of a rash) or arthritis and a previous tick bite from an area in which Lyme disease is endemic.

Republished with permission from Craven RB, Quan TJ, Bailey RE, et al. Improved serodiagnostic testing for Lyme disease: results of a multicenter serologic evaluation. *Emerg Infect Dis.* 1996;2:136–40.

Culture

The Lyme spirochete has been isolated from many different clinical specimens (33,37,43,45,48–50), but its isolation is rarely successful except when cultures are taken from the perimeter of an EM lesion. The organism grows readily in Barbour-Stoenner-Kelly medium, yielding positive results in 60% to 80% of patients when aspirates are taken from EM lesions (24,60). Attempts to culture the organism from other specimens are not usually successful. Unfortunately, Barbour-Stoenner-Kelly medium is not commercially available. Furthermore, the EM rash does not usually pose a diagnostic dilemma that requires further testing (59).

Enzyme-Linked Immunosorbent Assay, Indirect Immunofluorescence Assay, Western Blot, and Polymerase Chain Reaction

More than 20 commercially available serologic tests are available for diagnosing Lyme disease. There is great variability in the accuracy, reliability, and precision of these tests (58). The sensitivity and specificity of the enzyme-linked immunosorbent assay (ELISA) vary from 40% to 100% and 71% to 99.5%, respectively (58,59). Sensitivity of the assay is lowest early in Lyme disease, and increases in patients with late disease (3). Even with the best ELISA kit there are often false-negative and false-positive results. Early in Lyme disease, when EM is present, antibodies to the Lyme spirochete may not have developed, thus yielding negative serologic results (3,21,59). In areas endemic for the disease, seroprevalence for Lyme spirochetes can reach 8% in an asymptomatic population (61,62). Without a high degree of clinical suspicion for Lyme disease, serologic testing is more likely to yield a false-positive than a true-positive result (*see* Table 39.4) (59). Furthermore, false-positive results can occur in cases of syphilis, autoimmune disorders, or infectious mononucleosis. A positive Venereal Disease Research Laboratory test distinguishes syphilis from Lyme disease (3).

Because IgG antibodies to the Lyme spirochete remain present long after treatment, serology cannot distinguish inactive from active disease (61). Tests for IgM antibodies to the Lyme spirochete done with an ELISA may identify early infection, but the IgM antibodies are short lived, and the tests for IgM are even less accurate than those for IgG (8). A CSF/serum antibody ratio has been investigated as a method for diagnosing neurological involvement by Lyme disease. This method has not been well standardized, and is likely to have a low yield (8,59) The indirect immunofluorescence assay has a sensitivity and specificity similar to those of the ELISA, but is more difficult to automate and interpret. Moreover, the immunofluorescence assay is subject to the same limitations as the ELISA (59). A Western Blot can detect multiple antibodies to *B. burgdorferi*. It is best used to clarify indeterminate ELISA results or to confirm positive ELISA results (59).

The polymerase chain reaction (PCR) can be used to detect DNA from a small number of *B. burgdorferi* organisms. PCR has been used to detect spirochetes in blood, skin tissue, joint fluid, urine, and CSF. The specificity of PCR for *B. burgdorferi* DNA approaches 100% (59,63,64). However, because PCR cannot distinguish DNA from dead as opposed to live organisms, a positive PCR result does not necessarily indicate active infection (65). Furthermore, the sensitivity of PCR with synovial fluid or CSF used as a specimen is low (25%–35%) (59,63,64). PCR is therefore still under investigation for use in Lyme disease (66).

Treatment

A variety of antimicrobial agents are effective for treating Lyme disease. The duration and dosing of treatment depends on the stage and severity of the disease (Table 39.6) (66–68).

Table 39.6   Antibiotic Treatment Options for Lyme Disease*

Erythema Migrans
   Doxycycline 100 mg PO bid for 14–21 days[†]
   Tetracycline 250 mg PO qid for 14–21 days[†]
   Amoxicillin 500 mg PO tid for 14–21 days
   Cefuroxime axetil 500 mg PO bid for 14–21 days
   Erythromycin 250 mg PO qid for 14–21 days[‡]
   Azithromycin 500 mg PO on first day, then 250 mg PO qd for 4 days[‡]

Arthritis
   Mild
   Doxycycline 100 mg PO bid for 28 days[†]
   Amoxicillin 500 mg PO tid for 28 days
   Cefuroxime axetil 500 mg PO bid for 28 days
   Erythromycin 250 mg PO qid for 28 days[‡]

   Severe
   Ceftriaxone 2 gm/day for IV14 –28 days
   Penicillin G 20–24 MU IV qd for 14–28 days

Neurological Disease
   Facial Nerve Palsy
   Doxycycline 100 mg PO bid for 21–28 days[†]
   Amoxicillin 500 mg PO tid for 21–28 days
   Cefuroxime axetil 500 mg PO bid for 21–28 days
   Erythromycin 250 mg PO qid for 21–28 days[‡]

   Severe Neurological Disease
   Ceftriaxone 2 g IVqd for 14–28 days
   Cefotaxime 2 g IV q8h for 14–28 days
   Penicillin G 20–24 MU IV qd for 14–28 days

Carditis
   Mild
   Doxycycline 100 mg PO bid for 14–28 days[†]
   Amoxicillin 500 mg PO tid for 14–28 days
   Cefuroxime axetil 500 mg PO bid for 14–28 days
   Erythromycin 250 mg PO qid for 14–28 days[‡]

   Severe
   Ceftriaxone 2 g IV qd for 14–21 days
   Penicillin G 20–24 MU IV qd for 14–21 days

IV = intravenously; MU = million units; PO = orally
* Reduce dose for children
[†] Do not use in children <9 years or pregnant or lactating women.
[‡] For patients with severe penicillin allergy. May be less effective than other regimens
Republished with permission from references 63, 64, and 66.

For early localized infection limited to EM, a 14-day course of oral antimicrobial therapy with doxycycline at 100 mg twice daily, amoxicillin at 500 mg thrice daily, or cefuroxime axetil at 500 mg twice daily is effective. Erythromycin (or azithromycin) is an option for young children or pregnant women (in whom doxycycline is contraindicated) with severe penicillin allergies, but these agents may be less effective (66,69). The addition of probenecid to amoxicillin may increase the effectiveness of the latter drug by increasing its serum levels. When systemic symptoms are present, the duration of treatment should be extended to 3 weeks (66–68). Early treatment is nearly 100% effective at clearing EM lesions and preventing major late sequelae, but approximately 15% of patients will have prolonged fatigue and arthralgias, which can last up to 3 months (17,18,68).

Optimal treatment of severe Lyme arthritis, carditis, or meningitis requires intravenous antimicrobial therapy. Intravenous ceftriaxone at 2 g/d, or penicillin at 20 to 24 MU/d for 14 to 28 days, is recommended. When neurological involvement is limited to facial palsy, a trial of oral therapy with doxycycline at 100 mg twice daily or amoxicillin at 500 mg thrice daily for 3 to 4 weeks can be attempted. Likewise, mild carditis and arthritis can be treated with oral therapy (8,66,67). Approximately 15% of patients will develop a self-limited Jarisch-Herxheimer reaction, with increased fevers, chills, and myalgias on initiation of therapy (3,8,67).

Symptoms of Lyme disease may persist despite adequate antimicrobial therapy. This is especially common when treatment is begun later in the disease or when more severe symptoms are present. Prolonged or repeated antimicrobial therapy is not indicated. Instead, one should consider alternative reasons for persistent symptoms (*see* Table 39.3) (8,30,55,66).

Prevention

Tick avoidance is the best way to prevent Lyme disease. This can be done by applying insect repellent, particularly a repellant containing *N*-diethyl-m-toluamide (DEET), to exposed skin, and wearing long pants tucked into socks to prevent contact with the tick vector. In addition, since the Lyme disease tick requires more than 24 hours of attachment to the skin to transmit spirochetes, daily skin inspection with removal of ticks reduces the risk of disease. Large-scale insecticide applications in mid-May in geographic areas with significant tick populations can reduce the prevalence of the tick vector. Communities have also tried deer fencing, with some reduction in the risk of Lyme disease, but only after a 2-year exclusion of deer from the community (12,70).

The use of prophylactic antibiotic treatment for patients reporting a tick bite, or for routine prophylaxis after extended exposure in areas endemic for Lyme disease, has not been shown to be beneficial. Even with a known tick bite in an endemic community, the risk of infection with *B. burgdorferi* is sufficiently low that prophylaxis is not warranted (71–74). In an era of emerging antibiotic resistance, widespread use of antimicrobial drugs is not recommended.

A vaccine (LYMErix, Glaxo SmithKline) that uses recombinant antigen (outer surface protein A from *B. burgdorferi*) recently has been licensed by the FDA. The vaccine exerts its protective effect by eliciting antibodies that kill the spirochte within the tick gut. Vaccine should be administered intramuscularly as three doses at zero, one, and 12 months (72). Two large trials with over 10,000 participants each have shown vaccine efficacy of 49% to 68% in the first year (after two doses) and a vaccine efficacy of 76% to 98% in the second year (after three doses) in preventing clinical disease. The vaccine seems to be safe at 20 months of follow-up. The major adverse effects of vaccination include arm soreness, redness and swelling, and influenza-like illness (73,74). The necessity of booster vaccination is unclear. The vaccination is recommended for persons who reside, work, or recreate in an area endemic for Lyme disease and thus are at risk for exposure during daily activities. The vaccine is not licensed for use in children. There are no data on the safety of the vaccine in immunocompromised patients or in patients with chronic Lyme arthritis (72).

REFERENCES

1. **Centers for Disease Control and Prevention.** Case definitions for infectious conditions under public health surveillance. *MMWR Morb Mortal Wkly Rep.* 1997;46(RR-10):20–1.

2. **Steere AC, Malawista SE, Snydman DR, Shope RE.** Lyme arthritis: an epidemic of oligoarticular arthritis in children and adults in three Connecticut communities. *Arthritis Rheum.* 1977;20:7–17.

3. **Steere AC.** Lyme disease. N Engl J Med. 1989;321: 586–596.

4. **Burgdorfer W, Hayes SF, Benach JL, et al.** Lyme disease: a tick-borne spirochetosis? *Science.* 1982;216:1317–19.

5. **Barbour AG, Fish D.** The biological and social phenomenon of Lyme disease. *Science.* 1993;26:1610–16.

6. **Burgdorfer W, Kierans JE.** Ticks and Lyme disease in the United States. *Ann Intern Med.* 1983;99:121.

7. **Steere AC, Malawista SE.** Cases of Lyme disease in the United States: locations correlated with distribution of *Ixodes dammini. Ann Intern Med.* 1979;91:730–3.

8. **Steere AC.** *Borrelia burgdorferi* (Lyme disease, Lyme borreliosis). In Mandell, Douglas, Bennett (eds). *Principles and Practice of Infectious Diseases,* 4th ed. New York: Churchill Livingstone; 1995:2143–55.

9. **Benach JL, Coleman JL, Skinner RA, Bosler EM.** Adult *Ixodes dammini* in rabbits: a hypothesis for the development and transmission of *Borrelia burgdorferi. J Infect Dis.* 1987;155:1300–6.

10. **Piesman J, Mather TN, Sinsky RJ, Spielman A.** Duration of tick attachment and *Borrelia burgdorferi* transmission. *J Clin Microbiol.* 1987;25:557–8.

11. **Sood SK, Salza MB, Johnson BJB, et al.** Duration of tick attachment as a predictor of the risk of Lyme disease in an area in which Lyme disease is endemic. *J Infect Dis.* 1997;175:996–9.

12. **Fish D.** Environmental risk and prevention of Lyme disease. *Am J Med.* 1995; 98(Suppl 4A):2S–9S.

13. **Shadick NA, Phillips CB, Logigian EL, et al.** The long-term clinical outcomes of Lyme disease: a population-based retrospective cohort study. *Ann Intern Med.* 1994; 121:560–7.

14. **Logigian EL, Kaplan RF, Steere AC.** Chronic neurologic manifestations of Lyme disease. *N Engl J Med.* 1990;323:1438–1444.

15. **Asch ES, Bujak DI, Weiss M, et al.** Lyme disease: an infectious and postinfectious syndrome. *J Rheumatol.* 1994;21:454–461.

16. **Szer IS, Taylor E, Steere AC.** The long-term course of Lyme arthritis in children. *N Engl J Med.* 1991;325:159–63.

17. **Gerber MA, Shapiro ED, Burke GS, et al.** Lyme disease in children in southeastern Connecticut. *N Engl J Med.* 1996;335:1270–4.

18. **Reid CM, Schoen RT, Evans J, et al.** The consequences of overdiagnosis and overtreatment of Lyme disease: an observational study. *Ann Intern Med.* 1998;128: 354–62.

19. **Lyme disease–United States, 1996.** *MMWR Morb Mortal Wkly Rep.* 1997;46:531–5.

20. **Young JD.** Underreporting of Lyme disease. *N Engl J Med.* 1998;338:1692.

21. **Ciesielski CA, Markowitz LE, Horsley R, et al.** Lyme disease surveillance in the United States, 1983–1986. *Rev Infect Dis.* 1989;11(Suppl 6):1435S–41S.

22. **Anderson JF, Magnarelli LA, Burgdorfer W, Barbour AG.** Spirochetes in *Ixodes dammini* and mammals from Connecticut. *Am J Trop Med Hyg.* 1983;32:818–24.

23. **Anderson JF, Magnarelli LA.** Spirochetes in *Ixodes dammini* and *Babesia microti* on Prudence Island, Rhode Island. *J Infect Dis.* 1983;148:1124.

24. **Nadelman RB, Nowakowski J, Forseter G, et al.** The clinical spectrum of early Lyme borreliosis in patients with culture-confirmed erythema migrans. *Am J Med.* 1996;100: 502–8.

25. **Nadelman RB, Wormser GP.** Erythema migrans and early Lyme disease. *Am J Med.* 1995;98(Suppl 4A):15S–24S.

26. **Berger BW.** Dermatologic manifestations of Lyme disease. *Rev Infect Dis.* 1989; 11(Suppl 6):1475S–80S.

27. **Steere AC, Schoen RT, Taylor E.** The clinical evolution of Lyme arthritis. *Ann Intern Med.* 1987;107:725–31.

28. **Halperin JJ.** Neuroborreliosis. *Am J Med.* 1995;98(Suppl 4A):52S–9S.

29. **Fallon BAA, Nields JA.** Lyme disease: a neuropsychiatric illness. *Am J Psychiatry.* 1994;151:1571–83.

30. **Sigal LH.** Persisting complaints attributed to chronic Lyme disease: possible mechanisms and implications for management. *Am J Med.* 1994;96:365–74.

31. **Steere AC, Bartenhagen NH, Craft JE, et al.** The early clinical manifestations of Lyme disease. *Ann Intern Med.* 1983;99:76–82.

32. **Atlas E, Novack SN, Duray PH, Steere AC.** Lyme myositis: muscle invasion by *Borrelia burgdorferi* in a patient with Lyme disease. *Ann Intern Med.* 1988;109:245–6.

33. **Snydman DR, Schenkin DP, Berardi VP, et al.** *Borrelia burgdorferi* in joint fluid in chronic Lyme arthritis. *Ann Intern Med.* 1986;104:798–800.

34. **Pachner AR.** Early disseminated Lyme disease: Lyme meningitis. *Am J Med.* 1995; 98(Suppl 4A):30S–43S.

35. **Clark JR, Carlson R, Sasaki CT, et al.** Facial paralysis in Lyme disease. *Laryngoscope.* 1985;95:1341–5.

36. **Halperin JJ, Logigian EL, Finkel MF, Pearl RA.** Practice parameters for the diagnosis of patients with nervous system Lyme borreliosis (Lyme disease). *Neurology.* 1996;46:619–27.

37. **Preac-Murisc V, Wilske B, Schierx G, et al.** Repeated isolation of spirochetes from the cerebrospinal fluid of a patient with meningoradiculitis Bannwarth. *Eur J Clin Microbiol.* 1984;3: 564–5.

38. **Pachner AR, Duray P, Steere AC.** Central nervous system manifestations of Lyme disease. *Arch Neurol.* 1989;46: 790–5.

39. **Cox J, Krajden M.** Cardiovascular manifestations of Lyme disease. *Am Heart J.* 1991; 122:1449–55.

40. **Sigal, LH.** Early disseminated Lyme disease: cardiac manifestations. *Am J Med.* 1995; 98(Suppl 4A):25S–8S.

41. **McAlister HF, Klementowicz PT, Andrews C, et al.** Lyme carditis: an important cause of reversible heart block. *Ann Intern Med.* 1989;93:8–16.

42. **Gasser R, Dusleag J, Reisinger E, et al.** Reversal by ceftriaxone of dilated cardiomyopathy *Borrelia burgdorferi* infection. *Lancet.* 1992;339:1174–5.

43. **Stanek G, Klein J, Bittner R, Glogar D.** Isolation of *Borrelia burgdorferi* from the myocardium of a patient with longstanding cardiomyopathy. *N Engl J Med.* 1990;322: 249–252.

44. **Marcus LC, Steere AC, Duray PH, et al.** Fatal pancarditis in a patient with coexisting Lyme disease and babesiosis: demonstration of spirochetes in the myocardium. *Ann Intern Med.* 1985;103:374–6.

45. **de Koning J, Hoogkamp-Korstanje JA, van der Linde MR, Crijns HC.** Demonstration of spirochetes in cardiac biopsies of patients with Lyme disease. *J Infect Dis.* 1989;160:150–3.

46. **Sangha O, Phillips CB, Fleischmann KE, et al.** Lack of cardiac manifestations among patients with previously treated Lyme disease. *Ann Intern Med.* 1998;128: 346–53.

47. **Lesser, RL.** Ocular manifestations of Lyme disease. *Am J Med.* 1995;98(Suppl 4A): 60S–2S.

48. **Schlesinger P, Duray P, Burke B, et al.** Maternal-fetal transmission of the Lyme disease spirochete, *Borrelia burgdorferi. Ann Intern Med.* 1985;103:67–9.

49. **MacDonald A, Benach J, Burgdorfer W.** Stillbirth following maternal Lyme disease during pregnancy. *NY State J Med.* 1987;87:615–6.

50. **Silver HM.** Lyme disease during pregnancy. *Infect Dis Clin North Am.* 1997;11:43–7.

51. **Markowitz L, Steere A, Benach J, et al.** Lyme disease during pregnancy. *JAMA.* 1986;255:3394–6.

52. **Nadal D, Hunziker U, Bucher H, et al.** Infants born to mothers with antibodies against *Borrelia burgdorferi* at delivery. *Eur J Pediatr.* 1989;148:426–7.

53. **Strobino B, Williams C, Abid S, et al.** Lyme disease and pregnancy outcome: a prospective study of two thousand prenatal patients. *Am J Obstet Gynecol.* 1993;169: 367–74.

54. **Carlomagno G, Luksa V, Candussi G, et al.** Lyme *Borrelia*-positive serology associated with spontaneous abortion in an endemic Italian area. *Acta Eur Fertil.* 1988;19: 279–81.

55. **Sigal LH.** The Lyme disease controversy: social and financial costs of misdiagnosis and mismanagement. *Arch Intern Med.* 1996;156:1493–8.

56. **Bakken LL, Case KL, Callister SM, et al.** Performance of 45 laboratories participating in a proficiency testing program for Lyme disease serology. *JAMA.* 1992;268: 891–5.

57. **Luger SW, Krauss E.** Serologic tests for Lyme disease: interlaboratory variable. *Arch Intern Med.* 1990;150: 761–3.

58. **Craven RB, Quan TJ, Bailey RE, et al.** Improved serodiagnostic testing for Lyme disease: results of a multicenter serologic evaluation. *Emerg Infect Dis.* 1996;2:136–40.

59. **Tugwell P, Dennis DT, Weinstein A, et al.** Laboratory evaluation in the diagnosis of Lyme disease. *Ann Intern Med.* 1997;127:1109–23.

60. **Wormser GP, Forester G, Cooper D, et al.** Use of a novel technique of cutaneous lavage for diagnosis of Lyme disease associated with erythema migrans. *JAMA.* 1992;268: 1311–13.

61. **Steere AC, Taylor E, Wilson ML, et al.** Longitudinal assessment of the clinical and epidemiological features of Lyme disease in a defined population. *J Infect Dis.* 1986; 154: 295–300.

62. **Fahrer H, van der Linden SM, Sauvain MJ, et al.** The prevalence and incidence of clinical and asymptomatic Lyme borreliosis in a population at risk. *J Infect Dis.* 1991; 163: 305–10.

63. **Nocton JJ, Bloom BJ, Rutledge BJ, et al.** Detection of *Borrelia burgdorferi* DNA by polymerase chain reaction in cerebrospinal fluid in Lyme neuroborreliosis. *J Infect Dis.* 1996;174:623–7.

64. **Goodman JL, Bradley JF, Ross AE, et al.** Bloodstream invasion in early Lyme disease: results from a prospective, controlled, blinded study using the polymerase chain reaction. *Am J Med.* 1995;99:6–12.

65. **Sigal LH.** The polymerase chain reaction assay for *Borrelia burgdorferi* in the diagnosis of Lyme disease. *Ann Intern Med.* 1994;120:520–1.

66. **American Academy of Pediatrics.** Lyme disease. In Peter G (ed). *1997 Red Book: Report of the Committee on Infectious Diseases*, 24th ed. Elk Grove Village, IL: American Academy of Pediatrics; 1997:329–33.

67. Treatment of Lyme disease. *Med Lett.* 1997;39: 47–48.

68. **Rahn DW, Malawista SE.** Lyme disease: recommendations for diagnosis and treatment. *Ann Intern Med.* 1991;114:472–481.

69. **Luft BJ, Dattwyler RJ, Johnson RC, et al.** Azithromycin compared with Amoxicillin in the treatment of erythema migrans: a double-blind, randomized controlled trial. *Ann Intern Med.* 1996;124:785–91.

70. **Schulze TL, Jordan RA, Vasvary LM, et al.** Suppression of *Ixodes* (Acari: Ixodidae) *scapularis* nymphs in a large residential community. *J Med Entomol.* 1994;31:206–11.

71. **Shapiro ED, Gerber MA, Holabird NB, et al.** A controlled trial of antimicrobial prophylaxis for Lyme disease after deer-tick bites. *N Engl J Med.* 1992;327:1769–73.

72. **Magdid, D, Schwartz B, Craft J, Schwartz JS.** Prevention of Lyme disease after tick bites: a cost-effectiveness analysis. *N Engl J Med.* 1992;327:534–41.

73. **Fix, AD, Strickland T, Grant J.** Tick bites and Lyme disease in an endemic setting: problematic use of serologic testing and prophylactic antibiotic therapy. *JAMA.* 1998;279: 206–10.

74. **Warshafsky S, Nowakowski J, Nadelman RB, et al.** Efficacy of antibiotic prophylaxis for prevention of Lyme disease. *J Gen Intern Med.* 1996;11:329–33.

40

Malaria

Keith B. Armitage, MD
Charles H. King, MD

Epidemiology

Among parasitic infections, malaria is the leading cause of death worldwide. An estimated 500 million cases occur in the world per year, with one to two million deaths (1,2). Among immigrants and travelers returning from malarious areas, malaria should be considered a possible diagnosis in any individual with fever, and diagnostic steps should be promptly undertaken to exclude infection with the *Plasmodium* parasites that cause malaria. The four species of *Plasmodium* that cause malaria (i.e., *P. falciparum*, *P. vivax*, *P. ovale*, and *P. malariae*) are widely distributed throughout the world in tropical and subtropical areas where the insect vector of malaria, the anopheline mosquito, thrives (Table 40.1). Malaria is common in Africa, Southeast Asia, Papua New Guinea, the Pacific States, Haiti and parts of South America.

The post-World War II optimism about eliminating malaria by controlling its mosquito vectors and through mass treatment of human cases has given way to the reality of a world in which *Plasmodium* species are multiply drug-resistant (3,4). Today, there is an increasing resurgence of malaria in many parts of the world (2,5). Except for rare instances of limited outbreaks resulting from transmission of the disease by imported cases, malaria has been eliminated from the United States, Puerto Rico, Jamaica, Chile, Israel, Lebanon, North Korea, and Europe. On the other hand, malaria is found in varying degrees in all other areas of the world in which the climate is tropical or subtropical. In some parts of the world, notably sub-Saharan Africa, transmission

Table 40.1   Summary of *Plasmodium* Species

	Plasmodium falciparum	*P. vivax*	*P. ovale*	*P. malaria*
Geographic distribution	Central and South America, Haiti, Dominican Republic, Sub-Saharan Africa, India, Pakistan, Southeast Asia	Sub-Saharan Africa, Central and South America, Asia	Sub-Saharan Africa, Southeast Asia, New Guinea	Sub-Saharan Africa
Clinical features	High parasitemia, severe anemia, (often) daily spiking fevers, cerebral malaria, renal failure, jaundice, pulmonary edema, death	Anemia, splenic rupture	Anemia, splenic rupture	Persistent infection, nephritis
Chloroquine resistance	Yes	Yes, in Southeast Asia	No	No
Relapse	No	Yes	Yes	No
Incubation period	8–25 days (average 12 days)	8–27 days (average 14 days)	8–17 days (average 15 days)	15–30 days (average 15 days)
Appearance on thin film	Multiple infected RBCs, predominate rings, double nuclei, banana-shaped gametocytes	Enlarged RBCs with Schuffner's dots; trophozoite cytoplasm may be ameboid	Oval RBCs with fringed edges, compact cytoplasm	RBCs unchanged

RBC = red blood cells.

occurs in both urban and rural settings. In most of Central and South America, malaria is found primarily in rural areas.

Etiology

Malaria is transmitted by the bite of the female anopheline mosquito during the taking of a blood meal. The infectious sporozoite form of the *Plasmodium* parasite leaves the salivary glands of the mosquito and enters the host's skin. Sporozoites quickly enter the circulation to reach the liver. There, they invade hepatocytes and reproduce asexually for 10 to 14 days. After this asymptomatic incubation phase, *Plasmodium* merozoites emerge from the liver to infect host erythrocytes within the circulation. From this point forward, growth and reproduction of malaria parasites take place within the red cell. Two to 3 days after a red cell is infected, the parasite completes its growth and asexual division. A new generation of merozoites then matures and emerges into the plasma by rupturing the erythrocyte wall. Each merozoite is then capable of infecting a new red cell. In this cyclic manner, the level of infected erythrocytes grows geometrically. The process of parasite development within the erythrocyte cytoplasm takes 48 hours in the case of *P. falciparum*, *P. vivax*, and *P. ovale*, and 72 hours in the case of *P. malariae*.

Typically, cyclic systemic inflammation occurs in conjunction with the synchronous rupture of multiple infected erythrocytes, accounting for the periodicity of fever in malaria (6). In the case of *P. falciparum*, the merozoite is capable of infecting erythrocytes of all ages and stages of development, with the potential for massive hemolysis, severe anemia, and renal failure. Other *Plasmodium* species are not capable of infecting erythrocytes in all stages of development, and so do not cause massive hemolysis. Malaria caused by *P. vivax* and *P. ovale* is therefore not as clinically severe as malaria caused by *P. falciparum*.

The life cycle of malaria parasites is completed when a sub-population of merozoites develops into male and female gametocytes. When these are taken in a blood meal by a female anopheline mosquito, they mate (in sexual reproduction) within the insect abdomen and ultimately produce new sporozoites. These sporozoites migrate to the mosquito's salivary glands to initiate infection of a new host during the next blood meal. Without the continued presence of mosquitoes of the right vector species, endemic transmission of malaria cannot occur. In temperate areas such as the United States, brief epidemics may occur rarely in the summer months if anopheline mosquitoes flourish in a region where chronically infected humans are harboring asymptomatic malaria (7). This is extremely uncommon, and the great majority of malaria in the United States is seen in immigrants from or travelers to endemic areas. Other North American cases have been caused by blood-borne transmission of malaria parasites (i.e., by transfusion or by needle sharing among injection drug abusers). This is because merozoites in donor red cells can directly infect new red cells in the recipient's circulation. In transfusion-transmitted malaria, there is no initial stage of liver infection. Because of this, late recrudescence of malaria from dormant liver hypnozoites will not occur, as sometimes happens after initial treatment of mosquito-transmitted *P. vivax* and *P. ovale* malaria.

Clinical Manifestations

Infection with malaria parasites leads to hemolysis, anemia, tissue hypoxia, and secondary immunopathologic processes caused by the release of inflammatory cytokines (6). Together, these processes account for the clinical signs and symptoms of malaria, which in the case of *P. falciparum* malaria can be severe or fatal. The symptoms of acute malaria may be variable, depending on both parasite and host factors. High fevers and rigors are the hallmark of acute malaria, and malaria should be considered in any individual with an exposure history and any type of fever. In addition, malaise, headaches (often severe), myalgias, and fatigue often occur. Other symptoms, such as nausea, diarrhea, and cough may mimic abdominal disease or pneumonia. Patients may not have a synchronous infection, and the classic periodicity of fever (quartan or tertian fever) does not have to be present. In particular, patients with *P. falciparum* infection often present with daily spiking fevers. Patients may also have double infection with two or more species of malaria parasite (8). This frequently results in an inconstant pattern of fever spikes. Hepatosplenomegaly, pallor, and mild jaundice are common clinical signs in patients with acute malaria. Highly immune adults from endemic areas may be infected but asymptomatic. Such infection is often documented among refugee groups. If anopheline mosquitoes are present, there is the potential for local person-to-person transmission of malaria (*see* the Etiology section) (7).

Cerebral malaria is the most severe form of malaria, causing more than 80% of fatalities from malaria (9). It is caused only by *P. falciparum* infection and occurs in 0.5% to 1% of cases, with a mortality of approximately 50%. Patients with cerebral malaria often present with seizures, stupor, and focal neurological symptoms. The other severe complications of falciparum malaria include acute renal failure, pulmonary edema, hypoglycemia, and shock. Partly treated patients, or those with partial immunity, may have continued subclinical *P. falciparum* infection, and symptomatic relapse with falciparum malaria may occur for up to 1 year. Late relapses caused by a latent phase of infection in the liver are seen in *P. vivax* and *P. ovale* infection, but unlike *P. vivax* and *P. ovale*, *P. falciparum* does not have a latent liver phase, and will be eradicated if the red cell stage of disease is eliminated.

Diagnosis

The clinical gold-standard diagnosis of malaria rests on the demonstration of the parasites on Giemsa-stained blood smears. Thick blood smears are used as a sensitive screening test, whereas thin blood smears are necessary for species identification and estimation of the percentage of erythrocytes infected. This latter number gauges the severity of infection. The presence of the parasites in the blood may fluctuate, and multiple smears (separated by approximately 12 hours) should be done during the fever cycle before malaria can be ruled out. Even if blood smears are initially negative, treatment should not be delayed if the clinical suspicion of malaria is high.

Treatment

Antimalarial drugs are used for both the prophylaxis and treatment of infection caused by *Plasmodium* species. Therapeutic decisions are based on the suspicion of *P. Falciparum* as the causative organism, the severity of the infection, and known drug-resistance patterns for areas in which the patient has traveled. The use of a specific treatment agent depends on the species involved, local drug availability, and whether the patient is treated in the inpatient or outpatient setting. Resistance patterns of malaria parasites continue to evolve, and new therapeutic agents, such as the artemether compounds, are becoming generally available. It is imperative to have up-to-date information when treating malaria. The Centers for Disease Control and Prevention (CDC) Malaria Hotline (404-332-4555) and the CDC Internet site (www.cdc.gov) are good sources for up-to-date information.

Chloroquine Phosphate

Chloroquine phosphate is a 4-aminoquinoline used primarily for the treatment and prevention of infection by *P. vivax*, *P. malariae*, *P. ovale*, and sensitive strains of *P. falciparum*. Chloroquine-sensitive strains of *P. falciparum* are now rare, and are found in only a few geographic areas. Chloroquine can be given orally with food or injected parenterally. Parenteral dosing may be associated with respiratory depression, hypotension, cardiac arrest, and seizures, particularly after rapid administration of chloroquine. Parenteral therapy should be used for patients unable to take oral medicine, and patients should be switched to the oral route as soon as possible.

Oral doses of chloroquine are absorbed to an extent exceeding 90%, and intramuscular and subcutaneous doses are also rapidly absorbed. Because of the large volume of distribution of chloroquine, a loading dose is required. The drug undergoes extensive metabolism, and the kidney excretes approximately 50%. Renal failure does not change the therapeutic dose of chloroquine, but prophylactic doses should be reduced. The precise mechanism of action of chloroquine is unknown; it is known that chloroquine raises the pH of lysosomal vesicles of *Plasmodium*, and inhibits the proteolysis of hemoglobin.

In treating malaria, chloroquine is active against the asexual erythrocytic stages of sensitive strains of the causative parasites, and its administration leads to rapid clinical improvement. Chloroquine is therefore indicated for the erythrocytic stage of development of sensitive strains of *Plasmodium* species. Unfortunately, in most areas of the world *P. falciparum* is chloroquine-resistant, and may be resistant to second-line drugs as well; in addition, there have been isolated reports of *P. vivax* resistance in Papua New Guinea and Indonesia (3). Chloroquine has no exoerythrocytic activity and therefore is of no use against tissue stages of the life cycle of malarial parasites. When used to treat the erythrocytic stages of *P. vivax* and *P. ovale*, it must be followed with an agent such as primaquine, that is active against the tissue hepatic phase, to completely eradicate infection (*radical cure*).

Chloroquine phosphate (Aralen) is supplied as 250- and 500-mg (containing 150- and 300-mg base) tablets. Hydroxychloroquine sulfate (Plaquenil) is supplied in 200-mg tablets, and for dosing purposes, 400 mg of hydroxychloroquine sulfate is equal to 500 mg of chloroquine hydrochloride. Chloroquine hydrochloride for injection is supplied at a concentration of 50 mg/mL.

For prophylaxis, 500 mg of chloroquine is given once a week. Treatment is started 2 weeks before exposure and is continued for 6 weeks after exposure (Table 40.2).

Table 40.2   Prophylaxis of Malaria

Organism	Drug	Adult Dosage	Pediatric Dosage
Chloroquine-resistant *Plasmodium falciparum*	Mefloquine (Lariam)	250 mg/wk PO Begin 1 week before exposure Continue 4 weeks after exposure	5–9 kg: 1/8 tablet 10–19 kg: 1/4 tablet 20–30 kg: 1/2 tablet 31–45 kg: 3/4 tablet >45 kg: adult dosage
	Doxycycline (Vibramycin)	100 mg/d PO Begin 2 days before exposure Continue 28 days after exposure	Contraindicated in children >8 years of age
	Chloroquine + proguanil	Proguanil 200 mg/d PO plus chloroquine as below	<2 years: 50 mg/d 2–6 years: 100 mg/d 7–10 years: 150 mg/d >10 years: adult dose plus chloroquine as below
Chloroquine-sensitive *P. falciparum* and *P. vivax, P. ovale,* and *P. malaria*	Chloroquine (Aralen)	500 mg/wk chloroquine phosphate PO (300-mg base) Begin 2 weeks before exposure Continue 6 weeks after exposure	8.3 mg/kg/wk (5-mg base)
	Atavaquone + proguanil (Malarone)	1 tablet daily Begin 2 days before exposure Continue 7 days after exposure	11–20 kg: 1 pediatric tablet 21–30 kg: 2 pediatric tablets 31–40 kg: 3 pediatric tablets >40 kg: adult dosage

PO = orally.

The dose of chloroquine for treating acute infection is 1 g, followed by 500 mg from 6 to 8 hours later, and subsequent dosing at 500 mg/d for 2 days, for a total dose of 2.5 g. Parenteral dosing schedules are not as well established, but chloroquine can be given in a dose of 3.5 mg/kg every 6 hours to a total dose of 2.5 g. Children should not be given more than 10 mg/kg of chloroquine base per day regardless of the route of administration (Table 40.3), and their usual prophylactic dosage of chloroquine base is 5 mg/kg/wk (*see* Table 40.2).

Common side effects of the treatment dose of chloroquine (used in acute malaria attacks) include gastrointestinal upset, pruritus, headache, and visual effects. As noted above, intravenous preparations are available, but should be used cautiously, since rapid infusion of chloroquine can lead to cardiovascular collapse. The prophylactic dose is usually well tolerated, although prolonged use can lead to skin eruptions and changes in the fingernails. Prolonged use of chloroquine in high daily doses has been associated with more serious side effects such as myopathy and neuropathy. Chloroquine is contraindicated in severe hepatic disease, psoriasis, and porphyria.

Mefloquine

Mefloquine is a quinoline-carbinolamine compound active against chloroquine-resistant *P. falciparum* in most parts of the world, and is used for the prophylaxis and treatment of malaria where chloroquine resistance is likely. It is available only in oral form. Mefloquine has a long half-life, with an elimination time of 2 to 3 weeks. It is excreted in the feces, and dose adjustments do not need to be made in renal failure. The mechanism of action of mefloquine is unknown, but is probably similar to that of chloroquine. Like chloroquine, mefloquine is active only against the erythrocytic forms of *P. falciparum*. In the United States, mefloquine is sold under the trade name Lariam and is supplied as 250-mg tablets.

The most common prophylactic dosing schedule with mefloquine is 250 mg/week, beginning 1 week before travel. The drug should be continued for 4 weeks after the last exposure (*see* Table 40.2).

A single dose of 1000 to 1500 mg of mefloquine is used for treating chloroquine-resistant falciparum malaria. Side effects are uncommon at doses of less than 1000 mg; nausea, vomiting, abdominal pain and dizziness have been reported (*see* Table 40.3). Serious side effects on the central nervous system, such as seizures, hallucinations, psychosis, and depression, occur rarely at prophylactic doses (<0.5%) (10). Use of mefloquine in patients with cardiac conduction abnormalities or those taking beta-blockers for anti-arrhythmic indications has in rare cases been associated with sudden death, and its use should be avoided in these circumstances. Mefloquine is teratogenic in animals, and data are not currently available about its safety in pregnancy (11). The therapeutic dose for children is 25 mg/kg. Emergence of resistance to antimalarial drugs

Table 40.3   Treatment of Malaria

Organism	Drug	Adult Dosage	Pediatric Dosage
Chloroquine-resistant *Plasmodium falciparum*	Quinine sulfate *plus* Pyrimethamine–sulfadoxine	650 mg PO tid for 3–7 days 3 tablets on last day of quinine	25 mg/kg/d divided in three doses for 3–7 days Dosage by age: 2–11 months: 1/4 tablet 1–3 years: 1/2 tablet 4–8 years: 1 tablet 9–14 years: 2 tablets >14 years: adult dosage
	Or Quinine sulfate *followed by* Tetracycline *or* Oxycycline	See above 250 mg qid for 7 days 100 mg bid for 7 days	See above 20 mg/kg/d divided in four doses for 7 days* Contraindicated
	Or Quinine suflate *followed by* Clindamycin	See above 900 mg orally tid for 3 days	See above 20–40 mg/kg/d divided in three doses
	Mefloquine (Lariam)	1000–1500 mg PO as a single dose	25 mg/kg as a single dose
	Artemisinin (Quinghaosu)	50 mg/kg total dose administered over three days, with the first dose >10 mg/kg	Same as adult dosage
	Halofantrine	500 mg every 6 hours for three doses; repeat in 1 week	8 mg/kg every 6 hours for 3 doses; repeat in 1 week
	Parenteral Therapy		
	Quinidine gluconate	10 mg/kg loading dose (maximum 600 mg) infused in N/S over 1–2 hours, then 0.02 mg/kg/min for 72 hours†	Same as adult dosage
	Quinine dihydrochloride‡	20 mg salt/kg loading dose in D5W over 4 hours, followed by 10 mg salt/kg over 2–4 hours every 8 hours (maximum 1800 mg/d) for 72 hours or until patient is able to take oral medication	Same as adult dosage
Chloroquine-sensitive *P. falciparum* and *P. vivax, P. ovale,* and *P. malaria*	Chloroquine phosphate (Aralen) *and*	1000 mg chloroquine phosphate orally (600-mg base), followed by 500 mg 6 hours later and on days 2 and 3	15 mg/kg PO (10-mg base), followed by 7.5 mg/kg at 6 hours and on days 2 and 3
	Primaquine phosphate§	15-mg/d base PO (26.3 mg phosphate salt) for 14 days *or* 45-mg/wk base PO (79 mg salt) for 8 weeks for more resistant strains	0.3 mg/kg/d base (0.5 mg salt) for 14 days
	Atovaquone + proguanil (Malarone)	4 tablets per day for 3 days	11–20 kg: 1 adult tablet per day 21–30 kg: 2 adult tablets per day 31–40 kg: 3 adult tablets per day

D5W = 5% dextrose in water; N/S = normal saline; PO = orally.

* Contraindicated in children aged <8 years

† Cardiac monitoring is required; switch to oral therapy when patient is stable.

‡ Not available in the United States.

§ For the prevention of relapse due to *P. vivax, P. ovale,* and *P. malaria.*

may occur rapidly, and the most recent information about this may be obtained from the CDC Malaria Branch (404-488-4046). As of 1998, resistance to mefloquine was most often reported in parts of Thailand and West Africa.

Quinine

Quinine is an alkaloid extracted from the bark of the cinchona tree, and is highly active against blood forms of malarial parasites. It is more toxic and less efficacious than chloroquine, and its primary use is in treating resistant falciparum malaria. Quinine can be given by the oral, intravenous, or intramuscular route; it is metabolized in the liver and excreted by the kidney. The exact mechanism of action of quinine is unknown. The most commonly used preparation is quinine sulfate, the oral dose of which is 650 mg thrice daily, taken after meals, for 7 to 10 days; the duration of treatment with quinine can be decreased if other antimalarial drugs are used. Parenterally administered quinine is more toxic than the orally administered drug, and should be reserved for more severe cases of malaria; the dose is 20 mg of the salt/kg in 500 mL of either 5% dextrose-in-water (D5W) or saline, infused over a 4-hour period, with subsequent infusion at 10 mg/kg for 2 to 4 hours in every 8-hour period (*see* Table 40.3). Patients severely ill with falciparum malaria who have high levels of parasitemia (>5%10%) or massive hemolysis should be treated with exchange transfusion in combination with drug therapy.

Parenteral quinine is not available in the United States. Quinidine, a stereoisomer of quinine, can be used in place of the latter drug in patients who need parenteral therapy for malaria. Quinidine is given by continuous intravenous infusion. The most commonly used dosing schedule is 10 mg/kg in a loading dose, followed by 0.02 mg/kg/min (*see* Table 40.3). Quinidine undergoes hepatic metabolism and is excreted in the urine. Blood levels of this drug should be followed in patients with hepatic or renal failure.

Intravenous quinine and quinidine can cause hypotension and serious cardiac arrhythmias, particularly when given in bolus doses, and cardiac monitoring should be used during their administration. The fatal oral dose of quinine for adults is 2 to 8 g. Oral quinine is associated with a variety of side effects including nausea, vomiting, diarrhea, and hypoglycemia. Dosing with meals decreases gastrointestinal side effects. Dose-related side effects include tinnitus, headache, changes in vision, and vertigo. Tinnitus, optic neuritis, and hypersensitivity reactions are contraindications to the use of quinine.

Pyrimethamine

Pyrimethamine is a dihydrofolate-reductase inhibitor that is highly active against this enzyme in malaria parasites. It is used in the prophylaxis and treatment of resistant falciparum malaria. Pyrimethamine is well absorbed orally and has an extremely long tissue half-life (80–95 hours). It is particularly effective when used in combination with other folic acid antagonists, and such combination therapy delays the emergence of resistance. A common pyrimethamine/sulfa drug combination used for prophylaxis of malaria is Fansidar, which consists of pyrimethamine 25 mg and sulfadoxine 500 mg. In other countries, pyrimethamine in a dose of 12.5 mg is also available in combination with dapsone in a dose of 100 mg as Maloprim, but this formulation is not available in the United States.

Pyrimethamine in a single dose of 75 mg in combination with a sulfa drug is used for treating acute attacks of falciparum malaria. Resistance of *P. falciparum* to the pyrimethamine/sulfa combination has been encountered in some areas. In treating acute malaria, quinine is frequently used in combination with pyrimethamine, since pyrimethamine acts slowly in clearing parasitemia (*see* Table 40.3). The pediatric therapeutic dose of pyrimethamine is one fourth of a 25-mg tablet for children aged 2 to 11 months, one half of a tablet for children aged 1 to 3 years, one tablet for children aged 4 to 8 years, and two tablets for children 9 to 14 years old. Children over age 14 take the adult dose (three tablets).

Long-term prophylactic use of pyrimethamine/sulfa combinations (Fansidar) has been associated with severe cutaneous skin reactions, and mefloquine and doxycycline have largely supplanted the use of these combinations (12). Pyrimethamine/sulfa combinations have been used for individuals with prolonged exposure to resistant falciparum malaria and limited access to medical care who cannot tolerate mefloquine or doxycycline. The prophylactic dose is one Fansidar tablet taken weekly for 1 week before, each week during, and 6 weeks after exposure. The CDC now recommends that travelers not taking mefloquine or doxycycline and who are exposed to chloroquine-resistant malaria carry a therapeutic dose of pyrimethamine/sulfa, which is to be taken if a febrile illness develops and medical care is unavailable. There have been no reports of fatal cutaneous reactions to Fansidar when the drug is used only for acute febrile episodes of malaria. High doses of pyrimethamine lead to megaloblastic anemia, which can be prevented with concurrent use of folinic acid (leucovorin).

Proguanil (Chloroguanide)

Like pyrimethamine, proguanil (chloroguanide) is an inhibitor of protozoan dihydrofolate reductase. The drug is well absorbed orally and is readily excreted, and does not accumulate in the body. To be effective for prophylaxis of malaria it must be taken daily. Proguanil is used in the prophylaxis of resistant falciparum malaria (*see* Table 40.2), particularly as an alternative to pyrimethamine/sulfa in East Africa. For reasons that are not clear, proguanil is less effective in West Africa. The prophylactic dosage is 200 mg/d, and is associated with few side effects (occasional mouth ulcers, nausea, and diarrhea). In areas where *P. falciparum* is resistant to chloroquine, the combination of daily proguanil and weekly chloroquine is only approximately 75% effective in preventing falciparum malaria, as opposed to an efficacy of more than 95% for mefloquine. In addition, the need for a daily dose of proguanil (vs. weekly dosing with mefloquine) may lead to diminished compliance with its use.

Primaquine

Primaquine, an 8-aminoquinoline, is the prototype antimalarial drug with activity in tissue. The drug is well absorbed orally and extensively metabolized. Primaquine interferes with the mitochondrial function of *Plasmodium* species. It is primarily used to treat the liver phase of malaria caused by *P. vivax* and *P. ovale*. Patients treated for the blood phase of *P. vivax* or *P. ovale* malaria must receive treatment for the tissue phase to prevent relapse of their infection. By contrast, infection with *P. falciparum* occurs without a long-term hepatic stage, and primaquine is not needed when the blood phase is successfully treated. However, patients who acquire *P. falciparum* malaria and who are not taking chloroquine or other prophylaxis should be treated with primaquine, since coinfection with another species of malarial parasite is common, and relapses of this latter infection may occur without treatment of the hepatic stage of disease. The dose of primaquine is expressed in terms of the base. Primaquine is supplied in tablets containing 26.3 mg of the salt, which is equal to 15 mg of free primaquine base. Primaquine at 15 mg/d in combination with chloroquine cures malaria caused by sensitive strains of *P. vivax*. For more resistant strains, 45 mg of primaquine is given with chloroquine weekly for 8 weeks (*see* Table 40.3). Primaquine should always be given with a schizonticidal agent (preferably chloroquine) in acute malaria to prevent the development of resistance.

At higher doses, primaquine can cause gastrointestinal distress; however, the major toxicity is related to the drug's redox potential. In high doses primaquine can cause methemoglobinemia. In glucose-6-phosphate dehydrogenase (G6PD)-deficient individuals, primaquine at its usual doses provokes hemolysis, and patients should be screened for G6PD deficiency before such treatment. With higher doses of primaquine or in susceptible patients, the red blood cell count should be followed. Primaquine can rarely cause central nervous system toxicity. Agranulocytosis has also been reported, and primaquine is contraindicated in patients with neutropenia. Primaquine should also not be used during pregnancy (11).

Artemisinin (Qinghaosu)

Artemisinin (qinghaosu) is a member of a group of compounds, traditionally used to treat fever in China, that have recently been found to have anti-malarial activity. It is emerging as an alternative therapy for resistant falciparum malaria, and has been used extensively in China and Vietnam. Artemisinin and several related compounds (*see* next paragraph) are among the most rapidly schizonticidal drugs available. The mechanism of their action is not well understood, but is thought to be mediated by free radical damage to parasite membranes.

Artemisinin is commonly given orally or as a suppository. The total oral dose is 50 mg/kg given over a period of 3 days, with the first dose larger than 10 mg/kg. Suppository administration of artemisinin is used extensively in cases of severe malaria where parenteral therapy is not available. For this route of administration, a total of 2800 mg is given over a period of 3 days in five or six doses, with the first dose exceeding 10 mg/kg. Recently, experts have suggested the use of artemisinin along with mefloquine for treating of *P. falciparum* malaria in areas where mefloquine resistance is likely to be encountered. Two compounds similar to artemisinin, artemether and artesunate, have also been used. Artemether is given intramuscularly in an initial dose of 3.2 mg/kg, followed by 1.6 mg/kg every 12 to 24 hours for a total of six doses. Artesunate is given parenterally with a similar schedule. Severe toxicities with artemisinin and its related compounds are rare. Transient first-degree heart block, abdominal pain, diarrhea, fever, and cytopenias have been reported, but are uncommon, and artemisinin and its related compounds described here are generally well tolerated. However, their safety in pregnancy has not been established.

Halofantrine

Halofantrine is a 9-phenanthrenemethanol effective against chloroquine-sensitive and chloroquine-resistant falciparum malaria. The drug is available only in oral form; it is best absorbed when taken with a fatty meal. Halofantrine is excreted in the feces. The mechanism of action of this drug is not known. Like chloroquine and mefloquine, it is active only against the intraerythrocytic stages of *Plasmodium* species. Halofantrine is used in areas where there is resistance to chloroquine and mefloquine. There is some evidence of cross-resistance with mefloquine, which may limit the future usefulness of halofantrine. Administration consists of three 500-mg doses given at 6-hour intervals for adults and children weighing more than 40 kg, and 8 mg/kg given at the same 6-hour intervals for children under 40 kg. A second course of treatment after 7 days is recommended for patients not previously exposed to malaria. The most common side effects of halofantrine are headache, nausea, abdominal pain, diarrhea, and rash. The use of halofantrine is contraindicated in pregnancy and for lactating women.

Tetracycline

Members of the tetracycline family can be used to treat multiply-drug resistant falciparum malaria. They are slow to act and should be used with quinine. Tetracycline is given orally at a dosage of 250 mg four times daily. The equivalent dosage of doxycycline is 100 mg twice daily (*see* Table 40.3). Doxycycline can also be used for short-term prophylaxis of malaria at a dosage of 100 mg/d (*see* Table 40.2). Tetracyclines are associated with sun sensitization, and should not be used in children or during pregnancy (4,11,12).

Malarone

In April 2000, the combination of proguanil and the hydroxynaphthoquinone antimalarial agent atovaquone, was approved by the FDA for prophylaxis and therapy of malaria, including strains of *P. falciparum* that are resistant to chloroquine. The trade name for this combination of atovaquone 250 mg and proguanil 100 mg is Malarone. The pediatric-strength tablet contains 62.5 mg of atovaquone and 25 mg of proguanil. Malarone is generally well tolerated and should be taken with food. For prophylaxis, Malarone is given once daily, beginning two days before exposure and continuing 7 days after exposure. Malarone often is used as an alternative to mefloquine when there are concerns about neuropsychiatric side effects. Malarone also can be used in the therapy of resistant *P. falciparum* and other strains of malaria at a dosage of four pills per day for three consecutive days.

Choice of Therapy

In mild cases of malaria, oral quinine or pyrimethamine/sulfa should be used for treatment if falciparum malaria is suspected and is likely to be chloroquine-resistant. Severe infections, especially those marked by infection of more than 5% of erythrocytes, as determined on a thin blood smear, require parenteral treatment with quinidine or quinine (if available) and close monitoring (13). Chloroquine-sensitive falciparum malaria and malaria caused other *Plasmodium* species can be treated with oral or parenteral chloroquine (rare chloroquine-resistant *P. vivax* have been reported in Papua New Guinea, Indonesia, and Oceania). Patients with *P. vivax* and *P. ovale* should also be treated with primaquine for the latent liver phase of disease and to prevent relapse (*see* Table 40.3).

Prevention

Prevention of malaria is based on reducing mosquito exposure in endemic areas, and on the use of low-dose anti-malarial therapy to inhibit the progression of early, subclinical infection. Among people residing in endemic areas, research data indicate that reduction in the overall number of mosquito bites per annum will significantly alter the risk of mortality from malaria. The same is true for reducing the exposure of travelers in malaria-endemic zones.

Mosquito control may be achieved through the widespread or focused use of insecticides, by screening, and by the use of insect repellents. In the 1950s, many nations were able to significantly reduce their malaria prevalence through peridomestic spraying with dichlorodiphenyltrichloroethane (DDT). This approach proved to be environmentally toxic, however, and spraying programs have been significantly curtailed (14). In recent years, focused use of permethrin insecticide-impregnated bed nets has proven effective in reducing transmission of malaria in endemic populations. Personal use of insect repellent has also been shown to reduce the risk of infection in travelers (15,16).

In addition to vector avoidance, drug prophylaxis with chloroquine or mefloquine, as described above in the section on treatment of malaria, further reduces the risk of acquiring symptomatic malaria (15). Anti-malaria vaccines are under development, but are strictly investigational, and their usefulness for short-term travel to malaria-endemic regions may prove limited (17).

REFERENCES

1. **Greenwood BM.** The epidemiology of malaria. *Ann Trop Med Parasitol.* 1997;91:763–9.
2. **Krogstad DJ.** Malaria as a reemerging disease. *Epidemiol Rev.* 1996;18:77–89.
3. **Barat LM, Bloland PB.** Drug resistance among malaria and other parasites. *Infect Dis Clin North Am.* 1997;11:969–87.
4. **Longworth DL.** Drug-resistant malaria in children and travelers. *Pediatr Clin North Am.* 1995;42:649–64.
5. **Olliaro P, Cattani J, Wirth D.** Malaria, the submerged disease. *JAMA.* 1996;275: 230–3.
6. **Richards AL.** Tumour necrosis factor and associated cytokines in the host's response to malaria. *Int J Parasitol.* 1997;27:1251–63.
7. **Zucker JR.** Changing patterns of autochthonous malaria transmission in the United States: a review of recent outbreaks. *Emerg Infect Dis.* 1996;2:37–43.
8. **McKenzie FE, Bosser WH.** Mixed-species *Plasmodium* infections of humans. *J Parasitol.* 1997;83:593–600.
9. **World Health Organization.** Severe and complicated malaria. *Trans R Soc Trop Med Hyg.* 1990;84 (suppl 2):1–65.
10. **Croft A, Garner P.** Mefloquine to prevent malaria: a systematic review of trials. *Br Med J.* 1997;315:1412–6.

11. **Silver HM.** Malarial infection during pregnancy. *Infect Dis Clin North Am.* 1997;11: 99–107.

12. **White NJ.** The treatment of malaria. *N Engl J Med.* 1996;335:800–6.

13. **Lee LH, Caserta MT.** Malaria: update on treatment. *Pediat Infect Dis J.* 1998;17: 342–3.

14. **Greenwood BM.** What's new in malaria control? *Ann Trop Med Parasitol.* 1997;91: 523–31.

15. **Kain KC, Keystone JS.** Malaria in travelers. Epidemiology, disease, and prevention. *Infect Dis Clin North Am.* 1998;12:267–84.

16. **Fradin MS.** Mosquitoes and mosquito repellents: A clinician's guide. *Ann Intern Med.* 1998;128:931–40.

17. **Nussenzweig RS, Zavala F.** A malaria vaccine based on a sporozoite antigen. *N Engl J Med.* 1997;336:86–91.

Index

Note: *f* following page number indicates figure; *t* indicates table.